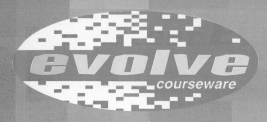

The Latest *Evolution* in Learning.

Evolve provides online access to free learning resources and activities designed specifically for the textbook you are using in your class. The resources will provide you with information that enhances the material covered in the book and much more.

Visit the Web address listed below to start your learning evolution today!

▶▶ **LOGIN:** *http://evolve.elsevier.com/Cameron*

Evolve Online Learning Resource for Cameron: *Physical Agents in Rehabilitation: From Research to Practice, 2nd Edition* offers the following features:

- **Frequently Asked Questions (FAQs)**
  Common questions related to the topics covered in the textbook.

- **Study Guide**
  Questions and answers to help you to increase your knowledge level.

- **Content Updates**
  Content is updated to stay current and fresh, optimizing learning and teaching.

- **WebLinks**
  Links to places of interest on the web specific to your classroom needs.

- **Links to Related Products**
  See what else Elsevier Science has to offer in a specific field of interest.

Think outside the book...*evolve.*

Physical Agents in Rehabilitation

From Research to Practice

Physical Agents in Rehabilitation

From Research to Practice

Second Edition

Michelle H. Cameron, PT, OCS
Guest Lecturer
Graduate Program of Physical Therapy
Samuel Merritt College
Oakland, California

Health Potentials, Owner
A Health Education and Consulting Company
Oakland, California

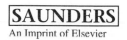
SAUNDERS
An Imprint of Elsevier

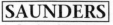

An Imprint of Elsevier

11830 Westline Industrial Drive
St. Louis, Missouri 63146

NOTICE

Rehabilitation is an ever-changing field. Standard safety precautions must be followed, but as new
research and clinical experience broaden our knowledge, changes in treatment and drug therapy may
become necessary or appropriate. Readers are advised to check the most current product information
provided by the manufacturer of each drug to be administered to verify the recommended dose, the
method and duration of administration, and contraindications. It is the responsibility of the licensed
prescriber, relying on experience and knowledge of the patient, to determine dosages and the best
treatment for each individual patient. Neither the Publisher nor the author assumes any liability for
any injury and/or damage to persons or property arising from this publication.

Previous edition copyrighted 1999

Acquisitions Editor: Marion Waldman
Developmental Editors: Sue Bredensteiner, Marjory Fraser
Publishing Services Manager: John Rogers
Project Manager: Kathleen L. Teal
Designer: Kathi Gosche
Cover Art: Kathi Gosche

Printed in the United States of America

Last digit is the print number: 9   8   7   6   5   4   3   2

This book is dedicated to the memory of
my husband and dearest friend
John Cameron
for encouraging me to aim high
and teaching me that I could do whatever I put my mind to.

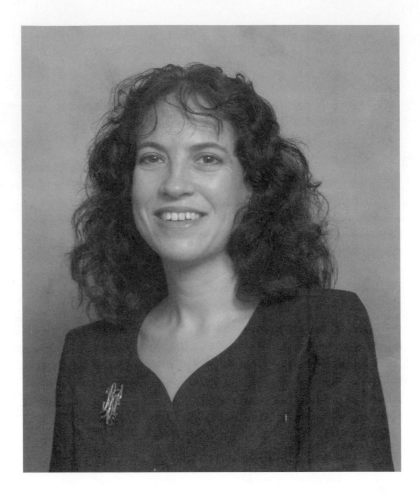

Michelle H. Cameron, PT, OCS, is the owner of Health Potentials, a health education and consulting company. She is a physical therapist clinician, a teacher, researcher, and author, and now also a full-time medical student at the University of California, San Francisco. She wrote the first edition and the current edition of this book, *Physical Agents in Rehabilitation: From Research to Practice*, published by Saunders. In addition, her research on phonophoresis is published in *Physical Therapy,* the Journal of the American Physical Therapy Association, and in *Clinical Management* mag-

azine, and earned her the California APTA Clinician Research Award. Michelle has also written and edited numerous articles on electrical stimulation, ultrasound and phonophoresis, and wound management, and wrote the section on ultrasound in Saunders' *Manual for Physical Therapy Practice*. Michelle's discussions of ultrasound, electrical stimulation, thermal agents, biofeedback, and wound management bring together current research and practice to provide the decision-making and hands-on tools that support optimal care within today's health care environment.

Acknowledgments

First and foremost, I want to thank the readers and purchasers of the first edition of this book. Without you, there wouldn't be a second edition. In particular, I would like to thank those readers who took the time to contact me with their comments, thoughts, and suggestions about what worked for them and what didn't. And, special thanks are due Dr. Marjorie Moore for her review and input on Figures 3–4 through 3–7 in the chapter on pain.

Thank you also to my friends, family, and colleagues. Your ongoing support, encouragement, and patience has kept me happy and relatively sane through this endeavor and the rest of my life. I would also like to give special thanks to:

Andrew Allen, publishing director at Elsevier Science, for his consistent support throughout this project;

As well as Marion Waldman, executive editor; Sue Bredensteiner, developmental editor; and Marjory Fraser, ancillary and website developer and editor, for their ongoing support.

The contributing authors to the first edition, including David Selkowitz, as well as those who have been part of both editions, and Sara Shapiro who is new to the team;

Sara, for her persistence and dedication with a job that turned out to be much more than she bargained for;

Julie Pryde, Diane Allen, and Gail Widener, who updated their respective chapters thoroughly and promptly; and

Linda Monroe for keeping this text in line with the APTA *Guide to Physical Therapist Practice*, second edition, and keeping my neck healthy through my hours at the computer.

Michelle H. Cameron

Contributors

Diane D. Allen, MS, PT
Adjunct Assistant Professor
Samuel Merritt College

Physical Therapist
Interim Health Care
San Jose, California
  Chapter 4: Tone Abnormalities

Linda G. Monroe, MPT, OCS
Physical Therapist
Private Practice
  Chapter 5: Motion Restrictions and Guide to Physical
  Therapist Practice (second edition content)

Suzana Otaño-Lata, MS
Biomedical Engineer
Boston Scientific Corp/Symbiosis
Miami, Florida
  Chapter 12: Electromagnetic Radiation (first edition)

Diana Perez, BSc, PT, MSc
Part-time Faculty & Course Coordinator
  Faculty of Medicine
School of Physical and Occupational Therapy
McGill University
Montreal, Quebec

Physical Therapist
Medi-Club Physiotherapy and Medical Wellness
  Center
  Chapter 12: Electromagnetic Radiation (first edition)

Julie A. Pryde, MS, PA-C, PT, OCS, SCS, ATC, CSCS
Adjunct Assistant Professor
Samuel Merritt College
Oakland, California

Physician Assistant
Muir Orthopaedic Specialists
Walnut Creek, California
  Chapter 2: Inflammation and Tissue Repair

Sara Shapiro, MPH, PT
Assistant Clinical Professor
University of California San Francisco
  Graduate Program in Physical Therapy
San Francisco, California

Owner
Apex Wellness & Physical Therapy
  Chapter 8: Electrical Currents

Gail L. Widener, PhD, PT
Associate Professor
Samuel Merritt College
Oakland, California
  Chapter 4: Tone Abnormalities

Preface to the Second Edition

In writing the first edition of this book I tried to meet a need that I believed existed—the need for a book on the use of physical agents in rehabilitation that covered the breadth and depth of this material in a readily accessible and easy to understand manner. I put together a text that leads the reader from the basic scientific and physiological principles underlying the application of physical agents, to the research evaluating their clinical use, and thence, to the practical details of selecting and applying each specific physical agent to optimize patient outcome. The enthusiasm with which the first edition of this book was received, including complimentary comments, adoption by many educational programs, and purchase by many clinicians, shows that the need was there and I met it.

Given how well the first edition of this book was received, I was leery to make too many changes for this second edition. I have done my best to keep all the positive aspects of the first edition while updating the information in all chapters. In addition, the concepts and language of the second edition of the American Physical Therapy Association's *Guide to Physical Therapist Practice* and the principles of evidence-based medicine have been incorporated into this new edition, and a few areas have been clarified or improved in other ways. Updates include consideration of the most recent research in all areas, with particular attention to meta-analyses and systematic reviews of the literature. Over 50 new illustrations have been added to clarify and update content. In addition, all aspects of the text, including the case studies, have been modified to be consistent with the *Guide to Physical Therapist Practice*, second edition.* The order of the chapters has been changed and, the

original chapter on traction and compression has been divided into two separate chapters, in order to reflect patterns of clinical practice rather than the physical properties of different physical agents. The electrical currents chapter has also been rewritten to make its style, content and level of detail more similar to that of the other chapters in section two of the book. This chapter has been slightly simplified and shortened while still thoroughly covering all aspects of the application of electrical currents in rehabilitation.

In addition to updating this book, there is now companion Evolve Online Learning Resources, which is available online at http://evolve.elsevier.com/Cameron The Student Resource Center provides a Study Guide with many boards-type multiple-choice questions to help students learn and assess their knowledge. Instructors' resources are available to instructors who adopt this book. The Instructors' Resource Center includes suggestions for laboratory activities, means to assess and document student competence in the selection and application of physical agents, and an electronic image collection of most of the figures in the text. Images in the collection can be copied into PowerPoint presentations.

The Preface to the First Edition states that this book was intended primarily for physical therapy students and physical therapists although I believed that it would also meet the needs of physical therapist assistants, occupational therapists, chiropractors and physicians, and students in these fields learning about the use of physical agents. Since the first edition was released it has come to my attention that many others, including athletic trainers, occupational therapy assistants, osteopaths, veterinarians and animal trainers also find this book to be a useful tool in their practice. I hope that this new edition continues to meet a wide range of professionals' needs for a readily accessible, clear, and thorough text on the application of physical agents in rehabilitation.

Michelle H. Cameron

---

*The Preferred Physical Therapist Practice PatternsSM are copyright 2002 American Physical Therapy Association and are taken from the *Guide to Physical Therapist Practice* (Guide to Physical Therapist Practice, 2nd Ed. *Phys Ther.* 2001;81:9-744). All rights reserved. Preferred Physical Therapist Practice PatternsSM is a trademark of the American Physical Therapy Association.

Preface to the First Edition

Teaching classes and courses on physical agents, I was frequently asked by my students, "Is there a book you would recommend that covers all this information?" and I would respond, "One of these days I'll write one." So, when the phone rang and the person on the other end of the line said, "I'm calling from the publisher W.B. Saunders. Will you write a new textbook on physical agents for us?" I immediately said "Yes, sure." Then came the shock, the work, the excitement, and now, here, a few years and a few life events later, is that book.

Although there are other texts on physical agents, I believe none cover the information with the same breadth and depth as this one. After reading this book the reader will be familiar with all the physical agents used by rehabilitation clinicians, including thermal agents, water, mechanical agents, and electrical agents. The reader will also understand the types of patient problems that can be treated effectively with physical agents and the physical properties and physiological effects of physical agents. Additionally, the reader will be able to apply this knowledge to select appropriate physical agents and treatment parameters and to use safe and effective application techniques in order to optimize patient outcome. The reader will also have a thorough understanding of why using physical agents benefits patients, the types of benefits that can be achieved by such interventions, and the mechanisms by which such interventions produce their effects.

This book provides rehabilitation students and practicing clinicians with a thorough understanding and firm basis for applying physical agents in rehabilitation. Although intended primarily for physical therapy students and physical therapists, this publication also meets the needs of physical therapist assistants, occupational therapists, chiropractors and physicians, and students in these fields learning about the use of physical agents. The book is structured to be used by students as a course text with outlines and objectives at the beginning of each chapter, lists that summarize content throughout the text, and chapter reviews; however, it can certainly be used by practicing clinicians as a reference. There is an accompanying instructor's manual and a study guide available to further facilitate the teaching and learning of the presented information.

This book is divided into three sections. The first includes chapters about the physiological processes most commonly affected by the application of physical agents, the second includes chapters about the specific different types of physical agents and their application, and the third includes chapters about integrating the application of physical agents with other treatment procedures and provides suggestions for future research on the application of physical agents in rehabilitation.

In *Section 1*, the reader learns about tissue inflammation and healing, pain, tone abnormalities, and motion restrictions. This information is presented first so that the information gained from assessment of a patient's presenting problems can be used in making decisions regarding the selection and application of physical agents.

In *Section 2*, the reader learns about the specific physical agents and their recommended clinical uses. Details of contraindications and precautions and specific guidelines for clinical application are presented in consistently formatted passages that are immediately recognizable and make the material easy to understand and review. The physical and physiological bases for the application of physical agents are described first, followed by an examination of the research on the effects of physical agents, in order to provide a basis for the recommended clinical application guidelines. This section includes chapters on thermal agents, hydrotherapy, traction and compression, ultrasound, electromagnetic fields and electrical currents.

Chapter 6, on thermal agents, describes the mechanisms and effects of decreasing or increasing tissue temperature and the clinical application of both cooling and heating agents.

Chapter 7, on hydrotherapy, describes the basis for the therapeutic application of water and provides guidelines for using water to cleanse open wounds or as an environment for exercise. Chapter 8 covers the application of mechanical force in the forms of traction and compression; the section on traction focuses on the application of mechanical traction to the spine, while the section focuses on the use of compression for controlling edema. Chapter 10, on electromagnetic agents, describes the electromagnetic spectrum and the physical agents, including ultraviolet, lasers, and diathermy, that apply electromagnetic radiation to achieve therapeutic effects. Chapter 11, on electrical currents, describes the types of electrical currents used in rehabilitation and their application to produce muscle contractions, modulate pain, promote tissue healing, and facilitate transdermal drug penetration. All chapters in Sections 1 and 2 include clinical case studies that illustrate the presented material within the context of patient care and demonstrate the clinical decision-making processes used in selection of the optimal physical agents and treatment parameters.

Section 3 integrates the information from the prior two sections. Chapter 12 discusses how physical agents may be used in conjunction with each other and with other types of interventions. A discussion of how physical agents may be used within the context of different health care delivery systems is also provided in this chapter. The final chapter explains why further research on the use of physical agents in rehabilitation is needed to validate and enable the progress of clinical practice and includes suggestions to direct such research.

This is the book on physical agents that I and my students have been looking for. The logical and consistent format of each chapter makes the presented information readily accessible, and the depth of information, complete referencing, and illustrative case studies facilitate the reader's understanding of how physical agents may be applied safely and effectively to enhance patient rehabilitation.

Michelle H. Cameron

Contents

APPENDICES

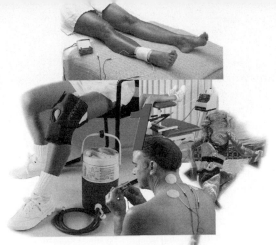

Introduction to Physical Agents

OBJECTIVES

Upon completion of this chapter, the reader will be able to:

1. Describe, categorize, and compare the types of physical agents used in rehabilitation.
2. Summarize the history of the clinical application of physical agents.
3. Explain the role of rehabilitation in patient care.
4. Explain the role of physical agents in rehabilitation.

5. Identify the physiologic effects of physical agents.
6. Outline the general contraindications and precautions for the use of physical agents.

This book is intended primarily as a course text for those learning to use physical agents in rehabilitation. It was written both to meet the needs of students learning about the theory and practice of applying physical agents and to assist practicing rehabilitation professionals in reviewing and updating their knowledge about the use of physical agents. This book describes the effects of physical agents, gives guidelines on when and how physical agents can be most effectively and safely applied, and describes the outcomes that can be expected from integrating physical agents within a program of rehabilitation. The theory underlying the application of each agent and the research concerning its effects are covered to provide a rationale for the treatment recommendations. Information is also provided on the physiologic processes influenced by physical agents in general, and regarding the specific effects produced by specific agents. After reading this book, the reader will be able to integrate the ideal physical agent(s) and treatment parameters within a complete program of rehabilitation care to promote optimal patient outcome.

This book uses a framework for describing the clinical use of physical agents based on the *Guide to Physical Therapist Practice*, 2nd edition (herein noted as the Guide).[1] However, this book presents more specific, research-based information regarding the theory, rationale, assessment process, and treatment parameters for the application of physical agents than provided by the Guide. It is important to note that the Guide is based on descriptions of preferred practice patterns for selected patient diagnostic groups. These practice patterns are not prescriptive, nor are they based on a review of available research evidence.

Following this introductory chapter, the book is divided into three sections. The first section covers the different types of musculoskeletal and neuromuscular problems that may be addressed by the use of physical agents. The second section describes the physical properties, physiologic effects, and application techniques for the different types of physical agents available. The third section integrates information from the first two and summarizes how different types of problems may be influenced by different physical agents, how treatments with physical agents may be integrated into a patient's complete plan of care, and how physical agents may be applied under different health care delivery systems. The final chapter discusses directions for future research on the use of physical agents in rehabilitation. A glossary of terms and abbreviations used in describing and documenting the application of physical agents is provided in Appendix A on pages 456-459.

DEFINITIONS AND EXAMPLES OF PHYSICAL AGENTS

Physical agents are various forms and means of applying of energy and materials to patients. Physical agents include heat, cold, water, pressure, sound, electromagnetic radiation, and electrical currents. The term *physical agent* can be used to describe the general type of energy, such as electromagnetic radiation or sound; a specific range within the general type, such as ultraviolet radiation or ultrasound and the actual means of applying the energy, such as an ultraviolet lamp or an ultrasound transducer. The terms *physical modality* and *modality* are also frequently used in place of the term *physical agent* and are used interchangeably in this book, with variation for ease of reading.

CATEGORIES OF PHYSICAL AGENTS

Physical agents are most readily categorized as *thermal, mechanical*, or *electromagnetic* (Table 1-1). Thermal agents include deep-heating agents, superficial heating agents, and superficial cooling agents. Mechanical agents include traction, compression, water, and sound. Electromagnetic agents include electromagnetic fields and electrical currents.

Thermal Agents

Thermal agents transfer energy to a patient to produce an increase or decrease in tissue temperature. Different thermal agents produce the greatest change in temperature in different types and areas of tissue. For example, a hot pack produces the greatest temperature increase in superficial tissues with high thermal conductivity in the area directly below it. In contrast, an ultrasound produces the most heat in tissues with high ultrasound absorption coefficients, such as tendon and bone. It produces this effect up to a depth of 5 cm but only in a small area, approximately twice that of the effective radiating area of the transducer.

TABLE **1-1**	Categories of Physical Agents	
Category	**Types**	**Clinical examples**
Thermal	Deep-heating agents	Diathermy
	Superficial heating agents	Hot pack
	Cooling agents	Ice pack
Mechanical	Traction	Mechanical traction
	Compression	Elastic bandage
	Water	Whirlpool
	Sound	Ultrasound
Electromagnetic	Electromagnetic fields	Ultraviolet
	Electric currents	TENS

Thermal agents that increase tissue temperature are most commonly applied when increasing of circulation, metabolic rate, and soft tissue extensibility, or the decrease of pain are expected to promote the goals of treatment. Thermal agents that decrease tissue temperature are most commonly applied when decreasing circulation, metabolic rate, or pain is expected to promote the treatment goals. A full discussion of the principles underlying the processes of heat transfer, the methods of heat transfer used in rehabilitation, and the effects, indications, and contraindications for applying superficial heating and cooling agents is provided in Chapter 6. The principles and practice of applying deep heating agents are discussed in Chapter 7 in the section on thermal applications of ultrasound and in Chapter 12 in the section on diathermy.

Ultrasound is a form of sound that cannot be heard by humans because of its high frequency. It is defined as sound with a frequency of greater than 20,000 cycles/second. Ultrasound a mechanical form of energy composed of alternating waves of compression and rarefaction. Ultrasound is used as a physical agent in rehabilitation to produce both thermal and nonthermal effects. Thermal effects, including increased deep and superficial tissue temperature, are produced by continuous ultrasound waves of a sufficient intensity, while nonthermal mechanical effects, including cavitation, microstreaming, and acoustic streaming, are produced by both continuous and pulsed ultrasound. Thermal-level ultrasound is used for the same purposes as other thermal agents when deep tissue is involved. These purposes include increasing circula-tion, metabolic rate, and soft tissue extensibility, and decreasing pain. Ultrasound is applied in a pulsed manner to optimize the nonthermal effects and facilitate tissue healing or promote transdermal drug penetration. Further information on the theory and practice of applying ultrasound can be found in Chapter 7.

Mechanical Agents

Mechanical agents apply mechanical force to increase or decrease pressure in or on the body. Water provides resistance to increase local pressure, hydrostatic pressure to increase circumferential pressure, and buoyancy to decrease pressure on weight-bearing structures. Traction decreases the pressure between structures, and compression increases the pressure between structures.

Water can be applied by immersion or nonimmersion techniques. The therapeutic application of water is known as *hydrotherapy*. Immersion in water produces pressure around the immersed area, provides buoyancy, and, if there is a difference in temperature between the area and the water, transfers heat to or from the area. Movement of the water produces local pressure, which can be used as resistance for exercise when an area is immersed and for cleansing or debriding open wounds with or without immersion. Further information on the theory and practice of hydrotherapy is provided in Chapter 9.

Traction is most commonly used to alleviate pressure on structures, such as nerves or joints that produce pain or other sensory changes or that become inflamed when compressed. Traction application can normalize sensation and prevent or reduce damage or inflammation of compressed structures. The pressure-relieving effects of traction may be temporary or permanent, depending on the nature of the underlying pathology and the force, duration, and means of traction application used. Further information on the theory and practice of applying traction is provided in Chapter 10.

Compression is used to counteract fluid pressure and control or reverse edema. The force, duration, and means of application of compression can be varied to control the magnitude of the effect and to accommodate different patient needs. Further information on the theory and practice of applying compression is provided in Chapter 11.

Electromagnetic Agents

Electromagnetic agents apply electromagnetic energy in the form of electromagnetic radiation or an electrical current. Variation of the frequency and intensity of electromagnetic radiation changes its effects and depth of penetration. For example, ultraviolet radiation, which has a frequency of 7.5×10^{14} to 10^{15} cycles/second, produces erythema and tanning of the skin but does not produce heat, whereas infrared radiation, which has a frequency of 10^{11} to 10^{14} cycles/second, produces heat only in superficial tissues. Continuous shortwave diathermy, which has a frequency of 10 million to 100 million cycles/second, produces heat in both superficial and deep tissues. When shortwave diathermy is pulsed to provide a low average intensity of energy, it does not produce heat; however, the electromagnetic energy is thought to modify cell membrane permeability and cell function by nonthermal mechanisms and thus acts to control pain and edema. Further information on the theory and practice of applying electromagnetic radiation is provided in Chapter 12.

The effects and clinical applications of electrical currents vary according to the waveform, intensity, duration, and direction of the current flow and according to the type of tissue to which the current is applied. Electrical currents of sufficient intensity and duration can depolarize nerves, causing sensory or motor responses that may be used to control pain or increase muscle strength and control. Electrical currents with an appropriate direction of flow can attract or repel charged particles and alter cell membrane permeability to control the formation of edema, promote

tissue healing, and facilitate transdermal drug penetration. Further information on the theory and practice of electrical current application is provided in Chapter 8.

HISTORY OF THE USE OF PHYSICAL AGENTS IN MEDICINE AND REHABILITATION

Physical agents have been a component of medical and rehabilitation treatment for many centuries and are used across a wide variety of cultures. For example, the remains of original bath houses with steam rooms and pools of hot and cold water that can still be seen in many major cities of the ancient Romans and Greeks provide evidence that these cultures used heat and water to maintain health and treat various musculoskeletal and respiratory problems.[2] The health benefits of soaking and exercising in hot water regained popularity many centuries later with the advent of health spas in Europe in the late 19th century in areas of natural hot springs. Today, the practices of soaking and exercising in water continue to be popular throughout the world because they provide resistance, thereby allowing the development of strength, endurance, and buoyancy, and reducing weight bearing on compression-sensitive joints.

Other examples of the historic use of physical agents include the use of torpedo fish, in approximately 400 B.C., to apply electric shocks to the head and feet to treat headaches and arthritis, and the use of amber in the 17th century to generate static electricity for the treatment of skin diseases, inflammation, and hemorrhage.[3] There are also reports from the 17th century of charged gold leaf being used to prevent scarring from smallpox lesions.[4]

Before the widespread availability of antibiotics and effective analgesic and antiinflammatory drugs, physical agents were commonly used to treat infection, pain, and inflammation. Examples of such applications include the use of sunlight for the treatment of tuberculosis, bone and joint diseases, and dermatologic disorders and infections, and the use of warm Epsom salt baths for the treatment of sore or swollen limbs.

Although physical agents have been used for their therapeutic benefits throughout history, over time, new uses, applications, and agents have been developed, and certain other agents and applications have fallen out of favor. New uses of physical agents have developed as a result of increased understanding of the biologic processes underlying disease, dysfunction, and recovery, and in response to the availability of advanced technology. For example, the use of transcutaneous electrical nerve stimulation (TENS) for the treatment of pain was developed based on the gate control theory of pain modulation, as proposed by Melzack and Wall. In contrast, the various modes of TENS application now available are primarily the result of the recent development of electrical current generators that allow fine control of the frequency, intensity, and pulse duration of the applied electrical current.

The use or specific application of a physical agent falling out of favor, usually occurs because the treatment is ineffective or because other, more effective treatments are developed. For example, infrared lamps were commonly used to treat open wounds because the superficial heat they provide can dry out the wound bed; however, these lamps are no longer used for this application because of the knowledge that wounds heal more rapidly when kept moist.[5,6] During the early years of the 20th century, sunlight was used to treat tuberculosis; however, since the advent of antibiotics, which are generally effective in eliminating bacterial infections, physical agents are now rarely used to treat tuberculosis or other infectious diseases. A number of physical agents have waned in popularity because they are cumbersome, have excessive associated risks, or interfere with other aspects of treatment. For example, the use of diathermy as a deep-heating agent was very popular 20 to 30 years ago, but because the machines are large and awkward to move around, can easily burn patients if not used appropriately, and the electromagnetic fields can interfere with the functioning of computer-controlled equipment nearby, diathermy is rarely currently used in the United States.

This book focuses on the physical agents most commonly used in the United States today. Physical agents that are not commonly of current use in the United States but were popular in the recent past, and those that are popular abroad or are expected to come back into favor as new delivery systems and applications are developed, are covered more briefly. Also included in this book is some discussion of modalities currently being used abroad that are awaiting approval by the Food and Drug Administration (FDA) for clinical use in the United States. The popularity of particular physical agents and applications is based on their history of clinical use and, in most cases,

research data supporting their efficacy; however, in some cases, their clinical application has continued despite the lack or limitations of supporting evidence. In most cases, more research is necessary to elucidate the ideal treatment and patient characteristics for optimal results and the precise nature of the outcomes to be expected from the application of physical agents in rehabilitation.

THE ROLE OF REHABILITATION IN PATIENT CARE

Rehabilitation is a goal-oriented treatment process designed to maximize independence in individuals who have compromised function as a result of underlying pathologic processes and secondary impairments. Rehabilitation generally addresses the sequelae of pathology rather than the pathology itself.

A number of classification schemes exist to categorize the sequelae of pathology. In 1980 the World Health Organization (WHO) published the first classification scheme known as the International Classification of Impairments, Disabilities and Handicaps (ICIDH).[7-9] This scheme, based primarily on the work of Wood, classifies the sequelae of pathology as impairments, disabilities, and handicaps.[10,11] Shortly thereafter, Nagi developed a model that classified the sequelae of pathology as impairments, functional limitations, and disabilities.[12] In 1993, the National Center for Medical Rehabilitation Research (NCMRR) published a classification scheme derived from a combination of the Nagi model and the original ICIDH model.[13] Most recently, in 2001, WHO further revised their classification scheme in their International Classification of Functioning, Disability and Health (ICIDH-2) scheme.[14]

The models of disability and the language used have been revised over time to reflect and create changes in perceptions of people with disabilities and to meet the needs of different groups of individuals. The original models were intended to differentiate disease and pathology from the limitations they produced. These models were developed primarily for use by rehabilitation professionals. The new, expanded models have a more positive perspective on the changes resulting from pathology and disease and are intended for use by a wide range of people, including community, national, and global institutions that create policy and allocate resources for persons with disabilities. Specifically, the NCMRR model added a category of societal limitations to the functional problems associated with disability, and it abandoned the previous linear modeling approach to reflect the frequently nonsequential nature of the relationships between categories. The ICIDH-2 has tried to change the perspective of disability from the negative focus of "consequences of disease" used in the 1980 model to a more positive focus on "components of health." Thus, while the first ICIDH used categories of impairments, disabilities, and handicaps to describe sequelae of pathology, ICIDH-2 uses categories of health conditions, body functions, activities, and participation to focus on abilities rather than on restrictions and limitations.

This book uses a scheme consistent with the terminology and framework of the *Guide to Physical Therapist Practice*, 2nd edition, which is based on the work of Nagi (Fig. 1-1), to evaluate clinical findings and determine a plan of care for the case studies presented.[1]

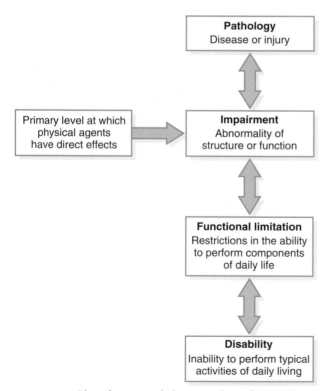

Figure 1-1. Classification of the sequelae of pathology. (Data from American Physical Therapy Association: *Guide to Physical Therapist Practice*, ed 2, Alexandria, VA, 2001, The Association.)

According to the Nagi scheme, the sequelae of pathology are classified as impairments, functional limitations, or disabilities.[7,12] *Pathology* refers to the alteration of anatomy or physiology due to disease or injury. Lumbar disc herniation and joint inflammation are examples of pathology.

Impairments are defined as alterations in anatomic, physiologic, or psychologic structures or functions as the result of some underlying pathology.[7,12] An impairment is a measure at the organ or organ system level and is equivalent to a sign or an objective measure. For example, decreased cervic mobility, diminished deep tendon reflexes, and absent sensation are all impairments. Impairments may lead to functional limitations or disabilities.

A functional limitation, as defined by the Nagi model, is a restriction in the ability to perform an activity in an efficient, typically expected, or competent manner. Examples of this classification include an inability to lift more than 20 lbs or a limitation in sitting tolerance. The Nagi model, then, defines a disability as the inability to perform activities required for self-care, home, work, or community roles. Examples of disability according to the Nagi model are the inability to lift one's child or to walk to the bathroom at home.

While medical treatment is generally directed at the underlying pathology or disease, rehabilitation focuses primarily on reversing or minimizing the associated impairments, functional limitations, and disabilities. Essentially, rehabilitation professionals must assess and set goals not only at the level of impairment, such as pain, decreased range of motion, or hypertonicity, but also at the level of functional limitation. These goals should include the patient's goals, such as being able to get out of bed, ride a bicycle, work, or compete in a marathon.

THE ROLE OF PHYSICAL AGENTS IN REHABILITATION

Physical agents are tools to be used, when appropriate, as components of rehabilitation. The American Physical Therapy Association's (APTA) position statement concerning the exclusive use of physical agents, published in 1995, states that "Without documentation which justifies the necessity of the exclusive use of physical agents/modalities, the use of physical agents/modalities, in the absence of other skilled therapeutic or educational intervention, should not be considered physical therapy."[15] This is a clear statement that the APTA believes that the use of physical agents alone does not generally constitute physical therapy, and that, in most cases, physical agents should be applied in conjunction with other interventions. The skilled application of physical agents that constitutes a component of physical therapy involves the integration of the appropriate intervention(s), which may include the application of a physical agent or agents or the education of the patient in such application, into the complete program of a patient's care to facilitate progress toward the functional goals of treatment.

The aim of this text is to give clinicians a better understanding of the theory and appropriate application of physical agents. Therefore the examples, documentation, and clinical case studies described focus on the physical agent being discussed. Inclusion of all possible goals and interventions for a given impairment or limitation is beyond the scope of this book.

Physical agents have direct effects primarily at the level of impairment. These effects can then promote improvements at the levels of functional limitation and disability. Physical agents are used primarily to reduce or eliminate soft tissue inflammation or circulatory dysfunction, increase the healing rate for soft tissue injury, modulate pain, modify tone, increase connective tissue extensibility and length, remodel scar tissue, or treat skin conditions. For example, thermal agents can be used to increase circulation and accelerate the metabolic rate to accelerate healing, and electrical currents can be used to stimulate sensory nerves to control pain or to stimulate motor nerves to produce muscle contractions.

Physical agents are frequently used in conjunction with, or in preparation for, other interventions such as therapeutic exercise, functional training, or manual mobilization to increase the efficacy of these interventions. For example, a hot pack may be applied before stretching to increase the extensibility of the superficial soft tissues and thus promote a more effective and safe increase in soft tissue length when the stretching force is applied.

When considering the application of a physical agent, one should begin the examination by checking the physician's referral, if one is required, for a diagnosis of the patient's condition and any precautions to be observed. The examination should include but not be limited to the patient's medical history; subjective complaints; review of systems, tests and measures;

functional status; and disabilities. The examination findings are then evaluated and, when possible, quantified. Following this analysis, a plan of care is established including anticipated goals. Given an understanding of the effects of different physical agents, the clinician can assess whether treatment using a physical agent may help the patient progress toward the anticipated goals. The clinician can then determine the treatment plan, including the ideal physical agent(s) and treatment parameters if indicated. The treatment plan is modified, as appropriate, when the patient's outcome is assessed. The sequence of examination, evaluation, and intervention is followed in the case studies in Section 2 of this book. Goals and interventions in this text primarily refer to treatment of impairment with the physical agent(s) being discussed.

EFFECTS OF PHYSICAL AGENTS

Modify inflammation and healing
Relieve pain
Alter collagen extensibility
Modify muscle tone

The application of physical agents primarily results in modification of tissue inflammation and healing, relief of pain, alteration of collagen extensibility, or modification of muscle tone. A brief review of these processes follows; more complete discussions of these processes are provided in Chapters 2 through 5.

Inflammation and Healing

When tissue is damaged by trauma or disease, it usually responds in a similar and predictable way. The first phase of recovery after damage has occurred is *inflammation*. This is followed by the proliferative phase of healing, which is completed during the maturation phase. Modification of inflammation and tissue healing can result in accelerated patient progress toward more active participation in rehabilitation and can expedite achievement of the therapy goals. Faster tissue repair can also reduce the risk and severity of the adverse effects of prolonged inflammation, pain, and disuse.

Thermal agents generally modify inflammation and healing by changing the rate of circulation and the rate of chemical reactions. Mechanical agents control motion and alter fluid flow, and electromagnetic agents alter cell function, particularly membrane permeability and transport. When selected and applied appropriately, physical agents can accelerate the completion and resolution of the phases of tissue healing, stimulate necessary processes to resume if they have stopped, accelerate recovery, and improve the final patient outcome. Physical agents can also minimize the risk of adverse effects from delayed or incomplete healing. However, if selected or applied inappropriately, physical agents may prolong inflammation, increase the severity of associated symptoms, prevent or delay healing, and increase the probability of adverse consequences and a poor outcome. A brief review of the processes of inflammation and healing and the factors that influence their progression follows; a more complete discussion of these processes is provided in Chapter 2.

During the inflammatory phase of healing, which generally lasts for 1 to 6 days, the cells necessary for removing debris and limiting bleeding enter the traumatized area. This phase is characterized by heat, swelling, pain, redness, and loss of function. The more quickly this phase is completed and resolved, the more quickly healing can proceed and the lower the probability of joint destruction, excessive pain, swelling, weakness, immobilization, and loss of function. Physical agents generally assist during the inflammatory phase by reducing circulation, reducing pain, reducing enzyme activity rate, controlling motion, and promoting progression to the proliferative phase of healing.

During the proliferative phase, which generally starts within the first 3 days after injury and lasts for approximately 20 days, collagen is deposited in the damaged area to replace tissue that was destroyed by the trauma; in addition, if necessary, myofibroblasts contract to accelerate closure, and epithelial cells migrate to resurface the wound. Physical agents generally assist during the proliferative phase of healing by increasing circulation, increasing enzyme activity rate, promoting collagen deposition, and promoting progression to the remodeling phase of healing.

During the maturation phase, which usually starts approximately 9 days after the initial injury and can last for up to 2 years, both deposition and resorption of collagen occur. The new tissue remodels itself to resemble the original tissue as closely as possible to best serve its original function. During this phase, the healing tissue changes both in shape and structure to allow for optimal functional recovery. The shape conforms more closely to the original tissue, often decreasing in size from the proliferative phase, and the structure becomes more organized; thus, greater strength is achieved with no change in tissue mass. Physical agents generally assist during the remodeling phase of healing by altering the balance of collagen deposition and resorption and improving the alignment of the new collagen fibers.

Pain Control

Pain is an unpleasant sensory and emotional experience associated with or described in terms of actual or potential tissue damage.[16–18] Pain usually protects individuals by preventing them from performing activities that would cause tissue damage; however, it may also interfere with normal activities and thus result in functional limitation and disability. For example, pain frequently interferes with an individual's ability to sleep, work, or exercise. Relieving pain can allow patients to participate more fully in normal activities of daily living and may accelerate the initiation of an active rehabilitation program, thereby limiting the adverse consequences of disuse and allowing more rapid progress toward the patient's functional goals.

Pain may be due to an underlying pathology, such as joint inflammation or pressure on a nerve that is in the process of resolution, or by a pathology, such as a malignancy, that is not expected to fully resolve. In either circumstance, relieving pain may facilitate resolution of the functional limitations and disability that result from the underlying pathology and can therefore assist the patient. The use of pain-relieving interventions, including physical agents, may be continued as long as pain persists and should be discontinued when the pain resolves.

Physical agents can control pain by modifying pain transmission or perception or by changing the underlying process causing the sensation. Physical agents may act by modulating transmission at the spinal cord level, changing the rate of nerve conduction, or altering the central or peripheral release of neurotransmitters. Physical agents can change the processes that cause pain by modifying tissue inflammation and healing, altering collagen extensibility, or modifying muscle tone. The processes of pain perception and pain control are explained in greater detail in Chapter 3.

Collagen Extensibility

Collagen is the main supportive protein of skin, tendon, bone cartilage, and connective tissue.[19] Tissues that contain collagen can become shortened as a result of being immobilized in a shortened position or being moved only through a limited range of motion. Immobilization may be the result of disuse as a result of debilitation or peripheral or central neural injury, or may be due to the application of an external device such as a cast, brace, or external fixator. Movement may be limited by internal derangement, pain, weakness, or poor posture or may be due to the application of an external device. Soft tissue shortening may cause impairment of restricted joint range of motion, shortened muscles, tendons, or joint capsules.

To return soft tissue to its normal functional length, thereby allowing full motion without damaging other structures, the collagen must be stretched. Collagen can be stretched most effectively and safely when it is most extensible. Since the extensibility of collagen is temperature dependent, increasing in response to increased temperature, thermal agents are frequently applied before soft tissue stretching to optimize the stretching process[20-24] (Fig. 1-2). The processes underlying the development and treatment of motion restrictions are discussed in detail in Chapter 5.

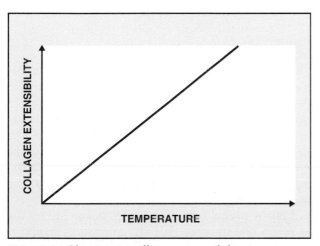

Figure 1-2. Changes in collagen extensibility in response to changes in temperature.

Muscle Tone

Muscle tone is the underlying tension that serves as a background for contraction in a muscle.[25] Muscle tone is affected by both neural and biomechanical factors and can vary in response to a pathology, expected demand, pain, and position.[26] Abnormal muscle tone is usually the direct result of nerve pathology or is a secondary sequela of pain due to injury of other tissues.[27]

Central nervous system injury, as may occur with head trauma or a stroke, can result in increased or decreased skeletal muscle tone in the affected area, whereas peripheral motor nerve injury, as may occur with nerve compression, traction, or sectioning, can decrease skeletal muscle tone in the affected area. For example, a patient who has had a stroke may have increased tone in the flexor muscles of the upper extremity and the extensor muscles of the lower extremity on the same side, whereas a patient who has had a compression injury to the radial nerve as it passes through the radial groove in the arm may have decreased tone in the wrist and finger extensors.

Pain may cause an increase or decrease in muscle tone. Muscle tone may be increased in the muscles surrounding a painful injured area in order to splint the area and limit motion, or tone in a painful area may be decreased as a result of inhibition. Although protective splinting may prevent further injury as a result of excessive activity, if prolonged it can also impair circulation, retarding or preventing healing. Decreased muscle tone as a result of pain—as occurs, for example, with the reflexive hypotonicity of the knee extensors—that causes buckling of the knee, when knee extension is painful, can limit activity and thus result in functional limitation.

Physical agents can alter muscle tone either directly, by altering nerve conduction or sensitivity or by altering the biomechanical properties of muscle, or indirectly, by reducing pain or the underlying problem causing pain. Normalizing muscle tone will generally reduce functional limitations and disability, allowing the individual to improve the performance of functional and therapeutic activities. Attempting to normalize muscle tone may also promote better outcomes from passive treatment techniques such as passive mobilization or positioning. The processes underlying changes in muscle tone are discussed fully in Chapter 4.

GENERAL CONTRAINDICATIONS AND PRECAUTIONS FOR THE USE OF PHYSICAL AGENTS

Pregnancy
Malignancy
Pacemaker
Impaired sensation
Impaired mentation

Restrictions on the use of particular treatment interventions are categorized as *contraindications* or *precautions*. Contraindications are conditions that render a particular form of treatment improper or undesirable, while precautions are conditions under which a particular form of treatment should be applied with special care or limitations.[6] The terms *absolute contraindications* and *relative contraindications* can be used in place of contraindications and precautions, respectively.

Although the specific contraindications and precautions for the application of particular physical agents vary, a number of conditions are contraindications or precautions for the use of most physical agents. Therefore caution should be used when considering application of a physical agent to a patient with any of these conditions. In patients with such conditions, the nature of the restriction, the nature and distribution of the physiologic effects of the physical agent, and the distribution of the energy produced by the physical agent must be considered. The conditions for which treatment with most physical agents are contraindicated or require caution are pregnancy, malignancy, the presence of a pacemaker, impaired sensation, and impaired mentation.

Pregnancy is generally a contraindication or precaution for the application of a physical agent if the energy produced by the agent or the physiologic effects of the agent may reach the fetus. These restrictions apply because the influences of these types of energy on fetal development are usually not known and because fetal development is adversely affected by many influences, some of which are subtle.

Malignancy is a contraindication or precaution for the application of physical agents if the energy produced by the agent or the physiologic effects of the agent may reach malignant tissue or alter the circulation to such tissue. Some physical agents accelerate the growth or metastasis of malignant tissue. These effects are thought to result from increased circulation or altered cellular function. Care must also be taken when considering treating any area of the body that currently has or previously had cancer cells, since malignant tissue can metastasize and may therefore be present in areas where it has not yet been detected.

The use of physical agents is generally contraindicated when the energy of the agent can reach a pacemaker because the energy produced by some of these agents may alter the functioning of the pacemaker and thus dangerously change the patient's heart rate.

Impaired sensation and mentation are contraindications or precautions for the use of many physical agents because the end limit for the application of these agents is the patient's report of how the treatment feels. For example, for most thermal agents, the patient's report of the sensation of heat being comfortable or painful is used as a guide to limit the intensity of the treatment. If the patient cannot feel heat or pain due to impaired sensation, or cannot report this sensation accurately and consistently due to impaired mentation or other factors affecting the ability to communicate, the application of the treatment would not be safe and is therefore contraindicated.

Specific contraindications and precautions, including questions to ask the patient and features to assess before before the application of each physical agent, are provided in Section 2 of this book in each of the chapters concerning the different types of physical agents.

CHAPTER REVIEW

Physical agents are various forms of energy and materials and their means of application as applied to patients. Physical agents include heat, cold, water, pressure, sound, electromagnetic radiation, and electrical currents. These agents can be categorized as thermal, mechanical, or electromagnetic. Physical agents have been used for many centuries and by many cultures and continue to be used today as a component of rehabilitation.

Rehabilitation focuses on the treatment of the sequelae of pathology, including impairments, functional limitations, and disabilities. Physical agents are included in rehabilitation care primarily to affect the impairments directly, thereby reducing functional limitation and disability. The use of physical agents is generally integrated into a program of patient treatment that includes other interventions to optimize the benefit and outcome.

When appropriately selected and applied, physical agents can promote the resolution of inflammation, accelerate tissue healing, relieve pain, increase soft tissue extensibility, and/or modify muscle tone. Most physical agents should not be applied when the energy provided by the agent or the physiologic effects produced can reach a fetus, malignant tissue, or a pacemaker. In addition, physical agents that use the patient's report as a guide for dosage or intensity should not be applied to patients with impaired sensation or mentation.

References

1. American Physical Therapy Association: *Guide to Physical Therapist Practice*, ed 2, Alexandria, VA, 2001, The Association.
2. Johnson EW: Back to water (or hydrotherapy), *J Back Musculoskel Med* 4(4):ix, 1994.
3. Baker LL, McNeal DR, Benton LA, et al: *Neuromuscular Electrical Stimulation: A Practical Guide*, ed 3, Downey, CA, 1993, Los Amigos Research & Education Institute.
4. Roberson WS: Digby's receipts, *Ann Med Hist* 7(3):216, 1925.
5. Hyland DB, Kirkland VJ: Infrared therapy for skin ulcers, *Am J Nurs* 80(10):1800-1801, 1980.
6. Cummings J: Role of light in wound healing. In Kloth L, McCulloch JM, Feedar JA, eds: *Wound Healing: Alternatives in Management*, Philadelphia, 1990, FA Davis.
7. Melvin JL, Nagi SZ: Factors in behavioral response to impairments, *Arch Phys Med Rehabil* 51:532-537, 1970.
8. Schenkman M, Butler RB: A model for multisystem evaluation, interpretation, and treatment of individuals with neurologic dysfunction, *Phys Ther* 69(7):538-547, 1989.
9. World Health Organization: *International Classification of Impairments, Disabilities and Handicaps (ICIDH)*, Geneva, 1980, The Organization.
10. Wood PHN: The language of disablement: A glossary relating to disease and its consequences, *Int Rehab Med* 2:86-92, 1980.
11. Wagstaff S: The use of the International Classification of Impairments, Disabilities and Handicaps in rehabilitation, *Physiotherapy* 68:548-553, 1982.
12. Nagi S: Disability concepts revisited. In Pope AM, Tarlov AR, eds: *Disability in America: Toward a National Agenda for Prevention*, Washington, DC, 1991, National Academy Press,
13. National Institutes of Health: *Research Plan for the National Center for Medical Rehabilitation Research*, Bethesda, MD, 1993, The Institutes.
14. World Health Organization: *International Classification of Functioning, Disability and Health (ICIDH-2)*, Geneva, 2001, The Organization.
15. American Physical Therapy Association: *Position on exclusive use of physical agents modalities*, Alexandria, VA 1995, House of Delegates Reference Committee, 25-95.
16. Sweet WH: *Pain:* In Field J, Magoun HW, and Hall WE: *Handbook of Physiology*, Section I, Neurophysiology, vol. 1, Washington DC, 1959, *Amer Physiol Soc,* pp. 459-506.
17. Bonica JJ: Pain: What is science doing about it? *Pain* 2:12-15, 1975.
18. Merskey H, ed: Classification of chronic pain: Description of chronic pain syndromes and definition of pain terms, *Pain* 13(Suppl 3):s1, 1986.
19. *Dorland's Illustrated Medical Dictionary,* ed 29, Philadelphia, 2000, WB Saunders.
20. Lentell G, Hetherington T, Eagan J et al: The use of thermal agents to influence the effectiveness of low load prolonged stretch, *J Orthop Sport Phys Ther* 16(5):200-207, 1992.
21. Warren C, Lehmann J, Koblanski J: Elongation of rat tail tendon: Effect of load and temperature, *Arch Phys Med Rehabil* 52:465-474, 484, 1971.
23. Warren C, Lehmann J, Koblanski J: Heat and stretch procedures: An evaluation using rat tail tendon, *Arch Phys Med Rehabil* 57:122-126, 1976.
24. Gersten JW: Effect of ultrasound on tendon extensibility, *Am J Phys Med* 34:362-369, 1955.
25. Lehmann J, Masock A, Warren C et al: Effect of therapeutic temperatures on tendon extensibility, *Arch Phys Med Rehabil* 51:481-487, 1970.
26. Keshner EA: Reevaluating the theoretical model underlying the neurodevelopmental theory: A literature review, *Phys Ther* 61:1035-1040, 1981.
27. Brooks VB: Motor control: How posture and movements are governed, *Phys Ther* 63:664-673, 1983.

Section One

Pathology and Patient Problems

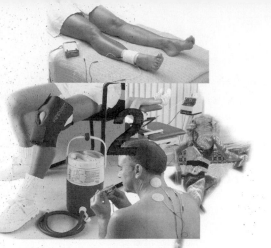

Inflammation and Tissue Repair

Julie A. Pryde, MS, PA-C, PT, OCS, SCS, ATC, CSCS

SUMMARY OF INFORMATION COVERED

Inflammation Phase (Days 1-6)
Proliferation Phase (Days 3-20)
Maturation Phase (Day 9 on)
Chronic Inflammation

Factors Affecting the Healing Process
Healing of Specific Musculoskeletal Tissues
Clinical Case Study
Chapter Review

OBJECTIVES

Upon completion of this chapter, the reader will be able to:

1. Define inflammation and identify its possible causes.
2. Identify the five cardinal signs of inflammation and their causes.
3. List the phases of tissue inflammation and repair and their relative time frames.
4. Describe the four responses of the inflammatory phase.
5. Discuss edema and its qualitative variability.
6. Describe the four processes that occur in the proliferation phase of healing.

7. Differentiate between the different types of collagen and their roles in tissue repair.
8. Describe the differences between the cellular responses in acute and chronic inflammation.
9. Identify local and systemic factors that can affect tissue healing.
10. Discuss how different types of musculoskeletal tissue heal.
11. List the physical agents that can affect or modify tissue healing.

Trauma or injury to vascularized tissue results in a coordinated, complex, and dynamic series of events collectively referred to as *inflammation and repair*. Although there are variations between the responses of different tissue types, overall the processes are remarkably similar. The sequelae depend on the source and site of injury, the state of local homeostasis, and whether the injury is acute or chronic. The ultimate goal of inflammation and repair is to restore function by eliminating the pathological or physical insult, replacing the damaged or destroyed tissue, and promoting regeneration of normal tissue structure.

Rehabilitation professionals treat a variety of inflammatory conditions resulting from trauma, surgical procedures, or problematic healing. The clinician who is called upon to manage such injuries needs to understand the physiology of inflammation and healing and how it can be modified. The clinician can enhance healing by the appropriate application of various physical agents, therapeutic exercises, or manual techniques. The foundation for a successful rehabilitation program requires an understanding of biomechanics, the phases of tissue healing, and the effects of immobilization and therapeutic interventions on the healing process.

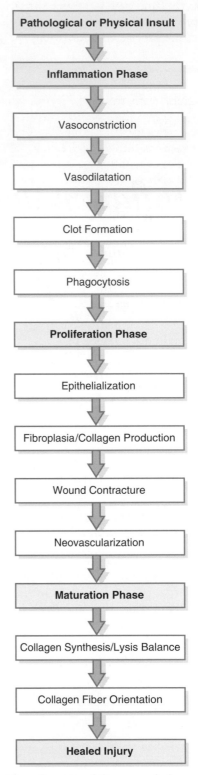

Figure 2-1. Flow diagram of the normal phases of inflammation and repair.

Common Causes of Inflammation
Soft tissue trauma (sprains, strains, and contusions)
Fractures
Foreign bodies (sutures)
Autoimmune diseases (rheumatoid arthritis)
Microbial agents (bacteria)
Chemical agents (acid, alkali)
Thermal agents (burns or frostbite)
Irradiation (UV or radiation)

This chapter will provide readers with information about the processes involved in inflammation and tissue repair so they can understand how physical agents may be used to modify these processes and improve patient outcome.

The process of inflammation and repair consists of three phases: inflammation, proliferation, and maturation. The inflammation phase prepares the wound for healing; the proliferation phase rebuilds the damaged structures and strengthens the wound; and the maturation phase modifies the scar tissue into its mature form (Fig. 2-1). The duration of each phase varies to some degree, and the phases generally overlap. Thus the timetables for the various phases of healing provided in this chapter are only general guidelines, not precise definitions (Fig. 2-2).

INFLAMMATION PHASE (DAYS 1-6)

Inflammation, from the Latin *inflamer,* meaning "to set on fire," begins when the normal physiology of tissue is altered by disease or trauma.[1] This immediate protective response attempts to destroy, dilute, or isolate the cells or agents that may be at fault. It is a normal and necessary prerequisite to healing. If there is no inflammation, healing cannot occur. Inflammation can also be harmful, particularly when it is directed at the wrong tissue or is overly exuberant. For example, inappropriately directed inflammatory reactions that underlie autoimmune diseases such as rheumatoid arthritis can cause excessive scarring, which can be disfiguring and limit joint mobility. Although the inflammatory process follows the same sequence regardless of the cause of injury, some causes result in exaggeration or prolongation of certain events.

Cornelius Celsus first described the inflammatory phase nearly 2000 years ago as being characterized by the four cardinal signs of *calor, rubor, tumor,* and *dolor* (Latin terms for heat, redness, swelling, and pain). *Functio laesa* (loss of function) was later added to this list by Virchow, bringing the number of cardinal signs of inflammation to five (Table 2-1).

An increase in blood in a given area, known as *hyperemia,* accounts primarily for the increased temperature and redness in the area of acute inflammation. The onset of hyperemia at the beginning of the inflammatory response is controlled by neurogenic and chemical mediators.[2] Local swelling results from increased permeability and vasodilatation of the local blood vessels and infiltration of fluid into the interstitial spaces of the injured area. Pain results from the pressure of the swelling and from irritation of pain-sensitive structures by chemicals released from damaged cells.[2] Both pain and swelling may result in loss of function.

There is some disagreement in the literature about the duration of the inflammation phase. Some investigators state that it is relatively short, lasting for less than 4 days,[3,4] and others believe it may last for up to 6 days.[5,6] This discrepancy may be the result of individual and injury-specific variation or the overlapping nature of phases of inflammation and tissue healing.

The inflammatory phase involves a complex sequence of interactive and overlapping events including vascular, cellular, hemostatic, and immune processes. Humoral and neural mediators act to control the inflammatory phase.

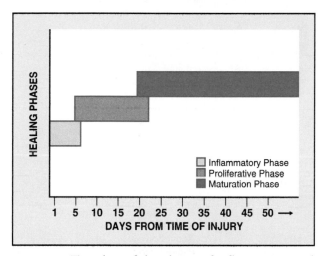

Figure 2-2. Time line of the phases of inflammation and repair.

TABLE 2-1 Cardinal Signs of Inflammation

Sign (English)	Sign (Latin)	Cause
Heat	*Calor*	Increased vascularity
Redness	*Rubor*	Increased vascularity
Swelling	*Tumor*	Blockage of lymphatic drainage
Pain	*Dolor*	Physical pressure and/or chemical irritation of pain-sensitive structures
Loss of function	*Functio laesa*	Pain and swelling

Vascular Response

Alterations in the anatomy and function of the microvasculature, including the capillaries, post-capillary venules and lymphatic vessels, are among the earliest responses in the inflammatory phase.[7] Trauma, such as a laceration, sprain, or contusion physically disrupts these structures and may produce bleeding, fluid loss, cell injury, and exposure of tissues to foreign material, including bacteria. The damaged vessels respond rapidly with transient constriction in an attempt to minimize blood loss. This response, which is mediated by norepinephrine, generally lasts for 5 to 10 minutes but can be prolonged in the small vessels by serotonin released from mast cells and platelets.

Following the transient vasoconstriction of injured vessels, the noninjured vessels near the injured area dilate. Capillary permeability is also increased by injury of the capillary walls and in response to chemicals released from injured tissues (Fig. 2-3). The vasodilation and increase in capillary permeability are initiated by histamine, Hageman factor, bradykinin, prostaglandins, and complement fractions. Vasodilation and increased capillary permeability last for up to 1 hour after tissue damage.

Histamine is released by mast cells, platelets, and basophils at the injury site.[8] Histamine causes vasodilation and increased vascular permeability in venules, which contributes to local edema (swelling) formation. Histamine also attracts leukocytes to the damaged tissue area.[9] Histamine is active for approximately 1 hour after tissue injury[10] (Fig. 2-4).

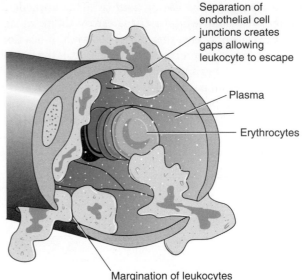

Figure 2-3. Vascular response to wound healing.

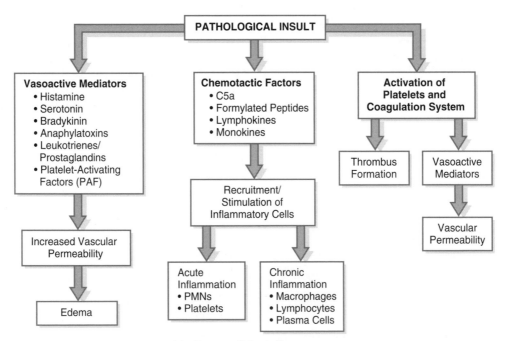

Figure 2-4. Mediators of the inflammatory response.

Hageman factor (also known as *clotting factor XII*), an enzyme found in the blood, is activated by contact with the negatively charged surfaces of the endothelial lining of vessels that are exposed when vessels are damaged. The role of Hageman factor is twofold. First, it activates the coagulation system to stop local bleeding. Second, it causes vasoconstriction and increased vascular permeability by activating other plasma proteins. It converts plasminogen to plasmin and prekallikrein to kallikrein, and it activates the alternative complement pathway[11] (Fig. 2-5).

Plasmin augments vascular permeability in both the skin and lungs by inducing breakdown of fibrin and by cleaving components of the complement system. Plasmin also activates Hageman factor, which initiates the cascade that generates bradykinin.

Plasma kallikrein attracts neutrophils and cleaves kininogen to generate several kinins such as bradykinin. The ability of a chemical to attract cells is known as *chemotaxis*. Kinins, such as bradykinin, are biologically active peptides that are potent inflammatory substances derived from plasma. Kinins function similarly to histamine, causing a marked increase in permeability of the microcirculation. They are most prevalent in the early phases of inflammation, after which they are rapidly destroyed by tissue proteases or kininases.[12]

Prostaglandins (PGEs) are produced by nearly all cells in the body and are released in response to any damage to the cell membrane. Two prostaglandins affect the inflammatory phase: PGE_1 and PGE_2. PGE_1 increases vascular permeability by antagonizing vasoconstriction, and PGE_2 attracts leukocytes and synergizes the effects of other inflammatory mediators such as bradykinin. Proinflammatory prostaglandins are also thought to be responsible for sensitizing pain receptors. In the early stages of the healing response, prostaglandins may regulate the repair process; they are also responsible for the later stages of inflammation.[13] Steroids and nonsteroidal antiinflammatory drugs inhibit prostaglandin synthesis. For example, acetylsalicylic acid (aspirin) and acetaminophen (Tylenol®) disrupt the production of prostaglandins but act at different points in their synthesis. Since prostaglandins are responsible for febrile states, these medications are effective in reducing fever.

The anaphylatoxins C3a, C4a, and C5a are important products of the complement system. These complement fractions cause increased vascular permeability and induce mast cell and basophil degranultaion, causing a further release of histamine and thus potentiating a further increase in vascular permeability (Table 2-2).

Aside from the chemically mediated vascular changes, changes in physical attraction between blood vessel walls also alter blood flow. During the initial vasoconstriction, the opposing walls of the small vessels become approximated, causing the lining of the blood vessels to stick together. Under normal physiologic conditions, the cell membranes of the inflammatory cells and the basement membranes have mutually repulsive negative charges; however, after injury, this repulsion decreases and the polarity may actually be reversed. This results in a decrease in the repulsion between the circulating inflammatory cells and the vessel walls and contributes to the adherence of inflammatory cells to the blood vessel linings.

As blood flow slows resulting from vasoconstriction of the postcapillary venules and increased permeability of the microvasculature, an increase in the cellular concentration occurs in the vessels, resulting in increased viscosity. In the normal physiological state, the cellular components of blood within the microvasculature are confined to a central axial column, and the blood in contact with the vessel wall

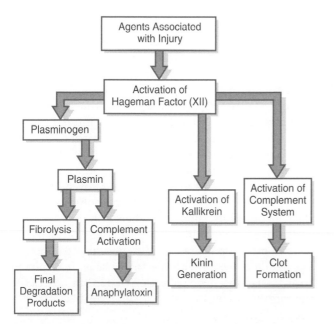

Figure 2-5. Hageman factor activation and inflammatory mediator production.

TABLE 2-2   Mediators of the Inflammatory Response

Response	Mediators
Vasodilation	Histamine Prostaglandins Serotonin
Increased vascular permeability	Bradykinin C3a, C5a PAF Histamine Serotonin Prostaglandins
Chemotaxis	Histamine C5a Monokines Kallikrein Lymphokines
Fever	Prostaglandins
Pain	Prostaglandins Hageman factor Bradykinin

is relatively cell-free plasma. Very early in the inflammatory response, neutrophils in the circulating blood begin migrating to the injured area. The sequence of events in the journey of these cells from inside the blood vessel to the tissue outside the blood vessel is known as *extravasation*. The neutrophils, which are a type of leukocyte (white blood cell), break away from the central cellular column of blood and start to roll along the blood vessel lining (the endothelium) and adhere. They line the walls of the vessels in a process known as *margination*. Within 1 hour, the endothelial lining of the vessels can be completely covered with leukocytes. As these cells accumulate, they lay down in layers in a process known as *pavementing*. Certain mediators control the adherence of leukocytes to the endothelium, either enhancing or inhibiting this process. For example, fibronectin, a glycoprotein present in plasma and basement membranes, has an important role in the modulation of cellular adherence to vessel walls. After injury to the vessels, increased amounts of fibronectin are deposited at the injury site. The adherence of the leukocytes to the endothelium or vascular basement membrane is critical for the recruitment of leukocytes to the site of the injury.

After margination occurs, leukocytes begin to squeeze through the vessel walls in a process known as *diapedesis*. The leukocytes insert their pseudopods into the junctions between the endothelial cells, crawl through the widened junctions, and assume a position between the endothelium and the basement membrane. Then, attracted by chemotactic agents, they escape to reach the interstitium. This process of leukocyte migration from the blood vessels into the perivascular tissues is known as *emigration* (Fig. 2-6).

Edema is an accumulation of fluid within the extravascular space and interstitial tissues. Edema is the result of increased capillary hydrostatic pressure, increased interstitial osmotic pressure, and an overwhelmed lymphatic system that is unable to accommodate this substantial increase in fluid and plasma proteins. Edema formation and control are discussed in detail in Chapter 11. The clinical manifestation of edema is swelling.

The fluid that first forms edema during inflammation has very few cells and very little protein. This fluid is known as *transudate*. Transudate is made up of predominantly dissolved electrolytes and water and has a specific gravity of less than 1.0. As the permeability of the vessels increases, more cells and lower molecular weight plasma proteins cross the vessel wall, making the extravascular fluid more viscous and cloudy. This cloudy fluid, known as *exudate,* has a specific gravity of greater than 1.0. It is also characterized by a high content of lipids and cellular debris. Exudate is often observed early in the acute inflammatory process and forms in response to such minor injuries as blisters and sunburns.

The loss of protein-rich fluid from the plasma reduces the osmotic pressure within the vessels and increases the osmotic pressure of the interstitial fluids, which, in turn, increases the outflow of fluid from the vessels, resulting in an accumulation of more fluid in the interstitial tissue. When the exudate's concentration of leukocytes increases, it is known as *pus* or *suppurative exudate*. Pus consists of polymorphonuclear neutrophils, liquefied digestion products of underlying tissue, fluid exudate, and very often bacteria if an infection is present. When localized suppurative exudate occurs within a solid tissue, it results in an abscess, a localized collection of pus buried in a tissue, organ, or confined space. Pyogenic bacteria produce abscesses.

Four mechanisms are responsible for the increased vascular permeability seen in inflammation. The first

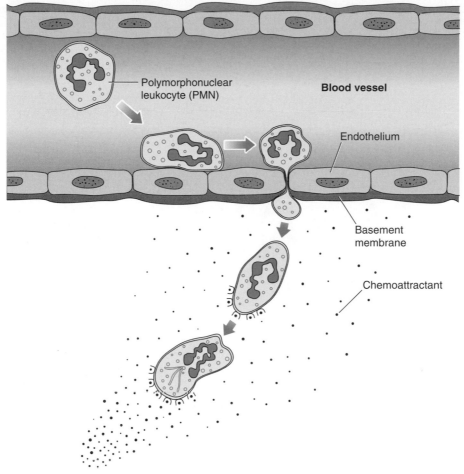

Polymorphonuclear
leukocyte (PMN)

Blood vessel

Endothelium

Basement
membrane

Chemoattractant

Source of injury

Figure 2-6. Illustration of leukocytic events in inflammation: margination, adhesion, diapedesis, and emigration in response to a chemoattractant emanating from the source of the injury.

and predominant mechanism is endothelial cell contraction, which leads to a widening of the intercellular junctions or gaps. This mechanism affects venules while sparing capillaries and arterioles. It is controlled by chemical mediators and is relatively short-lived, lasting for only 15 to 30 minutes.[14] The second mechanism is a result of direct endothelial injury and is an immediate, sustained response potentially affecting all levels of the microcirculation. This effect is often seen in severe burns or lytic bacterial infections, and is often associated with platelet adhesion and thrombosis or clot formation. Leukocyte-dependent endothelial injury is the third mechanism. Leukocytes bind to the area of injury and release various chemicals and enzymes that damage the endothelium and thus increase permeability. The final mechanism is leakage by regenerating capillaries that lack a differentiated endothelium and therefore do not have tight gaps. This may account for the edema characteristic of later healing inflammation (Fig. 2-7).

Hemostatic Response

The hemostatic response to injury controls the blood loss when vessels are damaged or ruptured. Platelets, the first cells at the site of the injury, enter the area and bind to the exposed collagen, releasing fibrin to stimulate clotting. Platelets also release a regulatory protein known as *platelet-derived growth factor (PDGF)*, which is chemotactic and mitogenic to fibroblasts

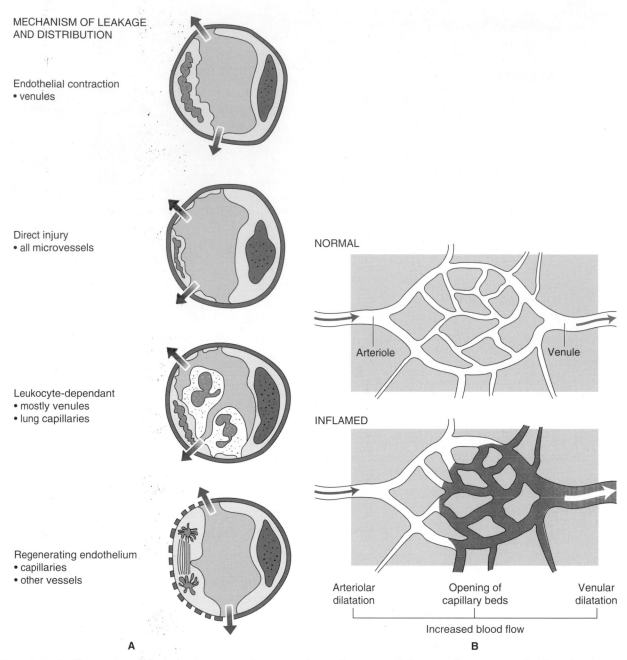

Figure 2-7. A, Illustration of four mechanisms of increased vascular permeability in inflammation. **B,** Vascular changes associated with acute inflammation.

and may also be chemotactic to macrophages, monocytes, and neutrophils.[15] Thus platelets play a role not only in hemostasis but also contribute to the control of fibrin deposition, fibroblast proliferation, and angiogenesis.

When fibrin and fibronectin enter the injured area they form cross-links with the collagen to create a fibrin lattice. This tenuous structure provides a temporary plug in the blood and lymph vessels, limiting local bleeding and fluid drainage. The lattice seals off damaged vessels and confines the inflammatory reaction to the area immediately surrounding the injury. The damaged, plugged vessels do not reopen until later in the healing process. The fibrin lattice serves as the wound's only source of tensile strength during the inflammatory phase of healing.[16]

Cellular Response

Circulating blood is composed of specialized cells suspended in a fluid known as *plasma*. These cells include erythrocytes (red blood cells), leukocytes (white blood cells), and platelets. Red blood cells play a minor role in the inflammatory process, although they may migrate into the tissue spaces if the inflammatory reaction is intense. The primary role of the red blood cells, oxygen transport, is carried out within the confines of the vessels. An inflammatory exudate that contains blood usually indicates severe injury to the microvasculature. The accumulation of blood in a tissue or organ is referred to as a *hematoma;* bloody fluid that is present in a joint is called a *hemarthrosis*. Hematomas in muscle can cause pain and limit motion or function; they can also increase scar tissue formation.

A critical function of inflammation is to deliver leukocytes to the area of injury via the circulatory system. Leukocytes are classified according to their structure into polymorphonucleocytes (PMNs) and mononuclear cells. PMNs have nuclei with several lobes and contain cytoplasmic granules. They are further categorized, by their preference for specific histological stains, as neutrophils, basophils, and eosinophils. Monocytes are larger than PMNs and have a single nucleus. In the inflammatory process, leukocytes play the important role of clearing the injured site of debris and microorganisms to set the stage for tissue repair (Fig. 2-8).

Migration of leukocytes into the area of injury occurs within hours of the injury. Each leukocyte is specialized and has a specific purpose. Some leukocytes are more prominent in early inflammation, whereas others become more important during the later stages. Initially the number of leukocytes at the injury site is proportional to their concentration in the circulating blood (Table 2-3).

Since neutrophils have the highest concentration in the blood, they predominate in the early phases of inflammation. Chemotactic agents released by other cells, such as mast cells and platelets, attract leuko-

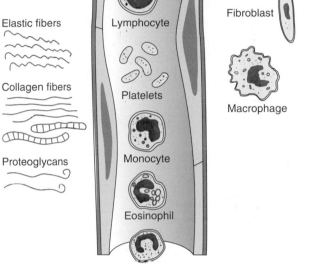

Figure 2-8. Intravascular cells, connective tissue matrix, and cells involved in the inflammatory response.

2-3 Concentration of Leukocytes in Adult Human Blood	
Type	**Concentration**
Polymorphonuclear Cells	
Neutrophils	62.0%
Eosinophils	2.3%
Basophils	0.4%
Mononuclear Cells	
Monocytes	5.3%
Lymphocytes	30.0%

cytes at the time of injury. Neutrophils rid the injury site of bacteria and debris by phagocytosis. When lysed, the lysosomes of the neutrophils release proteolytic enzymes (proteases) and collagenolytic enzymes (collagenases), which begin the debridement process. Neutrophils remain at the site of the injury for only 24 hours, after which time they disintegrate. However, they help to perpetuate the inflammatory response by releasing chemotactic agents to attract other leukocytes into the area.

Basophils release histamine after injury and contribute to early increased vascular permeability. Eosinophils may be involved in phagocytosis to some degree.

For 24 to 48 hours after an acute injury, monocytes predominate. Monocytes make up between 4% and 8% of the total white blood cell count. The predominance of these cells at this stage of inflammation is thought to result in part from their longer life span. Lymphocytes supply antibodies to mediate the body's immune response. They are prevalent in chronic inflammatory conditions.

Macrophage Products

Proteases
Elastase
Collagenase
Plasminogen activator
Chemotactic factors for other leukocytes
Complement components of the alternative and classical pathways
Coagulation factors
Growth-promoting factors for fibroblasts and blood vessels
Cytokines
Arachidonic acid metabolites

Monocytes are converted into macrophages when they migrate from the capillaries into the tissue spaces. The macrophage is considered the most important cell in the inflammatory phase and is essen-

tial for wound healing. Macrophages are important because they produce a wide range of chemicals. They play a major role in phagocytosis by producing enzymes such as collagenase (Fig. 2-9). These enzymes facilitate the removal of necrotic tissue and bacteria. Macrophages also produce factors that are chemotactic for other leukocytes.

Macrophages also probably play a role in localizing the inflammatory process and attracting fibroblasts to the injured area by releasing chemotactic factors such as fibronectin. Macrophages chemically influence the number of fibroblastic repair cells activated; therefore, in the absence of macrophages, fewer, less mature fibroblasts migrate to the injured site. Platelet derived growth factor (PDGF) released by platelets during clotting is also released by macrophages and can activate fibroblasts. In the later stages of fibroplasia, macrophages may also enhance collagen deposition by causing fibroblasts to adhere to fibrin.

As macrophages ingest microorganisms, they excrete products of digestion such as hydrogen peroxide, ascorbic acid, and lactic acid.[17] Hydrogen peroxide assists in the control of anaerobic microbial growth. The other two products signal the extent of the damage in the area, and their concentration is interpreted by the body as a need for more macrophages in the area.[18] This, in turn, causes increased production of by-products, which then results in an increased macrophage population and a more intense and prolonged inflammatory response.

Macrophages are most effective when oxygen is present in the injured tissues. However, they can tolerate low oxygen conditions, as is apparent by their presence in chronic inflammatory states. Adequate oxygen tension in the injured area is also necessary to minimize the risk of infection. Tissue oxygen tension

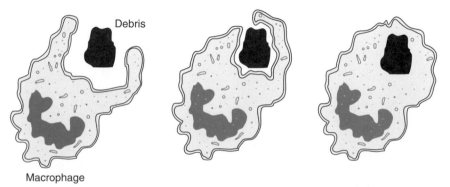

Debris

Macrophage

Figure 2-9. Diagrammatic representation of the process of phagocytosis.

depends on the concentration of atmospheric oxygen available for breathing, the amount of oxygen absorbed by the respiratory and circulatory systems, and the volume of blood available for transportation, as well as the state of the tissues. Local topical application of oxygen to an injured area does not influence tissue oxygen tension as much as the level of oxygen brought to the injured area by the circulating blood.[19-21]

Immune Response

The immune response is mediated by cellular and humoral factors. The roles of lymphocytes and phagocytic leukocytes in the immune response were discussed previously. The other mechanism involved in the immune response is the complement system which is an important source of vasoactive mediators. The complement system is one of the most important plasma protein systems of inflammation as its components participate in virtually every inflammatory response. The complement system can be activated by antigen-antibody complexes and by bacteria, foreign material, and other cellular products.

The complement system is a series of enzymatic plasma proteins that is activated by two different pathways, the classical and the alternative.[22] Activation of the first component of either pathway of the cascade results in the sequential enzymatic activation of the downstream components of the cascade (Fig. 2-10). The end product of the cascade, by either pathway, is a complex of C6, C7, C8, and C9, which form the membrane attack complex (MAC). The MAC creates pores in plasma membranes, thereby allowing water and ions into the cell. This causes loss of membrane integrity and cell lysis. The subcomponents generated earlier in the cascade also have important functions. Activation of components C1-C5 produces subunits that enhance inflammation by making bacteria more susceptible to phagocytosis (known as *opsonization*), attracting leukocytes by chemotaxis and acting as anaphylatoxins.

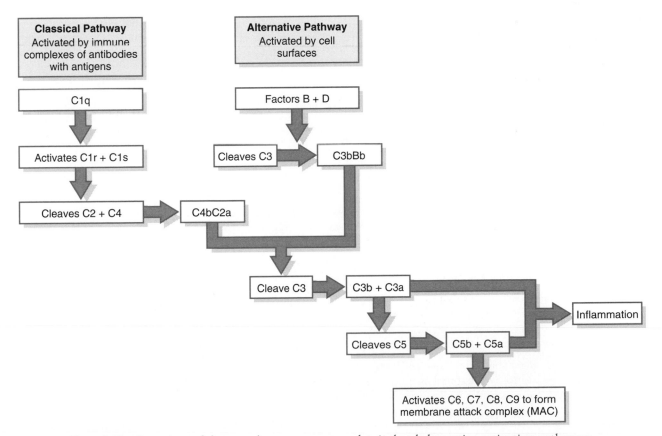

Figure 2-10. Overview of the complement system — classical and alternative activation pathways.

Anaphylatoxins induce mast cell and basophil degranulation, causing the release of histamine, platelet activating factor, and leukotrienes. These further promote increased vascular permeability.

The classical pathway of the complement cascade is activated by an antigen–antibody complex interacting with the first component of the complement cascade, C1. C1 consists of three proteins: C1q, C1r, and C1s. C1q binds to the antigen-antibody complex, resulting in a conformational change. C1r enzymatically activates C1s so that it can act on C4 and C2. C4 and C2 are cleaved to form C4bC2a, a complex that acts as a C3 convertase. C3 is cleaved into C3b and C3a by the C3 convertase. C3b then cleaves C5, producing C5a and C5b. C5b activates the production of the terminal products of the cascade, C6-C9.

The alternative pathway of the complement cascade is activated by a variety of cellular and microbial products and by foreign material. The binding of C3 with two plasma proteins, factors B and D, catalyzes the conversion of C3 to C3bBb which functions as a C3 convertase generating additional C3a and C3b in an amplification step. C3b then cleaves C5, resulting in the formation of the MAC, C6-C9. In contrast to the classical pathway, C1, C2, and C4 are not involved in the alternative pathway.

In summary, there are three major consequences of the inflammatory phase. First, fibrin, fibronectin, and collagen cross-link to form a fibrin lattice that limits blood loss and provides the wound with some initial strength. Then macrophages begin to remove damaged tissue. Finally, endothelial cells and fibroblasts are recruited and stimulated to divide. This sets the stage for the proliferation phase of healing (Table 2-4).

PROLIFERATION PHASE (DAYS 3-20)

The second phase of tissue healing is known as the *proliferation phase*. This phase generally lasts for up to 20 days and involves both epithelial cells and connective tissues.[16] Its purpose is to cover the wound and impart strength to the injury site.

Epithelial cells form the covering of mucous and serous membranes, and the epidermis of the skin. Connective tissue consists of fibroblasts, ground substance, and fibrous strands and provides the structure for other tissues. The structure, strength, and elasticity of connective tissue varies depending on the type of tissue it comprises. Four processes occur simultane-

---

TABLE 2-4 Summary of Events of the Inflammatory Phase

Response	Changes in the injured area
Vascular	Vasodilation followed by vasoconstriction at the capillaries, postcapillary venules, and lymphatics
	Vasodilation mediated by chemical mediators—histamine, Hageman factor, bradykinin, prostaglandins, complement fractions
	Slowing of blood flow
	Margination, pavementing, and ultimately emigration of leukocytes
	Accumulation of fluid in the interstitial tissues resulting in edema
Hemostatic	Retraction and sealing off of blood vessels
	Platelets form clots and assist in building of fibrin lattice, which serves as the wound's source of tensile strength in the inflammatory phase
Cellular	Delivery of leukocytes to the area of injury to rid the area of bacteria and debris by phagocytosis
	Monocytes, the precursors of macrophages, are considered the most important cell in the inflammatory phase
	Macrophages produce a number of products essential to the healing process
Immune	Mediated by both cellular and humoral factors
	Activation of the complement system via the alternative and classical pathways resulting in components that increase vascular permeability, stimulate phagocytosis, and act as chemotactic stimuli for leukocytes

ously in the proliferation phase to achieve coalescence and closure of the injured area: epithelialization, collagen production, wound contraction, and neovascularization.

Epithelialization

Epithelialization, the reestablishment of the epidermis, is initiated early in proliferation when a wound is superficial, often within a few hours of injury.[23] When a wound is deep, epithelialization occurs later, after collagen production and neovascularization. Epithelialization provides a protective barrier to prevent fluid and electrolyte loss and to decrease the risk of infection. Healing of the wound surface by epithelialization alone does not provide adequate strength to meet the mechanical demands placed on most tissues. Such strength is provided by the collagen produced during fibroplasia.

During epithelialization, uninjured epithelial cells from the margins of the injured area reproduce and migrate over the injured area, covering the surface of the wound and closing the defect. It is hypothesized that the stimulus for this activity is the loss of contact inhibition that occurs when epithelial cells are normally in contact with one another. The migrating epithelial cells stay connected to their parent cells, thereby pulling the intact epidermis over the wound edge. When epithelial cells from one edge meet migrating cells from the other edge, they stop moving due to contact inhibition (Fig. 2-11). Although clean, approximated wounds can be clinically resurfaced within 48 hours, larger open wounds take longer to resurface.[24] It then takes several weeks for this thin layer to become multilayered and to differentiate into the various strata of normal epidermis (Fig. 2-12).

Collagen Production

Fibroblasts make collagen. Fibroblast growth, known as *fibroplasia*, takes place in connective tissue. Fibroblasts develop from undifferentiated mesenchymal cells located around blood vessels and in fat. They migrate to the injured area along fibrin strands, in response to chemotactic influences, and are present throughout the injured area.[25] Adequate supplies of oxygen, ascorbic acid, and other cofactors such as zinc, iron, manganese, and copper are necessary for fibroplasia to occur.[26] As the number of fibroblasts increases, they begin to align themselves perpendicular to the capillaries.

The fibroblasts synthesize procollagen, composed of three polypeptide chains coiled and held together by weak electrostatic bonds into a triple helix. These chains undergo cleavage by collagenase to form tropocollagen. Multiple tropocollagen chains then coil together to form collagen fibrils, which then make up collagen filaments and ultimately combine to form collagen fibers (Fig. 2-13). Cross-linking between collagen molecules provides further tensile strength to the injured area.

Tissue containing the newly formed capillaries, fibroblasts, and myofibroblasts is referred to as *granulation tissue*. As the amount of granulation tissue increases, there is a concurrent reduction in the size of the fibrin clot, allowing for the formation of a more permanent support structure. These events are mediated by chemotactic factors that stimulate increased fibroblastic activity and by fibronectin that enhances migration and adhesion of the fibroblasts. The fibroblasts initially produce a thin, weak-structured collagen with no consistent organization known as *type III collagen*. This period is the most tenuous time during the healing process due to the limited tensile strength of the tissue. During the proliferation phase an injured area has the greatest amount of collagen, yet its tensile strength can be as low as 15% of that of normal tissue.[27]

Fibroblasts also produce hyaluronic acid, a glycosaminoglycan (GAG), which draws water into the area, increases the amount of intracellular matrix, and facilitates cellular migration. It is postulated that the composition of this substance is related to the number and location of the cross-bridges, thereby implying that the relationship between GAG and collagen dictates the scar architecture.[17,28]

The formation of cross-links allows the newly formed tissue to tolerate early, controlled movement without disruption. However, infection, edema, or excessive stress on the healing area may result in further inflammation and additional deposition of collagen. Excessive collagen deposition will result in excessive scarring that may limit the functional outcome.

By the seventh day after injury there is a significant increase in the amount of collagen, causing the tensile strength of the injured area to increase steadily. By day 12, the initial immature type III collagen starts to be replaced by type I collagen, a more mature and

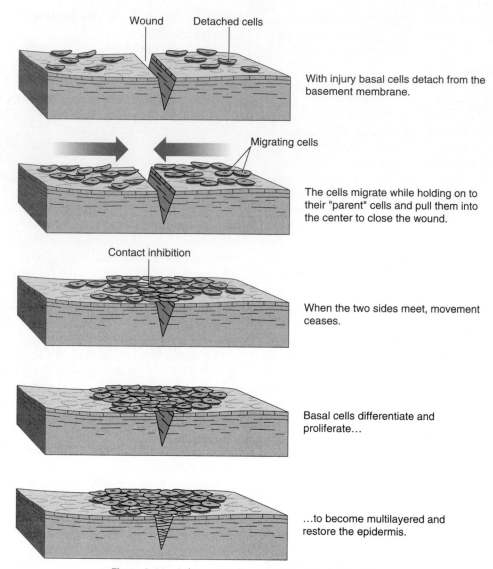

Wound   Detached cells

With injury basal cells detach from the basement membrane.

Migrating cells

The cells migrate while holding on to their "parent" cells and pull them into the center to close the wound.

Contact inhibition

When the two sides meet, movement ceases.

Basal cells differentiate and proliferate...

...to become multilayered and restore the epidermis.

Figure 2-11. Schematic diagram of epithelialization.

stronger form.[16,29,30] The ratio of type I to type III collagen increases steadily from this point on.

Wound Contraction

Wound contraction is the final mechanism for repairing an injured area. In contrast to epithelialization, which covers the wound surface, contraction pulls the edges of the injured site together, in effect shrinking the defect. Successful contraction results in a smaller area to be repaired by scar formation. Contraction of the wound begins approximately 5 days after injury

and peaks after about 2 weeks.[31] Myofibroblasts are the primary cells responsible for wound contraction. Myofibroblasts, identified by Gabbiani et al in 1971, are derived from the same mesenchymal cells as fibroblasts.[32] Myofibroblasts are similar to fibroblasts except that they also possess the contractile properties of smooth muscle. Myofibroblasts attach to the margins of the intact skin and pull the entire epithelial layer inward. The rate of contraction is proportional to the number of myofibroblasts at and under the cell margins and is inversely proportional to the lattice collagen structure.

HEALING BY PRIMARY INTENTION   HEALING BY SECONDARY INTENTION

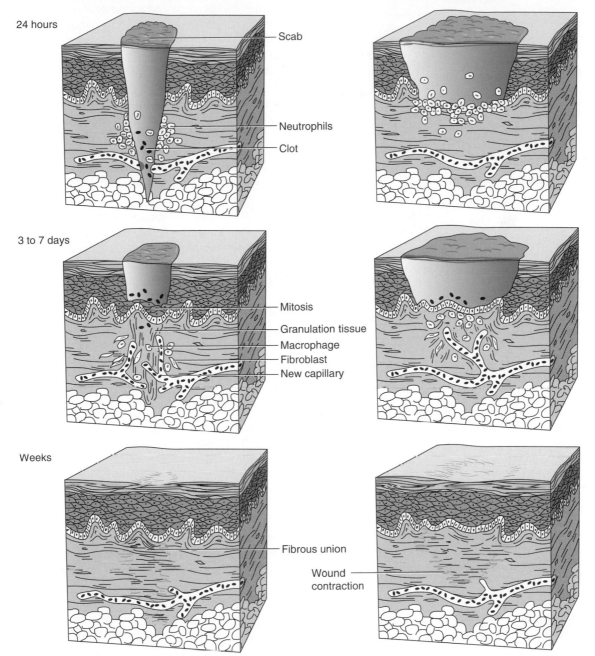

24 hours — Scab — Neutrophils — Clot

3 to 7 days — Mitosis — Granulation tissue — Macrophage — Fibroblast — New capillary

Weeks — Fibrous union — Wound contraction

Figure 2-12. Diagrammatic comparison of healing by primary intention (left) and secondary intention (right).

According to the "picture frame" theory, the wound margin beneath the epidermis is the location of myofibroblast action.[33] A ring of myofibroblasts moves inward from the wound margin. Although contractile forces are initially equal, the shape of the picture frame predicts the resultant speed of closure (Fig. 2-14). Linear wounds with one narrow dimension contract rapidly; square or rectangular wounds, with no close edges, progress at a moderate pace; and circular wounds contract most slowly.[34]

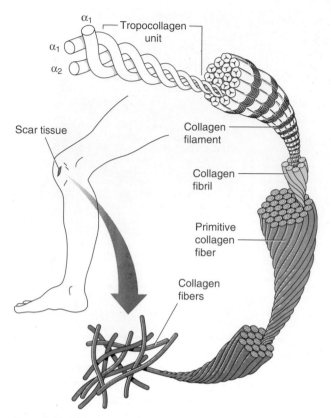

Figure 2-13. Diagrammatic representation of one tropocollagen unit joining with others to form collagen filaments and, ultimately, collagen fibers.

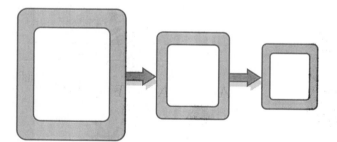

Figure 2-14. Illustration of the picture frame theory of wound contraction.

If wound contraction is uncontrolled it can result in the formation of contractures. Contractures are conditions of fixed high resistance to passive stretch that may result from fibrosis of tissues surrounding a joint.[35] Contractures may also result from adhesions, muscle shortening, or tissue damage. Contractures are discussed in greater depth in Chapter 5.

Wounds that are rapidly closed with sutures with minimal loss of tissue and minimal bacterial contamination can heal without wound contraction. This is known as *healing by primary union, primary intention,* or *first intention.* When there is significant loss of tissue or bacterial contamination, wound contraction is necessary to close the wound. Wound contraction is the feature that most clearly differentiates primary from secondary healing, also known as *healing by secondary intention* or *indirect union.*[36] Later approximation of a wound's edges with sutures or the application of skin grafts can reduce wound contraction and is known as *healing by delayed primary intention.*[37,38] To minimize contraction, grafts must be applied early in the inflammatory phase, before the process of contraction begins.[39]

As scar tissue matures, it develops pressure and tension-sensitive nerve endings to protect the immature vascular system, which is weak and can bleed easily with any insult. During the proliferation phase, the scar is red and swollen due to the increase in vascularity and fluid, the innervation of the healing site, and the relative immaturity of the tissue. The tissue can easily be damaged and is tender to tension or pressure.

Neovascularization

Neovascularization, the development of a new blood supply to the injured area, occurs as a result of angiogenesis, the growth of new blood vessels. Healing cannot occur without angiogenesis. These new vessels are needed to supply oxygen and nutrients to the injured and healing tissue. It is thought that macrophages signal the initiation of neovascularization. Angiogenesis can occur by three different mechanisms: generation of a new vascular network, anastomosis to preexisting vessels, or coupling of the vessels in the injured area.[40]

Vessels in the wound periphery develop small buds that grow into the wound area. These outgrowths eventually come in contact with and join other arterial or venular buds to form a capillary loop. These vessels fill the injured area, giving it a pinkish to bright red hue. As the wound heals, many of these capillary loops cease to function and retract, giving the mature scar a more whitish appearance than the adjacent tissues. Initially the walls of these capillaries are thin, making them prone to injury. Therefore immobilization at this stage may help to protect these vessels and permit further regrowth, whereas excessive early motion can cause microhemorrhaging and increase the likelihood of infection.

MATURATION PHASE (DAY 9 ON)

As the transition from the proliferation to the maturation stage of healing is made, changes occur in the size, form, and strength of the scar tissue. The maturation phase is the longest phase in the healing process. It can persist for over a year after the initial insult. During this time the number of fibroblasts, macrophages, myofibroblasts, and capillaries decrease and the water content of the tissue declines. The scar becomes whiter in appearance as the collagen matures and the vascularity decreases. The ultimate goal of this phase is restoration of the prior function of the injured tissue.

Several factors determine the rate of maturation and the final physical characteristics of the scar. These include fiber orientation and the balance of collagen synthesis and lysis.

Throughout the maturation phase, synthesis and lysis of collagen occur in a balanced fashion. Hormonal stimulation secondary to inflammation causes increased collagen destruction by the enzyme collagenase. Collagenase is derived from polymorphogranular leukocytes, the migrating epithelium, and the granulation bed. Collagenase is able to break the strong cross-linking bonds of the tropocollagen molecule, causing it to become soluble. It is then excreted as a waste by-product. Although collagenase is most active in the actual area of the injury, its effects can also be noticed, to a lesser extent, in areas adjacent to the injury site. Thus remodeling occurs through a process of collagen turnover.

Collagen, a glycoprotein, provides the extracellular framework for all multicellular organisms. Although more than 27 types of collagen have been identified, the following discussion is limited to types I, II, and III[41] (Table 2-5). All collagen molecules are made up of three separate polypeptide chains wrapped tightly together in a triple left-handed helix. Type I collagen is the primary collagen found in bone, skin, and tendon, and is the predominant collagen in mature scars. Type II collagen is the major collagen in cartilage. Type III collagen is found in the gastrointestinal tract, uterus, and blood vessels in adults. It is also the first type of collagen to be deposited during the healing process.

During the maturation phase, the collagen synthesized and deposited is predominantly type I. The balance between synthesis and lysis generally slightly favors synthesis. As type I collagen is stronger than the type III collagen deposited in the proliferation phase, tensile strength increases faster than mass. If the rate of collagen production is much greater than the rate of lysis, a keloid or hypertrophic scar can result. Both keloids and hypertrophic scars are the result of excessive collagen deposition due to inhibition of lysis. It is believed that this inhibition of lysis is due to a genetic defect. Keloids extend beyond the original boundaries of an injury and invade the surrounding tissue, whereas hypertrophic scars, although raised, remain within the margins of the original wound. The treatment of keloid scars through surgery, medications, pressure, and irradiation has only limited success.[42-44]

Collagen synthesis is oxygen dependent, while collagen lysis is not.[45] Thus, when oxygen levels are low, the process of maturation is weighted toward lysis, resulting in a softer, less bulky scar. Hypertrophic scars can be managed clinically with prolonged pressure, which causes a decrease in oxygen, resulting in decreased overall collagen synthesis while maintaining the level of collagen lysis.[37] This is one of the bases for the use of pressure garments in the treatment of patients suffering from burns, and for the use of elastomer in the management of scars in hand therapy. Eventually, balance is achieved when the scar bulk is flattened to approximate normal tissue.

TABLE 2-5	Collagen Types
Type	**Distribution**
I	Most abundant form of collagen: skin, bone, tendons, and most organs
II	Major cartilage collagen, vitreous humor
III	Abundant in blood vessels, uterus, skin
IV	All basement membranes
V	Minor component of most interstitial tissues
VI	Abundant in most interstitial tissues
VII	Dermal-epidermal junction
VIII	Endothelium
IX	Cartilage
X	Cartilage

Collagen synthesis and lysis may last for up to 12 to 24 months after an injury. The high rate of collagen turnover during this period can be viewed as both detrimental and beneficial. As long as the scar tissue appears redder than the surrounding tissue, remodeling is still occurring. Although a joint or tissue structure can lose mobility quickly during this stage, such a loss can still be reversed through appropriate intervention.

The physical structure of the collagen fibers is largely responsible for the final function of the injured area. Collagen in scar tissue is always less organized than collagen in the surrounding tissue. Scars are inelastic, so redundant folds are necessary to permit mobility of the structures to which they are attached. To understand this concept better, one may consider a spring, which, although made of an inelastic material, has a spiraled form that, like the redundant folds of a scar, allows it to expand and contract. If short, dense adhesions are formed, these will restrict motion because they cannot elongate.

Two theories have been proposed to explain the orientation of the collagen fibers in scar tissue: the induction theory and the tension theory. According to the induction theory, the scar attempts to mimic the characteristics of the tissue it is healing.[46] Thus a dense tissue induces a dense, highly cross-linked scar, whereas a more pliable tissue results in a loose, less cross-linked scar. Dense tissue types have a preferential status when multiple tissue types are in close proximity. Based on this theory, surgeons attempt to design repair fields that separate dense and soft tissues. If this is not possible, as in the case of repaired tendon left immobile over bone fractures, adhesions and poorly gliding tendons can result. In such cases, early controlled movement may be beneficial.

According to the tension theory, the internal and external stresses placed on the injured area during the maturation phase determine the final tissue structure.[40] Muscle tension, joint movement, soft tissue loading and unloading, fascial gliding, temperature changes, and mobilization are all forces that are thought to affect collagen structure. Thus the length and mobility of the injured area may be modified by the application of stress during the appropriate phases of healing. This theory has been supported by the work of Arem and Madden, which has shown that the two most important variables responsible for successful remodeling are the phases of the repair process in which mechanical forces were introduced

and the nature of the applied forces.[47] Scars need low-load, long-duration stretch during the appropriate phase for permanent changes to occur.

Studies have shown that the application of tension during healing causes an increase in tensile strength, and immobilization and stress deprivation reduce tensile strength and collagen structure. The recovery curves for tissue experimentally immobilized for between 2 and 4 weeks reveal that these processes can take months to reverse, and reversal is often never complete.

Each phase of the healing response is necessary and essential to the subsequent phase. In the optimal scenario, inflammation is a necessary aspect of the healing response and the first step toward recovery, setting the stage for the other phases of healing. If repeated insults or injury occur, however, a chronic inflammatory response may develop that can adversely affect the outcome of the healing process.

Acute inflammatory processes can have one of four outcomes. First, and most beneficial, is the complete resolution and replacement of the injured tissue with like tissue. Second, and most common, is healing by scar formation. The third is the formation of an abscess. Fourth is the possibility of progression to chronic inflammation.[10]

CHRONIC INFLAMMATION

Chronic inflammation is the simultaneous progression of active inflammation, tissue destruction, and healing. Chronic inflammation can arise in one of two ways. The first follows acute inflammation and can be due to the persistence of the injurious agent (such as a cumulative trauma) or to some other interference with the normal healing process. The second is a result of an immune response to either an altered host tissue or a foreign material, such as an implant or a suture, or is the result of an autoimmune disease such as rheumatoid arthritis.

The normal acute inflammatory process lasts for no more than 2 weeks. If it continues for more than 4 weeks, it is known as *subacute inflammation*.[3] Chronic inflammation is inflammation that lasts for months or years.

The primary cells present during chronic inflammation are mononuclear cells including lymphocytes, macrophages, and monocytes (Fig. 2-15). Occasionally eosinophils are also present.[48] The progression of the inflammatory response to a chronic state is a result of

Leukocyte	Characteristics / Functions
Monocyte/Macrophage Lysosome — Phagocytic vacuole	Associated with • chronic inflammation • phagocytosis Regulates coagulation/fibrolytic pathways Regulates lymphocyte response Monocytes are converted to macrophages when they emigrate from capillaries into the tissue spaces
Lymphocyte Lysosome — Sparse endoplasmic reticulum	Associated with • chronic inflammation Key cell in humoral and cell-mediated immune response
Eosinophil Granules	Associated with • allergic reactions • parasitic infections and associated inflammatory reactions Modulates mast cell-mediated reactions
Neutrophil	Associated with • acute inflammation • bacterial and foreign body phagocytosis
Basophil	• Not phagocytic • Contains histamine, which causes increased vascular permeability

Left vertical labels: Mononuclear cells (top two rows) · Polymorphonuclear cells (bottom two rows)

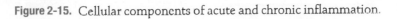

Figure 2-15. Cellular components of acute and chronic inflammation.

both immunologic and nonimmunologic factors. The macrophage is an important source of inflammatory and immunologic mediators and is an important component in the regulation of their actions. The role of eosinophils is much less clear, although they are often present in chronic inflammatory conditions that are caused by allergic reactions or parasitic infection.[48]

Chronic inflammation also results in increased fibroblast proliferation, which in turn increases collagen production and ultimately increases scar tissue and adhesion formation. This may lead to a loss of function as the delicate balance between optimal tensile strength and mobility of the involved tissues is lost.

FACTORS AFFECTING THE HEALING PROCESS

A number of factors, either local or systemic, can impact or modify the processes of inflammation and repair (Table 2-6). Local factors that can affect wound healing include the type, size, and location of the injury, infection, blood supply, and external physical forces.

Local Factors

Type, size, and location of the injury
Injuries located in well-vascularized tissue, such as the scalp, heal faster than those in poorly vascularized areas.[16] Injuries in areas of ischemia, such as those that may be caused by arterial obstruction or excessive pressure, heal more slowly.[16]

Smaller wounds heal faster than larger wounds, and surgical incisions heal faster than wounds caused by blunt trauma.[16] Soft tissue injuries over bones tend to adhere to the bony surfaces, preventing contraction and adequate opposition of the edges and delaying healing.[16]

Infection
Infection in an injured area is the most problematic local factor that can affect healing. Among the complications of wound healing, 50% are due to local infection.[11] Infections affect collagen metabolism, reducing collagen production and increasing lysis.[49] Infection often prevents or delays healing and encourages excessive granulation tissue formation.[16]

Vascular supply
The healing of injuries largely depends on the availability of a sufficient vascular supply. Nutrition, oxygen tension, and the inflammatory response all depend on the microcirculatory system to deliver their components.[50] Decreased oxygen tension resulting from a compromised blood supply can result in the inhibition of fibroblast migration and collagen synthesis, leading to decreased tensile strength of the injured area and increased susceptibility to infection.[20]

External forces
The application of physical agents including thermal agents, electromagnetic energy, and mechanical forces may also influence inflammation and healing. Cryotherapy (cold therapy), thermotherapy (heat), therapeutic ultrasound electromagnetic radiation, electrical currents, and mechanical pressure have all been used by rehabilitation professionals in an attempt to modify the healing process. The impact of these physical agents on tissue healing is discussed in Section 2 of this text, which describes each type of physical agent, its effects, and its clinical applications.

Movement
Early movement of a newly injured area may delay healing. Therefore immobilization may be used to aid early healing and repair. However, since immobility can result in adhesions and stiffness by altering collagen cross-linking and elasticity, continuous passive motion (CPM) with strictly controlled parameters is often used to remobilize and restore function safely.[51] The use of CPM in conjunction with short-

TABLE	**2-6**	**Factors Influencing Healing**

Local	Systemic
Type, size, and location of injury	Age
Infection	Infection or disease
Vascular supply	Metabolic status
Movement/excessive pressure	Nutrition
Temperature deviation	Hormones
Topical medications	Medication
Electromagnetic energy	Fever
Retained foreign body	Oxygen

term immobilization, compared to immobilization alone, has been shown to achieve a better functional outcome in some studies; however, other studies have found differences only in early range of motion.[52,53] It has also been reported that patients utilizing CPM during the inflammatory phase of soft tissue healing after anterior cruciate ligament reconstruction use significantly less pain-relieving narcotics than patients not using CPM[54] (Fig. 2-16).

Systemic Factors

Age

Age is a factor to be considered because of variations in healing between the pediatric, adult, and geriatric populations. In childhood, wound closure occurs more rapidly than in adulthood because the physiological changes and cumulative sun exposure that occur with aging can reduce the healing rate.[55] A decrease in the density and cross-linking of collagen, which results in reduced tensile strength, decreased numbers of mast cells and fibroblasts, and a lower rate of epithelialization, occurs in the elderly.[56,57] The poor organization of cutaneous vessels in older people also adversely affects wound healing.

Disease

A number of diseases can affect wound healing either directly or indirectly. For example, poorly controlled diabetes mellitus impairs collagen synthesis, increases the risk of infection due to a dampened immune response, and decreases phagocytosis due to alterations in leukocyte function.[50,58] Peripheral vascular compromise is also prevalent in this population,

leading to a decrease in local blood flow. Neuropathies, which are also common, can increase the potential for trauma and decrease the ability of soft tissue lesions to heal.

Patients who are immunocompromised, such as those with acquired immune deficiency syndrome (AIDS) or those taking immunosuppressive drugs after organ transplantation, are more prone to wound infections because they have an inadequate inflammatory response. AIDS also affects many other facets of the healing process through its impairment of phagocytosis, fibroblast function, and collagen synthesis.[59]

Problems involving the circulatory system, including atherosclerosis, sickle cell disease, and hypertension, can also have an adverse effect on wound healing since inflammation and healing depend on the cardiovascular system for the delivery of components to the local area of injury. Decreased oxygen tension resulting from a reduced blood supply can result in an inhibition of fibroblast migration and a decreased collagen synthesis, resulting in decreased tensile strength and making the injured area more susceptible to reinjury. Wounds with a decreased blood supply are also more susceptible to infection.[20,60]

Medications

Patients with injuries or wounds often take medications with systemic effects that alter tissue healing. For example, antibiotics can prevent or fight off infection, which can help to speed healing but may also have toxic effects that inhibit healing.

Corticosteroids, such as prednisone and dexamethasone, block the inflammatory cascade early on by blocking the release of arachidonic acid.[61] Corticosteroids have been shown to impair all phases of healing by stabilizing cell membranes and inhibiting the production of prostaglandins. They also decrease the margination, migration, and accumulation of monocytes at the site of inflammation.[62] They severely inhibit wound contracture, decrease the rate of epithelialization, and decrease the tensile strength of closed, healed wounds.[63-66] Corticosteroids that are administered at the time of injury have a greater impact because decreasing the inflammatory response at this early stage delays subsequent phases of healing and increases the incidence of infection.

In comparison with corticosteroids, nonsteroidal antiinflammatory drugs (NSAIDs) such as ibuprofen are less likely to impair healing. They act later in the

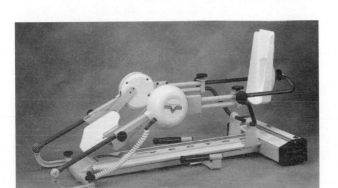

Figure 2-16. CPM machine. (Courtesy Thera-Kinetics Company, Cherry Hill, New Jersey.)

inflammatory cascade, interrupting the production of prostaglandins from arachidonic acid[61] (Fig. 2-17). They are not thought to adversely affect the function of fibroblasts or tissue macrophages.[67] NSAIDs can cause vasoconstriction and suppress the inflammatory response,[12] however, and some NSAIDs have been found to inhibit cell proliferation during tendon healing.[68]

Nutrition

Nutrition can have a profound effect on healing tissues. Deficiency of any of a number of important amino acids, vitamins, minerals, or water, as well as insufficient caloric intake, can result in delayed or impaired healing. This is because physiological stress from the injury induces a hypermetabolic state. Thus if insufficient "fuel" is available for the process of inflammation and repair, healing is slowed.

In most cases, healing abnormalities are associated with general protein-calorie malnutrition rather than depletion of a single nutrient.[69] Such is the case with patients with extensive burns who are in a prolonged hypermetabolic state. A protein deficiency can result in decreased fibroblastic proliferation, reduced proteoglycan and collagen synthesis, decreased angiogenesis, and disrupted collagen remodeling.[70] Protein deficiency can also adversely affect phagocytosis, which may lead to an increased risk of infection.[60]

Studies have shown that a deficiency of specific nutrients may also affect healing. Vitamin A deficiency can retard epithelialization, the rate of collagen synthesis, and cross-linking.[71] Thiamine (vitamin B_1) deficiency decreases collagen formation, and vitamin B_5 deficiency decreases the tensile strength of healed tissue and reduces the fibroblast number.[72,73] Vitamin C deficiency impairs collagen synthesis by fibroblasts, increases the capillary rupture potential, and increases the susceptibility of wounds to infection.[74]

Many minerals also play an important role in healing. Insufficient zinc can decrease the rate of epithelialization, reduce collagen synthesis, and decrease tensile strength.[75,76] Magnesium deficiency may also cause decreased collagen synthesis, and copper insufficiency may alter cross-linking, leading to a reduction in tensile strength.[74]

HEALING OF SPECIFIC MUSCULOSKELETAL TISSUES

The primary determinants of the outcome of any injury are the type and extent of the injury, the regenerative capacity of the tissues involved, the vascular supply of the injured site, and the extent of damage to the extracellular framework. The basic principles of inflammation and healing apply to all tissues; however, there is some tissue specificity to the healing response. For example, the liver can regenerate even

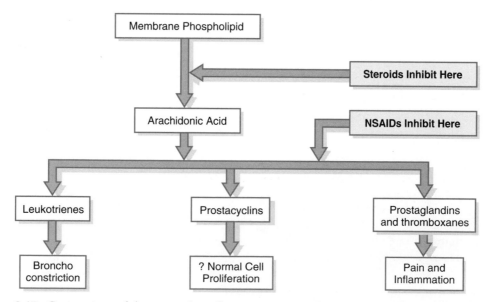

Figure 2-17. Comparison of the site in the inflammatory cascade acted on by NSAIDs and steroids.

when over half of it is removed, while even a thin fracture line in cartilage is unlikely to heal.

Cartilage

Cartilage has a limited ability to heal because it lacks lymphatics, blood vessels, and nerves.[77] However, cartilage reacts differently when injured alone than when injured in conjunction with the subchondral bone to which it is attached. Injuries confined to the cartilage do not form a clot or recruit neutrophils or macrophages, and the cells adjacent to the injury show a limited capacity to induce healing. This limited response generally fails to heal the defect, and these lesions seldom resolve.[78]

In injuries that involve both articular cartilage and subchondral bone, the vascularization of the subchondral bone allows for the formation of fibrin-fibronectin gel, giving access to the inflammatory cells and permitting the formation of granulation tissue. Differentiation of granulation tissue into chondrocytes can begin within 2 weeks. Normal-appearing cartilage can be seen within 2 months after the injury. However, this cartilage has a low proteoglycan content and is therefore predisposed to degeneration and erosive changes.[79]

Tendons and Ligaments

Tendons and ligaments pass through similar stages of healing. Inflammation occurs in the first 72 hours, and collagen synthesis occurs within the first week. Fibroplasia occurs from intrinsic sources such as adjacent cells, and from extrinsic sources such as those brought in via the circulatory system.

The repair potential of tendon is somewhat controversial. Both intrinsic cells such as epitendonous and endotendonous cells and extrinsic peritendonous cells participate in tendon repair. The exact role of these cells and the final outcome depend on several factors, including the type of tendon, the extent of damage to the tendon sheath, the vascular supply, and the duration of immobilization. The first two stages of tendon healing, inflammation and proliferation, are similar to the healing phases of other tissues. The third phase, scar maturation, is unique to tendons in that this tissue can achieve a state of repair close to regeneration.

During the first 4 days following an injury, the inflammatory phase progresses with an infiltration of both extrinsic and intrinsic cells. Many of these cells develop phagocytic capabilities, while others become fibroblastic. Collagen synthesis becomes evident by days 7 to 8, with fibroblasts predominating at around day 14. Early in this stage, both cells and collagen are oriented perpendicular to the tendon's long axis.[80] This orientation changes at day 10, when new collagen fibers begin to align themselves parallel to the old longitudinal axis of the tendon stumps.[81] For the following 2 months, there is a gradual transition of alignment, through remodeling and reorientation, parallel to the long axis. Ultimate maturation of the tissue depends on sufficient physiological loading.

If the synovial sheath is absent or uninjured, the relative contributions of the intrinsic and extrinsic cells are balanced and adhesions are minimal. If the synovial sheath is injured, the contributions of the extrinsic cells overwhelm the capacities of the intrinsic cells and adhesions are common.

Factors affecting the repair of tendons are different from those associated with the repair of ligaments.[82] Studies have shown that mobilization of tendons by controlled forces accelerates and enhances strengthening of tendon repair, but mobilization by active contraction of the attached muscle less than 3 weeks after repair generally results in a poor outcome. The poor results may be a result of the fact that high tension can lead to ischemia and tendon rupture. Recent studies have found no significant difference in tendon strength when tendons are exposed to controlled low or high levels of passive force after repair.[83,84] It appears that mechanical stress is needed to promote appropriate orientation of the collagen fibrils and remodeling of collagen into its mature form and to optimize strength, but the amount of tension necessary to promote the optimal clinical response is not certain.[85,86]

Many variables influence the healing of ligamentous tissue, the most important of which are the type of ligament, the size of the defect, and the amount of loading applied. For example, injuries to capsular and extracapsular ligaments generally stimulate an adequate repair response, while injuries to intracapsular ligaments often do not. In the knee, the medial collateral ligament often heals without surgical intervention, whereas the anterior cruciate ligament does not. These differences in healing may be due to the synovial environment, the limited neovascularization, or the fibroblast migration from surrounding tissues. Treatments that stabilize the injury site and maintain the apposition of the torn ligament can help the ligament heal in its optimal length and minimize scarring. However, mature ligamentous repair tissue is still 30% to 50% weaker than uninjured ligament.[87] This does not usually clinically significantly impair joint function because the repaired tissue is usually larger than the uninjured ligament. Early, controlled loading of healing ligaments can also promote healing, although excessive loading may delay or disrupt the healing process.[88,89]

Skeletal Muscle

Muscles may be injured by blunt trauma causing a contusion, by violent contraction or excessive stretch causing a strain, or by muscle-wasting diseases. Although skeletal muscle cells cannot proliferate, stem or reserve cells, known as *satellite cells*, can, under some circumstances, proliferate and differentiate to form new skeletal muscle cells after the death of adult muscle fibers.[79] Skeletal muscle regeneration has been documented in muscle biopsy specimens from patients with diseases such as muscular dystrophy and polymyositis; however, skeletal muscle regeneration in humans after trauma has not been documented. Following a severe contusion, a calcified hematoma, known as *myositis ossificans*, may develop. Myositis ossificans is rare following surgery if hemostasis is controlled.

Bone

Bone is a specialized tissue that is able to heal itself with like tissue. Bone can heal by two mechanisms: primary or secondary healing. Primary healing occurs with rigid internal fixation of the bone, while secondary healing occurs in the absence of such fixation.

Bone goes through a series of four histologically distinct stages in the healing process: inflammation, soft callus, hard callus, and bone remodeling. Some investigators also include the stages of impaction and induction before inflammation in this scheme.

Impaction is the dissipation of the energy from an insult. The impact of an insult is proportional to the energy applied to the bone and is inversely proportional to the volume of the bone. Thus a fracture is more likely to occur if the force is great or the bone is small. Energy dissipated by a bone is inversely proportional to its modulus of elasticity. Therefore the bone of a person suffering from osteoporosis, which has low elasticity, will sustain a fracture more easily.

Stages of Fracture Healing
1. **Impaction**
2. **Induction**
3. **Inflammation**
4. **Soft callus**
5. **Hard callus**
6. **Remodeling**

Young children have a more elastic bone structure that allows their bones to bend, accounting for the greenstick-type fractures seen in this population.

Induction is the stage when cells that possess osteogenic capabilities are activated. Induction is the least well-understood stage of bone healing. It is thought that the cells may be activated by oxygen gradients, forces, bone morphogenic proteins, or noncollagenous proteins. Although the timing of this process is not known exactly, it is thought to be initiated after the moment of impact. The duration of this stage is also not known, although the influence of the induction forces seems to lessen with time. Therefore optimizing the early conditions for healing to minimize the potential for delayed union or nonunion is imperative.

Inflammation begins shortly after impact and lasts until some fibrous union at the fracture site occurs. At the time of the fracture, there is disruption of the blood supply and formation of a fracture hematoma, as well as a decrease in oxygen tension and pH. This environment favors the growth of the early fibrous or cartilaginous callus. This callus forms more easily than bone and helps to stabilize the fracture site, decrease pain, and lessen the likelihood of a fat embolism. It also rapidly and efficiently provides a scaffold for further circulation, and for cartilage and endosteal bone production. The amount of movement at the fracture site influences the amount and quality of the callus. Small amounts of movement stimulate callus formation, while excessive movement can disrupt callus formation and inhibit bony union.

The soft callus stage begins when the pain and swelling subside and lasts until the bony fragments are united by fibrous or cartilaginous tissue. This period is marked by a great increase in vascularity, ingrowth of capillaries into the fracture callus, and increased cell proliferation. The tissue oxygen tension remains low, but the pH returns to normal. The hematoma becomes organized with fibrous tissue cartilage and bone formation; however, no callus is

> ▶ *Clinical Case Study* ◀

The following case study summarizes the concepts of inflammation and repair discussed in this chapter. Based on the scenario presented, an evaluation of the clinical findings and goals of treatment are proposed.

Case 1

JP is a 16-year-old high school student. She injured her right ankle 1 week ago playing soccer and was treated conservatively with crutches; rest, ice, compression, and elevation (RICE); and NSAIDs. She reports some improvement, although she is unable to play soccer due to continued complaints of right lateral ankle pain. Her x-ray films showed no fracture, and her family physician diagnosed the injury as a grade II lateral ankle sprain. She comes to your clinic with an order to "evaluate and treat."

JP sustained this injury during a cutting motion while dribbling a soccer ball. She noted an audible pop, immediate pain and swelling, and an inability to bear weight. She reports that her pain has decreased in intensity from 8/10 to 6/10 but that it increases with weight bearing and with certain demonstrated movements.

The objective exam reveals moderate warmth of the skin of the anterolateral aspect of the right ankle. Moderate ecchymosis and swelling are also noted, with a girth measurement of 34 cm on the right ankle compared with 30 cm on the left. Her range of motion is restricted to 0 degrees dorsiflexion, 30 degrees plantarflexion, 10 degrees inversion, and 5 degrees eversion,

with pain noted especially with plantarflexion and inversion. She exhibits a decreased stance phase on the right lower extremity. Pain and weakness occur on strength tests of the peroneals, gastrocnemius, and soleus muscles. JP also exhibits a marked decrease in proprioception, as evidenced by the single-leg balance test. Her anterior drawer test is positive, and her talar tilt is negative.

EVALUATION OF CLINICAL FINDINGS

The patient presents with impairments of pain, loss of subtalar and talocrual motion, decreased strength of the evertors and plantarflexors, increased girth of the right ankle, and decreased proprioception resulting in functional limitation of ambulation and sports activity. She performs home activities independently, without the use of adaptive equipment.

PREFERRED PRACTICE PATTERN

Impaired Joint Mobility, Motor Function, Muscle Performance, and Range of Motion Associated With Connective Tissue Dysfunction, (4D).

PLAN OF CARE

The goals of treatment at this time are to control the pain and edema, accelerate the resolution of the acute inflammatory phase of healing, and speed the recovery of JP's normal range of motion, strength, proprioception, and function.

visible radiographically. The callus is electronegative relative to the rest of the bone during this period. Osteoclasts remove the dead bone fragments.

The hard callus stage begins when a sticky, hard callus covers the ends of the fracture, and ends when new bone unites with the fragments. This period corresponds to the period of clinical and radiological fracture healing. The duration of this period depends on the fracture location and the patient's age, and can range from 3 weeks to 4 months.

The remodeling stage begins when the fracture is both clinically and radiologically healed. It ends when the bone has returned to its normal state and the patency of the medullary canal is restored. The fibrous bone is converted to lamellar bone, and the medullary canal is revised. This process can take several months to several years to complete.[90]

CHAPTER REVIEW

The processes of inflammation and tissue repair involve a complex and dynamic series of events, the ultimate goal of which is the restoration of normal function. In these events the involved tissue progresses through three stages: inflammation, proliferation, and maturation. The inflammation phase involves interaction of hemostatic, vascular, cellular, and immune responses mediated by a number of neural and chemical factors. The proliferation phase is characterized by epithelialization, fibroplasia, wound contraction, and neovascularization. The maturation phase involves balanced collagen synthesis and lysis to ultimately remodel the injured area.

This series of events follows a similar timely and predictable course. If the normal healing process is interfered with however, healing may be delayed or chronic inflammation may result. Various local and systemic factors can influence the progression of inflammation and tissue repair, including physical agents utilized by clinicians to facilitate the healing process. The rehabilitation specialist must assess the state of inflammation and repair to determine the appropriate agent to incorporate into the treatment plan for an optimal outcome. The reader is referred to the Evolve Website at http://evolve.elsevier.com/Cameron for study questions pertinent to this chapter.

References

1. *Stedman's Medical Dictionary,* ed 25, Baltimore, 1990, Williams & Wilkins.
2. Price SA, Wilson LM: Pathophysiology: *Clinical Concepts of Disease Processes,* ed 2, New York, 1982, McGraw Hill.
3. Kellett J: Acute soft tissue injuries—a review of the literature, *Med Sci Sports Exerc* 18:489-500, 1986.
4. Garrett WE Jr, Lohnes J: Cellular and matrix responses to mechanical injury at the myotendinous junction. In Leadbetter WB, Buckwalter JA, Gordon SL, eds: *Sports-Induced Inflammation,* Park Ridge, IL, 1990, American Academy of Orthopaedic Surgeons.
5. Andriacchi T, Sabiston P, DeHaven K et al: Ligament: Injury and repair. In Woo SL-Y, Buckwalter JA, eds: *Injury and Repair of the Musculoskeletal Soft Tissues,* Park Ridge, IL, 1988, American Academy of Orthopaedic Surgeons.
6. Garrett WE Jr: Muscle strain injuries: Clinical and basic aspects, *Med Sci Sports Exerc* 22:436-443, 1990.
7. Fantone JC, Ward PA: Inflammation. In Rubin E, Farber JL, eds: *Pathology,* Philadelphia, 1988, JB Lippincott.
8. Wilkerson GB: Inflammation in connective tissue: etiology and management. *Athl Training* 20:298-301, 1985.
9. Christie AL: The tissue injury cycle and new advances toward its management in open wounds, *Athl Training* 26:274-277, 1991.
10. Robbins SL, Kumar V, Cotran RS et al: *Robbins Pathologic Basis of Disease,* ed 5, Philadelphia, 1994, WB Saunders.
11. Fantone JC: Basic concepts in inflammation. In Leadbetter WB, Buckwalter JA, Gordon SL, eds: *Sports-Induced Inflammation,* Park Ridge, IL, 1990, American Academy of Orthopaedic Surgeons.
12. Peacock EE: *Wound Repair,* ed 3, Philadelphia, 1984, WB Saunders.
13. Salter RB, Simmons DF, Malcom BW et al: The biological effects of continuous passive motion on the healing of full thickness defects in articular cartilage, *J Bone Joint Surg* 62-A:1232-1251, 1980.
14. Majno G, Palade GE: Studies on inflammation. I. The effect of histamine and serotonin on vascular permeability: an electron microscopic study, *J Biophys Biochem Cytol* 11:571, 1961.
15. Pierce GF, Mustoe TA, Senia RM et al: In vivo incisional wound healing augmented by PDGF and recombinant c-sis gene homodimeric proteins, *J Exp Med* 167:975-987,1988.
16. Martinez-Hernandez A, Amenta PS: Basic concepts in wound healing. In Leadbetter WB, Buckwalter JA, Gordon SL, eds: *Sports-Induced Inflammation,* Park Ridge, IL, 1990, American Academy of Orthopaedic Surgeons.
17. Hardy M: The biology of scar formation, *Phys Ther* 69:1014-1024, 1989.
18. Rutherford R, Ross R: Platelet factors stimulate fibroblasts and smooth muscle cells quiescent in plasma serum to proliferate, *J Cell Biol* 69:196-203, 1976.
19. Mathes S: Roundtable discussion: problem wounds, *Perspect Plastic Surg* 2:89-120, 1988.
20. Whitney JD, Heiner S, Mygrant BI et al: Tissue and wound healing effects of short duration postoperative oxygen therapy, *Biol Res Nurs* Jan;2(3):206-215, 2001.
21. Davidson JD, Mustoe TA: Oxygen in wound healing: more than a nutrient, *Wound Repair Regen* May-Jun;9(3):175-177, 2001.
22. Bellanti JA, ed: *Immunology III,* ed 3, Philadelphia, 1985, WB Saunders.
23. Werb A, Gordon S: Elastase secretion by stimulated macrophages, *J Exp Med* 142:361-377, 1975.
24. Madden JW: Wound healing: biologic and clinical features. In Sabiston DC, ed: *Davis-Christopher Textbook of Surgery,* ed 11, Philadelphia, 1997, WB Saunders.
25. Clark RAF: Overview and general considerations of wound repair. In Clark RAF, Henson PM, eds: *The Molecular and Cellular Biology of Wound Repair,* New York, 1988, Plenum Press.
26. Stotts NA, Wipke-Tevis D: Co-factors in impaired wound healing, *Ostomy* 42(2):44-56, 1996.
27. Levenson S: Practical applications of experimental studies in the care of primary closed wounds, *Am J Surg* 104:273-282, 1962.
28. Nemeth-Csoka M, Kovacsay A: The effect of glycosaminoglycans (GAG) on the intramolecular bindings of collagen, *Acta Biol* 30(4):303-308, 1979.
29. Lachman SM: *Soft Tissue Injuries in Sports,* St. Louis, 1988, Mosby.
30. Hunt TK, Van Winkle W Jr: Wound healing. In Heppenstall RB, ed: Fracture Treatment and Healing, Philadelphia, 1980, WB Saunders.
31. Daly T: The repair phase of wound healing: re-epithelialization and contraction. In Kloth L, McCulloch J, Feeder J, eds: *Wound Healing: Alternatives in Management,* Philadelphia, 1990, FA Davis.
32. Gabbiani G, Ryan G, Majeno G: Presence of modified fibroblasts in granulation tissue and their possible role in wound contraction, *Experientia* 27:549-550, 1971.
33. Watts GT, Grillo HC, Gross J: Studies in wound healing: II. The role of granulation tissue in contraction, *Ann Surg* 148:153-160, 1958.

34. McGrath MH, Simon RH: Wound geometry and the kinetics of the wound contraction, *Plast Reconstr Surg* 72:66-73, 1983.

35. *Taber's Cyclopedic Medical Dictionary,* ed 15, Philadelphia, 1985, FA Davis.

36. Billingham RE, Russell PS: Studies on wound healing, with special reference to the phenomena of contracture in experimental wounds in rabbit skin, *Ann Surg* 144:961, 1956.

37. Sawhney CP, Monga HL: Wound contracture in rabbits and the effectiveness of skin grafts in preventing it, *Br J Plast Surg* 23:318-321, 1970.

38. Stone PA, Madden JW: Biological factors affecting wound contraction, *Surg Forum* 26:547-548, 1975.

39. Rudolph R: Contraction and the control of contraction, *World J Surg* 4:279-287, 1980.

40. Alvarez OM: Wound healing. In Fitzpatrick T, ed: *Dermatology in General Medicine,* ed 3, New York, 1986, McGraw-Hill.

41. Eyre DR: The collagens of musculoskeletal soft tissues. In Leadbetter WB, Buckwalter JA, Gordon SL, eds: *Sports-Induced Inflammation,* Park Ridge, IL, 1990, American Association of Orthopaedic Surgeons.

42. McPherson JM, Piez KA: Collagen in dermal wound repair. In Clark RAF, Henson PM, eds: *The Molecular and Cellular Biology of Wound Repair,* New York, 1988, Plenum Press.

43. Kosaka M, Kamiishi H: New concept of balloon-compression wear for the treatment of keloids and hypertrophic scars, *Plast Reconstr Surg* Oct;108(5):1454-1455, 2001.

44. Uppal RS, Khan U, Kakar S et al: The effects of a single dose of 5-fluorouracil on keloid scars: a clinical trial of timed wound irrigation after extralesional excision, *Plast Reconstr Surg* Oct;108(5):1218-1224, 2001.

45. Hunt TK, Van Winkle W: *Wound Healing: Normal Repair — Fundamentals of Wound Management in Surgery*, South Plainfield, NJ, 1976, Chirurgecom, Inc.

46. Madden J: Wound healing: the biological basis of hand surgery, *Clin Plast Surg* 3:3-11, 1976.

47. Arem AJ, Madden JW: Effects of stress on healing wounds: I. Intermittent noncyclical tension, *J Surg Res* 20:93-102, 1976.

48. Fantone JC: Basic concepts of inflammation. In Leadbetter WB, Buckwalter JA, Gordon SL, eds: *Sports-Induced Inflammation,* Park Ridge, IL, 1990, American Academy of Orthopaedic Surgeons.

49. Irvin T: Collagen metabolism in infected colonic anastomoses, *Surg Gynecol Obstet* 143:220-224, 1976.

50. Carrico T, Mehrhof A, Cohen I: Biology of wound healing, *Surg Clin North Am* 64:721-733, 1984.

51. Woo SL, Gelberman RM, Cobb NG et al: The importance of controlled passive mobilization on flexor tendon healing: a biochemical study, *Acta Orthop Scand* 52:615-622, 1981.

52. Gelberman RH, Woo SL, Lothringer K et al: Effects of early intermittent passive immobilization on healing canine flexor tendons, *J Hand Surg* 7:170-175, 1982.

53. Lau SK, Chiu KY: Use of continuous passive motion after total knee arthroplasty, *J Arthroplasty* Apr;16(3):336-339, 2001.

54. McCarthy MR, Yates CK, Anderson MA et al: The effects of immediate continuous passive motion on pain during the inflammatory phase of soft tissue healing following anterior cruciate ligament reconstruction, *JOSPT* 17(2):96-101, 1993.

55. Thomas DR: Age-related changes in wound healing, *Drugs Aging* 18(8):607-620, 2001.

56. Holm-Peterson P, Viidik A: Tensile properties and morphology of healing wounds in young and old rats, *Scand J Plast Reconstr Surg* 6:24-35, 1972.

57. van de Kerkhoff PCM, van Bergen B, Spruijt K et al: Age-related changes in wound healing, *Clin Exerc Dermatol* 19:369-374, 1994.

58. Goodson W, Hunt T: Studies of wound healing in experimental diabetes mellitus, *J Surg Res* 22:221-227, 1997.

59. Peterson M, Barbul A, Breslin R et al: Significance of T-lymphocytes in wound healing, *Surgery* 2:300-305, 1987.

60. Gogia PP: The biology of wound healing, *Ostomy* 38(9):12-22, 1992.

61. Leadbetter WB: Corticosteroid injection therapy in sports injuries. In Leadbetter WB, Buckwalter JA, Gordon SL, eds: *Sports-Induced Inflammation,* Park Ridge, IL, 1990, American Academy of Orthopaedic Surgeons.

62. Behrens TW, Goodwin JS: Oral corticosteroids. In Leadbetter WB, Buckwalter JA, Gordon SL, eds: *Sports-Induced Inflammation,* Park Ridge, IL, 1990, American Academy of Orthopaedic Surgeons.

63. Ehlrich H, Hunt T: The effect of cortisone and anabolic steroids on the tensile strength of healing wounds, *Ann Surg* 170:203-206, 1969.

64. Baker B, Whitaker W: Interference with wound healing by the local action of adrenocortical steroids, *Endocrinology* 46:544-551, 1950.

65. Howes E, Plotz C, Blunt J et al: Retardation of wound healing by cortisone, *Surgery* 28:177-181, 1950.

66. Stephens F, Dunphy J, Hunt T: The effect of delayed administration of corticosteroids on wound contracture, *Ann Surg* 173:214-218, 1971.

67. Abramson SB: Nonsteroidal anti-inflammatory drugs: mechanisms of action and therapeutic considerations. In Leadbetter WB, Buckwalter JA, Gordon SL, eds: *Sports-Induced Inflammation,* Park Ridge, IL, 1990, American Academy of Orthopaedic Surgeons.

68. Riley GP, Cox M, Harrall RL et al: Inhibition of tendon cell proliferation and matrix glycosaminoglycan synthesis by non-steroidal anti-inflammatory drugs in vitro, *J Hand Surg* [Br] Jun;26(3):224-228, 2001.

69. Albina JE: Nutrition in wound healing, *J Parenter Enteral Nutr* 18(4):367-376, 1994.
70. Pollack S: Wound healing: a review. III. Nutritional factors affecting wound healing, *J Dermatol Surg Oncol* 5:615-619, 1979.
71. Freiman M, Seifter E, Connerton C: Vitamin A deficiency and surgical stress, *Surg Forum* 21:81-82, 1970.
72. Alverez OM, Gilbreath RL: Thiamine influence on collagen during granulation of skin wounds, *J Surg Res* 32:24-31, 1982.
73. Grenier JF, Aprahamian M, Genot C et al: Pantothenic acid (vitamin B$_5$) efficiency on wound healing, *Acta Vitaminol Enzymol* 4:81-85, 1982.
74. Pollack S: Systemic drugs and nutritional aspects of wound healing, *Clin Dermatol* 2:68-80, 1984.
75. Sandstead HH, Henriksen LK, Grefer JL et al: Zinc nutriture in the elderly in relation to taste acuity, immune response, and wound healing, *Am J Clin Nutr* 36(Suppl 5):1046-1059, 1982.
76. Maitra AK, Dorani B: Role of zinc in post-injury wound healing, *Arch Emerg Med* Jun;9(2):122-124, 1992.
77. Athanasiou KA, Shah AR, Hernandez RJ et al: Basic science of articular cartilage repair, *Clin Sports Med* Apr;20(2):223-247, 2001.
78. Gelberman R, Goldberg V, An K-N et al: Tendon. In Woo SL-Y, Buckwalter JA, eds: *Injury and Repair of Musculoskeletal Soft Tissues,* Park Ridge, IL, 1988, American Academy of Orthopaedic Surgeons.
79. Caplan A, Carlson B, Faulkner J et al: Skeletal muscle. In Woo SL-Y, Buckwalter JA, eds: *Injury and Repair of Musculoskeletal Soft Tissues,* Park Ridge, IL, 1988, American Academy of Orthopaedic Surgeons.
80. Strickland JW: Flexor tendon injuries, *Orthop Rev* 15(10):21, 1986.
81. Lindsay WK: Cellular biology of flexor tendon healing. In Hunter JM, Schneider LH, Mackin EJ, eds: *Tendon Surgery of the Hand,* St Louis, 1987, Mosby.
82. Akeson WH, Frank CB, Amiel D et al: Ligament biology and biomechanics. In Finnerman G, ed: *American Academy of Orthopaedic Surgeon's Symposium on Sports Medicine,* St Louis, 1985, Mosby.
83. Ketchum LD: Primary tendon healing: a review, *J Hand Surg* 2:428-435, 1977.
84. Goldfarb CA, Harwood F, Silva MJ et al: The effect of variations in applied rehabilitation force on collagen concentration and maturation at the intrasynovial flexor tendon repair site, *J Hand Surg* [Am] Sep;26(5):841-846, 2001.
85. Peacock EE Jr: Biological principles in the healing of long tendons, *Surg Clin North Am* 45:461-476, 1965.
86. Potenza AD: Tendon healing within the flexor digital sheath in the dog, *J Bone Joint Surg* 44A:49-64, 1962.
87. Frank C, Woo SL-Y, Amiel D et al: Medial collateral ligament healing: a multidisciplinary assessment in rabbits, *Am J Sports Med* 11:379-389, 1983.
88. Fronek J, Frank C, Amiel D et al: The effects of intermittent passive motion (IPM) in the healing of medial collateral ligaments, *Trans Orthop Res Soc* 8:31, 1983.
89. Long M, Frank C, Schachar N et al: The effects of motion on normal and healing ligaments, *Trans Orthop Res Soc* 7:43, 1982.
90. McKibben B: The biology of fracture healing in long bones, *J Bone Joint Surg* (BR) 60:150-162, 1978.

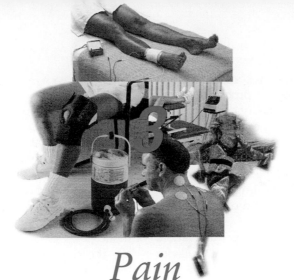

Pain

OBJECTIVES

Upon completion of this chapter, the reader will be able to:

1. Differentiate acute, chronic, and referred pain.
2. Discuss the peripheral and central mechanisms of nociception and pain transmission.
3. Appraise current theories of pain control.
4. Select and apply appropriate methods and tools to quantify and qualify pain.
5. Compare and contrast various medical and physical therapies used to control pain.
6. Evaluate the use of physical agents for controlling pain.

Pain is an experience based on a complex interaction of physical and psychological processes. It has been defined as an unpleasant sensory and emotional experience associated with actual or potential tissue damage or described in terms of such damage.[1-3] Pain usually serves as a warning to protect the body from damage and thus, although unpleasant, serves an essential function in survival.[4] It is important to realize that pain is not just the activation of receptors of noxious stimuli, known as *nociception*, but also the sensory experiences associated with such activation, as well as the suffering and alterations in behavior associated with such activation.

Pain is the most common symptom prompting patients to seek medical attention and is also a predominant symptom leading patients to receive rehabilitation.[5] Many patients with musculoskeletal or neurological impairments present with complaints of pain, and most of these individuals consider pain control or relief to be the primary goal of treatment.[6] Pain may also contribute to physical impairment and disability, limiting participation in home, work, and recreational activities.[7] The pain complaints encountered by rehabilitation professionals are generally related to inflammation of musculoskeletal or neurological structures caused by injury, trauma, or degenerative disease. These structures can be sources of pain and can increase the responsiveness of peripheral pain receptors to other painful stimuli.[8-10]

The goals of pain treatment include resolving the underlying pathology causing the pain, when possible; modifying the patient's perception of the discomfort; and maximizing function within the limitations imposed by the source of pain, whether or not the source of pain can be modified. The final goal of treatment is resolution of the underlying condition. However, even when the source of pain can be modified by treatment, for example, in the case of structural malalignment because of poor posture or imbalanced muscle length, or when the pain is caused by a self-limiting condition such as inflammation after an acute soft tissue injury, it is beneficial to control pain during recovery so that the patient can participate more fully in a rehabilitation program to correct the underlying deficit. When the pain is caused by a condition that cannot be directly modified, such as phantom limb pain or rheumatoid arthritis, pain control may facilitate increased participation in a rehabilitation program, increased patient function, and decreased disability.

TYPES OF PAIN

Pain can be categorized according to its duration or source as *acute, chronic*, or *referred*. Acute pain is generally defined as pain of less than 6 months' duration for which an underlying pathology can be identified.[11] Acute pain is felt in response to actual or potential tissue damage that resolves when tissue damage or the threat of damage passes. Chronic pain, also known as persistent pain, persists beyond the normal time for tissue healing.[10] Chronic pain conditions are generally the result of activation of dysfunctional neurological or psychological responses that cause the individual to continue to experience the sensation of pain even when no damaging or threatening stimulus is present. Referred pain is the experience of pain in one area when the actual or potential tissue damage is in another area. Knowing whether a patient's pain is acute, chronic, or referred will help the clinician determine the mechanisms and processes that may be contributing to the sensation and facilitate selection of the most appropriate intervention to control or relieve this symptom.

Acute Pain

Acute pain consists of a complex combination of unpleasant sensory, perceptual, and emotional experiences with associated autonomic, psychological, emotional, and behavioral reactions that occur in response to a noxious stimulus provoked by acute injury or disease.[12,13] Acute pain is generally viewed as biologically meaningful, useful, and time-limited. Acute pain is mediated through rapidly conducting pathways and is associated with increases in muscle tone, heart rate, blood pressure, skin conductance, and other manifestations of increased sympathetic nervous system activity.[14] The intensity and location of the pain are usually related to the degree of tissue inflammation, damage, or destruction in the area in which the pain is felt. Acute pain is generally well-localized and defined, although its degree of localization varies to some extent with the type of tissue involved. Pain sensations from the skin are localized with great accuracy, whereas muscle pain is frequently more diffuse.[15,16] Acute pain lasts as long as the noxious stimulation persists. Acute pain serves a protective function following an injury by limiting activity to prevent further damage and promote tissue healing and recovery; however, it may also adversely affect an individual's quality of life and impair the ability to function.

Treatment of acute pain resulting from musculoskeletal injury generally attempts to facilitate resolution of the underlying disorder, reduce inflammation, and modify the transmission of pain from the periphery to the central nervous system.

Chronic Pain

Chronic pain starts as acute pain. Most authors and organizations define chronic pain as pain that does not resolve in the usual time it takes for the disorder to heal or that continues beyond the duration of noxious stimulation.[17] However, some authors and organizations use time-based definitions, defining chronic pain as any pain lasting longer than 3 months or 6 months.[18,19] The use of time-based definitions is not recommended because they do not take into account the variable course and duration of different pathologies and therefore do not differentiate long-term pain caused by chronic or progressive diseases or pathological states, such as rheumatoid arthritis, cancer, or neural entrapments, from pain that persists after the pathology has resolved. Chronic pain generally continues even after noxious stimuli are no longer active and when there is no longer any tissue damage or threat of tissue damage, whereas pain from a long-term disorder is generally associated with a long-term noxious stimulus. It has been estimated that approximately one third of the American population has chronic pain and 14% of the U.S. population suffers from chronic pain related to the joints and the musculoskeletal system.[20,21]

Chronic persistent pain is generally associated with physical, psychological, and social dysfunction (see box). Patients with chronic pain generally have been physically inactive for a prolonged period, resulting in loss of strength, skill, and endurance and thus progressive disability. They often dramatize their complaints, reporting that their pain is unbearable or incapacitating, and frequently receive excessive treatment, which is ineffective but can result in drug misuse or abuse and progressive dependence on others, including health care practitioners and family members. These patients also often show signs of depression, including delayed sleep onset and frequent awakening, altered eating habits, and social isolation.[22] The pain behavior of the patient with chronic persistent pain may be perpetuated by financial gain.[23,24]

Common Features of Patients with Chronic Pain

Have pain of several months' or years' duration.

Have pain similar to the initial pain that is associated with a medical problem or injury.

History of many treatment failures provided in great detail.

Many medications tried, with a minimal to poor response.

Continuous use of analgesics and tranquilizers, despite patients' testimony that the medications offer no notable or long-lasting relief.

Pain described as being unbearable and incapacitating.

Strong belief that pain has an unidentified organic cause.

Desire and willingness expressed to undergo "any treatment" for pain relief.

Claim that everything will be fine if only the "doctor would treat my pain."

Pain not relieved by any medical or surgical treatment.

Substantial psychosocial changes present, especially depression, although patients vehemently deny the label; they frequently do admit to feeling frustrated, angry, and irritable, with disturbed sleep, altered moods, weight changes, decreased energy, decreased physical, social, recreational, and sexual activities, and increased family stresses and economic difficulties.

From Gildenberg PL, DeVaul RA: *The Chronic Pain Patient: Evaluation and Management,* New York, 1985, Karger.

Chronic persistent pain may be the result of changes in sympathetic nervous system and adrenal activity, reduced production of endogenous opioids, or sensitization of primary afferent and spinal cord neurons. Decreased levels of enkephalins and increased numbers and sensitivity of nociceptors have been observed in individuals with chronic pain.[25] These individuals frequently have increased sensitivity to both noxious (hyperalgesia) and nonnoxious (allodynia) stimuli.[26] These changes in pain perception may be the result of a process known as *wind-up* or *central hypersensitization,* whereby the pathways that transmit pain continue to discharge after the discontinuation of intense or repeated stimulation. Then, even a small additional stimulus exceeds the threshold that is perceived as painful.[27-30] Thus for an individual with a painful condition that is severe or long-lasting, the noxious stimulation may result in increased pain receptor activity and a consequent reduced tolerance for other noxious or nonnoxious stimuli. Understanding of this sensitization mechanism has led to increased study and use of preemptive analgesia before procedures that are known to be painful in an attempt to reduce postprocedural pain and reduce recovery time.[31-33]

Psychological and social factors have also been implicated in the etiology and maintenance of chronic pain.[34] The disturbed sleep associated with depression may cause musculoskeletal pain, and the decreased activity may perpetuate pain by causing weakness and deconditioning.[22] Individuals with chronic pain also frequently adopt the dependent sick patient role and behaviors of the chronic invalid, which result in progressively reduced functional activity.[35] These behaviors may be unintentionally encouraged by the individual's family members, who, in an attempt to help, actually promote the dependent role.[24]

Ideally, the development of chronic pain should be prevented by early identification of individuals at risk. Patients with prolonged, severe, or very disabling acute pain are at increased risk of developing chronic pain. Therefore, to reduce this risk, pain-controlling interventions, such as physical agents or medications, should be applied during the acute stage of an injury and during the later recovery phases, when pain is still the result of pain receptor activation.[36] Should chronic pain develop, successful treatment usually requires that all components of the dysfunction be addressed. Multidisciplinary treatment programs based on a biopsychosocial model of pain have been specifically developed to address these problems.[4] These treatment programs are described below in the section on pain management.

Referred Pain

Referred pain is felt at a location distant from its source. Pain may be referred from one joint to another, from a peripheral nerve to a distal area of innervation, or from an internal organ to an area of musculoskeletal tissue. For example, hip joint pathology occasionally refers pain to the knee, particularly in children, and compression of the spinal nerve roots at the L5–S1 level as they exit through the spinal foramen may cause pain in the lateral leg because this is the area of sensory innervation.[37,38] Common referral patterns from internal organs to musculoskeletal

tissue include the pain associated with myocardial infarction or angina caused by cardiac ischemia that is felt in the upper chest, left shoulder, jaw and arm, and pain originating from the central portion of the diaphragm that is frequently felt in the lateral tip of either shoulder. The gallbladder also frequently refers pain to the right shoulder or the inferior angle of the right scapula, and the spleen refers pain to the left shoulder.

It is proposed that pain is referred in one of three ways: from a nerve to its area of innervation, from one area to another derived from the same dermatome, or from one area to another derived from the same embryonic segment, because the peripheral neural pathways from these different areas converge on the same or similar areas of the spinal cord and synapse with the same second-order neurons to ascend the spinal cord and reach the central cortex.[39] For example, pain is referred from the diaphragm to the tip of the shoulder because both of these areas initially develop in the neck region during embryonic development, causing them both to have efferent innervation from the phrenic nerve and afferent innervation to the second through fourth levels of the cervical spine. When pain that may be of either visceral or musculoskeletal origin converges on the same neuron in the spinal cord, it is usually interpreted to be of musculoskeletal origin. This may be because musculoskeletal injury and pain are so much more common that the brain "learns" that activity arriving along that pathway is associated with pain stimulus in a particular musculoskeletal area.

Clinicians who treat neuromusculoskeletal dysfunction must be aware of the potential for pain referral and be familiar with common pain referral patterns to determine the source of a patient's complaints and select appropriate treatment methods. Therefore when a patient with pain in a musculoskeletal area seeks treatment, the clinician should first determine if the source of the pain is located in the area of this sensation. Pain of musculoskeletal origin generally varies with position or movement of the painful area, whereas pain caused by dysfunction in other systems generally varies with stress on those systems. For example, shoulder pain that is aggravated by raising the arm is likely to originate in the shoulder, whereas left shoulder pain that is aggravated by all forms of strenuous exercise may be caused by a cardiac condition. When assessing pain that is determined to be of musculoskeletal origin, it is also important to accurately determine the structure(s) at fault to provide the most effective treatment. This can be done by performing provocative tests to reproduce the patient's chief complaint. Physical agents may effectively relieve referred pain; however, they should not be used as a substitute for determining the true source of the pain or for treating its underlying cause. They may be used for pain relief while the source of the pain is being investigated, during the recovery process, and for controlling referred pain where the underlying cause cannot be directly treated.

MECHANISMS OF PAIN RECEPTION AND TRANSMISSION

> **Specificity and pattern theories**
> **Pain receptors**
> **Peripheral nerve pathways**
> **Central pathways**
> **Sympathetically mediated pain**
> **The role of substance P**

Pain is generally felt in response to stimulation of peripheral nociceptive structures. The stimulus is transmitted along peripheral nerves to the central nervous system, from where it can reach the cortex and consciousness. The sensation of pain and the individual's response to the sensation are influenced by a variety of factors, including the physiological mechanisms of the pain receptors, the anatomy of pain-transmitting structures, neurotransmitter levels, and the motivation, behavior, and physiological and emotional state of the individual. Variations in any of these factors can alter the individual's perception of pain severity, type, location, and duration.

Specificity and Pattern Theories

Over the years, various theories regarding the nature of peripheral pain reception and transmission have been proposed. The primary early theories were the specificity theory and the pattern theory. Current theories integrate components of both of these with more recent findings and observations. According to the specificity theory, as described by Von Frey and others, the sensation of pain depends on the stimulation of specific nerve endings that are specialized for each type of sensation.[40-42] Thus a specific type of

nerve fiber will always transmit the same sensation, no matter how intensely or frequently it is stimulated. According to this theory, specific pain fibers are responsible for the transmission of the sensation of pain (Fig. 3-1, *A*). Von Frey supported this theory with his identification of free nerve endings widely distributed in the skin that caused a sensation of pain when stimulated. He proposed that these free nerve endings were specific pain receptors.[42] Although the specificity theory is consistent with Von Frey's findings, it has since been found that the sensation of pain does not have the precise one-to-one relationship with the type of receptor stimulated that would be predicted by the specificity theory. The specificity theory also fails to account for the fact that many types of stimuli are perceived as painful and that pain can be modulated by input from the spinal cord or brain. The limitations of the specificity theory led to the development of an alternative explanation of pain perception, the pattern theory.

According to the pattern theory, the sensation of pain results from an appropriate intensity or frequency of stimulation of receptors that also respond to other stimuli such as touch, pressure, or temperature.[43] Neural impulses from the periphery are combined and modified to summate in central nervous system structures, where the pain is then localized and interpreted. According to the pattern theory, temporal and spatial summation of impulses along the pathways from the skin to the cerebral levels determines the individual's sensation of pain (Fig. 3-1, *B*). This theory accounts for the fact that a wide variety of stimuli cause the sensation of pain and also suggests a role for central influence by pain summation; however, it fails to consider the role of the identified specialized pain receptor structures and to account for affective or central pain modulation.

Current theories integrate components of the specificity theory and the pattern theory with other, more recent findings regarding neural anatomy and the functions of endogenous neurotransmitters. Current findings indicate that specific nerve endings called *nociceptors,* respond to all painful stimuli, and specific nerve types, small myelinated A-delta fibers and unmyelinated C fibers, transmit the sensation of pain from these nerve endings to the spinal cord and thence, within specific tracts, to the brain. The quality of the pain depends on the type of tissue from which the stimulus originates and on which of the two nerve

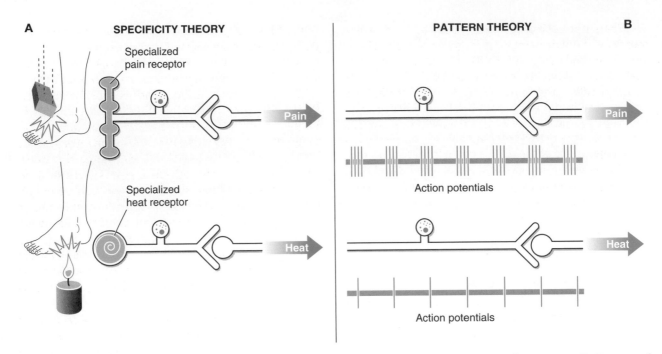

Figure 3-1. Specificity versus pattern theory of pain. **A,** Specific receptors for each type of sensation. **B,** Pattern of action potentials resulting in sensation of pain.

types transmits the pain; the intensity of the pain is related to the firing rate of the nerves. Pain from cutaneous noxious stimulation is usually perceived as sharp, pricking, or tingling and is easy to localize, whereas pain from musculoskeletal structures is usually dull, heavy, or aching and is harder to localize.[44] Visceral pain has an aching quality similar to that of musculoskeletal pain but tends to refer superficially rather than deeply.[15] Pain transmitted by C fibers is usually dull, long-lasting, and aching, whereas pain transmitted by A-delta fibers is generally sharp. The intensity of the pain and the responses to it are thought to be more severe when the relative intensity of nociceptive receptor stimulation is greater than that of nonnociceptive receptor stimulation, when levels of endogenous opioids are low, and with certain variations in the individual's psychological state.[45]

Pain Receptors

Nociceptors are free, noncorpuscular peripheral nerve endings consisting of a series of spindle-shaped, thick segments linked by thin segments to produce a "string-of-beads" appearance. The beads and end bulbs contain mitochondria, glycogen particles, vesi-

cles, and bare areas of axolemma that are not covered by Schwann cell processes.[46] Nociceptors are present in almost all types of tissue. However, no nociceptors are present in the nucleus pulposus and the inner part of the annulus fibrosus of the spinal discs.[47-50]

Nociceptors can be activated by intense thermal, mechanical, or chemical stimuli from exogenous or endogenous sources. For example, intense mechanical stimulation, such as that caused by a brick falling on someone's foot or a piece of broken bone compressing a nociceptor, will result in nociceptor activation. Chemical stimulation by exogenous substances such as acid or bleach, or by endogenously produced substances such as bradykinin, histamine, and arachidonic acid, which are released as part of the inflammatory response to tissue damage, can also activate nociceptors. Because these chemical mediators remain after the initial physical stimulus has passed, they generally cause pain to persist beyond the duration of the initial noxious stimulation. It is important to note that chemical mediators of inflammation also sensitize nociceptors, reducing their activation threshold to other stimuli.[51,52] This is the reason that, clinically, many activities and stimuli to recently injured areas are perceived as painful even when they are not damaging.

When nociceptors are activated, they release a variety of neuropeptides from their peripheral terminals, including substance P and a number of breakdown products of arachidonic acid such as prostaglandins and leukotrienes.[25] Nociceptors also convert the initial stimulus into electrical activity, in the form of action potentials, by a process known as *transduction*[25] (Fig. 3-2). It is thought that the released neuropeptides may initiate or participate in transduction because they sensitize nociceptors.[53] The action potentials resulting from the process of transduction propagate from the nociceptors along afferent nerve pathways toward the spinal cord.

Peripheral Nerve Pathways

Nociceptors give rise to two types of first-order afferent nerve fibers, C fibers and A-delta fibers. The activity in both types of fibers increases in response to peripheral noxious stimulation, including that associated with acute inflammation or muscle ischemia.[54-56] Eighty percent of afferent pain-transmitting fibers are C fibers, and the remaining 20% are A-delta fibers.[57] Generally, about 50% of the sensory fibers in a cutaneous nerve have nociceptive functions.[45]

C fibers, also known as *group IV afferents,* are small, unmyelinated nerve fibers that transmit action potentials quite slowly, at the rate of 1.0 to 4.0 meters/second.[58] They respond to noxious levels of mechanical, thermal, and chemical stimulation, causing pain that is generally described as dull, throbbing, aching, or burning and may also be reported as tingling or tapping[59,60] (Fig. 3-3). The pain sensations transmitted by these fibers have a slow onset after the initial painful stimulus, are long-lasting, emotionally difficult for the individual to tolerate, and tend to be diffusely localized, particularly when the stimulus is intense.[61,62] They can be accompanied by autonomic responses such as sweating, increased heart rate and blood pressure, or nausea.[63] The pain associated with C-fiber activation can be reduced by opiates, and this pain relief is blocked by the opiate antagonist naloxone.[64]

A-delta fibers, also known as *group III afferents,* are also small-diameter fibers; however, they transmit more rapidly than C fibers, at a rate of about 30 meters/second, because they are myelinated.[58,65] They are most sensitive to high-intensity mechanical stimulation, although they can also respond to stimulation by heat or cold and are capable of transmitting

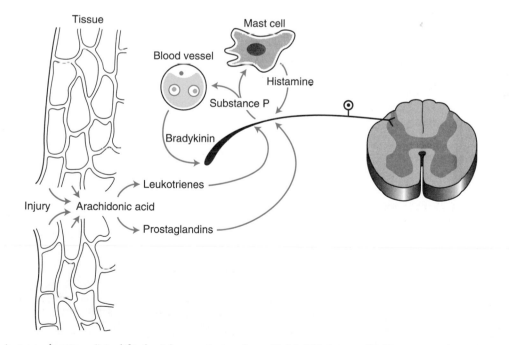

Figure 3-2. Pain transduction. (Modified with permission from Fields HL, Levine JD: Pain—mechanisms and management [medical progress], *West J Med* 141:347-357, 1984.)

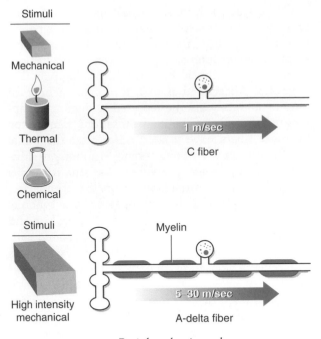

Figure 3-3. Peripheral pain pathways.

nonnoxious information.[66] The sensations associated with A-delta fiber activity are generally described as sharp, stabbing, or pricking.[45] The pain sensations transmitted by these fibers have a quick onset after the painful stimulus, last only for a short time, are generally localized to the area from which the stimulus arose, and are not generally associated with emotional involvement. The pain associated with A-delta fiber activation is generally not blocked by opiates.[67]

Mechanical trauma usually activates both C and A-delta fibers. Take the example of a brick landing on someone's foot. Almost immediately the individual feels a sharp sensation of pain. The initial pain is followed by a deep ache that may last for several hours or days. The initial sharp pain is transmitted by the A-delta fibers and is produced in response to the high-intensity mechanical stimulation of the nociceptors as a result of the impact of the brick. The later, deep ache is transmitted by the C fibers and is produced in response to stimulation by chemical mediators of inflammation released by the tissue after the initial injury.

Central Pathways

The peripheral first-order C and A-delta afferents project from the periphery to the gray matter of the spinal cord. The C and A-delta fibers synapse, either directly or via interneurons, with second-order neurons in the superficial dorsal horn of the gray matter (the substantia gelatinosa).[58,68-71] Some A-delta fibers penetrate more deeply into the dorsal horn to terminate at the normal termination sites of A-beta afferents. The second-order neurons in the dorsal horn are known as *transmission* or *T cells* (Fig. 3-4).

T cells make local connections within the spinal cord, either with efferent neurons as part of spinal cord reflexes or with afferent neurons that project toward the cortex. Continued or repetitive C-fiber activation can sensitize the T cells, causing them to fire more rapidly and to increase their receptor field size, and input from other interneurons originating in the substantia gelatinosa of the spinal cord or from descending fibers originating in higher brain centers can inhibit T-cell activity.[72] Inhibitory interneurons in the substantia gelatinosa are activated by input from large-diameter, myelinated, low-threshold sensory neurons (primarily A-beta nerves) that respond to nonpainful stimuli.[73,74] These inhibitory interneurons release various neurotransmitters, including norepinephrine, serotonin, and enkephalins, to modulate the flow of the afferent pain pathways.[75-77] Thus the transmission cells receive excitatory input from the C fibers and A-delta nociceptor afferents and inhibitory

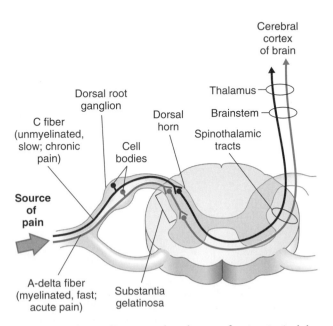

Figure 3-4. Ascending neural pathway of pain via A-delta and C fibers.

input from large-diameter, nonnociceptor sensory afferents and from descending fibers from higher brain centers[45] (Fig. 3-5). The balance of these excitatory and inhibitory inputs influences whether or not the individual feels pain and how severe the pain sensation is.[73] The inhibition of pain by inputs from nonnociceptor afferents is known as *pain gating,* and is discussed in greater detail below in the section on pain modulation and control theories.

Transmission cell activation can also increase muscle spasm via a spinal cord reflex in which the transmission cell synapses with anterior horn cells to cause muscle contractions. The ongoing muscle contractions can then cause accumulation of fluid and tissue irritants. The contracting muscles may also directly become initiators of further nociceptive impulses by mechanically compressing the nociceptors. In this way the combination of ongoing chemical and mechanical stimuli can set up a self-sustaining cycle of pain causing muscle spasm, which then causes more pain. This is known as the *pain-spasm-pain cycle* (Fig. 3-6). Many interventions indirectly reduce pain, even after their direct analgesic effect has passed, because they reduce muscle spasms and thereby interfere with this self-perpetuating cycle.

Ascending second-order nerves carry stimuli within the spinal cord toward the higher brain centers (Fig. 3-7). The second-order pathways that carry pain stimuli are located primarily in the anterolateral aspect of the cord.[78] This area of the spinal cord also

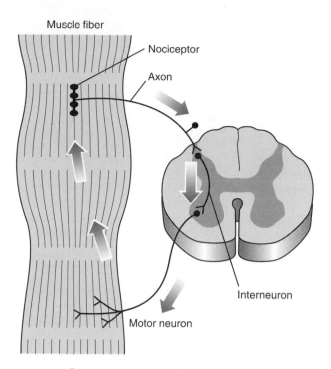

Figure 3-6. Pain-spasm-pain cycle: nociceptor activation resulting in T-cell activation stimulating an anterior horn cell to cause a muscle fiber to contract, resulting in accumulation of fluid and tissue irritants and mechanical compression of the nociceptor and increasing nociceptor activation.

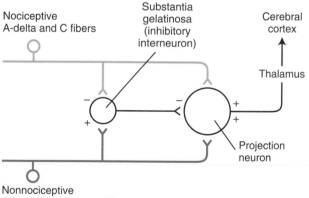
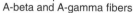

Figure 3-5. Simple diagram showing the gate control mechanism of pain modulation through the activation by A-delta and C-fiber input and gating/inhibition by nonnociceptor A-beta sensory nerves and higher center input.

transmits information about temperature and touch. Most axons in the anterolateral system cross midline in the spinal cord to ascend contralaterally. Information regarding pain is transmitted within the anterolateral cord via both the lateral spinothalamic tract and the larger anterospinothalamic tract to project to the thalamus. The lateral spinothalamic tract projects directly to the medial area of the thalamus, whereas the anterospinothalamic tract separates from the lateral spinothalamic tract in the brain stem to synapse with neurons in the reticular formation and the hypothalamic and limbic systems to then project to lateral, ventral, and caudal areas of the thalamus. The anterospinothalamic tract also relays information to the periaqueductal gray matter, where there is a large concentration of opiate receptors, and is thought, thereby, to be associated with pain modulation. Impulses relayed via the lateral spinothalamic tract are involved in transmission of sharp pain and in localization of the painful stimulus, whereas those sent via the anterospinothalamic tract are involved in

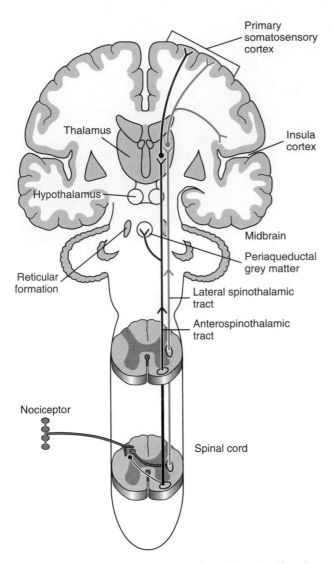

Figure 3-7. Central pain pathways from the spinal level to the higher brain centers.

of smooth and cardiac muscles and with glandular secretion. This contrasts with most of the nervous system, which is concerned with voluntary activation of the skeletal muscles or with transmission of sensory impulses from the periphery[79,80] (Fig. 3-8). The sympathetic nervous system is considered to be primarily involved in producing effects that prepare the body for "fight or flight," such as increasing heart rate and blood pressure, constricting cutaneous blood vessels, and increasing sweating in the palms of the hands. Although it is normal for the sympathetic nervous system to be activated by acute pain or injury, stimulation of the sympathetic nervous system efferents does not usually cause pain.[81] However, abnormal sympathetic activation, caused by a hyperactive response of the sympathetic nervous system to an acute injury or by a failure of its response to subside, can increase pain severity and cause exaggerated signs and symptoms of sympathetic activity such as excessive vasomotor or sweating reactions. In patients with such signs and symptoms, pain relief can often be achieved by interrupting sympathetic nervous system activity by chemical or surgical means.[82-84] In addition, stimuli that evoke sympathetic discharges, such as the startle reflex or emotional events, frequently exacerbate pain. It has therefore been proposed that excessive sympathetic nervous system activation may increase or maintain pain.[80,79]

Pain that is believed to involve sympathetic nervous system overactivation has a variety of names, including causalgia, reflex sympathetic dystrophy (RSD), shoulder-hand syndrome, posttraumatic dystrophy, Sudeck's atrophy, and sympathetically maintained pain.[85] Currently, the International Association for the Study of Pain (IASP) recommends the use of the term *complex regional pain syndrome (CRPS)*.[86] CRPS involving tissue damage without nerve damage is categorized as type I, and CRPS associated with nerve involvement is categorized as type II.[86]

CRPS generally includes the following signs and symptoms: severe pain that is out of proportion to the inciting injury or disease, hyperesthesia (excessive reaction to painful stimuli), and allodynia (the sensation of pain in response to stimuli that are not usually painful). CRPS frequently also includes trophic changes such as skin atrophy and hyperhidrosis, edema, stiffness, increased sweating, and decreased hair growth.[86] These symptoms generally result in decreased function and, if the syndrome is prolonged, spotty osteoporosis in the affected area.[87] Other sen-

transmission of more prolonged, aching pain and are thought to have stronger association with the disturbing emotions that accompany the pain sensation. The second-order neurons synapse in the thalamus with third-order neurons to project to the cortex, from where the sensation of pain can reach consciousness.

Sympathetic Nervous System Influences

The sympathetic nervous system is a component of the autonomic nervous system. The autonomic nervous system consists of the sympathetic and parasympathetic systems and is concerned with the activities

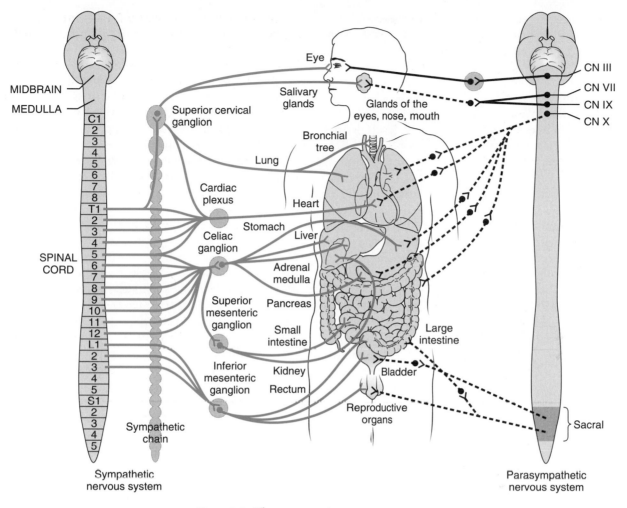

Figure 3-8. The autonomic nervous system.

sory, vasomotor, and skeletal motor abnormalities have also been associated with this syndrome.[88] CRPS can occur in any area of the body but is most common in the hand and, in such cases, is frequently associated with ipsilateral restriction of shoulder motion. CRPS may develop as a consequence of major or minor trauma, after visceral disease or central nervous system lesions, or without any known antecedent event.

The mechanism by which the sympathetic nervous system affects pain is not well understood; however, it may be the result of direct excitation of the nociceptors by the sympathetic efferent fibers or by the neurotransmitters released by the sympathetic nerves. The normal activation of sympathetic activity caused by pain may in some cases activate the afferent C fibers, further increasing pain, which could then

increase sympathetic activation, creating a self-sustaining vicious cycle. This cycle could amplify the sensation of pain and the signs of sympathetic activity, causing them to persist long after an injury or disease has resolved.[73] It has also been proposed that faulty sympathetic effector mechanisms that cause inappropriate vasoconstriction, vasodilation, increased capillary permeability, or smooth muscle tone may indirectly cause or exacerbate pain.[45]

The Role of Substance P

Substance P is a chemical mediator that is thought to be involved in the transmission of neuropathic and inflammatory pain. It is abundant in the central nervous system and is found in approximately 20% of C fibers.[89] It is also released from peripheral nociceptors and has been detected in inflammatory exudate.[90-92] Substance P release has been shown to excite pain-transmitting neurons in the dorsal horn of the spinal cord, and to be involved in nociceptive processing at the spinal cord level.[93-95] Although less than 5% of the neurons in the dorsal horn express substance P receptors, the majority of pain-transmitting neurons express these receptors. Substance P levels in the spinal cord increase in response to induction of joint inflammation and in response to movement of inflamed joints. Highly elevated levels of substance P have also been found in the cerebrospinal fluid of patients with persistent pain. Substance P receptor activation appears to be involved in the sensitization of pain-transmitting neurons and in the development of hyperalgesia.[95-98] Substance P release and receptor activation is thought to be a response to tissue injury and stress.

A number of mechanisms have been proposed for the action of substance P on pain transmission. Substance P may facilitate excitation of afferent pain fibers by activating the neurokinin-1 receptors in the spinal cord.[99,100] When released into the periphery, substance P increases the production of the inflammatory mediator prostaglandin E2 and the release of cytokines from macrophages and neutrophils.[101] Both prostaglandins and cytokines sensitize primary afferent nociceptors.[102]

Treatments to control pain based on the inhibition of substance P release or on the use of specific substance P antagonists are currently being researched.[92] Opiates may in part exert an analgesic effect by inhibiting the release of substance P from peripheral nerves; however, studies indicate that substance P receptor-expressing neurons are not the major site of action of opiates.[96,103]

PAIN MODULATION AND CONTROL

Gate control theory
The endogenous opioid system

A number of observations make it apparent that pain transmission and perception are subject to inhibition and modification. For example, rubbing or shaking an area that hurts can relieve pain in that area, and stress can cause pain not to be felt at the time an injury occurs. A number of mechanisms have been proposed to explain pain control and modulation. These proposed mechanisms attempt to correlate what is known regarding people's experience of pain with the structures and physiological processes thought to be involved in pain transmission. According to the gate control theory, pain is modulated at the spinal cord level by inhibitory effects of nonnoxious afferent input. According to the theory of endogenous opiates, pain is modulated at the peripheral, spinal cord, and cortical levels by endogenous neurotransmitters that have the same effects as opiates. Psychological central control mechanisms are also thought to affect pain perception and control.

Various physical, chemical, and psychological interventions have been developed based on the current understanding of the mechanisms underlying pain modulation. For example, transcutaneous electrical nerve stimulation (TENS) devices were developed based on the gate control theory of pain modulation. Also, the efficacy of a number of established treatment approaches is now better understood because the underlying mechanisms of pain control have become clearer. For example, it is now thought that thermal agents, which have been used to control pain for centuries, may be effective for this purpose because they gate pain transmission at the spinal cord.

Gate Control Theory

The gate control theory of pain modulation was first proposed by Melzack and Wall in 1965.[73] According to this theory, severity of the pain sensation is determined by the balance of excitatory and inhibitory inputs to the T cells in the spinal cord. These cells receive excitatory input from C and A-delta nociceptor afferents and inhibitory input, via the substantia gelatinosa, from large-diameter A-beta nonnociceptor sensory afferents. Increased activity of the nonnociceptor sensory afferents causes presynaptic inhibition of the T cells, and thus effectively closes the spinal gate to the cerebral cortex and decreases the sensation of pain (see Fig. 3-5).

Many physical agents and interventions are thought to control pain in part by activating nonnociceptive sensory nerves, thereby inhibiting activation of pain transmission cells and closing the gate to the transmission of pain.[104,105] For example, electrical stimulation, traction, compression, and massage can all activate low-threshold, large-diameter, nonnociceptive sensory nerves and therefore may inhibit pain transmission by closing the gate to pain transmission at the spinal cord level.

Although the gate control theory explains many observations regarding pain control and modulation, it fails to account for recent findings that descending controls from higher brain centers, in addition to ascending input from sensory afferents, can affect pain perception.[106,107] Therefore the gate theory has been modified to include influences from descending neurons from the limbic system, the raphe nucleus, and the reticular systems, which affect pain perception, the emotional aspects of pain, and motor responses to pain.[108]

The Endogenous Opioid System

Pain perception has also been shown to be modulated by endogenous opiate-like peptides. These peptides are known as *opiopeptins* (previously known as *endorphins*). Opiopeptins control pain by binding to specific opiate receptors in the nervous system.

An endogenous system of analgesia was first discovered by three independent groups of researchers who were investigating the mechanisms of morphine-induced analgesia. In 1973 they discovered specific opiate-binding sites in the central nervous system.[109-111] In 1975, two peptides, met-enkephalin (methionine-enkephalin) and leu-enkephalin (leucine-enkephalin), which were isolated from the central nervous system of a pig, were shown to produce physiological effects similar to those of morphine.[112] These peptides also bind specifically to the opiate receptors and have their action and binding blocked by naloxone, an opiate antagonist.[113] These findings demonstrated that these endogenous peptides are similar to exogenous opiates such as morphine. Consequently, researchers identified and isolated other similar-acting endogenous peptides, such as beta-endorphin and dynorphin A and B.[114]

Opiopeptins and opiate receptors have been localized in many peripheral nerve endings and in neurons in several regions of the nervous system.[115] Concentrations of opiopeptins and opiate receptors have been identified in various areas of the brain, including the periaqueductal gray matter (PAGM) and the raphe nucleus of the brain stem, which are structures that induce analgesia when electrically stimulated, and in various areas of the limbic system. Opiopeptins are also found in high concentrations in the superficial layers of the dorsal horn of the spinal cord (layers I and II) and in the enteric nervous system as well as in the nerve endings of C fibers. It has been proposed that opiate receptors inhibit the release of substance P from C fiber terminals because local opiate application to C fiber terminals depresses pain transmission at the spinal cord level.[116]

Opioids and opiopeptins always have an inhibitory action. They cause presynaptic inhibition by suppressing the inward flux of calcium and cause postsynaptic inhibition by activating an outward potassium current. In addition, opiopeptins indirectly inhibit pain transmission by inhibiting the release of gamma aminobutyric acid (GABA) in the PAGM and the raphe nucleus.[117] GABA inhibits the activity of various pain-controlling structures, including A-beta afferents, the PAGM, and the raphe nucleus, and can thus increase pain transmission in the spinal cord (Fig. 3-9).

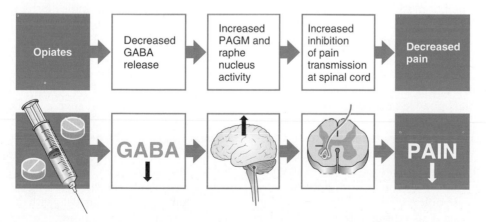

Figure 3-9. Indirect inhibition of pain by application of opiates to opiate receptors.

Electrical stimulation of areas with high levels of opiopeptins, such as the PAGM and the raphe nucleus, has been found to strongly inhibit the transmission of pain messages by some spinal dorsal horn neurons, thereby causing analgesia.[118,119] Electrical stimulation of these areas of the brain can also relieve intractable pain in humans and increase the amount of beta-endorphin in their cerebrospinal fluid (CSF).[120] Since these effects are reversed by the administration of naloxone, they have been attributed to the release of opiopeptins.[121] The concentration of opiate receptors and opiopeptins in the limbic system, an area of the brain largely associated with emotional phenomena, also provides an explanation for the emotional responses to pain, and for the euphoria and relief of emotional stress that is associated with use of morphine and the release of opiopeptins.[122]

The release of opiopeptins is thought to play an important role in the modulation and control of pain during times of emotional stress. Levels of opiopeptins in the brain and CSF become elevated, and pain thresholds increase in both animals and humans when stress is induced experimentally by the anticipation of pain.[123,124] Experimentally, animals have been shown to experience a diffuse analgesia when placed under stress. Humans demonstrate a naloxone-sensitive increase in pain threshold and a parallel depression of the nociceptive flexion reflex when subjected to emotional stress.[124,125] These findings indicate that pain suppression by stress is most likely caused by increased opiopeptin levels at the spinal cord and higher central nervous system centers.

The endogenous opiate system also provides an explanation for the paradoxical pain-relieving effects of painful stimulation and acupuncture. Bearable levels of painful stimulation, such as topical preparations that cause the sensation of burning, or noxious TENS that causes the sensation of pricking or burning, have been shown to reduce the intensity of less bearable preexisting pain in the area of application and in other areas.[125] Painful stimuli have also been shown to reduce the nociceptive flexion reflex of the lower limb.[126] Because these effects of painful stimulation are blocked by naloxone, they are thought to be mediated by opiopeptin.[124,125,127,128] Pain may be relieved because the applied painful stimulus causes neurons in the PAGM regions of the midbrain and thalamus to produce and release opiopeptins.[128]

Placebo analgesia is also thought to be mediated in part by opiopeptins. This claim is supported by the observation that the opiate antagonist naloxone can reverse placebo analgesia and that placebos can also produce respiratory depression, a typical side effect of opioids.[129,130]

MEASURING PAIN

> **Visual analog and numeric scales**
> **Comparison with a predefined stimulus**
> **Semantic differential scales**

To determine the most appropriate treatment for a patient's pain and to assess the efficacy of such treatment, it is helpful to assess the nature and severity of the patient's experience of pain. Such an assessment should attempt to ascertain the causes and sources of pain, the intensity and duration of pain, and the degree to which the pain results in disability or handicap. Various methods and assessment tools have been developed to quantify and qualify both experimentally induced and clinical pain. These methods are based on patients rating their pain on a visual analog or numeric scale, comparing their present pain with that experienced in response to a predefined, quantifiable pain stimulus, or selecting words from a list to describe their present experience of pain. Different tools provide different amounts and types of information and require differing amounts of time and cognitive ability to complete.

Visual Analog and Numeric Scales

Visual analog and numeric scales assess pain severity by asking the patient to indicate the present level of pain on a drawn line or to rate the pain numerically on a scale of 1 to 10 or 1 to 100.[131] With a visual analog scale, the patient marks a position on a horizontal or vertical line, where one end of the line represents no pain and the other end represents the most severe pain possible or the most severe pain the patient can imagine (Fig. 3-10). With a numeric rating scale, 0 is no pain and 10 or 100, depending on the scale used, is the most severe pain possible or the most severe pain the patient can imagine.

Scales similar to the visual analog or numeric scales have been developed for use with individuals who have difficulty using numeric or standard visual analog scales. For example, children who understand

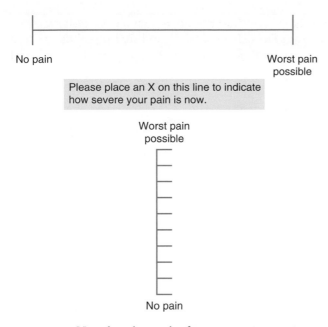

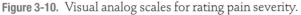

Figure 3-10. Visual analog scales for rating pain severity.

These types of scales are frequently used to assess the severity of a patient's clinical pain because they are quick and easy to administer, are easily understood, and provide readily quantifiable data.[131] However, visual analog and numeric scales provide only a single measure of the patient's pain complaint and fail to provide information about the patient's affective response to pain or the effect of the pain on his or her functional activity level. Also the reliability of visual analog and numeric rating varies between individuals and with the patient group examined, although the two scales have a high degree of agreement between them.[132] These types of measures are most useful in the clinical setting when a quick estimate of a patient's perceived progress or change in symptoms over time, or in response to different activities or treatment interventions, is desired.

Comparison with a Predefined Stimulus

Pain quantification methods that involve comparison with a predefined painful stimulus are intended to provide a greater degree of intersubject reliability than visual analog and numeric scales. For this type of assessment, the individual compares the severity of his or her symptoms with the same predefined stimulus, causing their rating scales to be more similar. Stimuli used for comparison include the application of a tourniquet to the upper extremity to produce ischemia and the application of electrical, thermal, or fingertip pressure stimuli.[133,134] The tourniquet pain test is reported to correlate well with pain assessments using a visual analog scale.[135] Matching the

words or pictures but are too young to understand numeric representations of pain can use a scale with faces with different expressions to represent different experiences of pain, as shown in Fig. 3-11. This type of scale can also be used to assess pain in patients with limited comprehension because of language barriers or cognitive deficits. Pain scales are also available for rating pain in very young children and infants. These are based on describing the child's expression and behavior (Table 3-1).

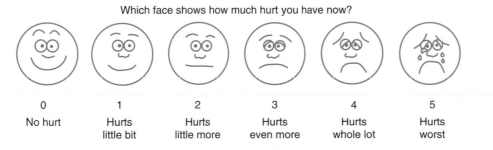

Figure 3-11. Face scale for rating pain severity in children age 3 years and older and others with limited numeric communication ability. The patient uses this tool by pointing to each face and using the brief word instructions under it to describe pain intensity. (From Wong DL, Perry SE, Hockenberry MJ: *Maternal Child Nursing Care,* ed 2, St. Louis, 2002, Mosby.)

TABLE 3-1 Neonatal Infant Pain Scale (NIPS) Operational Definitions

Behavior and score	Description
Facial Expression	
0 – Relaxed muscles	• Restful face, neutral expression
1 – Grimace	• Tight facial muscles, furrowed brow, chin, jaw (negative facial expression – nose, mouth, and brow)
Cry	
0 – No cry	• Quiet, not crying
1 – Whimper	• Mild moaning, intermittent
2 – Vigorous cry	• Loud screams, rising, shrill, continuous (Note: Silent cry may be scored if baby is intubated, as evidenced by obvious mouth, facial movement.)
Breathing Patterns	
0 – Relaxed	• Usual pattern for this baby
1 – Change in breathing	• Indrawing, irregular, faster than usual, gagging, breath holding
Arms	
0 – Relaxed/restrained	• No muscular rigidity, occasional random movements of arms
1 – Flexed/extended	• Tense, straight arms, rigid or rapid extension, flexion
Legs	
0 – Relaxed/restrained	• No muscular rigidity, occasional random leg movement
1 – Flexed/extended	• Tense, straight legs, rigid or rapid extension, flexion
State of Arousal	
0 – Sleeping/awake	• Quiet, peaceful, sleeping, or alert and settled
1 – Fussy	• Alert, restless, and thrashing

Neonatal Infant Pain Scale © 1989, Children's Hospital of Eastern Ontario. Used with permission.
Score 0 = no pain likely, maximum score 7 = severe pain likely.

intensity of clinical pain with electrical, thermal, or fingertip pressure stimuli has also been reported to correlate well with other measures of pain and has been reported to have a high degree of intrasubject reliability.[136,137] However, these types of pain assessment tools also have a number of limitations. They require that the patient experience clinical pain at the time at which the comparison stimulus is applied to make an accurate comparison. Also if a patient has severe pain, it may be both impractical and ethically unacceptable to induce a sufficiently intense pain to provide a comparison with the clinical pain. For patients with pain that is different in quality from the pain of the experimental stimulus; for example, burning or tingling rather than the ache of ischemic pain, a quantitative comparison may not be possible or meaningful. This type of pain measure also fails to take into account, or report on, the emotional, behavioral, or motivational components of a patient's clinical condition. Thus although comparison pain measures may allow for a reliable gauge of some types of pain, particularly experimentally induced pain or clinical acute pain that is moderate or less severe, they are not well-suited for measuring clinical pain that is severe or chronic, or that has a quality different from that of the comparison stimulus.

Semantic Differential Scales

Semantic differential scales consist of word lists and categories that represent various aspects of the patient's pain experience. The patient is asked to select, from these lists, words that best describe his or her present experience of pain. These types of scales are designed to collect a broad range of information about the patient's pain experience and to provide quantifiable data for intra- and intersubject comparisons. The semantic differential scale included in the McGill pain questionnaire, or variations of this scale, are commonly used to assess pain[138-140] (Fig. 3-12). This scale includes descriptors of sensory, affective, and evaluative aspects of the patient's pain and groups the words into various categories within each of these aspects. The categories include temporal, spatial, pressure, and thermal to describe the sensory aspects of the pain; fear, anxiety, and tension to describe the affective aspects of the pain; and the cognitive experience of the pain based on past experience and learned behaviors to describe the evaluative aspects of the pain. The patient circles the one word in each of the applicable categories that best describes the present pain.[138,140]

Semantic differential scales have a number of advantages and disadvantages compared with other types of pain measures. They allow assessment and quantification of various aspects of the pain's scope, quality, and intensity. Counting the total number of words chosen provides a quick gauge of the pain severity. A more sensitive assessment of pain severity can be obtained by adding the rank sums of all the words chosen to produce a pain rating index (PRI). For greater specificity with regard to the most problematic area, an index for the three major categories of the questionnaire can also be calculated.[140] The primary disadvantages of this scale are that it is time-consuming to administer, and it requires the patient to have an intact cognitive state and a high level of literacy. Given these advantages and limitations, the most appropriate use for this type of scale is when detailed information about a patient's pain is needed, such as in a chronic pain treatment program or in clinical research.

Other Measures

Other measures or indicators of pain that may provide additional useful information about the individual's pain complaint and clinical condition include daily activity/pain logs indicating which activities ease or aggravate the pain, body diagrams on which the patient can indicate the location and nature of the pain (Fig. 3-13), and open-ended, structured interviews.[141,142] A physical examination that includes observation of posture and assessment of strength, mobility, sensation, endurance, response to func-

tional activity testing, and soft tissue tone and quality can also add valuable information to the evaluation of the severity and cause(s) of a patient's pain complaint.

In selecting the measures to be used to assess pain, one should consider the duration of the symptoms, the cognitive abilities of the patient, and the amount of time appropriate to assess this aspect of the patient's complaint. In many situations, a simple visual analog scale may be sufficient to provide information regarding a progressive decrease in pain as the patient recovers from an acute injury. However, in more complex or prolonged cases, more detailed measures such as semantic differential scales or a combination of several measures are more appropriate.

PAIN MANAGEMENT APPROACHES

Pharmacological approaches
    Systemic analgesics
    Spinal analgesia
    Local injections to painful structures
Physical agents
Multidisciplinary pain treatment programs

Once the severity and nature of an individual's pain has been evaluated and, ideally, its source and nature determined, the goals of treatment include eliminating the cause of pain, controlling the nociceptor input, and reducing the degree of patient impairment. A wide range of pain management approaches may be used to help achieve these goals. These approaches are based on our current understanding of pain transmission and control mechanisms. They may act by controlling inflammation, altering nociceptor sensitivity, increasing binding to opiate receptors, modifying nerve conduction, modulating pain transmission at the spinal cord level, or altering higher-level aspects of pain perception. In addition, some treatment approaches also address the psychological and social aspects of pain. Different approaches are appropriate for different situations and clinical presentations and are frequently most effective when used together.

The primary intervention used to alleviate pain is the administration of pharmacological agents. Although pharmacological agents are often effective for this purpose, they can also produce a variety

What does your pain feel like?

Some of the words below describe your *present* pain. Indicate which words describe it best. Leave out any word group that is not suitable. Use only a single word in each appropriate group—the one that applies *best*.

1	2	3	4
1 Flickering	1 Jumping	1 Pricking	1 Sharp
2 Quivering	2 Flashing	2 Boring	2 Cutting
3 Pulsing	3 Shooting	3 Drilling	3 Lacerating
4 Throbbing		4 Stabbing	
5 Beating		5 Lancinating	
6 Pounding			

5	6	7	8
1 Pinching	1 Tugging	1 Hot	1 Tingling
2 Pressing	2 Pulling	2 Burning	2 Itchy
3 Gnawing	3 Wrenching	3 Scalding	3 Smarting
4 Cramping		4 Searing	4 Stinging
5 Crushing			

9	10	11	12
1 Dull	1 Tender	1 Tiring	1 Sickening
2 Sore	2 Taut	2 Exhausting	2 Suffocating
3 Hurting	3 Rasping		
4 Aching	4 Splitting		
5 Heavy			

13	14	15	16
1 Fearful	1 Punishing	1 Wretched	1 Annoying
2 Frightful	2 Gruelling	2 Blinding	2 Troublesome
3 Terrifying	3 Cruel		3 Miserable
	4 Vicious		4 Intense
	5 Killing		5 Unbearable

17	18	19	20
1 Spreading	1 Tight	1 Cool	1 Nagging
2 Radiating	2 Numb	2 Cold	2 Nauseating
3 Penetrating	3 Drawing	3 Freezing	3 Agonizing
4 Piercing	4 Squeezing		4 Dreadful
	5 Tearing		5 Torturing

Figure 3-12. Semantic differential scale from the McGill Pain Questionnaire. (Reprinted from Melzack R: The McGill Pain Questionnaire: major properties and scoring methods. In *Pain*, Amsterdam, 1975, Elsevier Science.)

of adverse effects. Therefore the use of physical agents, which also effectively control pain in many cases while producing fewer adverse effects, may be more appropriate. Some patients, particularly those with persistent pain, may need integrated multidisciplinary treatment, which includes psychological as well as physiological therapies, to achieve pain relief or a return to a more normal functional activity level.

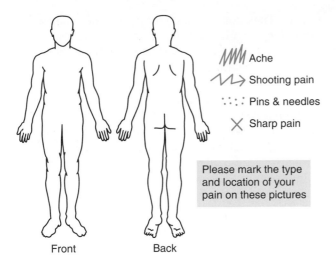

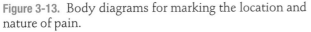

Front   Back

Figure 3-13. Body diagrams for marking the location and nature of pain.

Pharmacological Approaches

Pharmacological analgesic agents control pain by modifying inflammatory mediators at the periphery, altering pain transmission from the periphery to the cortex, or altering the central perception of pain. The selection of a particular pharmacological analgesic agent depends on the cause of the pain, the length of time the individual is expected to need the agent, and the side effects of the agent. Pharmacological agents may be administered systemically by mouth or injection, or locally by injection into structures surrounding the spinal cord or into painful or inflamed areas. These different routes of administration allow concentration of the drug at different sites of pain transmission to optimize the control of symptoms with varying distributions.

Systemic analgesics

Administration of a systemic analgesic is usually the primary method of pain management. This type of treatment is easy to administer and inexpensive, and can be an effective and appropriate pain-relieving intervention for many patients. A wide range of analgesic medications can be systemically administered orally or by other routes. These medications include nonsteroidal antiinflammatory drugs (NSAIDs), acetaminophen, opiates and opioids, and antidepressants.

Nonsteroidal antiinflammatory drugs

NSAIDs have both analgesic and antiinflammatory properties and can therefore relieve pain from both inflammatory and noninflammatory sources. They inhibit peripheral pain and inflammation by inhibiting the conversion of arachidonic acid to prostaglandins by cyclooxygenase; however, much lower doses and blood levels are required to reduce pain than to reduce inflammation.[143] NSAIDs have been shown to reduce both spontaneous and mechanically evoked activity in C and A-delta fibers in acute and chronic models of joint inflammation. Evidence also exists that NSAIDs exert central analgesic effects at the spinal cord and at the thalamus.[144-148]

Although NSAIDs have excellent short- to medium-term application for the control of moderately severe pain caused by musculoskeletal disorders, particularly when the pain is associated with inflammation, side effects can limit their long-term use. The primary long-term complication of most NSAIDs is gastrointestinal irritation and bleeding.[149,150] NSAIDs also cause decreased platelet aggregation and thus prolonged bleeding time. They can cause kidney damage, bone marrow suppression, rashes and anorexia, and decreased renal blood flow in dehydrated patients.[151,152] Using different NSAIDs together increases the risk of side effects.

The first NSAID was aspirin. Many other NSAIDs, such as ibuprofen (Motrin), naproxen sodium (Naprosyn, Aleve), and piroxicam (Feldene), are now available both over the counter (OTC) and by prescription. The principal advantages of these newer NSAIDs over aspirin are that some have a longer duration of action, allowing less frequent dosing and better compliance, and some cause fewer gastrointestinal side effects. However, for most patients, aspirin effectively relieves pain at considerably less expense, although with a slightly higher risk of gastrointestinal bleeding, than the newer NSAIDs. Recently, specific cyclooxygenase type 2 (COX2) inhibitor NSAIDs, such as celecoxib (Celebrex) and rofecoxib (Vioxx), have been developed. Prior NSAIDs inhibited both cyclooxygenase types 1 and 2. Cyclooxygenase type 1 catalyzes the production of prostaglandins associated with joint inflammation while cyclooxygenase type 2 catalyzes the production of prostaglandins that protect the gut mucosa. Thus COX2 inhibitors have more specific antiinflammatory effects and a lower risk of gastrointestinal irritation and bleeding. NSAIDs are primarily administered orally, although one, ketorolac (Toradol®), is available for administration by injection.[153] The mode of administration does not alter the analgesic or adverse effects of these drugs.

Acetaminophen

Acetaminophen (Tylenol®) is an effective analgesic for mild to moderately severe pain; however, unlike an NSAID, it has no clinically significant antiinflammatory activity.[154] Taken in the same dosage as aspirin, it has analgesic and antipyretic effects comparable to those of aspirin.[154] Acetaminophen is administered primarily by the oral route, although administration by suppository is effective for patients who are unable to take medications by mouth. Acetaminophen is useful for patients who cannot tolerate NSAIDs because of gastric irritation or when prolonged bleeding time caused by NSAIDs would be a disadvantage. Prolonged use or large doses of acetaminophen can cause liver damage; this risk is elevated in the chronic alcoholic. Skin rashes are also an occasional side effect of this medication.

Opiates

Opiates are narcotic drugs that contain opium, derivatives of opium, or any of several semisynthetic or synthetic drugs with opium-like activity. Morphine, hydromorphone, fentanyl, and meperidine are examples of opiates commonly used for clinical applications. Although these opiate drugs have slightly different mechanisms of action, they all bind to opiate-specific receptors, and the effects of all of them are reversed by naloxone.[155] The opiates differ primarily in their potency, duration of action, and restriction of use as a result of variations in pharmacodynamics and pharmacokinetics.

It has been proposed that opiates provide analgesia by mimicking the effects of endorphins and binding to opiate-specific receptor sites in the central nervous system.[156] They may also relieve pain by inhibiting the release of presynaptic neurotransmitters and inhibiting the activity of interneurons early in the nociceptive pathways to reduce or block C-fiber inputs into the dorsal horn.[116]

When given in sufficient doses, opiates will control even the most severe acute pain with tolerable side effects. They control pain that cannot be relieved by nonnarcotic agents and are most effective when the pain is dull and poorly localized. The side effects of opiates, including nausea, vomiting, sedation, suppression of cough, gastrointestinal mobility, and respiration, as well as their propensity to cause physical dependence and depression with long-term use, limit their application for the long-term management of musculoskeletal pain. Respiratory depression also limits the dose that can be used even for short-term administration. Tolerance causes drug doses to maintain pain control and to experience withdrawal, and causes a consequent rebound increase in pain when use of the drug is decreased or discontinued after long-term use. Opiates are generally used clinically to relieve postoperative pain or pain due to malignancy. Unfortunately, concerns about tolerance and side effects frequently result in the administration of insufficient doses of these medications to patients with severe pain, resulting in unnecessarily high levels of pain.[157,158] The risk of psychological addiction or habituation should not prevent the appropriate use of opiate medications, particularly in the management of terminal illness.

Opiates can be delivered by mouth, intravenously, or by direct intraarticular injection.[159,160] A popular and effective means of administration, particularly for hospitalized patients, is patient-controlled analgesia (PCA). With PCA, patients use a pump to self-administer small, repeated intravenous doses. The amount of medication delivered is limited by preestablished dosing intervals and maximum doses within a defined period. Pain control is more effective and adverse effects are less common with this means of administration than with more conventional physician-controlled opiate administration methods.[161,162]

Antidepressants

Antidepressants, particularly the tricyclics such as amitryptiline (Elavil®), have been found to be an effective adjunctive component of chronic pain treatment, with smaller doses being effective for this application than those typically used for the treatment of depression.[163,164] The efficacy of these drugs for the treatment of chronic pain is thought to be related to their effects on sleep, nerve function, and mood. Studies have shown that patients with chronic pain who are also depressed report much higher levels of pain and show more pain-related behaviors than those who are not depressed.[165,166] Although it is not certain if the higher level of pain in such patients is the cause or the product of their depression, the use of antidepressants in either situation may prove beneficial.

Spinal analgesia

Pain relief may be achieved by the administration of drugs such as opiates, local anesthetics, and corticosteroids into the epidural or subarachnoid space of the spinal cord.[167] This route of administration provides analgesia to the areas innervated by the segments of the cord receiving the drug and is therefore most effective when the pain has a spinal distribution, such as a dermatomal distribution in a single limb. The primary advantages of this route of administration are that the drug bypasses the blood-brain barrier and that high concentrations reach the spinal cord at opiate receptors at sites of nociceptive transmission, thus increasing the analgesic effects while reducing adverse side effects.

Opiates administered spinally exert their effects by stimulating opiate receptors in the dorsal horn of the spinal cord.[168] When administered spinally, fat-soluble opiates have a rapid onset and a short duration of action, whereas water-soluble opiates have a slow onset and a more prolonged duration of action.[169] Local anesthetics delivered spinally have the unique ability to completely block nociceptive transmission; however, with increasing concentration, these drugs also block sensory and then motor transmission, causing numbness and weakness.[170] High doses of these drugs can also cause hypotension. These side effects of local anesthetics limit their application to the short-term control of pain and diagnostic purposes. Catabolic corticosteroids, such as cortisone and dexamethasone, can be administered to the epidural or subarachnoid space to relieve pain due to inflammation of the spinal nerve roots or surrounding structures. These drugs inhibit the inflammatory response to tissue injury; however, because of the side effects of repeated or prolonged use, including fat and muscle wasting, osteoporosis, and symptoms of Cushing's syndrome, these drugs are not suitable for long-term application.

Local injection

Local injection of a corticosteroid, opiate, or a local anesthetic can be particularly effective for relieving pain associated with local inflammation.[159] Such injections can be administered into joints, bursae, trigger points, or around tendons and can be used for therapeutic purposes, to relieve pain, or for diagnostic purposes in identification of the structure(s) at fault.[171] Although this type of treatment can be very effective, repeated local injections of corticosteroids are not recommended because they can cause tissue breakdown and deterioration. Local injections of corticosteroids directly after acute trauma are also not recommended because these drugs reduce the inflammatory response and may thus impair healing. Local injections of anesthetics generally provide only short-term pain relief and are therefore used primarily during painful procedures or diagnostically.

Physical Agents

Many physical agents effectively control or relieve pain. They are thought to exert these effects by moderating the release of inflammatory mediators, modulating pain at the spinal cord level, altering nerve conduction, or increasing endorphin levels. They may also indirectly reduce pain by decreasing the sensitivity of the muscle spindle system, thereby reducing muscle spasms, or by modifying vascular tone and the rate of blood flow, thereby reducing edema or ischemia.[172-174] In addition, physical agents may reduce pain by helping to resolve the underlying cause of the painful sensation.

Different physical agents control pain in different ways. For example, cryotherapy, the application of cold, controls acute pain in part by reducing the metabolic rate and thus reducing the production and release of inflammatory mediators such as serotonin, histamine, bradykinin, substance P, and prostaglandins.[175] These chemicals cause pain directly by stimulating nociceptors and indirectly by impairing the local microcirculation and, in so doing, can damage tissue and impair tissue repair. Reducing the release of inflammatory mediators can thus directly relieve pain caused by acute inflammation and may indirectly limit pain by controlling edema and ischemia. These short-term benefits can also optimize the rate of tissue healing and recovery.

Cryotherapy, thermotherapy, electrical stimulation, and traction, which provide thermal, mechanical, or other nonnociceptive sensory stimuli, are thought to alleviate pain in part by inhibiting pain transmission at the spinal cord. Physical agents that act by this mechanism can be used for the treatment of acute and chronic pain because they do not generally produce significant adverse effects or adverse interactions with drugs, and they do not produce physical dependence with prolonged use. They are also effective and appropriate for pain caused by conditions that cannot be directly modified, such as pain caused by malignancy or a recent fracture, and for pain caused by peripheral nervous system pathology, such as phantom limb pain and peripheral neuropathy.[176]

Electrical stimulation is also thought to control pain in part by stimulating the release of opiopeptins at the spinal cord and at higher levels.[128] Studies have shown that pain relief by certain types of electrical stimulation is reversed by naloxone.[128]

Physical agents have many advantages over other pain-modifying interventions. They are associated with fewer, and generally less severe, side effects than pharmacological agents. The adverse effects from using physical agents to control pain are generally localized to the area of application and are easily avoided with care in applying the treatment. When used appropriately, attending to all contraindications and dose recommendations, the risk of further injury from the use of physical agents is minimal. For example, an excessively warm hot pack may cause a burn in the area of application, but this risk can be minimized by carefully monitoring the hot pack's temperature, using adequate insulation between the hot pack and the patient, not applying hot packs to individuals with impaired sensation or an impaired ability to report pain, and by checking with the patient for any sensation of excessive heat. Patients also do not develop dependence on physical agents, although they may wish to continue to use them even after they are no longer effective because they enjoy the sensation or attention associated with their application. For example, patients may wish to continue to be treated with ultrasound even though they have reached a stage of recovery where they would benefit more from active exercise. Physical agents also do not generally cause a degree of sedation that would impair an individual's ability to work or drive safely.

Many physical agents have the additional advantage of being readily used independently by patients to treat themselves. For example, a patient can be educated to apply a pain-controlling agent, such as heat, cold, or electrical stimulation, when needed, and so becomes more independent of the health care practitioner and pharmacological agents. The application of such physical agents at home can be an effective component of the treatment of both acute and chronic pain.[177] This type of self-treatment can also assist in containing the costs of medical care.

Physical agents, used either alone or in conjunction with other interventions, such as pharmacological agents, manual therapy, or exercises, can also help remediate the underlying cause of pain while controlling the pain itself. For example, cryotherapy applied to an acute injury controls pain; however, this treatment also controls inflammation, limiting further tissue damage and pain. In this case, the use of NSAIDs, rest, elevation, and compression, in conjunction with cryotherapy, could also prove beneficial, although it may make assessment of the benefits of any one of these interventions more difficult. The selection of physical agents and their specific mechanisms of action and modes of application for controlling pain are discussed in detail in Section 2 of this book regarding the different types of physical agents.

Multidisciplinary Pain Treatment Programs

Over the past 2 to 3 decades, multidisciplinary programs have been developed specifically for the treatment of chronic pain.[4,178] These programs are based on a biopsychosocial model of pain and attempt to address the multiple facets of chronic pain with a multidisciplinary, coordinated program of care.[4,179] These programs attempt to address not only the physical and physiological aspects of the patients' pain but also the behavioral, cognitive-affective, and environmental factors contributing to their symptoms by the use of medical, psychological, and physical interventions.[180,181]

Psychological intervention is focused on improving the coping skills of patients and modifying their behavior, whereas physical activities are focused on reversing the adverse effects of the sedentary lifestyle adopted by most patients with chronic pain. Coping skills can be improved with relaxation training, activity pacing, distraction techniques, cognitive restructuring, and problem solving.[182,183] Behavior modification using the principles of operant conditioning can also alter the patient's perception of and response to pain.[184] Graded activation and exercise programs, in which the patient learns the difference between hurt and harm, can help patients with chronic pain return to a more functional, active lifestyle.[185] The patients' family members are generally involved in these programs by learning appropriate coping skills for themselves and the patient. Such involvement can assist the family members to help individuals with chronic pain more effectively rather than reinforce pain-related behaviors.

In contrast with traditional treatment approaches to acute pain, in which the goal of care is to eliminate the sensation of pain, the goals of care in most multidisciplinary pain treatment programs also include learning to cope and function with pain that may not resolve, although frequently patients also report a reduction in pain after completing these programs.[186,187] Goals of treatment also generally include decreasing dependence on health care personnel and pain-relieving medications, particularly habit-forming opiates or other narcotics; increasing physical activities; and returning patients to their usual social roles. If necessary, narcotic medications are replaced with non–habit-forming drugs or with nonchemical modes of pain relief such as exercise or physical agents.[4] Many studies have shown that multidisciplinary pain treatment programs do result in increased functional activity levels while reducing pain behaviors and the use of medical interventions in patients with chronic pain.[188-191] These programs have also been shown to be cost effective.[181,192-194]

▶ *Clinical Case Studies* ◀

The following case studies summarize the concepts of pain discussed in this chapter. Based on the scenario presented, an evaluation of the clinical findings and goals of treatment are proposed. This is followed by a discussion of the factors to be considered in treatment selection.

Case 1

MP is a 45-year-old female who has been referred to physical therapy with a diagnosis of low back pain and a physician's order to evaluate and treat. MP complains of severe central low back pain that is aggravated by any movement, particularly forward bending. She reports no radiation of pain or other symptoms into her extremities. Pain disturbs her sleep, and she is unable to work at her usual secretarial job or perform her usual household tasks such as grocery shopping and cleaning. She reports that the pain started about 4 days ago, when she reached to pick up a suitcase, and has gradually decreased since its initial onset from a severity of 8, on a scale of 1 to 10, to a severity of 5 or 6. Her only current treatment is 600 mg ibuprofen, which she is taking 3 times a day. The objective exam is significant for restricted lumbar range of motion in all planes. Forward bending is restricted to approximately 20% of normal, backward bending is restricted to approximately 50% of normal, and side bending is restricted to approximately 30% of normal in both directions. Palpable muscle guarding and tenderness in the lower lumbar area occur when the patient is standing or prone. All neurological testing, including straight leg raise and lower extremity sensation, strength, and reflexes are within normal limits.

EVALUATION OF CLINICAL FINDINGS

This patient seeks medical treatment for the impairments of low back pain and restricted lumbar range of motion. These impairments have resulted in difficulties with her normal functional activities of sleeping, working, shopping, and cleaning. Although further analysis may help identify the specific structures causing this patient's pain, its recent onset related to a specific event using the painful area and its gradual resolution over the last few days indicate that her pain is acute and is the result of local musculoskeletal injury and probable inflammation.

PREFERRED PRACTICE PATTERN

Impaired Joint Mobility, Motor Function, Muscle Performance, Range of Motion, and Reflex Integrity Associated With Spinal Disorders, (4F).

PLAN OF CARE

The goals of treatment at this time include controlling pain to allow MP to sleep and return to other functional activities as soon as it is safe for her to do so. The anticipated goals of treatment would also include regaining normal lumbar range of motion and, ideally, preventing a recurrence of the present symptoms.

Continued

◗ *Clinical Case Studies—cont'd* ◖

ASSESSMENT REGARDING SELECTION OF THE OPTIMAL TREATMENT

The optimal intervention would ideally address the acute symptom of pain and the underlying inflammation and, if possible, would help to resolve any underlying structural tissue damage or changes. Although a single treatment may not be able to address all of these issues, treatments that address as many of these issues as possible and that do not adversely affect the patient's progress are recommended. As is explained in greater detail in Part 2 of this book, a number of physical agents, including cryotherapy and electrical stimulation, may be used to control this patient's pain and reduce the probable acute inflammation of the lumbar structures, and lumbar traction may also help to relieve her pain while modifying the underlying spinal dysfunction.

Case 2

TJ is a 45-year-old female who has been referred for therapy with a diagnosis of low back pain and an order to evaluate and treat, with a focus on developing a home program. TJ complains of stiffness and general aching of her lower back that is aggravated by sitting for more than 30 minutes. She reports occasional radiation of pain into her left lateral leg but no other symptoms in her extremities. She states that the pain occasionally disturbs her sleep, and she is unable to work at her usual secretarial job because of her limited sitting tolerance. She can perform most of her usual household tasks, such as grocery shopping and cleaning, although she frequently receives help from her family. She reports that the pain started about 4 years ago, when she reached to pick up a suitcase, and although it was initially severe, at a level of 10 on a scale of 1 to 10, and subsided to some degree over the first few weeks, it has not changed significantly in the past 2 to 3 years and is now usually at a level of 9 or greater. She has had multiple diagnostic tests that have not revealed any significant anatomical pathology, and she has received multiple treatments, including narcotic analgesics and physical therapy consisting primarily of hot packs, ultrasonography, and massage, without significant benefit. Her only current treatment is 600 mg of ibuprofen, which she is taking 3 times a day. The objective exam is significant for restricted lumbar range of motion in all planes. Forward bending is restricted to approximately 40% of normal, backward bending is restricted to approximately 50% of normal, and side bending is restricted to approximately 50% of normal in both directions. Palpation reveals stiffness of the lumbar facet joints at L3 through L5 and tenderness in the lower lumbar area. All neurological testing, including lower extremity sensation, strength, and reflexes are within normal limits, although straight leg raising is limited to 40 degrees bilaterally by hamstring tightness and prone knee bending is limited to 100 degrees bilaterally by quadriceps tightness. TJ is 5 feet 3 inches tall and reports her weight to be 180 pounds. She reports that she has gained 50 pounds since her initial back injury 4 years ago.

EVALUATION OF CLINICAL FINDINGS

This patient seeks medical treatment for the impairments of low back pain and restricted lumbar range of motion. These impairments have resulted in difficulties with her normal functional activities of sleeping, working, shopping, and cleaning. Although further analysis may help identify the specific structures causing this patient's pain, the long duration of the pain is well beyond the normal time needed for a minor back injury to resolve. The lack of change in her pain over the previous years and its lack of response to multiple treatments indicate that her pain may have a variety of contributory factors beyond local tissue damage, including deconditioning, psychological dysfunction, or social problems.

PREFERRED PRACTICE PATTERN

Impaired Posture, (4B).

PLAN OF CARE

The proposed goals of treatment at this time may include controlling pain and regaining normal lumbar range of motion. However, the primary goals of treatment would be to return TJ to her maximal functional level and minimize her dependence on medical personnel and further medical treatment.

ASSESSMENT REGARDING SELECTION OF THE OPTIMAL TREATMENT

The optimal intervention would ideally address the functional limitations caused by this patient's chronic pain and provide her with independent means to manage her symptoms without adverse consequences. Thus the probable focus of care would be on teaching TJ coping skills and improving her physical condition, including strength and flexibility. The use of physical agents would probably be restricted to independent use for pain management or as an adjunct to promote progression toward more functional goals. As is explained in greater detail in Section 2 of this book, a number of physical agents, including cryotherapy, thermotherapy, and electrical stimulation, may be used by patients independently to control pain, while thermotherapy may also be used to help increase the extensibility of soft tissues to allow for more effective and rapid recovery of flexibility.

CHAPTER REVIEW

Pain is the result of a complex interaction of physical and psychological processes that occur when tissue is damaged or at risk of being damaged. The sensation and experience of pain varies with the duration and source of the painful stimulus to produce acute, chronic, or referred pain. Pain is generally perceived when specialized pain receptors (nociceptors) at the periphery are stimulated by noxious thermal, chemical, or mechanical stimuli. Nociceptors cause transmission of the sensation of pain along C fibers and A-delta fibers to the dorsal horn of the spinal cord and thence, via the thalamus, to the cortex. Pain transmission may be inhibited at the spinal cord level by activity of A-beta fibers that transmit nonnoxious sensations, or at the periphery, spinal cord, or higher levels by endogenous opiates. Pain may also be modified indirectly by disruption of the pain-spasm-pain cycle. The severity and quality of an individual's pain can be assessed using a variety of measures, including visual analog and numeric scales, comparison with a predefined stimulus, or selection of words from a given list. These measures can help to direct care and indicate patient progress. A number of approaches can be used to relieve or control pain. These include pharmacological agents, physical agents, and multidisciplinary treatment programs. Pharmacological agents may alter inflammation or peripheral nociceptor activation or may act centrally to alter pain transmission. Physical agents can also modify nociceptor activation and may alter endogenous opiate levels. Multidisciplinary treatment programs integrate pharmacological, physical, and other medical approaches with psychological and social interventions to address the multifaceted dysfunction of chronic pain. A good understanding of the mechanisms underlying pain transmission and control, the tools available for measuring pain, and the various approaches available for treating pain is required to select and direct the use of physical agents appropriately within a comprehensive treatment program for the patient with pain. The reader is referred to the Evolve website http://evolve.elsevier.com/Cameron for study questions pertinent to this chapter.

References

1. Sweet WH: In Field J, Magoun HW, Hall VE eds: *Handbook of Physiology. Section 1: Neurophysiology, Volume I.* Washington, DC, 1959, American Physiological Society.
2. Bonica JJ: Pain: what is science doing about it? *Pain* 2:12-15, 1975.
3. Merskey H, ed: Classification of chronic pain: description of chronic pain syndromes and definition of pain terms, *Pain* (Suppl 3) 3(Suppl):S1, 1986.
4. Vasudevan SV, Lynch NT: Pain centers: organization and outcome, *West J Med* 154(5):532-535, 1991.
5. Vasudevan SV: Rehabilitation of the patient with chronic pain: is it cost effective? *Pain Digest* 2:99-101, 1992.
6. Kazis LE, Meenan RF, Anderson J: Pain in the rheumatic diseases: investigations of a key health status component, *Arthritis Rheum* 4(Suppl 2):10-13, 1983.
7. Strang P: Emotional and social aspects of cancer pain, *Acta Oncol* 31(3):323-326, 1992.
8. Stubble HG, Grubb BD: Afferent and spinal mechanisms of joint pain, *Pain* 55:5-54, 1993.
9. Sluka KA: Pain mechanisms involved in musculoskeletal disorders, *J Orthop Sport Phys Ther* 24(4):240-254, 1996.
10. Grigg P, Stubble HG, Schmidt RF: Mechanical sensitivity of group III and IV afferents from posterior articular nerve in normal and inflamed cat knee, *J Neurophysiol* 55:635-643, 1986.
11. Bonica JJ: *The Management of Pain,* ed 2, Philadelphia, 1990, Lea & Febiger.
12. Bonica JJ: Importance of the problem. In Aronoff GM, ed: *Evaluation and Treatment of Chronic Pain,* Baltimore, 1985, Urban & Schwarzenberg.
13. Vasudevan SV: Management of chronic pain: what have we achieved in the last 25 years? In Ghia JN, ed: *The Multidisciplinary Pain Center: Organization and Personnel Functions for Pain Management,* Boston, 1988, Kluwer.
14. Melzack R, Dennis SG: Neurophysiological foundations of pain. In Sternbach RA, ed: *The Psychology of Pain,* New York, 1978, Raven Press.
15. Kellgren JH: Observations on referred pain arising from muscle, *Clin Sci* 3:175-190, 1938.
16. Staff PH: Clinical consideration in referred muscle pain and tenderness—connective tissue reactions, *Eur J Appl Physiol* 57:369-372, 1988.
17. Black RG: Evaluation of the pain patient, *J Disabil* 1:85-97, 1990.
18. International Association for the Study of Chronic Pain, Subcommittee on Taxonomy: Classification of Chronic Pain, *Pain* (Suppl);3:S1-S225, 1986.
19. Crue BL, ed: *Pain: Research and Treatment,* New York, 1974, Academic Press.
20. Osterweis M, Kleinman A, Mechanic D, eds: *Pain and Disability - Clinical Behavioral and Public Policy Perspective: Committee on Pain, Disability and Chronic Illness Behavior,* Washington, DC, 1987, National Academy Press.
21. Magni G, Caldieron C, Luchini SR et al: Chronic musculoskeletal pain and depressive symptoms in the general population: an analysis of the 1st national health and nutrition examination survey data, *Pain* 43:299-307, 1990.

22. Braky AJ, Klerman GL: Overview: hypochondriasis, bodily complaints, and somatic styles, *Am J Psychol* 140:273-283, 1983.

23. Brena SF: The Mystery of Pain: Is Pain a Sensation? In Brena SF, Chapman SL: *Management of Patients with Chronic Pain,* New York, 1983, SP Medical & Scientific Books, a division of Spectrum Publications.

24. Gildenberg PL, DeVaul RA: *The Chronic Pain Patient: Evaluation and Management,* New York, 1985, Karger.

25. Leavitt F, Garron DC: Psychological disturbance and pain report differences in both organic and non-organic low back pain patients, *Pain* 7:65-68, 1979.

26. Nichols ML, Allen BJ, Rogers SD et al: Transmission of chronic nociception by spinal neurons expressing the substance P receptor, *Science* 286:1558-1561, 1999.

27. Dickenson AH: NMDA receptor agonists as analgesics. In Fields HL, Liebeskind JC, eds: *Pharmacologic Approaches to the Treatment of Chronic Pain: New Concepts and Critical Issues: Progress in Pain Research,* vol 1, Seattle, 1994, IASP Press.

28. Price DD, Hayes RL, Ruda M et al: Spatial and temporal transformation of input to the spinothalamic tract neurons and their relationship to somatic sensations, *J Neurophysiol* 41:933-947, 1978.

29. Woolf CJ: Evidence for a central component of post-injury pain hypersensitivity, *Nature* 41:686-688, 1983.

30. Dickenson AH, Sullivan AF: Evidence for a role of the NMDA receptor in the frequency dependent potentiation of deeper dorsal horn neurons following c-fiber stimulation, *Neuropharmacology* 26:1235-1238, 1987.

31. Gottschalk A, Smith DS, Jobes DR et al: Preemptive epidural analgesia and recovery from radical prostatectomy: a randomized controlled trial, *JAMA* 279:1076-1082, 1998.

32. Carr DB: Preempting the memory of pain, *JAMA* 279:1114-1115, 1998.

33. Ji RR, Baba H, Brenner GJ et al: Nociceptive-specific activation of ERK in spinal neurons contributes to pain hypersensitivity, *Nat Neurosci* 2:1114-1119, 1999.

34. Wooley S, Blackwell B, Winger C: A learning theory model of chronic illness behavior: theory, treatment, and research, *Psychosom Med* 40:379-401, 1978.

35. Brena SF, Chapman SL: *Management of Patients with Chronic Pain,* New York, 1983, SP Medical & Scientific Books, a division of Spectrum Publications

36. Blackwell B, Galbraith JR, Dahl DS: Chronic pain management, *Hosp Community Psychiatry* 35:999-1008, 1984.

37. Tippett SR: Referred knee pain in a young athlete: a case study, *J Orthop Sports Phys Ther* 19(2):117-120, 1994.

38. Kendall FP, McCreary EK: *Muscles, Testing and Function,* ed 3, Baltimore, 1983, Williams & Wilkins.

39. Willis WD, Coggeshall RE: *Sensory Mechanisms of the Spinal Cord,* New York, 1991, Plenum Press.

40. Von Frey J: Beitrage zur physiologica des schmerzsinns, *Ber Kgl Sachs Ges Wis* 46:185, 1894.

41. Perl ER: Pain and nociception. In Brookhart JM, Mountcastle VB, Darian-Smith I, Geiger SR: *Handbook of Physiology. Section 1: The Nervous System. Volume III. Sensory Process, Part 2.* Bethesda, MD, 1984, American Physiological Society.

42. Willis WD: *The Pain System: The Neural Basis of Nociceptive Transmission in the Mammalian Nervous System,* Basel, 1985, Karger.

43. Goldscheider A: *Veber den Schmertz in Physiologischer und Klinischer Hensicht,* Berlin, 1894, Hirschwald.

44. Torebjork HE, Schady W, Ochoa J: Sensory correlates of somatic afferent fibre activation, *Hum Neurobiol* 3:15-20, 1984.

45. Zimmerman M: Basic concepts of pain and pain therapy, *Drug Res* 34(2):1053-1059, 1984.

46. Heppleman B, Meslinger K, Neiss WF et al: Ultrastructural three-dimensional reconstruction of group III and IV sensory nerve endings ("free nerve endings") in the knee joint capsule of the cat: evidence for multiple receptive sites, *J Comp Neurol* 292:103-116, 1990.

47. Polacek P: Receptors of joints: their structure, variability and classification, *Acta Facultat Med Univesitat Brunensis* 23:1-107, 1966.

48. Freeman MAR, Wyke B: The innervation of the knee joint: an anatomical and histological study in the cat, *J Anat* 101:505-532, 1967.

49. Halata Z, Groth HP: Innervation of the synovial membrane of the cat's joint capsule, *Cell Tissue Res* 169:415-418, 1976.

50. Halata Z, Badalamente ME, Dee R et al: Ultrastructure of sensory nerve endings in monkeys' knee joint capsule, *J Orthop Res* 2:218-226, 1984.

51. Beck PW, Handwerker HO: Bradykinin and serotonin effects on various types of cutaneous nerve fibers, *Pflugers Arch* 347:209-222, 1974.

52. Berberich P, Hoheisel U, Mense S: Effects of a carrageenan-induced myositis on the discharge properties of group III and IV muscle receptors in the cat, *J Neurophysiol* 59:1395-1409, 1988.

53. Gilfoil TM, Klavins I: 5-Hydroxytryptamine, bradykinin and histamine as mediators of inflammatory hyperesthesia, *J Physiol* 208:867-876, 1965.

54. Stubble H, Schmidt RF: Effects of an experimental arthritis on the sensory properties of fine articular afferent units, *J Neurophysiol* 54:1109-1122, 1985.

55. Stubble H, Schmidt RF: Time course of mechanosensitivity changes in articular afferents during a developing experimental arthritis, *J Neurophysiol* 60:2180-2194, 1988.

56. Mense S, Stahnke M: Responses in muscle afferent fibres of slow conduction velocity to contraction and ischemia in the cat, *J Physiol* (Lond) 342:383-387, 1983.

57. Fields HL, Levine JD: Pain—mechanisms and management, *West J Med* 141:347-357, 1984.

58. Elliott KJ: Taxonomy and mechanisms of neuropathic pain, *Semin Neurol* 14(3):195-205, 1994.

59. Ochoa JL, Torebjork HE: Sensations by intraneural microstimulation of single mechanoreceptor units innervating the human hand, *J Physiol* (Lond) 342:633-654, 1983.

60. Torebjork HE, Ochoa JL, Schady W: Referred pain from intraneuronal stimulation of muscle fascicles in the median nerve, *Pain* 18:145-156, 1984.

61. Marchettini P, Cline M, Ochoa JL: Innervation territories for touch and pain afferents of single fascicles of the human ulnar nerve, *Brain* 113:1491-1500, 1990.

62. Gybels J, Handwerker HO, Van Hees J: A comparison between the discharges of human nociceptive fibers and the subject's rating of his sensations, *J Physiol* (Lond) 186:117-132, 1979.

63. Wood L: Physiology of pain. In Kitchen S, Bazin S, eds: *Clayton's Electrotherapy*, ed 10, London, 1996, WB Saunders.

64. Watkins LR, Mayer D: Organization of endogenous opiate and nonopiate pain control systems, *Science* 216:1185-1192, 1982.

65. Heppleman B, Heuss C, Schmidt RF: Fiber size distribution of myelinated and unmyelinated axons in the medial and posterior articular nerves of the cat's knee joint, *Somatosens Res* 5:267-275, 1988.

66. Nolan MF: Anatomic and physiologic organization of neural structures involved in pain transmission, modulation, and perception. In Echternach JL, ed: *Pain,* New York, 1987, Churchill Livingstone.

67. Grevert P, Goldstein A: Endorphins: Naloxone fails to alter experimental pain or mood in humans, *Science* 199:1093-1095, 1978.

68. Lamotte C: Distribution of the tract of Lissauer and the dorsal root fibers in the primate spinal cord, *J Comp Neurol* 72:529-561, 1977.

69. Light AR, Perl ER: Spinal termination of functionally identified primary afferent neurons with slowly conducting myelinated fibers, *J Comp Neurol* 186:133-150, 1979.

70. Light AR, Perl ER: Re-examination of the dorsal root projection to the spinal dorsal horn including observations on the differential termination of course and fine fibers, *J Comp Neurol* 186:117-132, 1979.

71. Light AR, Perl ER: Differential termination of large-diameter and small-diameter primary afferent fibers in the spinal dorsal gray matter as indicated by labeling with horseradish peroxidase, *Neurosci Lett* 6:59-63, 1977.

72. Besson JM, Charouch A: Peripheral and spinal mechanisms of nociception, *Physiol Rev* 67(1):67-186, 1988.

73. Melzack JD, Wall PD: Pain mechanisms: a new theory, *Science* 150:971-979, 1965.

74. Hillman P, Wall PD: Inhibitory and excitatory factors influencing the receptive fields of lamina 5 spinal cord cells, *Exp Brain Res* 9:161-171, 1969.

75. Belcher G, Ryall RW, Schaffner R: The differential effects of 5-hydroxytryptamine, noradrenaline, and raphe stimulation on nociceptive and non-nociceptive dorsal horn interneurons in the cat, *Brain Res* 151:307-321, 1978.

76. Fleetwood-Walker SM, Mitchell R, Hope PJ et al: An A_2 receptor mediates the selective inhibition by noradrenaline of nociceptive responses of identified dorsal horn neurons, *Brain Res* 334:243-354, 1985.

77. Unnerstall JR, Kopajtic TA, Kuhar MJ: Distribution of A_2 agonist binding sites in the rat and human central nervous system: analysis of some functional autonomic correlates of the pharmacologic effects of clonidine and related adrenergic agents, *Brain Res* 319:69-101, 1984.

78. Willis WD: Control of nociceptive transmission in the spinal cord. In Autrum H, Ottoson D, Perl ER, Schmidt RF, eds: *Progress in Sensory Physiology,* vol 3, Berlin, 1982, Springer-Verlag.

79. Janig W, Kollmann W: The involvement of the sympathetic nervous system in pain, *Drug Res* 34(2):1066-1073, 1984.

80. Gilman AG, Goodman L, Rall TW et al, eds: *Goodman and Gilman's The Pharmacologic Basis of Therapeutics*, ed 7, New York, 1985, Macmillan.

81. Janig W, McLachlan EM: The role of modification in noradrenergic peripheral pathways after nerve lesions in the generation of pain. In Fields HL, Liebeskind JC, eds: *Pharmacologic Approaches to the Treatment of Chronic Pain: New Concepts and Critical Issues: Progress in Pain Research and Management,* vol 1, Seattle, 1994, IASP Press.

82. Bonica JJ, Liebeskind JC, Albe-Fessard DG: *Advances in Pain Research and Therapy,* vol 3, New York, 1979, Raven Press.

83. Kleinert HE, Norberg H, McDonough JJ: Surgical sympathectomy: upper and lower extremity. In Omer GE, ed: *Management of Peripheral Nerve Problems*, Philadelphia, 1980, WB Saunders.

84. Campbell JN, Raja SN, Selig DK, et al: Diagnosis and management of sympathetically maintained pain. In Fields HL, Liebeskind JC, eds: *Pharmacological Approaches to the Treatment of Chronic Pain: New Concepts and Critical Issues: Progress in Pain Research and Management*, vol 1, Seattle, 1994, IASP Press.

85. Price DD, Long S, Huitt C: Sensory testing of pathophysiological mechanisms of pain in patients with reflex sympathetic dystrophy, *Pain* 49:163-173, 1992.

86. Stanton-Hicks M, Janig W, Hassenbusch S et al: Reflex sympathetic dystrophy: changing concepts and taxonomy, *Pain* 63:127-133, 1995.

87. Fields HL: *Pain: Mechanisms and Management,* New York, 1987, McGraw Hill.

88. Selkowitz DM: The sympathetic nervous system in neuromotor function and dysfunction and pain: a brief review and discussion, *Funct Neurol* 7:89-95, 1992.

89. White DM, Helme RD: Release of substance P from peripheral nerve terminals following electrical stimulation of the sciatic nerve, *Brain Res* 336:27-31, 1985.

90. Larsson J, Ekblom A, Henriksson K et al: Concentration of substance P, neurokinin A, calcitonin gene-related peptide, neuropeptide Y and vasoactive intestinal polypeptide in synovial fluid from knee joints in patients suffering from rheumatoid arthritis, *Scand J Rheumatol* 20:326-335, 1991.

91. Marshall KW, Chiu B, Inman RD: Substance P and arthritis: analysis of plasma and synovial fluid levels, *Arthritis Rheum* 33:87-90, 1990.

92. Gamse R, Holzer P, Lembeck F: Decrease of substance P in primary afferent neurons and impairment of neurogenic plasma extravasation by capsaicin, *Br J Pharmacol* 68:207-213, 1980

93. Neugebauer V, Wieretter F, Stubble HG: Involvement of substance P and neurokinin-1 receptors in hyperexcitability of dorsal horn neurons during development of acute arthritis in rat's knee joint, *J Neurophysiol* 73:1574-1583, 1995.

94. Randic M, Miletic V: Effect of substance P in cat dorsal horn neurons activated by noxious stimuli, *Brain Res* 128:164-169, 1977.

95. Stubble HG, Jarrott B, Hope PJ et al: Release of immunoreactive substance P in the spinal cord during development of acute arthritis in the knee joint of the cat: a study with antibody microprobes, *Brain Res* 529:214-223, 1990.

96. Oku R, Satoh M, Tagaki H: Release of substance P from the spinal dorsal horn is enhanced in polyarthritic rats, *Neurosci Lett* 74:315-319, 1987.

97. Russell IJ, Orr MD, Littman B et al: Elevated cerebrospinal fluid levels of substance P in patients with the fibromyalgia syndrome, *Arthritis Rheum* 37(11): 1593-1601, 1994.

98. Vaeroy H, Helle R, Forre O et al: Elevated CSF levels of substance P and high incidence of Raynaud phenomenon in patients with fibromyalgia: new features for diagnosis, *Pain* 32:21-26, 1988.

99. Radharkrishnan V, Henry JL: Antagonism of nociceptive responses of cat spinal dorsal horn neurons in vivo by the NK-1 receptor antagonists CP-96,345 and CP-99,994, but not by CP-96,344, *Neuroscience* 64: 943-958, 1995.

100. Slake KA, Milton MA, Westlund KN et al: Involvement of neurokinin receptors in the joint inflammation and heat hyperalgesia following acute inflammation in unanesthetized rats, *J Physiol* (Lond) 483P:152-153, 1995.

101. Khalil Z, Hleme RD: Sequence of events in substance P mediated plasma extravasation in rat skin, *Brain Res* 500:256-262, 1989.

102. Vasko MR, Campbell WB, Waite KJ: Prostaglandin E2 enhances bradykinin-stimulated release of neuropeptides from rat sensory neurons in culture, *J Neurosci* 14:4987-4997, 1994.

103. Jessell TM, Iversen LL: Opiate analgesics inhibit substance P release from rat trigeminal nucleus, *Nature* 268:549-551, 1977.

104. Nathan PW, Wall PD: Treatment of post-herpetic neuralgia by prolonged electrical stimulation, *Br Med J* 3:645-657, 1974.

105. Wall PD, Sweet WH: Temporary abolition of pain in man, *Science* 155:108-109, 1967.

106. Nathan PW, Rudge P: Testing the gate control theory of pain in man, *J Neurol Neurosurg Psychiatry* 3:645-657, 1974.

107. Kerr FWL: Pain: A central inhibitory balance theory, *Mayo Clin Proc* 50:685-690, 1975.

108. Melzack R, Casey KL: Sensory, motivational, and central control determinants of pain. In Kenshalo DR, ed: *The Skin Senses,* Springfield, IL, 1968, Charles C Thomas.

109. Pert CB, Pasternak G, Snyder SH: Opiate agonists and antagonists discriminated by receptor binding in the brain, *Science* 182(119):1359-1361, 1973.

110. Simon EJ: In search of the opiate receptor, *Am J Med Sci* 266(3):160-168, 1973.

111. Terenius L: Characteristics of the "receptor" for narcotic analgesics in synaptic plasma membrane fraction from rat brain, *Acta Pharmacol Toxicol* (Copenh) 33(5):377-384, 1973.

112. Huges J, Smith TW, Kosterlitz HW et al: Identification of two related pentapeptides from the brain with potent opiate agonist activity, *Nature* 258:577-579, 1975.

113. Mayer DJM, Price DD: Central nervous system mechanisms of analgesia, *Pain* 2:379-404, 1976.

114. Simon EJ, Hiller JM: The opiate receptors, *Annu Rev Pharmacol Toxicol* 18:371-377, 1978.

115. Willer JC: Endogenous, opioid, peptide-mediated analgesia, *Int Med* 9(8):100-111, 1988.

116. Mao J, Price DD, Mayer DJ: Mechanisms of hyperalgesia and morphine tolerance: a current view of their possible interactions: review article, *Pain* 62:259-274, 1995.

117. Hao JX, Xu XJ, Yu YX et al: Baclofen reverses the hypersensitivity of dorsal horn wide dynamic range neurons to mechanical stimulation after transient spinal cord ischemia: implications for a tonic GABAergic

inhibitory control of myelinated fiber input, *J Neurophysiol* 68:392-396, 1992.

118. Balagura S, Ralph T: The analgesic effect of electrical stimulation of the diencephalon and mesencepahlon, *Brain Res* 60:369-381, 1973.

119. Duggan AW, Griersmith BT: Inhibition of spinal transmission of nociceptive information by supraspinal stimulation in the cat, *Pain* 6:149-161, 1979.

120. Adams JE: Naloxone reversal of analgesia produced by brain stimulation in the human, *Pain* 2:161-166, 1976.

121. Akil H, Mayer DJ, Liebeskind JC: Antagonism of stimulation-produced analgesia by naloxone, a narcotic antagonist, *Science* 191:961-962, 1976.

122. Snyder SH: Opiate receptors and internal opiates, *Sci Am* 240(3):44-56, 1977.

123. Terman GW, Shavit Y, Lewis JW et al: Intrinsic mechanisms of pain inhibition: activation by stress, *Science* 226:1270-1277, 1984.

124. Willer JC, Dehen H, Cambrier J: Stress-induced analgesia in humans: endogenous opioids and naloxone-reversible depression of pain reflexes, *Science* 212:689-691, 1981.

125. Willer JC, Roby A, Le Bars D: Psychophysical and electrophysiological approaches to the pain-relieving effects of heterotopic nociceptive stimuli, *Brain Res* 107:1095-1112, 1984.

126. Tricklebank MD, Curzon G: *Stress-Induced Analgesia*, Chichester, England, 1984, Wiley.

127. Mayer DJ, Price DD, Barber J et al: Acupuncture analgesia: evidence for activation of a pain inhibitory system as a mechanism of action. In Bonica JJ, Albe-Fessard D, eds: *Advances in Pain Research and Therapy*, New York, 1976, Raven Press.

128. Bassbaum AI, Fields HL: Endogenous pain control mechanisms: review and hypothesis, *Ann Neurol* 4:451-462, 1978.

129. Levine JD, Gordon NC, Fields HL: The mechanism of placebo analgesia, *Lancet* 2:654-657, 1978.

130. Bendetti F, Amanzio M, Baldi S et al: Inducing placebo respiratory depressant responses in humans via opioid receptors, *Eur J Neurosci* 11:625-631, 1999.

131. Downie W, Leatham PA, Rhind VM et al: Studies with pain rating scales, *Ann Rheum Dis* 37:378-388, 1978.

132. Grossman SA, Shudler VR, McQuire DB et al: A comparison of the Hopkins Pain Rating Instrument with standard visual analogue and verbal description scales in patients with chronic pain, *J Pain Symptom Mgmt* 7:196-203, 1992.

133. Sternbach RA: *Pain Patients: Traits and Treatment*, New York, 1974, Academic Press.

134. Posner J: A modified submaximal effort tourniquet test for evaluation of analgesics in healthy volunteers, *Pain* 19:143-151, 1984.

135. Sternbach RA: The tourniquet pain test. In Melzack R, ed: *Pain Measurement and Assessment*, New York, 1983, Raven Press.

136. Kast EC: An understanding of pain and its measurement, *Med Times* 94:1501-1503, 1966.

137. Hardy JD, Wolff HG, Goodell H: *Pain Sensations and Reactions*, New York, 1952, Hafner.

138. Melzack R: The McGill Pain Questionnaire: major properties and scoring methods, *Pain* 1:277-299, 1975.

139. Byrne M, Troy A, Bradley LA et al: Cross-validation of the factor structure of the McGill Pain Questionnaire, *Pain* 13(2):193-201, 1982.

140. Prieto EJ, Hopson L, Bradley LA et al: The language of low back pain: factor structure of the McGill Pain Questionnaire, *Pain* 8(1):11-19, 1980.

141. Ransford AO, Cairns D, Mooney V: The pain drawing as an aid to the psychological evaluation of patients with low-back pain, *Spine* 1(2):127-134, 1976.

142. Grieve GP: Common patterns of clinical presentation. In Grieve GP: *Common Vertebral Joint Problems*, ed 2, New York, 1988, Churchill Livingstone.

143. Tuman KJ, McCarthy RJ, March RJ et al: Effects of epidural anesthesia and analgesia on coagulation and outcome after major vascular surgery, *Anesth Analg* 73:696-704, 1991.

144. Heppleman B, Pfeffer A, Stubble HG et al: Effects of acetylsalicylic acid and indomethacin on single groups III and IV sensory units from acutely inflamed joints, *Pain* 26:337-351, 1986.

145. Grubb BD, Birrell J, McQueen DS et al: The role of PCE2 in the sensitization of mechanoreceptors in normal and inflamed ankle joints of the rat, *Exp Brain Res* 84:383-392, 1991.

146. Malmberg AB, Yaksh TL: Hyperalgesia mediated by spinal glutamate or substance P receptor block by cyclo-oxygenase inhibition, *Science* 257:1276-1279, 1992.

147. Carlsson KH, Monzel W, Jurna I: Depression by morphine and the non-opioid analgesic agents, metamizol (dipyrone), lysine and acetylsalicylate, and paracetomol, of activity in rat thalamus neurons evoked by electrical stimulation of nociceptive afferents, *Pain* 32:313-326, 1988.

148. Jurna I, Spohrer B, Bock R: Intrathecal injection of acetylsalicylic acid, salicylic acid and indomethacin depresses C-fibre-evoked activity in the rat thalamus and spinal cord, *Pain* 49:249-256, 1992.

149. Semble EL, Wu WC: Anti-inflammatory drugs and gastric mucosal damage, *Semin Arthritis Rheum* 16:271-286, 1987.

150. Griffin MR, Piper JM, Daugherty JR et al: Nonsteroidal anti-inflammatory drug use and increased risk for peptic ulcer disease in elderly persons, *Ann Intern Med* 114:257-259, 1991.

151. Ali M, McDonald JWD: Reversible and irreversible inhibition of platelet cyclo-oxygenase and serotonin release by nonsteroidal anti-inflammatory drugs, *Thromb Res* 13:1057-1065, 1978.

152. Patronon C, Dunn MJ: The clinical significance of inhibition of renal prostaglandin synthesis, *Kidney Int* 31:1-12, 1987.

153. Package insert: Toradol. Nutley, NJ: Hoffmann-La Roche; July 1995.

154. Ameer B, Greenblatt DJ: Acetaminophen, *Ann Intern Med* 87:202-209, 1977.

155. Hyleden JLK, Nahin RL, Traub RJ et al: Effects of spinal kappa-aged receptor agonists on the responsiveness of nociceptive superficial dorsal horn neurons, *Pain* 44:187-193, 1991.

156. Hudson AH, Thomson IR, Cannon JE et al: Pharmacokinetics of fentanyl inpatients undergoing abdominal aortic surgery, *Anesthesiology* 64:334-338, 1986.

157. D'Amours RH, Ferrante FM: Postoperative pain management, *J Orthop Sport Phys Ther* 24(4):227-236, 1996.

158. Dickey NW: Pain management at the end of life, *J Orthop Sport Phys Ther* 24(4):237-239, 1996.

159. Stein C, Comisel K, Haimerl E et al: Analgesic effect of intraarticular morphine after arthroscopic surgery, *N Engl J Med* 325:1123-1126, 1991.

160. Likaar R, Schafer M, Paulak F et al: Intra-articular morphine analgesia in chronic pain patients with osteoarthritis, *Anesth Analg* 84:1313-1317, 1997.

161. Camp JF: Patient-controlled analgesia, *Am Fam Physician* 44:2145-2149, 1991.

162. Egbert AM, Parks LH, Short LM et al: Randomized trial of postoperative patient-controlled analgesia vs. intramuscular narcotics in frail elderly men, *Arch Intern Med* 150:1897-1903, 1990.

163. Watson CP, Evans RJ, Reed K et al: Amitryptaline versus placebo in postherpetic neuralgia, *Neurology* (NY) 32:671-673, 1983.

164. Von Korff M, Wagner EH, Dworkin SF et al: Chronic pain and use of ambulatory health care, *Psychosom Med* 53(1):61-79, 1991.

165. Parmalee PA, Katz IB, Lawton MP: The relation of pain to depression among institutionalized aged, *J Gerontol* 46:15-21, 1991.

166. Keefe FJ, Wilkins RH, Cook WA et al: Depression, pain, and pain behavior, *J Consult Clin Psychol* 54:665-669, 1986.

167. Coombs DW, Danielson DR, Pagneau MG et al: Epidurally administered morphine for postceasarean analgesia, *Surg Gynecol Obstet* 154:385-388, 1982.

168. Yaksh TL, Noveihed R: The physiology and pharmacology of spinal opiates, *Ann Rev Pharmacol* 25:443-462, 1975.

169. Sjostrum S, Hartvig P, Persson MP et al: The pharmacokinetics of epidural morphine and meperidine in humans, *Anesthesiology* 67:877-888, 1987.

170. Gissen AJ, Covino BG, Gregus J: Differential sensitivity of fast and slow fibers in mammalian nerve. III. Effect of etidocaine and bupivicaine on fast/slow fibres, *Anesth Analg* 61:570-575, 1982.

171. McAfee JH, Smith DL: Olecranon and prepatellar bursitis: diagnosis and treatment, *West J Med* 149:607-612, 1988.

172. Ernst E, Fialka V: Ice freezes pain? A review of the clinical effectiveness of analgesic cold therapy, *J Pain Symptom Mgmt* 9(1):56-59, 1994.

173. Crockford GW, Hellon RF, Parkhouse J: Thermal vasomotor response in human skin mediated by local mechanisms, *J Physiol* 161:10-15, 1962.

174. McMaster WC, Liddie S: Cryotherapy influence on posttraumatic limb edema, *Clin Orthop Relat Res* 150:283-287, 1980.

175. Hocutt JE, Jaffe R, Ryplander CR: Cryotherapy in ankle sprains, *Am J Sports Med* 10:316-319, 1982.

176. Winnem MF, Amundsen T: Treatment of phantom limb pain with transcutaneous electrical nerve stimulation, *Pain* 12:299-300, 1982.

177. Bigos S, Bowyer O, Braen G et al: Acute Low Back Problems in Adults, Clinical Practice Guideline No 14. AHCPR Publication No. 95-0642, Rockville, MD, 1994, Agency for Health Care Policy and Research, Public Health Service, US Dept of Health and Human Services.

178. Aronoff AM: *Pain Centers: A Revolution in Health Care*, New York, 1988, Raven Press.

179. Fordyce WE: The biopsychosocial model revisited. Paper presented at the annual meeting of the American Pain Society, Los Angeles, November 1995.

180. Tollison CD, Kriegel ML, Satherwaite JR et al: Comprehensive pain center treatment of low back workers compensation injuries—an industrial medicine clinical outcome follow-up comparison, *Orthop Res* (Suppl 8):1115-1126, 1989.

181. Cicala RS, Wright H: Outpatient treatment of patients with chronic pain: an analysis of cost savings, *Clin J Pain* 5:223-226, 1989.

182. Keefe FJ, Beaupre PM, Gil KM: Group therapy for patients with chronic pain. In Turk DC, Gatchel RJ, eds: *Psychological Factors in Pain: Critical Perspectives*, New York, 1999, Guildford Press.

183. Keefe FJ, Kashikar-Zuck S, Opiteck J et al: Pain in arthritis and musculoskeletal disorders: the role of coping skills training and exercise interventions, *J Orthop Sport Phys Ther* 24(4):279-290, 1996.

184. Wickramaskerra I: Biofeedback and behavior modification for chronic pain. In Echternach HL, ed: *Pain*, New York, 1987, Churchill Livingstone.

185. Linton IJ, Bradley LA, Jensen I et al: The secondary prevention of low back pain: a controlled study with follow up, *Pain* 36:197-207, 1989.

186. Keefe FJ, Caldwell DS, Williams DA et al: Pain coping skills training in the management of osteoarthritic knee pain: a comparative study, *Behav Ther* 21:49-62, 1990.

187. Keefe FJ, Caldwell DS, Williams DA et al: Pain coping skills training in the management of osteoarthritic knee pain: follow-up results, *Behav Ther* 21:435-448, 1990.

188. Swanson DW, Swenson WM, Maruta T et al: Program for managing chronic pain. Program description and characteristics of patients, *Mayo Clin Proc* 51:401-408, 1976.

189. Seres JL, Newman RI: Results of treatment of chronic low-back pain at the Portland Pain Center, *J Neurosurg* 45:32-36, 1976.

190. Guck TP, Skultety FM, Meilman DW et al: Multidisciplinary pain center follow-up study: evaluation with no-treatment control group, *Pain* 21:295-306, 1985.

191. Keefe FJ, Caldwell DS, Queen KT et al: Pain coping strategies in osteoarthritis patients, *J Consult Clin Psychol* 55:208-212, 1987.

192. Mayer TG, Gatchel RJ, Mayer H et al: A prospective two-year study of functional restoration in industrial low back injury—an objective assessment procedure, *JAMA* 258:1763-1767, 1987.

193. Stieg RL, Williams RC, Timmermans-Williams G et al: Cost benefits of interdisciplinary chronic pain treatment, *Clin J Pain* 1:189-193, 1986.

194. Simmons JW, Avant WS Jr, Demski J et al: Determining successful pain clinic treatment through validation of cost effectiveness, *Spine* 13:342-344, 1988.

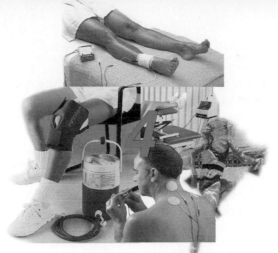

Tone Abnormalities

Diane D. Allen, MS, PT, and Gail L. Widener, PhD, PT

SUMMARY OF INFORMATION COVERED

Muscle Tone Defined

Terminology for Tone Abnormalities

Measuring Muscle Tone

The Anatomical Bases of Muscle Tone and Muscle Activation

Abnormal Muscle Tone and It's Consequences

Clinical Case Studies

Chapter Review

OBJECTIVES

Upon completion of this chapter, the reader will be able to:

1. Define muscle tone and identify tone changes in the normal adult.
2. Use appropriate terminology to describe abnormal muscle tone.
3. Describe quantitative and qualitative methods used to measure muscle tone, determining when each is appropriate.
4. Identify the active and passive elements of muscle that contribute to muscle tone.
5. Describe the function of the alpha motor neuron and its conduction of electrochemical signals.
6. Identify peripheral, spinal, and supraspinal sources of input to the alpha motor neuron.
7. Describe muscle tone differences resulting from changes in excitatory and inhibitory input to alpha motor neurons.
8. Discuss various pathologies that might result in abnormal muscle tone, including the type of tone abnormality that is likely to occur.
9. Identify clinically relevant consequences of increased, decreased, or fluctuating muscle tone.
10. Determine appropriate management of patients with abnormal muscle tone, stating the expected effect of various treatments.

Significant problems in both muscle tone and muscle activation severely limited Mrs. H's function. While she sat in her wheelchair, her thorax was kyphotic, her head was exaggeratedly extended forward, her left arm writhed, her left leg danced, and her right arm hugged her right knee to her chest. Her mouth and tongue worked continuously. The constant involuntary motion, or dyskinesia, was probably a result of large doses of medication used to control the lack of motion, or akinesia, typical of her Parkinson's disease. Her dyskinesia alternated with a "freeze state" in which her left arm and leg would slow and then stop; she would let go of her right leg and become still in her chair, sitting with a masked face and both feet on the floor like a sedate statue. In the akinetic freeze state, even the simplest functional movements became nearly impossible for her.

Mrs. H's dyskinesia and freezes represent fluctuations in the tone and activation of her muscles. Muscle activation, or contraction, is readily understandable because it is usually visible through movements and can be measured by the force or torque generated around a joint. In contrast, muscle tone is a quality that is difficult to define or quantify. It is observable in its extreme states and even in its normal fluctuations. The difficulty lies in the perpetually changing nature of muscle tone and in the many factors that affect it. This chapter describes accepted definitions of muscle tone and its related concepts, ways of measuring muscle tone, the anatomic bases for muscle tone, and some of the issues that arise when tone is abnormal. Examples and problems are drawn from both neurorehabilitation and orthopedic settings. The focus, as in the rest of this text, is on problems that may be affected by physical agents.

MUSCLE TONE DEFINED

Muscle tone is variously described as muscle tension at rest, readiness to move or hold a position, priming or tuning of the muscles,[1] or the degree of activation before movement. Muscle tone is the underlying tension in the muscle that serves as a background for contraction. To define it more concretely, muscle tone is the passive resistance to the stretch of a muscle. The subject must be instructed not to resist the stretch applied so that whatever resistance is noted can be attributed to the various components of muscle tone rather than to voluntary muscle contraction. The components of muscle tone include the active resistance generated by neurally activated muscle fibers and the passive, biomechanical tension inherent in the connective tissue and muscle at the length at which the muscle is tested.[2] Physical agents used in physical therapy may affect the neural or the biomechanical components of muscle tone, or both.

The following example may help clarify some concepts. A runner's quadriceps muscles have lower tone when the runner is relaxed and sitting, with feet propped up, than when those same muscles are lengthened over a flexed knee and preparing for imminent contraction at the starting block of a race (Fig. 4-1). The difference between the lower tone and the higher tone can be palpated as a qualitative difference in the resistance to finger pressure over the muscle in each instance. In the relaxed condition, a palpating finger will sink into the muscle slightly because the muscle provides so little resistance to that deforming pressure, which is a type of stretch on the surface muscle fibers. The finger will register relative softness compared with the hardness or resistance to deformation that is felt in the "ready" condition. In the ready condition, both the biomechanical and the neural components contribute to a greater resistance to deformation, or increased muscle tone. From a biomechanical standpoint, the muscle is stretched over the flexed knee, so any slack in the soft tissue is taken up, and the contractile elements are positioned for most efficient muscle shortening when the nerves signal the muscle to contract. From a neural standpoint, when the runner is poised at the starting block, the neural activity increases in anticipation of the beginning of the race. This neural activation of the quadriceps is greater than when the runner was sitting and relaxed; it presets the muscle for imminent contraction.

Note that the same qualitative difference in resistance to finger pressure could be palpated if the runner relaxed and then contracted the quadriceps voluntarily. One of the difficulties with tone identification and description is the overlap between how a muscle looks and feels when it is subconsciously being prepared to move or hold, and how it looks and feels when it is consciously ordered to contract. A key to the assessment of muscle tone is that no active resistance to the muscle stretch occurs. If a subject is unable to avoid actively resisting, then the tonal quality assessed when the muscle is stretched will be a combination of tone and voluntary contraction. Even people who have normal control over their muscles sometimes have difficulty relaxing at will; therefore, one can see

High tone in quadriceps muscle

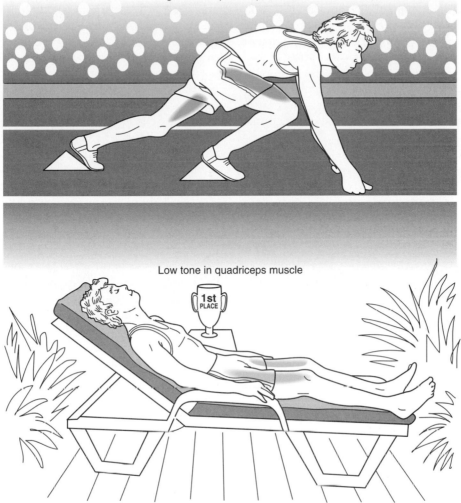

Low tone in quadriceps muscle

Figure 4-1. Normal variations in muscle tone.

why the differentiation between muscle tone and voluntary muscle contraction might be difficult.

The continually changing nature of muscle tone can also lead to problems with its identification. Despite the differences in tone between the relaxed and imminent-contraction, or ready states, the runner in the example described above is considered to have normal muscle tone in both instances. Normal, then, is a spectrum rather than a precise point on a scale. Abnormal muscle tone may overlap normal muscle tone at either end of the span (Fig. 4-2), but it has the following distinction: with abnormal tone, the individual has a restricted ability to change that tone to prepare to move readily or to hold a position. In other words, slow movement is not abnormal unless an

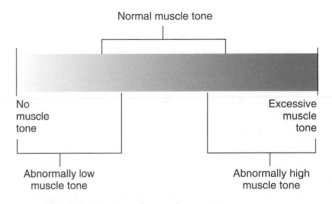

Figure 4-2. Normal muscle tone is a spectrum.

individual can *only* move slowly. Lower tone is not abnormal unless an individual cannot increase it sufficiently to prepare for movement or holding. Higher tone is not abnormal unless the individual cannot alter it at will, or unless it occurs uncomfortably as muscle spasms, cramps, or inefficient use of energy. Normal muscle tone, then, is not a particular amount of passive resistance to stretch, but rather is a controllable range of appropriate tensions to support normal movement and posture.

TERMINOLOGY FOR TONE ABNORMALITIES

Flaccidity is the term used to denote lack of tone or zero resistance to passive movement within the middle range of the muscle's length, and is usually concurrent with total paralysis of the muscle. *Hypotonicity* is the term used to describe decreased resistance to stretch compared with normal muscles. Flaccidity is an extreme case of hypotonicity.

Hypertonicity, the term for high tone, may be either spastic, defined as velocity-dependent resistance to stretch (quick stretch),[3] or rigid, like the muscles in Mrs. H's freeze state, which are resistant to stretch that is applied quickly or slowly. A hypertonic or hypotonic muscle may or may not have some degree of voluntary contractility. Mrs. H, for example, has both rigidity and akinesia during a freeze, which means that she also has difficulty initiating voluntary movement.

The term *spasticity* has had wide clinical use but causes confusion unless it is narrowly defined (Table 4-1). The term has sometimes been paired with *paralysis*, which is the loss of voluntary movement, and has shared the blame for the loss of function noted in patient conditions labeled *spastic paralysis* or *spastic hemiplegia*.[4,5] Muscle tone and voluntary muscle contraction, however, are distinct from each other, as are spasticity and loss of function. Muscle tone and posture are also different entities. For example, an individual who presents with an adducted and internally rotated shoulder, a flexed elbow, and flexed wrist and fingers, holding the hand close to the chest, can be said to have a flexed posture of the arm. He or she cannot be said to have spasticity until the passive resistance to stretch is assessed at different velocities for each of the involved muscle groups. Spasticity coexists with hyperactive stretch reflexes in its typical clinical presentation,[4,6] but because patients with rigidity can also have hyperactive stretch reflexes,[7] the two terms should not be equated. In addition, some confusion has arisen regarding the term *spasticity* because it has been applied to abnormal muscle tone having different underlying neural pathologies, such as spinal cord injury versus stroke or cerebral palsy. To clarify use in this text, *spasticity* will be applied only to a particular type of abnormal muscle response, whatever the pathology, in which quicker passive muscle stretches elicit greater resistance than slower stretches.[3]

Clonus is the term used to describe multiple rhythmic oscillations or beats in the resistance of a muscle responding to quick stretch, observed particularly with stretch to ankle plantar flexors or wrist flexors. The clasp-knife phenomenon consists of initial resistance followed by a sudden release of resistance in response to a quick stretch of a hypertonic muscle, much like the resistance felt when closing a pocketknife. A muscle spasm is an involuntary, strong contraction of a muscle, typically as the result of a painful

---

TABLE 4-1   What Spasticity Is and Is Not

Spasticity is:	Spasticity is not:
A type of abnormal muscle tone	Paralysis
One type of hypertonicity	Abnormal posturing
Velocity-dependent resistance to passive muscle stretch	A particular diagnosis or neural pathology
	Hyperactive stretch reflex
	Muscle spasm
	Voluntary movement restricted to movement in flexor or extensor synergy

Note: Spasticity, when present, is not always the cause of motor dysfunction.

stimulus. A client who has pain in the low back may have muscle spasms in the paraspinal musculature that cannot be relaxed voluntarily.

For those who, like Mrs. H in the example described earlier, have fluctuating abnormal tone, qualitative descriptions are applied. Mrs. H's tone varies between rigidity of the muscles on both sides of her joints during a freeze, and alternating higher and lower tone in agonists and antagonists about the joints during her dyskinetic states. Muscle tone is especially difficult to assess when it is fluctuating wildly, so it is common to describe visible movement rather than the tone itself. The common term used to describe any type of abnormal movement that is involuntary and has no purpose is *dyskinesia*. Some specific terms used to describe various types of dyskinesia are *choreiform movements* or *chorea* (dance-like, sharp, jerky movements), *ballismus* (ballistic or large throwing-type movements), *tremor* (low-amplitude, high-frequency, oscillating movements), *athetoid movements* (worm-like writhing motions), and *dystonia* (involuntary sustained muscle contraction). One example of dystonia is seen in the condition called *spasmodic torticollis*, or *wry neck*, in which the individual's neck musculature is continuously contracted on one side and the individual holds the head asymmetrically.[8]

MEASURING MUSCLE TONE

Several quantitative and qualitative methods have been used to assess muscle tone. Its variability with subtle intrasubject or environmental changes, however, limits the usefulness of static measures of muscle tone. In addition, measuring tone at one point in time during one movement or state of the muscle (at rest or during contraction) provides little information about how the muscle tone enhances or limits a different movement or state.[9] Therefore examiners must be careful to record the specific state of contraction or relaxation of the muscle group in question when they assess muscle tone, and not interpret the results as true for all other states of the muscle group. In other words, ankle plantar flexor hypertonicity assessed at rest cannot be said to limit ankle dorsiflexion during the swing phase of gait unless testing is completed while the client is upright and moving the leg forward. The methods described in this section for measuring muscle tone, then, should be used with two caveats in mind. First, the examiner should avoid generalizing the results of a single test, or even multi-

ple tests, to all conditions of the muscle. Second, the examiner should include measures of movement or function to obtain a more complete picture of the subject's ability to use muscle tone appropriately.

Quantitative Measures

Passive resistance to stretch provided by muscle tone can be measured by tools similar to those used to measure the force generated by a voluntarily contracting muscle. When a voluntary contraction is measured, a subject is asked to "push against the device with all your strength." When muscle tone is measured, a subject is asked to "relax, and let me move you." Such measures are restricted to the assessment of muscles that are both reasonably accessible to the examiner and easy to isolate by the subject to contract or relax on command. Muscles at the knee, elbow, wrist, and ankle, for example, are easier to position and to isolate than trunk muscles.

One protocol for quantifying muscle tone in the ankle plantar flexors was described by Boiteau et al and utilizes a hand-held dynamometer or myometer.[10] The subjects were seated and positioned so that their feet were unsupported. The head of the dynamometer was placed at the metatarsal heads of the foot. The examiner passively dorsiflexed the ankle to a neutral position with pressure through the dynamometer, several times at different velocities. The examiner controlled the velocities by counting seconds: completing the movement in 3 seconds for a slow velocity and in less than half a second for a fast velocity. The authors reported high reproducibility (intraclass correlation coefficients = .79 and .90) for both the high- and low-velocity conditions.[10] Comparing high- and low-velocity conditions enables the examiner to distinguish between neural and biomechanical components of spasticity.

A diagnostic tool frequently used for quantifying muscle tone in research is electromyography (EMG) (Fig. 4-3). EMG is a record of the electrical activity sampled from muscles at rest and during contraction, using surface, fine wire, or needle electrodes (Fig. 4-4). During voluntary muscle contraction, the record will show deviations away from a straight isoelectric line (Fig. 4-5). The number and size of the deviations (peaks and valleys) give a measure of the amount of muscle tissue that is electrically active during the contraction. When a supposedly relaxed muscle demonstrates electrical activity when stretched, that activity is a measure of the neurally derived muscle tone at that moment.

There are several advantages to using EMG to evaluate muscle tone. One advantage is its sensitivity to low levels of muscle activity that may not be readily palpable by an examiner. In addition, precise timing of muscle activation or relaxation can be picked up by EMG and matched to a command to contract or relax. Because of these benefits, EMG can be used to provide biofeedback to a subject who is trying to learn how to initiate contraction or relaxation in a particular muscle group.[11] Another advantage of EMG is that

in some cases it can differentiate between the neural and biomechanical components of muscle tone, which palpation alone is unable to do. If a relaxed muscle shows no electrical activity via EMG when stretched, but still provides resistance to passive stretch, then its tone can be attributed to the biomechanical properties rather than the neural components of the muscle involved.

Disadvantages of EMG include its restriction to monitoring only a local area of muscle tissue directly adjacent to the electrode. It also requires specialized equipment, and sometimes training, that is beyond the budget of many clinical facilities. In addition, muscle tone and active muscle contraction cannot be distinguished from each other by looking at an EMG record. A label of some kind must state when the subject was told to contract and relax and when the muscle was stretched. Although EMG is capable of recording the amount of muscle activation, it measures force only indirectly via a complex relationship between activity and force output.[12]

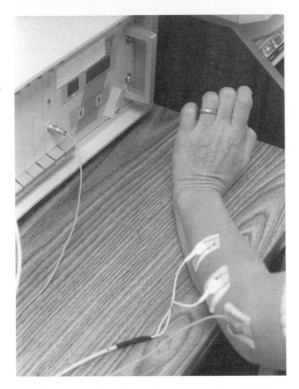

Figure 4-3. Setup for performing surface EMG.

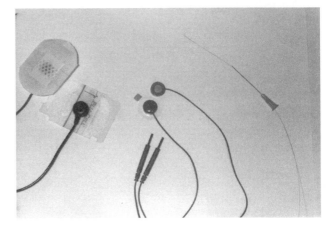

Figure 4-4. Disposable (small), surface, and fine wire EMG electrodes.

Figure 4-5. Example of an EMG tracing from the extensor pollicis longus *(upper tracing)* and flexor pollicis muscles *(lower tracing)* during an isometric contraction of the flexor pollicis longus muscle. The *middle tracing* is the force output produced with a 60% maximum voluntary contraction (MVC). (Reprinted with permission from Basmajian JV, De Luca CJ: *Muscles Alive: Their Functions Revealed by Electromyography,* ed 5, Baltimore, 1985, Williams & Wilkins.)

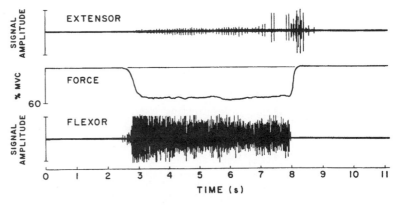

Some measures of muscle tone have been developed to test particular types of abnormalities, not just tone in general. One of these is called the *pendulum test*, which is intended to test spasticity. The test consists of holding an individual's limb so that when it is dropped, gravity provides a quick stretch to the spastic muscle. The resistance to that quick stretch will stop the limb from falling before it reaches the end of its range. The measurement of spasticity, via an electrogoniometer[13] or isokinetic dynamometer,[14] is the difference between the angle at which the spastic muscle "catches" the movement and the angle the limb would reach at the end of its normal range. Bohannon reported the test-retest reliability as high when the quadriceps muscle was tested consecutively in 30 patients who had spasticity after experiencing a stroke or head injury.[14] A limitation of the pendulum test is that some muscle groups cannot be tested by dropping a limb and watching it swing, specifically, the muscles of the trunk and neck.

Qualitative Measures

Muscle tone is more often assessed qualitatively than quantitatively. One clinical measure in common use is a 5-point ordinal scale that places normal tone at 2+. No tone and hypotonia are given scores of 0 and 1+, respectively, and moderate and severe hypertonia are given scores of 3+ and 4+, respectively.[15] The clinician obtains an impression of the muscle tone relative to normal by passively moving the patient at varying speeds. When muscle tone is normal, movement is light and easy. When muscle tone is decreased, movement is still easy or unrestricted but the limbs are heavy, as if they are dead weight. When tone is increased for a particular muscle, the movement that mechanically stretches that muscle is stiff or unyielding. Various movements must be made at multiple joints to distinguish between the differences in muscle tone of the flexors versus the extensors, for instance.

Another common qualitative way to assess muscle tone is to observe the response elicited by tapping on its tendon, activating the muscle stretch reflex. As with the clinical tone scale, in this 5-point scale, 2+ is considered normal, 0 is absent reflexes, 1+ is diminished, 3+ is brisker than average, and 4+ is very brisk or hyperactive.[16] The normal responses for different tendons differ. For example, a tap on the patellar tendon will normally result in a slight swing of the free lower leg from the knee. In contrast, a biceps or triceps tendon tap is still considered normal if a small twitch of the muscle belly is observed or palpated; actual movement of the whole lower arm would generally be considered hyperactive. Normal responses are determined by what is typical for that tendon reflex. In addition, symmetry of reflexes, assessed by comparing the responses to stimulation of the left and right sides of the body, determines the degree of normalcy of the response.

The Ashworth Scale[17] and the Modified Ashworth Scale[18] were developed to specifically measure spasticity. Five ordinal grades are defined, from 0 (no increase in muscle tone) to 4 (rigidly held in flexion or

TABLE 4-2 Modified Ashworth Scale for Grading Spasticity

Grade	Description
0	No increase in muscle tone
1	Slight increase in muscle tone, manifested by a catch and release or by minimal resistance at the end of the range of motion when the affected part(s) is moved in flexion or extension
1+	Slight increase in muscle tone, manifested by a catch, followed by minimal resistance throughout the remainder (less than half) of the ROM
2	More marked increase in muscle tone through most of the ROM, but affected part(s) easily moved
3	Considerable increase in muscle tone, passive movement difficult
4	Affected part(s) rigid in flexion or extension

ROM, range of motion.
Reprinted with permission of the American Physical Therapy Association. From Bohannon RW, Smith MB: Interrater reliability of a Modified Ashworth Scale of Muscle Spasticity, *Phys Ther* 67:207, 1987.

extension). An intermediate grade of 1+ distinguishes the original Ashworth Scale and the Modified Ashworth Scale, and is defined by a slight catch and continued minimal resistance through the range (Table 4-2). Bohannon and Smith reported 86.7% interrater agreement when testing 30 patients who had spasticity in the elbow flexor muscles.[18]

General Considerations When Measuring Muscle Tone

The relative positions of the limb, body, neck, and head with respect to one another and to gravity can all affect muscle tone. For example, the asymmetric and symmetric tonic neck reflexes (ATNR and STNR, respectively) are known to influence the tone of the flexors and extensors of the arms and legs, depending on the position of the head (Fig. 4-6), both during infancy and in subjects who have neurological deficits.[19] Subtle differences in muscle tone due to these reflexes can be palpated when the head position changes even in subjects with mature and intact nervous systems. Likewise, the pull of gravity on a limb to stretch muscles, or on the vestibular system to trigger responses to keep the head upright, will change muscle tone according to the position of the head and body. The testing position, therefore, must be reported for accurate interpretation and replication of any measurement of tone.

Additional general rules for measuring muscle tone include standardization of touch and consideration of the muscle length at which a group of muscles is to be tested. The examiner must be aware that touching the subject's skin, either with a hand or with an instrument, can influence muscle tone. The handholds and instrument placement must therefore be consistent for accurate interpretation and replication. The length at which a specific muscle's tone is tested must also be standardized. Because muscle tone differs with passive biomechanical differences at the extremes of range, and range of motion (ROM) can be altered as a result of long-term changes in tone, the most consistent length to measure muscle tone is at the midrange of the available length of the muscle tested.

THE ANATOMICAL BASES OF MUSCLE TONE AND MUSCLE ACTIVATION

Muscle tone and muscle activation originate from interactions between nervous system input and the biomechanical and biochemical properties of the muscle and its surrounding connective tissue. The practitioner must have an understanding of the anatomical bases for both tone and activation to determine appropriate physical agents to apply when either is dysfunctional. The anatomical contributions to muscle tone and activation are reviewed in this section.

Muscular Contributions to Muscle Tone and Activation

Muscle is composed of (1) contractile elements in the muscle fibers, (2) cellular elements providing structure, (3) connective tissue providing coverings for the fibers and the entire muscle, and (4) tendons attaching muscle to bone. When neural input signals the muscle to contract or relax, biochemical activity of the contractile elements shortens and lengthens muscle fibers. As the contractile elements work, they slide against each other, facilitated by the cellular elements to maintain structure and the connective tissue coverings to provide support and lubrication while the muscle changes length.

The myofilaments, actin and myosin, are the contractile elements of muscle. With neural stimulation of the muscle fiber, storage sites in the muscle release calcium ions that allow the actin and myosin molecules to bind together. The binding occurs at particular sites to form cross-bridges (Fig. 4-7). Breaking of these cross-bridges, so that new bonds can be formed at different sites, is mediated by energy derived from adenosine triphosphate (ATP). As bonds are formed, broken, and reformed, the length of the contractile unit, or sarcomere, changes. The cycle of binding and releasing continues as long as calcium ions and ATP are present. Calcium ions are taken back into storage when activation of muscle ceases. Sources within the muscle supply an adequate amount of ATP for short-duration activities, but the muscle must depend on fuel delivered by the circulatory system for longer-duration activities.

Actin and myosin myofilaments must overlap for cross-bridge formation to occur (Fig. 4-8). When the muscle is stretched too far, cross-bridges cannot be formed because there is no overlap. When the muscle is in its most shortened position, actin and myosin run into the structural elements of the muscle fiber and no further cross-bridges can be formed. In the midrange of the muscle, actin and myosin can form the greatest number of cross-bridges. The midrange, then, is the length at which that muscle can generate the greatest amount of force, or tension. This length-tension relationship is one of the biomechanical properties of muscles.

SYMMETRICAL TONIC NECK REFLEX (STNR)

STIMULUS
Neck flexed

RESPONSE
Tone changes so arms flex, legs extend

STIMULUS
Neck extended

RESPONSE
Arms extend, legs flex

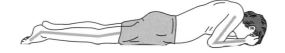

ASYMMETRICAL TONIC NECK REFLEX (ATNR)

STIMULUS
Neck rotation to one side

RESPONSE
Tone changes so jaw limbs extend
and skull limbs flex

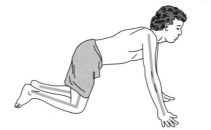

SYMMETRICAL TONIC LABYRINTHINE REFLEX (TLR OR STLR)

STIMULUS
Prone or supine position
noted by labyrinths in head

RESPONSE
Tone changes toward total flexion
or total extension

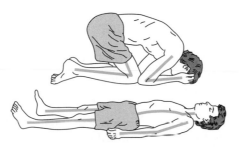

Figure 4-6. Reflex responses to head or neck position.

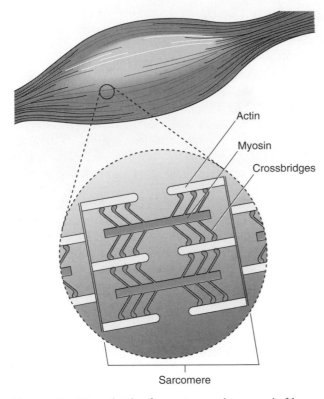

Actin

Myosin

Crossbridges

Sarcomere

Figure 4-7. Cross-bridge formation within muscle fibers.

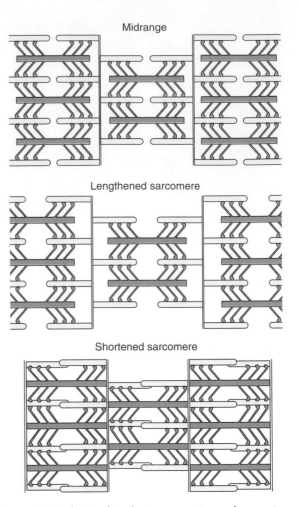

Midrange

Lengthened sarcomere

Shortened sarcomere

Figure 4-8. Relationship between actin and myosin at three different sarcomere lengths.

Other biomechanical properties of muscles include friction and elasticity. Friction between connective tissue coverings as they slide past one another may be affected by pressure on the tissues and by the viscosity of the tissues and fluids in which they reside. Elasticity of connective tissue results in varying responses to stretch at different muscle lengths. When tissue becomes taut, as it is when a muscle is fully lengthened, connective tissue contributes more to the overall resistance of the muscle to stretch. When connective tissue is slack, it contributes very little to a muscle's tension. In fact, when muscle is stimulated to contract while it is shortened, there is a delay before movement can occur or force can be generated while the slack in the connective tissue is taken up. The runner's crouch in Fig. 4-1 takes up some initial slack in the quadriceps before the start of the race to reduce any delay in activation.

Both active contractile elements and passive properties of the tissues contribute to muscle tone and activation. However, muscle tone can be generated from the passive elements alone, whereas muscle activation requires both active and passive elements.

Physical agents, such as heat and cold, can change both muscle tone and activation by altering the accessibility of ATP to the myofilaments through improved circulation and by changing the elasticity or friction of the tissues. Physical agents can also change the amount of neural stimulation of the muscle fibers.

Neural Contributions to Muscle Tone and Activation

Neural sources of input that contribute to muscle tone and muscle activation come from the periphery, the spinal cord, and supraspinal brain centers (Fig. 4-9). Even though multiple areas of the nervous system may participate, all of them must work through the final common pathway, the alpha motor neuron,

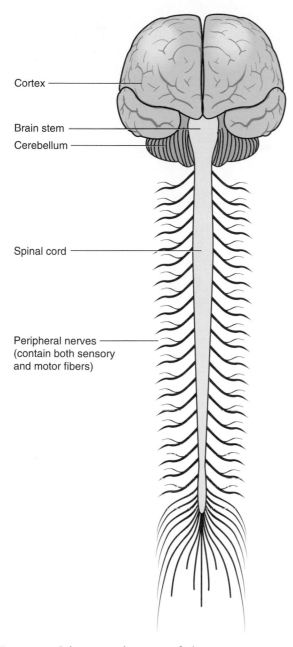

Cortex

Brain stem

Cerebellum

Spinal cord

Peripheral nerves
(contain both sensory
and motor fibers)

Figure 4-9. Schematic drawing of the nervous system, front view.

which ultimately stimulates muscle fibers to contract (Fig. 4-10). The generation, summation, and conduction of an activating signal in alpha motor neurons are critical components of muscle tone and activation. In this section, discussion of nerve structure and function will be followed by an account of some significant influences on the alpha motor neuron. See a

major neurophysiological text for a more complete description of known input to alpha motor neurons.

Structure and function of nerves

Nerve cells, or neurons, include most of the components of other cells, including cell bodies with a cell membrane, nucleus, and multiple internal organelles that keep the cell alive. The distinguishing features of a neuron include the multiple projections, called *dendrites,* that receive stimuli—usually from other nerve cells—and the single axonal projection that conducts stimuli toward a destination. The axon ends in multiple synaptic boutons (Fig. 4-11). These boutons transmit stimuli across the narrow gap, or synapse, between a bouton and its target muscle fibers, bodily organs, glands, or other neurons. Although a few specialized neurons can receive electrical, mechanical, chemical, or thermal stimuli, most neurons respond to and transmit signals via chemicals known as *neurotransmitters.*

Neurotransmitter molecules are manufactured and stored in the synaptic boutons (Fig. 4-12). An electrical signal conducted down an axon causes the release of these molecules into the synaptic cleft. The molecules cross the cleft and, if the postsynaptic cell is another neuron, bind to one of the chemically specific receptor sites covering the dendrites, cell body, or axon (Fig. 4-13).

The neurotransmitter dopamine exemplifies the specificity of neurotransmitters and is significant to the study of muscle tone and activation. Dopamine is normally found in high quantities in the neurons of the substantia nigra, one of the basal ganglia, which is discussed later in this chapter. Deficits in the production or use of dopamine result in rigidity, resting tremors, and difficulty initiating and executing movement,[20] all manifestations of Parkinson's disease.[21]

The binding of a specific neurotransmitter with its receptor site tends either to excite or inhibit the postsynaptic cell. Whether the postsynaptic cell responds, by transmitting the signal from the receptor site to the rest of the cell, depends on summation, or adding together, of many excitatory and inhibitory signals. Summation may be spatial or temporal (Fig. 4-14). Input to receptor sites from many different synaptic boutons at one time results in spatial summation, and sequential stimulation through the same receptor sites results in temporal summation. Excitatory input must exceed inhibitory input if the sum is to cause signal conduction down an axon. A single neuron

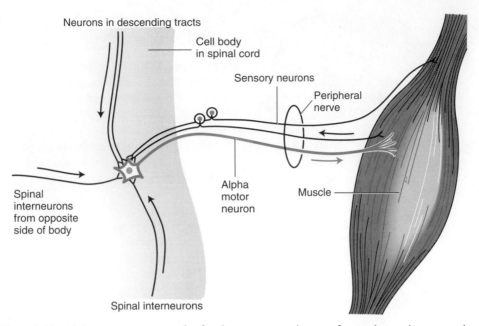

Figure 4-10. Alpha motor neuron: the final common pathway of neural signals to muscles.

typically receives input from hundreds or thousands of other neurons.

Once excitatory stimulation reaches a particular threshold level, the signal is conducted down the axon in an action potential (having the potential to cause an action). The action potential rapidly transforms the membrane of the neuron from its electrochemical state at rest. Membrane transformation occurs in a wave of electrochemical current that progresses rapidly from the cell body down the axon to the synaptic boutons.

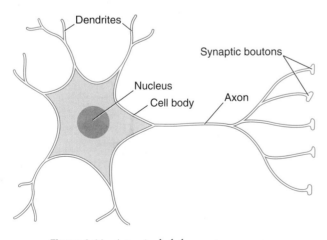

Figure 4-11. A typical alpha motor neuron.

At rest, the neuronal membrane separates the concentration of sodium (Na^+), chloride (Cl^-), and potassium (K^+) ions on the inside of the cell from the concentration on the outside. Na^+ and Cl^- are in greater concentration outside the cell, and K^+ and negatively charged protein molecules are in greater concentration inside the cell. In addition to the chemical difference across the membrane, an overall electrical difference exists immediately adjacent to the membrane of approximately -70 mV, with the inside of the membrane more negative than the outside. Biological systems with a difference in charge or concentration between two areas will come to equilibrium if possible. Because of the electrochemical difference, the membrane is said to have a resting potential, which is the potential for movement of ions toward equilibrium if the membrane allowed it.

Channels or holes in the membrane allow selective movement of ions from one side of the membrane to the other. Allowing movement of only some ions makes the membrane semipermeable. Potassium ions move freely across the membrane when the neuron is at rest. Some membrane channels open and close at specific times to allow certain other ions to move according to their electrochemical gradients. Still other ions are actively moved through the membrane from one side to the other in a biochemical pumping process. This process requires energy because these ions are

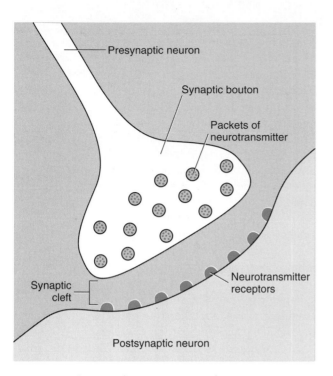

Figure 4-12. Synapse between pre- and postsynaptic neurons at rest.

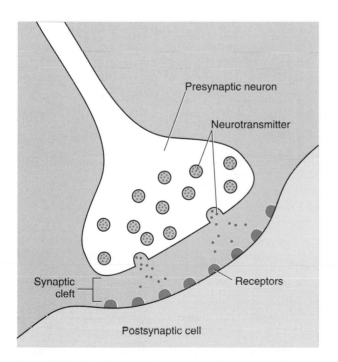

Figure 4-13. Synapse between pre- and postsynaptic neurons when activated.

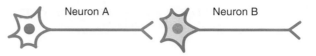

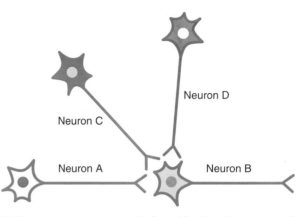

1. Multiple discharges from neuron A will activate neuron B temporally, or in time

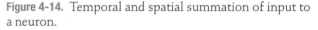

2. Discharges from neurons A, C, and D will activate neuron B spatially, or from multiple spaces on neuron B

Figure 4-14. Temporal and spatial summation of input to a neuron.

moved against their electrochemical gradient; that is, they move farther away from equilibrium of charge or concentration on the two sides of the membrane.

When an action potential sweeps down an axon, channels in the membrane open, allowing Na^+ ions to rush into the cell, thereby altering both the concentration and the electrical differences between the inside and outside of the membrane. During the action potential, the polar difference between the electrical charge inside and outside the membrane changes in that location; that is, that section of membrane has depolarized, with an increase in positive charge on the inside. A sodium-potassium pump quickly restores the electrochemical difference between the inside and outside by transporting Na^+ ions back outside the cell and K^+ ions back inside. The end result of the sodium-potassium pump is repolarization of that section of the cell membrane.

The successive depolarization and repolarization of membrane sections continues down the axon until those changes stimulate the release of neurotransmitters from all of the axon's synaptic boutons (see Fig. 4-13). The speed of conduction of an action potential depends on the diameter of the neuron and the insulation available along the axon. Neurons with smaller diameters have slower conduction velocities. Larger-diameter neurons have faster conduction velocities.

Insulation speeds the transmission of a depolarizing wave by increasing the speed with which the ions move across the membrane. A fatty tissue called *myelin*, provided by Schwann cells in the peripheral nervous system (PNS) and oligodendrocytes in the central nervous system (CNS), is the source of insulation for neurons. Myelin wraps around the axons of neurons, leaving gaps at regular intervals (Fig. 4-15). When a depolarizing wave travels down an axon, it moves quickly down sections with myelin on them and slows at gaps where no myelin is present, at the nodes of Ranvier. Because the signal slows at the nodes and travels very quickly between nodes, it appears to jump from one node to the next in rapid succession all the way to the end of all the axonal branches.[22] This jumping is referred to as *saltatory conduction* (Fig. 4-16).

The fastest conduction velocities recorded in human nerves are up to 70-80 m/sec.[23] Temperature changes can alter these velocities. When axons are cooled, as with the application of ice packs, nerve conduction velocity slows by approximately 2 m/sec for every 1°C decrease in temperature.[24]

Once the signal reaches the synaptic boutons and neurotransmitters are released, there is a slight delay for the molecules to move across the synaptic cleft. Even at 200 Ångstrom units (200×10^{-10} m), it takes time for diffusion and then reception by the next neuron or target tissue. In addition, the receiving neuron must sum all of its input, both excitatory and inhibitory, before an action potential can develop. Therefore, larger numbers of connections between neurons take longer to transmit a signal than do smaller numbers. The shortest connection known is the *single monosynaptic connection* of the muscle stretch reflex, observable when certain tendons are tapped (Fig. 4-17). It is so called because there is only one synapse between the sensory neuron receiving the stretch stimulus and the motor neuron transmitting the signal to the muscle fibers to contract.

Monosynaptic transmission, as recorded from muscle stretch (tap) to initiation of muscle stretch reflex contraction, has been recorded in as little as 25 milliseconds at the arm.[25] The length of time between stimulus and response when multiple synapses are involved is longer. For example, when the arm is working to move a load and visual input indicates a sudden change in the load, it takes approximately 300 milliseconds for the arm muscles to respond to that input.[25] If a person unexpectedly saw a ball begin to drop off a shelf 1 meter above her, the ball would fall approximately 44 centimeters before she could start to move to catch it.

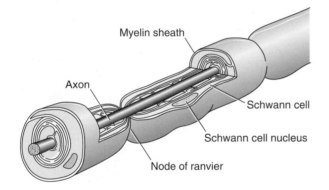

Figure 4-15. Myelin formed by Schwann cells on a peripheral neuron.

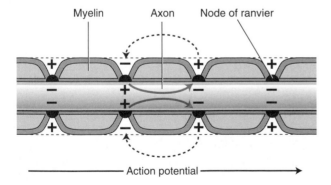

Figure 4-16. Saltatory conduction along a myelin-wrapped axon.

Sources of Neural Stimulation of Muscle

The alpha motor neuron

Muscle tone and activation depend on alpha motor neurons for neural stimulation. An alpha motor neuron, which is sometimes called an *anterior horn cell*, transmits signals from the CNS to muscles. With its cell body in the ventral or anterior gray matter or horn of the spinal cord (Fig. 4-18), its axon exits the spinal cord, and thus the CNS, through the ventral nerve root. Each axon eventually reaches muscle, where it branches and innervates between 6 (in the eye muscles) and 2000 (in the gastrocnemius muscle) muscle fibers at motor endplates.26 The muscle fibers innervated by a single axon with its branches, which is one motor unit (Fig. 4-19), all contract at once whenever an action potential is transmitted down that axon. A sin-

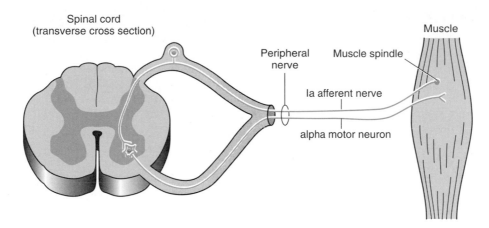

Figure 4-17. Monosynaptic muscle stretch reflex.

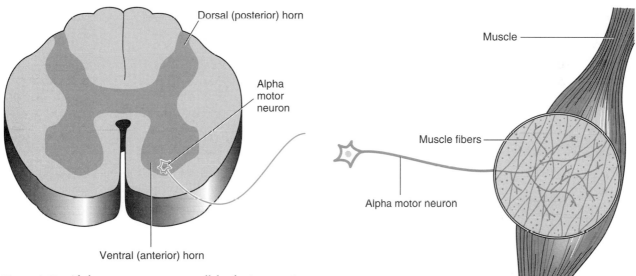

Figure 4-18. Alpha motor neuron: cell body in anterior horn of spinal cord, axon exiting spinal cord.

Figure 4-19. One motor unit: alpha motor neuron and muscle fibers innervated by it.

gle action potential generated by the alpha motor neuron cannot provide its motor unit with a graded signal; each action potential is "all or none." When sufficient motor units are recruited, the muscle contracts. More forceful contraction of the muscle requires an increased number or rate of action potentials down the same axons, or recruitment of additional motor units.

Activation of a particular motor unit depends on the sum of excitatory or inhibitory input to that alpha motor neuron (Fig. 4-20). Excitation or inhibition, in turn, depends on the sources and amounts of input via the thousands of neurons that synapse on that one particu-

lar alpha motor neuron. An understanding of the sources of input to alpha motor neurons is essential when attempting to control motor unit activation or alter muscle tone via physical agents or other means (Table 4-3).

Input from the periphery
The PNS includes all of the neurons that project outside of the CNS even if the cell bodies are located within the CNS. The PNS is composed of the alpha motor neurons, gamma motor neurons, some

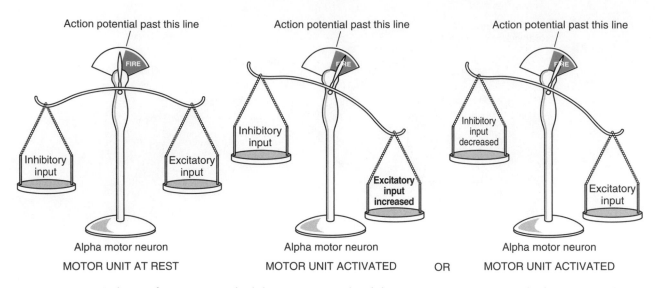

Figure 4-20. Balance of excitatory and inhibitory input to the alpha motor neuron at rest and when activated.

TABLE 4-3   Input to Alpha Motor Neurons (Simplified)

From peripheral receptors	From spinal sources	From supraspinal sources
Muscle spindles via Ia sensory neurons	Propriospinal interneurons	Cortex, basal ganglia via corticospinal tract
GTOs via Ib sensory neurons		Cerebellum, red nucleus via rubrospinal tract
Cutaneous receptors via other sensory neurons		Vestibular system, cerebellum via vestibulospinal tracts
		Limbic system, autonomic nervous system via reticulospinal tracts

autonomic nervous system effector neurons, and all of the sensory neurons that carry information from the periphery to the CNS. In this section, discussion will focus on sensory input from muscles, joints, and skin to alpha motor neurons.

Sensory neurons can stimulate neurons in the spinal cord directly (Fig. 4-21), so they can have a quicker and less modulated effect on alpha motor neurons than some other sources of input that must traverse the brain. Quick, relatively stereotyped motor responses, called *reflexes*, commonly result from unmodulated peripheral input. At its simplest, a reflex involves only one synapse between a sensory neuron and a motor neuron; that is, the monosynaptic stretch reflex defined previously (see Fig. 4-17). In the monosynaptic case, for every action potential in the sensory neuron, the motor neuron receives the same unmodu-lated input. Most reflexes, however, involve multiple interneurons in the spinal cord between the sensory and motor neurons. Because of the volume of input from multiple neurons and sources, the actual motor response to a specific sensory input can be modulated according to the context of the action.[27]

The presumed objective of many peripheral sources of input in the normally functioning nervous system is to protect the body, counter obstacles, or adapt to unexpected occurrences in the environment during volitional movement. Because of its direct connections in the spinal cord, peripheral input can assist function even before the brain has received or processed information about the success or failure of the movement. Peripheral input also influences muscle tone and is frequently the medium through which physical agents effect change.

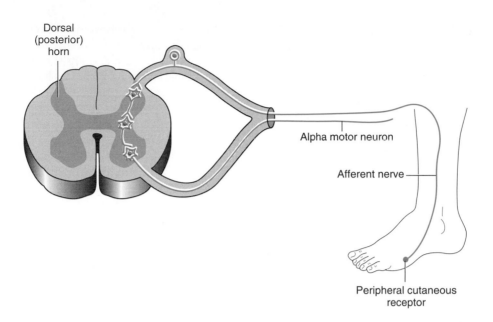

Figure 4-21. Sensory input into spinal cord to alpha motor neurons.

Muscle spindle

Inside the muscle, lying parallel to muscle fibers, are sensory organs called *muscle spindles* (Fig. 4-22). When a muscle is stretched, as it is when a tendon is tapped to stimulate a stretch reflex, the muscle spindles also are stretched. Receptors wrapped around the equatorial regions of the spindles sense the lengthening and send an action potential through sensory neurons, specified as *type Ia*, into the spinal cord. A primary destination of this signal is the pool of alpha motor neurons for the muscle that was stretched (homonymous muscle). If the excitatory input of the Ia sensory neurons is sufficiently greater than any inhibitory input from elsewhere, the alpha motor neurons will generate a signal to contract their associated muscle fibers. Several traditional facilitation techniques for increasing muscle tone use the stretch reflex: quick stretch, tapping, resistance, high-frequency vibration, and positioning a limb so that gravity can provide stretch or resistance.

Another destination for signals transmitted by type Ia sensory neurons from the muscle spindle is the pool of alpha motor neurons for the antagonist muscle to inhibit activity on the opposite side of the joint. In other words, signals from the muscle spindles in the biceps tend to excite alpha motor neurons of the biceps and to inhibit those of the triceps (Fig. 4-23). This is an example of reciprocal inhibition,

which helps ensure that a muscle is not working against its antagonist when it is activated.

Because muscles shorten as they contract, and muscle spindles register lengthening of muscles only if they are taut, spindles must be continually reset to eliminate sagging in the center portion of the spindles. Gamma motor neurons innervate muscle spindles at the end regions and, when stimulated, cause the equatorial region of the spindle to tighten (see Fig. 4-22). In other words, gamma motor neurons sensitize the spindles to changes in muscle length.[28] Gamma motor neurons are typically activated at the same time as alpha motor neurons during voluntary movement, a process called *alpha-gamma coactivation*.[29] In addition, gamma motor neurons can be activated separately from alpha motor neurons to prepare the muscle spindle to sense expected changes in length that might occur during voluntary movement. A good example of this occurs when someone walks across an icy sidewalk, knowing that a slip is probable. Gamma motor neurons are activated to increase spindle sensitivity so that muscles can respond very quickly if one foot starts to slip on the ice.

Golgi tendon organs

Golgi tendon organs (GTOs) are sensory organs located in the connective tissue at the junction

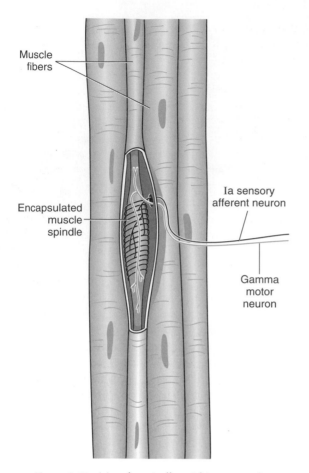

Muscle
fibers

Encapsulated
muscle
spindle

Ia sensory
afferent neuron

Gamma
motor
neuron

Figure 4-22. Muscle spindle within a muscle.

Because of their location at the musculotendinous junction, GTOs have been shown to signal a maximal stretch of the muscle and are thus thought to protect against muscle damage.[30] GTOs have also been shown to be extremely sensitive to active contraction, particularly small amounts of muscle tension.[31] Houk and Henneman estimated that these sensory receptors can respond to activation of one or two single muscle fibers that are in series with that GTO.[31] GTOs are limited in their ability to sense steady or larger levels of muscular tension, however, so they must be supplemented by many other types of peripheral input in signaling overall muscle contraction.[32]

GTOs transmit signals via type Ib sensory neurons to the alpha motor neuron pools of both the homonymous and antagonist muscles. The input to homonymous muscles is inhibitory, to stop signaling the muscle fibers to contract. This spinal reflex response is called *autogenic inhibition*. The input to alpha motor neurons of antagonist muscles is excitatory, to signal contraction. The purpose of the GTOs is regulatory during active muscle contraction, possibly to help put on the brakes during activation.

Note that muscle stretch can provide contradictory input to an alpha motor neuron. Quick stretch stimulates the spindles to register a change in length, facilitating muscle contraction. Prolonged stretch may initially facilitate contraction but ultimately inhibits contraction as the GTOs register tension at the tendon and signal inhibition to the homonymous alpha motor neurons. Prolonged stretch is thus traditionally used to inhibit abnormally high tone in agonists and facilitate antagonist muscle groups. Inhibitory

between muscle fibers and tendons (Fig. 4-24). They function in series with muscle fibers, which is in contrast to muscle spindles, which function in parallel.

Figure 4-23. Reciprocal inhibition: muscle spindle input excites agonist muscles and inhibits antagonist muscles.

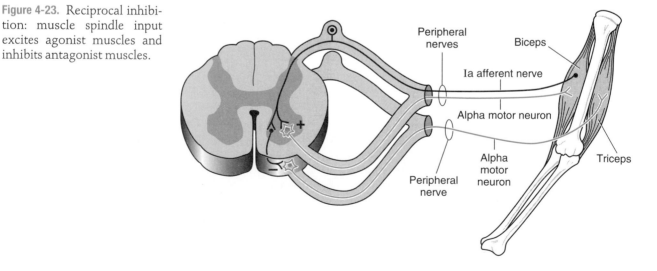

Peripheral
nerves

Biceps

Ia afferent nerve

Alpha motor neuron

Alpha
motor
neuron

Triceps

Peripheral
nerve

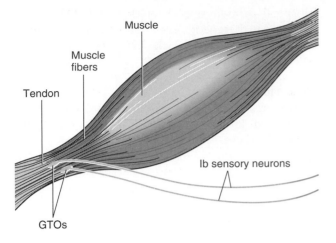

Figure 4-24. GTOs within a muscle.

pressure on the tendon of a hypertonic muscle is also thought to stimulate the GTOs to inhibit abnormal muscle tone in the agonists while facilitating antagonists.[33] These techniques should be considered when positioning a patient for application of physical agents or other modalities.

Cutaneous receptors

Stimulation of cutaneous sensory receptors occurs with every interaction of a person's skin with the external world. Temperature, texture, pressure, pain, and touch are all transmitted through these receptors. Cutaneous reflex responses tend to be more complex than muscle and tendon responses, involving multiple muscles. Painful stimuli at the skin, like stepping on a tack or touching a hot iron, will ultimately facilitate alpha motor neurons of withdrawal muscles. In a flexor withdrawal reflex, the hip and knee flexors or elbow flexors are signaled to pull the foot or hand away from the painful stimulus. If the body is upright when the painful stimulus occurs, a crossed extension reflex is likely. Alpha motor neurons of the opposite leg's hip and knee extensor muscles will be facilitated so that when the foot is withdrawn from the painful stimulus, the other leg can support the individual's weight (Fig. 4-25).

Because muscles are linked to each other neurally via spinal interneurons for more efficient functioning, traditional antagonists on opposite sides of joints are frequently inhibited when a particular agonist is facilitated. For example, when the biceps muscle is facilitated during a withdrawal reflex, the triceps

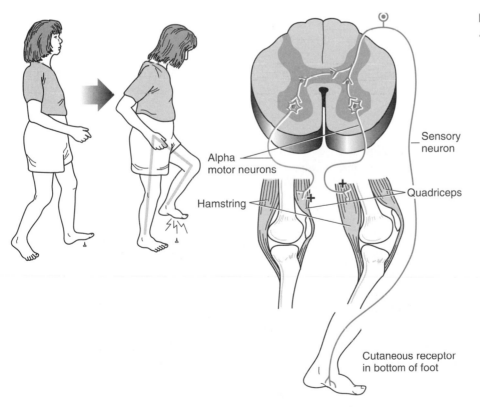

Figure 4-25. Flexor withdrawal and crossed extension reflexes.

muscle of the same arm is inhibited. Likewise, if a muscle is contracting strongly, many of its synergists will also be facilitated to contract to help the function of the original muscle.

Treatment techniques that use cutaneous receptors to increase muscle tone include quick, light touch; manual contacts; brushing; and quick icing. Techniques that use cutaneous receptors to decrease muscle tone include slow stroking, maintained holding, neutral warmth, and prolonged icing.[33] The facilitative techniques probably direct attention to the part of the body that the patient is about to activate, and the cutaneous receptors register changes in input. The brain seems to alert itself when changes are occurring, preparing itself to respond with movement, which necessitates increases in muscle tone. The inhibitory techniques begin in a similar way to the facilitative techniques by directing attention to the relevant part of the body. Because of the slow, repetitive, or maintained nature of the stimuli, however, the cutaneous receptors adapt to the input. The brain ignores what it already knows is there, and general relaxation is possible, with a diminution of muscle tone.

Because cutaneous receptors can alter muscle tone, any physical agent that touches the skin can change tone, whether the touch is intentional or incidental. Thus it is necessary to consider the location and type of cutaneous input provided whenever using physical agents, especially because the effect on muscle tone may be counter to the effect desired from the agent itself.

Input from spinal sources

In addition to the sensory information from the periphery that signals alpha motor neurons, circuits of neurons within the spinal cord also contribute to excitation and inhibition. These circuits are composed of interneurons, neurons that connect two other neurons. Propriospinal pathways are one type of neural circuit that communicate intersegmentally, between different levels within the spinal cord. They receive input from peripheral afferents, as well as from many of the descending pathways that are discussed below, and help produce synergies or particular patterns of movements.[34]

For example, when a client flexes the elbow forcefully against resistance, propriospinal pathways assist in the communication between neurons at multiple spinal levels. The result is coordinated recruitment of synergistic muscles that add force to the movement. That same resisted arm movement also facilitates flexor muscle activity in the opposite arm via the propriospinal pathways. Both of these principles have been used in therapeutic exercises to increase the tone and force output from muscles in persons with neurological dysfunction.[35-37]

Supraspinal sources of input

Supraspinal refers to CNS areas that originate above the spinal cord in the upright human (see Fig. 4-9). Ultimately these brain areas influence alpha motor neurons by sending signals down axons in a variety of descending pathways. Any voluntary, subconscious, or pathological change in the amount of input from descending pathways alters the excitatory and inhibitory input to alpha motor neurons. Such changes, in turn, alter muscle tone and activation, depending on the individual and the pathway or tract involved. Several of the major descending pathways and their influence on motor neurons are discussed in relation to the brain areas to which they are most closely related.

Sensorimotor cortical contributions

Volitional movement originates in response to a sensation, an idea, a memory, or an external stimulus to move, act, or respond. The decision to move is initiated in the cortex, with signals moving rapidly among neurons in various brain areas until they reach the motor cortex. Axons from many of the neurons in the motor cortex form a corticospinal tract (from cortex to spinal cord) that runs through the brain, mostly crosses at the pyramids at the base of the brain stem, and descends to synapse on appropriate alpha motor neurons on the opposite side of the spinal cord (Fig. 4-26). When the alpha motor neurons have sufficient excitatory input, action potentials signal all the associated muscle fibers to contract. Corticospinal input to alpha motor neurons in the spinal cord is primarily responsible for voluntary contraction and contributes less to muscle tone.

Cerebellum

For every set of instructions that descend through the corticospinal tract to signal posture or movement, a copy is routed to the cerebellum (see Fig. 4-26). The neuronal activity of the cerebellum functions to compare the intended movement with the sensory input it receives about the actual movement. The cerebellum registers any discrepancies between the signal from the motor cortex and the accumulated sensory input from muscle spindles, tendons, joints, and skin of the body during the movement. Cerebellar output helps

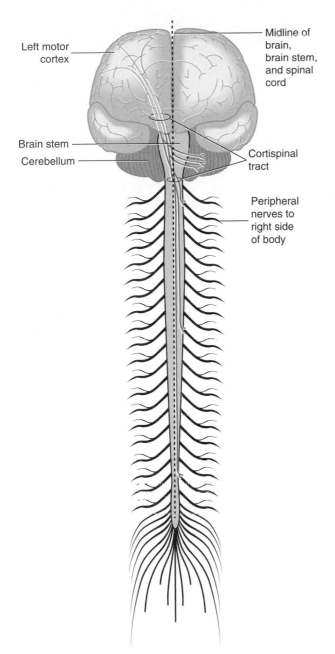

Left motor cortex

Midline of brain, brain stem, and spinal cord

Brain stem

Cerebellum

Cortispinal tract

Peripheral nerves to right side of body

Figure 4-26. Corticospinal tract: schematic pathway from cortex to cerebellum and spinal cord.

correct for movement errors or unexpected obstacles to movement via the cortex and the red nuclei in the brain stem. The red nuclei, in turn, can send signals to the alpha motor neurons through the rubrospinal tracts (RuSTs). Ongoing correction is successful only during slower movements; if a movement is completed too quickly to alter, information about the suc-

cess or failure of the movement can improve subsequent trials. Both corticospinal and rubrospinal inputs to alpha motor neurons function primarily to activate musculature. Direct influences of the cerebellum on muscle tone and posture are mediated through connections with the vestibulospinal tracts (VSTs).

Basal ganglia

The basal ganglia function as a movement- and tone-modulating system. Any volitional movement involves processing through connections in these five nuclei, or groups of neurons: putamen, caudate, globus pallidus, subthalamic nucleus, and substantia nigra (Fig. 4-27). Multiple chains of neurons looping through these nuclei and back to motor cortical areas influence the planning and postural adaptation of motor behavior. Dysfunction of any of the nuclei of the basal ganglia is associated with abnormal tone and disordered movement. In the example from the beginning of the chapter, Mrs. H's tone and movement patterns exemplify two of the extreme forms of abnormality seen in basal ganglia disorders: the rigidity and akinesia of a freeze state and the wildly fluctuating tone and dyskinesia associated with high levels of the medication used to treat Parkinson's disease.

Other descending input

The VSTs help to regulate posture by transmitting signals from the vestibular system to the alpha motor neuron pools in the spinal cord. The vestibular system receives ongoing information about the position of the head and the way it moves in space with respect to gravity. The vestibular nuclei also integrate and transmit responses to information received about the movement of the head via the joint, muscle, and skin receptors of the head and neck. The VSTs and related tracts generally facilitate the extensor (antigravity) alpha motor neurons of the lower extremity and trunk to keep the body and head upright against gravity. The muscle tone of antigravity muscles tends to be higher than the tone of other muscle groups when a person has a neurological deficit, partly because of the stretch that gravity places on them and partly because of the increased effort required to stay upright.

The reticulospinal tracts (RSTs) transmit signals from the reticular system, which is a group of neuron cell bodies located in the central region of the brain stem, to the spinal cord. The reticular system receives a rich supply of input from multiple sensory systems, including vision, auditory, vestibular, and

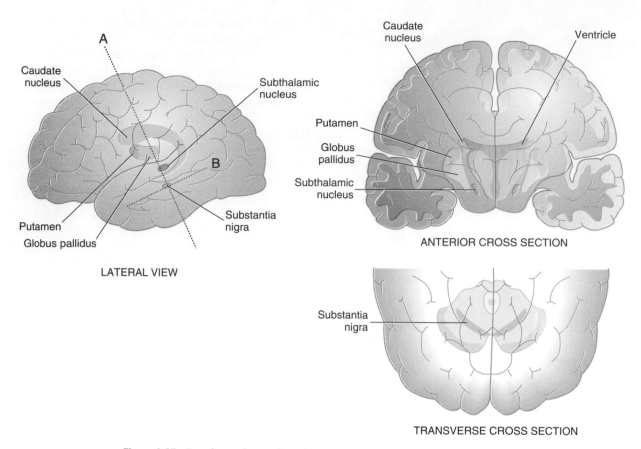

Figure 4-27. Basal ganglia within the brain: side and cross-sectional views.

somatosensory, and the motor cortex. In addition, it receives input from the autonomic nervous system (ANS) and hypothalamus, reflecting the individual's emotions, motivation, and alertness. Muscle tone differences between someone who is slumped due to sadness or lethargy and someone who is happy and energetic is mediated through these tracts. The RSTs can also help regulate responses to reflexes according to the context of the current movement. For example, while walking, someone may step on a sharp object with the right foot, noticing it only as the left foot is leaving the ground. Instead of allowing the expected flexor withdrawal reflex on the right (which would cause the person to fall), the RSTs help increase input to the alpha motor neurons of extensor muscles on the right, momentarily permitting weight bearing on that sharp object until the left foot can be positioned to bear weight.

Limbic system

The limbic system influences movement and muscle tone via the RSTs and through connections with the basal ganglia. Circuits of neurons in the limbic system provide the ability to generate memories and attach meaning to them. Changes in muscle tone or activation can occur as a result of emotions recalled with particular memories of real or imagined events. For example, fear may heighten one's awareness when walking into a dark parking lot, activating the sympathetic nervous system (SNS) to start planning for fight or flight. The SNS activates the heart and lungs to work faster, dilates the pupils, and decreases the amount of blood pulsing through the internal organs, diverting that blood flow to the muscles. Muscle tone is increased to get ready to fight or flee from any potential danger in the parking lot. Muscle tone may further increase with a sudden unexpected noise, but then decrease again to an almost limp state when the noise is quickly identified as two good friends approaching from behind. Patients may have similar changes in muscle tone with emotional responses to fears of falling or of increased pain.

Summary

Muscle tone and muscle activation depend on the normal composition and functioning of the muscles, the PNS, and the CNS. Although both biomechanical and neural factors influence muscular responses, neural stimulation through the alpha motor neurons is a powerful influence on both muscle tone and activation, especially when the muscle is in the midrange of its length. Multiple sources of neural input, both excitatory and inhibitory, are required for normal functioning of the alpha motor neurons (see Table 4-3). Ultimately the sum of all the input determines the amount of neurally derived muscle tone and activation seen in the associated muscles.

The assumption in this section has been that the body is intact. The motor units, with both the alpha motor neurons and the muscle fibers, have all been functioning normally and receiving normal input from all sources. When pathology or injury affects the muscles, alpha motor neurons, or any of the sources of input to the alpha motor neurons, abnormalities in muscle tone and activation may result.

ABNORMAL MUSCLE TONE AND IT'S CONSEQUENCES

Many types of injuries or pathologies can result in abnormal muscle tone, some of which are considered in this section. One example of such a pathology is depicted in

Fig. 4-28, with possible consequences to muscle tone and function (see also Fig. 1-1).[38,39] When present, abnormal muscle tone is considered an impairment that may or may not lead to functional changes. Evaluation of muscle tone before and after a treatment can indicate the effectiveness of the treatment in reducing muscle tone or in changing its precipitating condition. Treatment decisions will depend on the role abnormal muscle tone plays in exacerbating functional limitations or disability, or whether it is likely to result in future problems such as adverse shortening of soft tissue.

In this section, some of the consequences of muscle tone abnormalities are listed and rehabilitative treatments are discussed. The consequences of abnormal tone depend on circumstances, each of which must be assessed along with the evaluation of muscle tone. Circumstances could include any additional impairments the patient has, as well as the psychological, physiological, and environmental resources available to the patient. A young, active, optimistic patient tends to have less severe functional limitations than an older, sedentary, depressed patient with the same degree of impairment.

Note that any observed changes in muscle tone consequent to a pathological condition depend on the remaining input available to that muscle's alpha motor neurons. The remaining input may include partial or aberrant information from sources damaged by the pathology, normal information from undamaged sources, and altered input from undamaged sources in

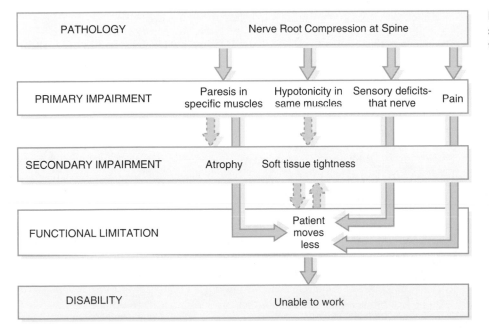

Figure 4-28. Classification scheme for pathologies and their consequences.

response to the pathology. When an individual has a movement problem, he or she will use whatever neural resources are most available to solve it. For example, high muscle tone may be useful for some patients if increased quadriceps tone allows weight bearing on an otherwise weak leg.

Low Muscle Tone

Abnormally low muscle tone results from loss of the normal alpha motor neuron input to otherwise normal muscle fibers. Although some muscle or motor endplate diseases may also result in low muscle tone, this discussion is limited to neuronal pathologies. Losses may result from damage to the alpha motor neurons themselves, so that the related motor units cannot be activated. Loss of neuronal stimulation of the muscles may also result from conditions that either increase inhibitory input or prevent adequate excitatory input from reaching the alpha motor neurons (Fig. 4-29).

Low muscle tone means there is insufficient activation of the motor units to prepare for holding or movement. Consequences include (1) difficulty developing adequate force output for posture or movement, with secondary problems resulting from lack of movement, and (2) poor posture caused by frequent supporting of weight through taut ligaments, as in a hyperextended knee. Poor posture results in cosmetically undesirable changes in appearance, especially with a slumped spine or drooping facial muscles. Stretched ligaments cancompromise joint integrity and lead to pain (Table 4-4).

Alpha motor neuron damage

If alpha motor neurons are damaged, electrochemical impulses will not reach the muscle fibers of those motor units. If all the motor units of a particular muscle are involved, the muscle tone is flaccid and muscle activation is not possible; the muscle is paralyzed. Sometimes the term *flaccid paralysis* is used to describe such a muscle's tone and loss of activation. When disease or injury of the alpha motor neurons removes neuronal input from the muscle, denervation results. Denervation of a muscle or group of muscles may be whole or partial. Examples of processes that may result in symptoms of denervation include poliomyelitis, which affects the cell bodies; Guillain-Barré syndrome, which attacks the Schwann cells so that the axons are essentially demyelinated; crush or cutting types of trauma to the nerves; and nerve compression.

When poliomyelitis eliminates functioning alpha motor neurons, recovery is limited by the number of intact motor units remaining. Each remaining alpha motor neuron may increase the number of muscle fibers it innervates by increasing its number of axonal branches. This process is known as *rearborizing*. Intact neurons may thereby reinnervate muscle fibers that lost their innervation with the destruction of associated alpha motor neurons (Fig. 4-30). Such muscles would be expected to have larger-than-normal motor units, with more muscle fibers being innervated by a single alpha motor neuron.[40] Denervated muscle fibers that are not close enough to an intact alpha motor neuron for reinnervation will die, and loss of muscle bulk (atrophy) will be evident. Maintaining the length and viability of the muscle fibers while any possible rearborization takes place is advocated.[40,41]

Recovery after injury to the axons of alpha motor neurons includes the possibility of regrowth of the axons from an intact cell body, through any remaining myelin sheaths toward the muscle fibers.[20]

Figure 4-29. Inhibition of alpha motor neuron: inhibitory input exceeds excitatory input.

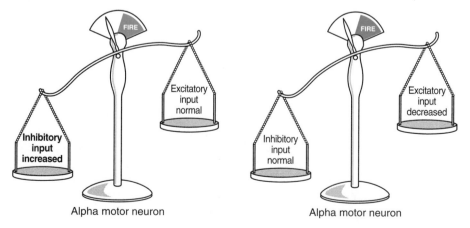

TABLE 4-4 Consequences of Abnormally Low Muscle Tone

1. Difficulty developing adequate force output for normal posture and movement
   a. Motor dysfunction
   b. Secondary problems resulting from lack of movement, e.g., pressure sores, loss of cardiorespiratory endurance

2. Poor posture
   a. Reliance on ligaments to substitute for muscle holding—eventual stretching of ligaments, compromised joint integrity, pain
   b. Cosmetically undesirable changes in appearance, e.g., slumping of spine, drooping of facial muscles
   c. Pain

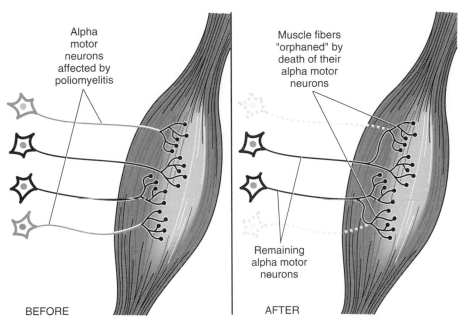

Alpha motor neurons affected by poliomyelitis

Muscle fibers "orphaned" by death of their alpha motor neurons

Remaining alpha motor neurons

BEFORE

AFTER

Figure 4-30. Rearborization of remaining axons to innervate orphaned muscle fibers after polio eliminates some alpha motor neurons.

Regrowth is slow, however, proceeding at a rate of 1-8 mm/day,[41] and may not be able to continue if the distance is too far. Again, maintaining the viability of muscle fibers while regrowth takes place is advocated.[40] Recovery following Guillain-Barré syndrome depends both on remyelination of the axons, which can be fairly rapid, and on regrowth of any axons that were secondarily damaged during the demyelinated period.[42]

Rehabilitation following alpha motor neuron damage

Rehabilitation of patients who have denervation includes treatments that facilitate activation of alpha motor neurons. In the past, physical agents included electrical stimulation to facilitate muscle fiber viabil-ity while axons regrew or rearborized. Electrical stimulation for this purpose has become controversial, with evidence that the quiescence of denervated muscle may actually trigger regrowth of neurons (see Chapter 8). Additional physical agents that are used after alpha motor neuron damage include hydrotherapy and quick ice.[33,43]

Because of buoyancy, hydrotherapy may be used to support the body or limbs and resist movement with range-of-motion exercises in the water.[43] The combination of buoyancy and resistance can help strengthen remaining or returning musculature (see Chapter 9). Quick ice (see Chapter 6) or light touch on the skin over a particular muscle group adds excitatory input to any intact alpha motor neurons via cutaneous sensory neurons.[33]

Other treatment options include range-of-motion exercise and therapeutic exercise to maintain muscle length and joint mobility and to strengthen the remaining musculature. Treatment also includes functional training that teaches patients to compensate for the movement losses they have experienced. Orthotic devices may be prescribed to support a limb for function while the muscle is flaccid or to protect the nerve from being overstretched.

Note that excitatory input to an alpha motor neuron that is not intact will be ineffective. The alpha motor neuron that is not intact cannot transmit information to its related muscle fibers, either to change tone or to contract voluntarily. Also, if alpha motor neurons are damaged in a cut or crush injury or by compression, local sensory neurons bringing information in the same nerve would also be damaged and unable to provide sensory input.

Insufficient excitation of alpha motor neurons

If a pathology affects peripheral, spinal, or supraspinal sources of input to alpha motor neurons, but does not affect the alpha motor neurons or muscle fibers themselves, low muscle tone may result. The alpha motor neurons may be stimulated to transmit information to muscle fibers to contract if excitatory input can be raised to a higher level than inhibitory input. Any condition, however, that prohibits alpha motor neurons from receiving sufficient excitatory input to activate the muscle fibers will result in decreased muscle tone.

Immobilization

One condition that alters peripheral sources of input to the alpha motor neuron is application of a cast to maintain a position during healing of a fracture. The cast applies a fairly constant stimulus to cutaneous receptors but inhibits reception of the variety of cutaneous input ordinarily encountered. The cast also inhibits movement at one or more joints, restricting lengthening or shortening of the local muscles. Alpha motor neurons are thus deprived of normal alterations in muscle spindle, GTO, or joint receptor input. When the cast is removed, the result is typically a measurable loss of strength in the muscles and a loss of ROM in the joints. Muscle tone is also affected, with decreased activation of the motor units and increased biomechanical stiffness. Because the neural and biomechanical components of muscle tone counter one another in this case, the actual change in resistance to passive stretch must be carefully

assessed. The known effects of immobilization in decreasing muscle tone have been used deliberately to lower hypertonicity in severe cases.[44]

Stroke or head injury

Other ways to affect supraspinal input to the alpha motor neurons are through loss of blood supply or direct injury to cortical or subcortical neurons, as occurs with strokes or head injuries. The resulting muscle tone changes depend on the remaining proportion of excitatory and inhibitory input to the alpha motor neurons. For example, if the descending tracts are destroyed on one side, volitional movement and muscle tone may be lost in the associated muscles. However, most of the alpha motor neuron groups that receive input from multiple descending tracts will not lose all descending input. Those alpha motor neurons must adapt to a new proportion of excitatory and inhibitory input when the input from the damaged tracts is lost. The usual progression from flaccidity to increased tone after a stroke[36] may be a result of adaptation to new levels of inhibitory and excitatory input.

The prediction of muscle tone changes in a particular individual after a stroke is complicated by the fact that lesions within the supraspinal areas do not always completely eliminate the corticospinal tract. The portion of the tract that remains can still be used to signal volitional movement. In addition, although most of the fibers of the corticospinal tract cross to synapse on the opposite side of the body from the origin of those axons, some of the fibers do not cross. Therefore even if all of one corticospinal tract is destroyed, some fibers of the opposite corticospinal tract may provide enough input to alpha motor neurons for the tone in some of the muscles to remain relatively normal.

Rehabilitation to increase muscle tone

Physical agents are not often associated with the rehabilitation of patients who have had a stroke, head injury, or other supraspinal lesions. However, they can be a valuable adjunct to the therapeutic exercises, orthotics, and functional training of traditional neurorehabilitation.[5,36] Electrical stimulation, biofeedback, hydrotherapy, and quick ice may all be used.[33] The intent of any treatment choice is to affect the alpha motor neurons via the remaining intact peripheral, spinal, and supraspinal sources of input. Quick icing and tapping, for example, are facilitative techniques that can increase tone via cutaneous and muscle spindle receptors, respectively, and, when paired with voluntary movement, can increase functional motor output. Electrical stimulation might be combined with resistance of the muscle being stimulated or of synergistic muscles to increase tone and activation via interneurons of the spinal cord. Many authors have described in much more detail the treatment choices available to the rehabilitation specialist for increasing muscle tone and motor output in patients who have had a stroke or head injury.[5,33,36,45,46] The box below summarizes treatment suggestions to increase low muscle tone for improved functional activation.

Treatment Suggestions for Low Muscle Tone

Hydrotherapy
Quick ice
Electrical stimulation (when muscle fibers are
   innervated)
Biofeedback
Light touch
Tapping
Resistive exercises
Range-of-motion exercises
Therapeutic exercises
Functional training
Orthotics

High Muscle Tone

Many pathological conditions result in abnormally high muscle tone. Any of the supraspinal lesions mentioned in the previous section could ultimately result in hypertonicity, even though they begin with some form of low muscle tone. Only the loss of alpha motor neurons themselves will be restricted to a hypotonic presentation; hypertonicity does not occur as a result of lesions limited to the alpha motor neurons. Instead, hypertonicity is a result of abnormally high excitatory input compared to the inhibitory input to an otherwise intact alpha motor neuron, whatever the source of that input (see Fig. 4-20).

Researchers have argued about the effects of hypertonicity, particularly spasticity, on function. Some have pointed out that spasticity of the antagonist does not necessarily interfere with voluntary movement of the agonist.[4] During walking, for example, it has been assumed that spasticity in the ankle plantar flexors prevents adequate dorsiflexion during the swing phase of gait, resulting in toe drag.

However, EMG studies of patients with hypertonicity have shown essentially absent activity in the plantar flexors during swing, as in normal gait.[7] Another study of upper extremity function found deficits due to inadequate recruitment of the agonists, not by increased activity in the spastic antagonist muscles.[47] Instead, voluntary movement is hindered by slowed and inadequate recruitment of the agonist and delayed termination of agonist contraction.[4]

On the other hand, some researchers have shown that coactivation of spastic antagonists increases with faster movements, substantiating the claim that abnormal activation inhibits voluntary motor control.[48] Additionally, a review of multiple drug studies has revealed improved function in 60% to 70% of patients receiving intrathecally administered baclofen, a drug that reduces spasticity. The authors state that "spasticity reduction *can* be associated with improved voluntary movement," although it is also possible that a decrease in tone will have no measurable effect or even a negative effect on function.[49]

Because of the controversy, it cannot be stated unequivocally that hypertonicity itself inhibits voluntary movement. However, other effects of hypertonicity must not be ignored. These include (1) muscle spasms that contribute to discomfort; (2) hypertonicity in a muscle group on one side of a joint that can result in contractures (shortened resting length) or other soft tissue changes; (3) abnormal postures resulting from hypertonicity that can lead to skin breakdown or pressure ulcers; (4) resistance to passive movement of a nonfunctioning limb that results in caregiver difficulties during assisted dressing, transfers, hygiene, and other activities; and (5) possibly a stereotyped movement pattern that could inhibit alternative movement solutions (Table 4-5).

Pain, cold, and stress

An example of a peripheral source of input that might lead to hypertonicity is input from sensory receptors registering pain. Cutaneous reception of painful stimuli, and the consequent withdrawal or crossed extension reflexes, have already been discussed. Painful stimuli to the muscles or joints commonly result in increased muscle tension. This muscle tension is a form of hypertonicity and may be seen as muscle spasms in the paraspinal musculature of a person with back pain, for example. Such muscle spasms are known as *guarding* and are thought to be a mechanism

---

TABLE **4-5**   **Consequences of Abnormally High Muscle Tone**

1. Discomfort or pain from muscle spasms

2. Contractures

3. Abnormal posture

4. Skin breakdown

5. Increased effort by caregivers to assist with bathing, dressing, transfers

6. Development of stereotyped movement patterns that may inhibit development of movement alternatives

7. May or may not inhibit function

---

used to avoid further pain. Guarding probably has a supraspinal component as well as a peripheral component, because the emotions and thus the limbic system are so heavily involved in the interpretation of and response to pain.

The human body also responds to cold via peripheral and supraspinal systems. When homeostasis is threatened, muscle tone increases and the body may begin to shiver. Muscle tone also tends to increase with other threats, registered as stress. Hypertonicity may be palpable in various muscle groups, such as those in the shoulders and neck, when an individual registers more general pain or perceives a situation as threatening to the body or to self-esteem. The muscles are preparing for fight or flight, and the rest of the body is engaged in other SNS responses.

Treatment for reducing high tone

Patients with hypertonicity due to pain, cold, or stress can be treated in several ways. The first and most effective measure is to remove the source of the hypertonicity; treat the biomechanical cause of the pain, warm the patient, or alleviate the stress. When these measures are not possible, not applicable, or otherwise ineffective, treatment to decrease muscle tone may include education in relaxation techniques, EMG biofeedback, the use of neutral warmth or heat (see Chapter 6), or hydrotherapy (see Chapter 9).

Knott and Voss describe a twofold approach to relaxation of a particular muscle group.[35] Muscles can be approached directly, with verbal cues to relax or application of cold towels to elicit muscle relaxation. Alternatively, muscles can be approached indirectly, by stimulating the antagonists, which results in reciprocal inhibition of agonists and lowers agonist muscle tone.

Antagonists can be stimulated with resisted exercise or electrical stimulation (see Chapter 8).

Spinal cord injury

Following a spinal cord injury (SCI), the alpha motor neurons below the level of the lesion lack both inhibitory and excitatory input from supraspinal sources. They still receive input from propriospinal and other neurons below the level of the lesion. Immediately following the injury, however, the nervous system is typically in a state called *spinal shock,* in which it shuts down at and below the level of the injury. The condition may last for hours or weeks, and is marked by the flaccid tone of the affected muscles and the loss of spinal level reflex activity like the muscle stretch reflex. When spinal shock resolves, the lack of inhibitory input from supraspinal areas as a result of the SCI allows alpha motor neurons below the level of the injury to respond especially easily to muscle spindle, GTO, or cutaneous input. The hypertonicity thus apparent is known as spasticity since quick stretch elicits greater resistance than slow stretch.

Quick stretch may occur not only when the muscles are specifically tested for tone, but also whenever the patient moves and the weight of a limb suddenly exerts a different pull on the muscles. For example, a patient who has a complete thoracic-level injury may use his arms to pick up his legs and place his feet on the foot pedals of his wheelchair. When the leg is lifted, the foot hangs down with the ankle plantar-flexed. When the leg is placed, the weight lands on the ball of the foot and the ankle moves passively into relative dorsiflexion. If the foot placement is quick, the plantar flexors are quickly stretched and clonus may be seen.

Frequently, the hypertonicity is greater on one side of a joint than on the other because the force of gravity is unidirectional on the mass of a limb. Because the patient with SCI has no active movement that can counter the hypertonicity, muscle shortening tends to occur in the muscles that are relatively more hypertonic. The biomechanical stiffness of the hypertonic muscles thus increases, and contractures can develop. Such contractures can inhibit functions such as dressing, transfers, and positioning for pressure relief.

Treating hypertonicity following SCI

Selective range-of-motion exercises,[50,51] prolonged stretch,[33] positioning or orthotics to maintain functional muscle length, local or systemic medications, and surgery[51] have been used to counter either the hypertonicity or the contractures interfering with function. Heat could be used before before stretching of shortened muscles (see Chapter 6), but it must be carefully monitored because of the patient's potential insensitivity to pain or decreased sensation below the level of the spinal cord injury. Other locally applied tone-inhibiting therapies, such as prolonged icing, could theoretically alleviate hypertonicity in patients with SCI. However, research is lacking either to confirm or to reject the usefulness of these agents in this population. Functional electrical stimulation (FES) has also been used to increase the function of paretic muscles in this population (see Chapter 8) but not for changing muscle tone.

Patients with SCI may also have muscle spasms, generally attributable to painful stimuli, except that patients may be unaware of the pain because sensory signals arising from below the level of the injury do not reach the cerebral cortex. Muscle spasms may also be attributed to visceral stimuli such as a urinary tract infection, distended bladder, or some other internal irritation.[51] Identification and removal of the painful stimuli are the first steps in alleviating muscle spasms. When muscle spasms are persistent, frequent, or inhibit function, and are without identifiable and removable causes, systemic or locally injected medications are sometimes prescribed to alleviate them.[51] Careful evaluation of the source of a muscle spasm must occur before any physical agent or treatment is applied.

Cerebral lesions

Lesions from cerebral vascular disorders or stroke, cerebral palsy, tumors, CNS infection, or head injury may result in hypertonicity. In addition, conditions that affect transmission of neural impulses in the CNS, like multiple sclerosis (MS) can result in hypertonicity. Hypertonicity in patients following all of these pathologies is the result of a change in input to alpha motor neurons (see Fig. 4-20). The extent of the pathology determines whether many muscle groups are affected or only a few, and whether alpha motor neurons to a particular muscle group lose all or only some of a particular source of supraspinal input.

Hypertonicity: primary impairment or adaptive response?

The neurophysiological mechanism of hypertonicity is in some dispute. A variety of treatment approaches address hypertonicity based on assumptions about the way the nervous system functions. In one approach, developed by Bobath,[5] the nervous system is assumed to function as a hierarchy in which the supraspinal centers control the spinal centers of movement, and "abnormal tonus" results from loss of inhibitory control from higher centers. The resultant therapeutic sequence is to normalize the hypertonicity before before facilitating normal movement. In another approach, the task-oriented approach, which is based on a systems model of the nervous system, each movement is a product of sensorimotor, motivational, biomechanical, and environmental input.[9,52-54] The primary goal of the nervous system in producing movement is to accomplish the desired task. After a lesion develops, the nervous system uses its remaining resources to perform movement tasks. Hypertonicity, then, may be the best adaptive response the nervous system can make given its available resources after injury rather than a primary result of the injury itself.

An example of task-oriented reasoning is as follows: patients with paresis are sometimes able to use trunk and lower extremity extensor hypertonicity to hold an upright posture. In this case, hypertonicity is an adaptive response to accomplish the task of maintaining an upright posture.[54,55] Eliminating the hypertonicity in such a case would decrease function unless concurrent increases in controlled voluntary movement are elicited. On the other hand, controlled movement is always preferable to hypertonicity if it can be elicited. Control implies the ability to make changes in a response according to environmental demands, whereas the hypertonic extensor response mentioned above is relatively stereotyped. The use of a stereotyped hypertonic response for function seems to block spontaneous development of more normal control.[5,56]

Evidence that hypertonicity may be an adaptive response includes the fact that it is not an immediate sequela of injury but instead develops over time. Following a cortical stroke, recovery of muscle tone and voluntary movement follows a fairly predictable course.[36,44] At first, muscles are flaccid and paralyzed on the side of the body opposite the lesion, without elicitable stretch reflexes. The next stage of recovery is characterized by increasing response of the muscles to quick stretch and the beginning of voluntary motor output that is limited to movement in flexor or extensor patterns, called *synergies.* Because muscle tone and synergy patterns of movement appear at approximately the same time, clinicians tend to equate the two, but spasticity and synergy are distinct from each other (see Table 4-1). Further recovery stages include progression to full-blown spasticity and ultimately the gradual normalization of muscle tone. At the same time, voluntary movement shows full-blown synergy dependence, progressing to the mixing of synergies, and finally resolving to controlled movement of isolated musculature.[36] A particular patient's course of recovery may stall, skip, or plateau anywhere along the way, but it does not regress.

Rehabilitation to decrease muscle tone

Rehabilitation to address hypertonicity after a stroke depends on whether the clinician believes that hypertonicity inhibits function or instead is a product of adaptive motor control. In either case, the emphasis is on return of independent function, whether that necessitates tone reduction or the reeducation of controlled voluntary movement patterns.

Treatment to reduce hypertonicity in preparation for functional movement could include prolonged icing, inhibitory pressure, prolonged stretch,[33] inhibitory casting,[57] or positioning. Reeducation of controlled voluntary movement patterns could include weight bearing to facilitate normal postural responses or training with directed practice of functional movement patterns.[45] Reduction of hypertonicity may, in fact, be a product of improved motor control in the following example. If a patient feels insecure standing upright, muscle tone will increase commensurate with the anxiety level. If balance and motor control are improved such that the patient feels more confident in the upright position, hypertonicity will also be reduced.[45] Positioning for comfort and to reduce anxiety is a critical adjunct to any treatment intended to reduce muscle tone.

If a patient has severe hypertonicity or if many muscle groups are affected, techniques that influence the ANS to decrease arousal or calm the individual generally might be used. Such techniques include soft lighting or music, slow rocking, neutral warmth, slow stroking, maintained touch,[33] rotation of the trunk, or hydrotherapy (see Chapter 9), as long as the patient feels safely supported. For example, hydrotherapy in a cool water pool is particularly advocated for patients with MS to reduce spasticity. Stretching and cold packs are also of benefit in temporarily reducing the spasticity of MS, but they lack hydrotherapy's added benefit of allowing gentle range-of-motion exercises with a diminished pull of gravity.[55]

Rigidity: a consequence of CNS pathology

Some cerebral lesions are associated with rigidity instead of spasticity. Head injuries, for example, may result in one of two specific patterns of rigidity that may be either constant or intermittent. Both patterns include hypertonicity in the neck and back extensors, the hip extensors, adductors, and internal rotators, the knee extensors, and the ankle plantar flexors and invertors. The elbows are held rigidly at the sides, with the wrists and fingers flexed in both patterns, but in decorticate rigidity the elbows are flexed, and in decerebrate rigidity they are extended. The two types of rigidity are thought to indicate the level of the lesion: above or below the red nucleus in the brain stem, respectively. In most patients with head injury, however, the lesion is diffuse, and this designation is unhelpful. Two positioning principles can diminish rigidity in either case and should be considered along with any other therapies: (1) reposition the patient in postures opposite to those listed, with emphasis on slight neck and trunk flexion and hip flexion past 90 degrees, and (2) avoid the supine position, which promotes extension in the trunk and limbs via the symmetrical tonic labyrinthine response (see Fig. 4-6).

Rigidity, like spasticity, can result in biomechanical muscle stiffness after long-term placement in the shortened position. The longer the period of time without range-of-motion exercises or positioning to elongate a muscle group, the greater the biomechanical changes that occur. Prevention is the best cure for biomechanical components of hypertonicity, but orthotics[58] or serial casting[57] have also been useful in reducing the muscle stiffness related to hypertonicity. Heat may be used to increase ROM temporarily before applying a cast or orthotic.

Parkinson's disease usually includes rigidity, which occurs throughout the skeletal musculature rather than being limited to a particular extensor pattern. In addition to pharmaceutical replacement of dopamine,[59] treatment can include temporary reduction of hypertonicity through heat and other general inhibiting techniques to allow patients to accomplish particular functions. The following box summarizes treatment suggestions to decrease high muscle tone.

Treatment Suggestions for High Muscle Tone Associated with Pain, Cold, or Stress

Remove source
- **Eliminate pain**
- **Warm patient**
- **Alleviate stress**

Relaxation techniques
EMG biofeedback
Neutral warmth
Heat
Hydrotherapy
Cold towels
Stimulation of antagonists
- **Resisted exercise**
- **Electrical stimulation**

Associated with Spinal Cord Injury
Selective range-of-motion exercises
Prolonged stretch
Positioning
Orthotics
Medication
Surgery
Heat
Prolonged ice

Associated with Cerebral Lesions
Prolonged ice
Inhibitory pressure
Prolonged stretch
Inhibitory casting
Positioning
Reeducation of voluntary movement patterns
General relaxation techniques
- **Soft lighting or music**

- **Slow rocking**
- **Neutral warmth**
- **Slow stroking**
- **Maintained touch**
- **Rotation of the trunk**
- **Hydrotherapy**

Associated with Rigidity
Positioning
Range-of-motion exercises
Orthotics
Serial casting following head injury
Heat
Medication
General relaxation techniques (as listed above)

Fluctuating Muscle Tone

Commonly, pathology of the basal ganglia results in disorders of muscle tone and activation. Not only is voluntary motor output difficult to initiate, execute, and control, but the variations in muscle tone seen in this population can be so extreme as to be visible with movement. The resting tremors of a patient with Parkinson's disease and the dyskinesias seen in the example with Mrs. H while she is medicated are examples of fluctuating tone that result in involuntary movement. A child with athetoid-type cerebral palsy, for whom movement is a series of involuntary writhings, also demonstrates fluctuating tone.

When an individual has fluctuating tone that moves the limbs through large ranges of motion, contractures are usually not a problem, but inadvertent self-inflicted injuries sometimes occur. As a hand or foot flails around, it will sometimes run into a hard, immovable object. Patients and caregivers can be educated to alter the environment, padding necessary objects or removing unnecessary ones to avoid harm. If the fluctuating tone does not result in movement of large amplitude, then positioning and range-of-motion treatments should be considered. Neutral warmth has been advocated to reduce excessive movement resulting from muscle tone fluctuations in athetosis.[60]

▶ *Clinical Case Studies* ◀

The following case studies summarize the concepts of tone abnormalities discussed in this chapter and are not intended to be exhaustive. Based on the scenarios presented, an evaluation of the clinical findings and goals of treatment are proposed. These are followed by a discussion of the factors to be considered in treatment selection. Note that any technique used to alter tone abnormalities must be followed with functional use of the musculature involved if the patient is to improve the ability to hold or move.

Case 1

GM is a 37-year-old businessman who said that the first signs of his Bell's palsy appeared after a long airplane flight when he slept with his head against the window. He'd had a cold, but whether or not this factor and his nap on the plane precipitated his unilateral facial paralysis, he did not know. A noticeable droop was visible on the left side of his face, and he was having trouble with lip closure to control saliva and eat properly.

What is the muscle tone in the left facial muscles? What techniques would be appropriate for changing the tone for this patient?

EVALUATION OF THE CLINICAL FINDINGS
Bell's palsy is any disorder of the facial nerve, usually only on one side, with varied etiologies. The sudden onset of GM's symptoms may indeed have been instigated by the chilling of the side of his face while on the airplane or by his cold virus. If the entire facial nerve is affected on the left, then none of the muscle fibers on the left side of the face will be able to receive signals from any alpha motor neurons, and the muscles will be flaccid. If the facial nerve is only partially affected, then some muscles might be hypotonic. GM noted that the entire left side of his face felt as though it was being pulled downward.

PREFERRED PRACTICE PATTERN
Impaired Motor Function and Sensory Integrity Associated With Nonprogressive Disorders of the Central Nervous System—Acquired in Adolescence or Adulthood, (5D).

PLAN OF CARE
Fortunately, reinnervation of the muscle fibers is common following a facial palsy, usually within 1 to 3 months. Muscle tone can be expected to normalize as reinnervation occurs if the muscle and connective tissues have been maintained so that secondary biomechanical changes do not interfere. Therefore anticipated goals of treatment would include prevention of overstretching of soft tissues, eye protection (while the blink reflex is lost), and strengthening of muscles once reinnervation occurs.

PROPOSED TREATMENT PLAN AND RATIONALE
Gentle passive movement of the facial musculature may be indicated to counter soft tissue changes resulting from lack of active movement. Otherwise, GM may be left with a cosmetically unacceptable facial droop when the muscles are reinnervated. A patch or other form of protection over the left eye may be required to prevent eye injury while the motor component of the corneal reflex is paralyzed. As the muscle fibers are reinnervated, the emphasis will be on exercises to elicit voluntary contraction rather than on improving muscle tone. Quick icing or light touch on the skin over a particular muscle that is beginning to be innervated may help GM to isolate a muscle to move it voluntarily. Practice of facial movements while looking in a mirror may provide extra feedback for GM while he is attempting to reestablish normal activation of the facial muscles. Electrical stimulation with biofeedback may be used to help the patient resume function once muscles are reinnervated.

Case 2

EL was young, only in her 40s, for the severity of arthritic damage to her right hip. The damage was most likely the result of abnormal use of the right leg following a case of polio when she was an infant. Several surgeries in childhood to stabilize the foot and to transfer a hamstring tendon anteriorly to function for the quadriceps had allowed her independent ambulation, but her limp had worsened over the last several years. The head of the femur had slipped out of the acetabulum and moved farther up toward her trunk; EL had to walk on her right toes since the right leg was functionally several inches shorter than the left. After a successful total hip replacement that evened the leg lengths, EL was learning to walk again. Her gait training was more complex than is typical following total hip replacement surgery because of her complications. During supine passive ROM of her right leg (within the limits allowed by her postoperative total hip precautions), the ankle plantar flexors resisted stretch. Her hip and knee moved very easily but the leg felt heavy, almost like dead weight.

Based on the information presented, how should EL's muscle tone be described in the hip flexors? The knee extensors? The ankle plantar flexors? What treatment techniques would be appropriate to alter the muscle tone labeled in the preceding question?

EVALUATION OF CLINICAL FINDINGS

Both the hip flexors and knee extensors are hypotonic, a 1 on the clinical tone scale, with decreased activation of the alpha motor neurons. The ankle plantar flexor would be expected to have biomechanical shortening, causing stiffness and resistance to muscle stretch at the end of a diminished ROM, a result of habitual toe walking. If passive movement resulted in resistance in the middle of the available range, then the ankle plantar flexor would be labeled *hypertonic*, a 3 on the clinical tone scale. Neurally mediated hypertonicity is unlikely with this diagnosis since no spinal or supraspinal neural lesions are evident.

The hip flexor alpha motor neurons may be temporarily inhibited because of pain in the incision area lateral to the hip. If this hypothesis is correct, normalization of muscle tone and voluntary contraction will progress as pain resolves.

The quadriceps muscle was presumably affected by the polio since the hamstring tendon was transferred many years ago. The quadriceps would have been hypotonic following loss of the affected alpha motor neurons: no activation would have been possible via those neurons, either for passive resistance to stretch or for voluntary contraction. EL's present knee extensor, the hamstring muscle, is probably normal in tone, which will be apparent once the hip heals further and pain resolves.

Having no information about EL's muscle tone or strength before the total hip replacement surgery, the clinician must palpate for activation of the muscles during voluntary contraction. EMG testing of the quadriceps, hip flexors, ankle plantar flexors, and hamstrings may also provide information about the number and size of active motor units in each muscle group. Such information could differentiate between muscles that were more or less affected by poliomyelitis. Muscles that were more affected do not have the same capacity for motor unit recruitment during strength training as muscles that were less affected. The goals for strengthening would be reduced in muscles that were more affected.

PREFERRED PRACTICE PATTERN

Impaired Joint Mobility, Motor Function, Muscle Performance and Range of Motion Associated With Joint Arthroplasty, (4H), or Impaired Motor Function and Sensory Integrity Associated With Acute or Chronic Polyneuropathies, (5G).

PLAN OF CARE

Anticipated goals include pain alleviation at the hip, incision healing, and improvement of hip muscle activation, recruitment, and timing to improve functions such as gait and transfers. Increasing the ROM at the ankle will also be necessary.

PROPOSED TREATMENT PLAN AND RATIONALE

Pain control could be accomplished with physical agents, soft tissue mobilization, and positioning. (See Chapter 6 for instructions on the use of heat or cold, or see Chapter 8 for instructions on the use of electrical stimulation.) Gait training and functional training with appropriate feedback and practice will be necessary. Gait training in a pool will take advantage of buoyancy and the resistance the water provides against movement and could begin as soon as the surgical incision is well healed (see Chapter 9). The hypotonicity is expected to become less apparent as EL's pain decreases and she is better able to contract at will.

Treatment of the ankle plantar flexors must include prolonged stretch, preferably with prior heat or thermal-level ultrasound (see Chapters 6 and 7) for soft tissue remodeling. Stretch could be accomplished with exercise or weight bearing on the whole foot. Some would advocate serial casting if functional dorsiflexion range of motion cannot be obtained in any other way.

Case 3

SP, a 24-year-old female, had noticed intermittent back pain over the last several months. Her lifestyle had changed significantly from that of an athlete, training regularly, to that of a student, sitting for long periods. The pain increased dramatically yesterday, however, while she was bowling for the first time in a couple of years. One of her problems at this point is the palpable muscle spasm in the paraspinal muscles at the lumbar level.

What is the underlying stimulus causing the muscle spasm? What treatment is appropriate to alleviate the spasm?

EVALUATION OF CLINICAL FINDINGS

Muscle spasms typically originate from painful stimuli, even if the stimuli are subtle. Possible stimuli in SP's case include injury to muscle fibers or other tissue while engaging in vigorous but unaccustomed activity, pain signals from a facet joint, or nerve root irritation. The consequent tension in the muscle may hold or splint the injured area to avoid local movement that could irritate and exacerbate the pain. If persistent, the muscle spasm itself can contribute to the pain and discomfort by inhibiting local circulation and setting up its own painful feedback loop.

POSSIBLE PREFERRED PRACTICE PATTERNS

Impaired Joint Mobility, Motor Function, Muscle Performance, and Range of Motion Associated with Connective Tissue Dysfunction, (4D), or Impaired Joint Mobility, Motor Function, Muscle Performance, and Range of Motion Associated with Localized

Continued

▶ Clinical Case Studies—cont'd ◀

Inflammation, (4E), or Impaired Joint Mobility, Motor Function, Muscle Performance, Range of Motion, and Reflex Integrity Associated with Spinal Disorders, (4F), or Impaired Posture, (4B).

PLAN OF CARE

The anticipated goals of treatment would include identifying and removing the cause of the painful stimulus. Frequently, temporarily easing the muscle spasm first allows more accurate identification of the underlying pathology.

PROPOSED TREATMENT PLAN AND RATIONALE

Diagnosing the source of the painful stimulus is beyond the scope of this chapter, but many texts are devoted to the subject.[61-63] Once stimulus identification and removal occurs, the muscle spasm may diminish by itself or it may require separate treatment. Heat, ultrasound, or massage can increase local circulation (see Chapters 6 and 7). Prolonged icing, neutral warmth, or slow stroking could be used to diminish the hypertonicity directly and thus allow restoration of more normal local circulation. Once the painful feedback loop of the muscle spasm is broken, patient education is necessary. Education should include instructions on preventive strengthening of local musculature and avoidance of postures and movements that reaggravate the initial injury. Other stretching and strengthening exercises have been identified but will not be discussed in this text on physical agents.

Case 4

RB had a left hemiplegia following a stroke. He had progressed from an initial flaccid paralysis to his current status of hypertonicity in the biceps brachii and ankle plantar flexors. When asked to lift his left arm, he was unable to do so without elevating and retracting his scapula, abducting and externally rotating his shoulder, and flexing and supinating at the elbow, all consistent with a flexor synergy. When standing, he tended to rotate internally and adduct his left hip, with a retracted pelvis and a hyperextended knee, consistent with the lower extremity extensor synergy pattern. He was dependent in bed mobility and transfers because of lack of controlled movement of the left side of his body. The hypertonicity in the arm and leg increased when he attempted to keep his balance in a standing position or take steps with a quad-cane.

What measures of muscle tone are appropriate in evaluating Mr. B? What treatment is appropriate considering Mr. B's hypertonicity?

EVALUATION OF CLINICAL FINDINGS

Muscle tone would most likely be assessed using stretch reflexes, the clinical tone scale or the Modified Ashworth Scale, and clinical observation. Mr. B was found to have a hyperactive stretch reflex in both the biceps and the triceps, but muscle tone in the triceps was hypotonic, with a 1 on the clinical tone scale. The biceps and plantar flexors were given a 1+ on the Modified Ashworth Scale which equaled a 3 on the clinical tone scale. During quick stretch of the plantar flexors, clonus was apparent, lasting for three beats. During clinical observation, Mr. B rested his left forearm in his lap while sitting with his back supported, but when he stood, gravity quick-stretched his biceps once the weight of his forearm was unsupported, and the elbow flexed to approximately 80 degrees. During bed mobility, transfers, or standing, full elbow extension was never observed. His left ankle bounced with plantar flexion clonus when he first stood up, ending with weight mostly on the ball of his foot unless care was taken to position the foot before standing to facilitate weight bearing through the heel.

Other possible tests for Mr. B's muscle tone include the pendulum test for the biceps, a dynamometer or myometer test for the plantar flexors, or EMG studies to compare muscle activity on the two sides of Mr. B's body. These quantitative measures would be especially useful for research that requires more precise measurement than the qualitative measures described above.

PREFERRED PRACTICE PATTERN

Impaired Motor Function and Sensory Integrity Associated With Nonprogressive Disorders of the Central Nervous System—Acquired in Adolescence or Adulthood, (5D).

PLAN OF CARE

Goals are focused on improving Mr. B's function and preventing secondary problems.

PROPOSED TREATMENT PLAN AND RATIONALE

Appropriate treatment techniques for Mr. B may come from multiple sources and theoretical backgrounds. Only a few techniques that influence muscle tone will be discussed here. Prolonged stretch of the biceps or the plantar flexors may be incorporated into functional activities like standing or weight bearing on the hand to normalize muscle tone. Prolonged icing (see Chapter 6) may be added if soft tissue shortening is inhibiting full passive ROM. Exercises to facilitate activity of the antagonists to inhibit the biceps or plantar flexors may be used. Electrical stimulation of the triceps and dorsiflexors would have the dual benefit of inhibiting hypertonic musculature and strengthening muscles that are currently weak (see Chapter 8). EMG biofeedback might be used during a specific task to train Mr. B in more appropriate activation patterns for the biceps or plantar flexors.

The hypertonicity increase seen during standing could be alleviated with techniques to increase Mr. B's alignment, balance, and confidence while standing. If he is better able to relax in this posture, his muscle tone will decrease as well. Discussion of specific therapeutic exercises to enhance Mr. B's balance is beyond the scope of this chapter.

Case 5

Mrs. H was eager to tell her story. Her Parkinson's disease had progressed, with increasing tremor and harder and longer freezes of her limbs between dyskinetic states that led to the gradual loss of handwriting, reading ability, and other functions. She had taken increasing doses of a dopamine replacement drug with decreasing benefit. Because of her good health otherwise, she was deemed a good candidate for a surgical procedure called a *pallidotomy* and had a 3- to 4-inch recent incision visible in the left side of her scalp. Now she could sign her name with her right hand and read print on an exercise sheet. But she still froze a few times each day, when she would find any movement difficult, although not impossible with sufficient effort, until her muscle tone diminished after an hour or so.

EVALUATION OF CLINICAL FINDINGS

Mrs. H, described at the beginning of this chapter, is an example of a patient with fluctuating muscle tone during her dyskinetic periods and rigid hypertonicity during her freeze states. Her limbs have such large movements during her dyskinetic periods that loss of motion will probably not be a problem. Her trunk and neck muscles, routinely positioned with a thoracic kyphosis and forward-extended head, however, could tighten.

PREFERRED PRACTICE PATTERN

Impaired Motor Function and Sensory Integrity Associated With Progressive Disorders of the Central Nervous System, (5E).

PLAN OF CARE

Anticipated goals of treatment include avoiding injury, preventing secondary problems like soft tissue shortening, and promoting independent function.

PROPOSED TREATMENT PLAN AND RATIONALE

Mrs. H's environment should be assessed and her wheelchair footplates padded to avoid injury when her flailing limbs knock against objects. Posture training, active and passive ROM, locally applied heat, and supine positioning can help maintain her trunk and neck tissue integrity. In Mrs. H's case, since her dyskinesia is a result of massive doses of a dopamine replacement drug, one might ask why she does not have the dose reduced or the drug eliminated to decrease the fluctuation of her muscle tone. Her response is that she prefers dyskinesia to a freeze: it is easier to initiate movement and therefore function in the former condition. The patient's preference takes precedence, although reports of specific, effective therapy for dyskinesia are rare. Neutral warmth, as is used in athetosis, and hydrotherapy, for its resistance to limb movement in all directions, have potential effectiveness but require further study.

CHAPTER REVIEW

Muscle tone is defined as a muscle's passive resistance to stretch. The resistance has both a neural component, from the activation of motor units via alpha motor neurons, and biomechanical and biochemical components, from the properties of the muscle fibers and connective tissue surrounding them. Neurally-derived tone abnormalities result from abnormal changes in the inhibitory and excitatory input to the alpha motor neuron. Abnormal changes may occur as a result of peripheral, spinal, or supraspinal pathologies that affect either the alpha motor neuron itself or any of the sources of input to the alpha motor neuron.

If the result is hypotonicity, the goal of rehabilitation is to increase the muscle tone to promote easier activation of motor output, improve posture, and restore an acceptable cosmetic appearance. If the result of abnormal input to the alpha motor neuron is hypertonicity, the goal of rehabilitation is to decrease the muscle tone to decrease discomfort, ease ROM and caregiving activities, allow normal positioning, and prevent contractures. If the result of abnormal input is an uncontrollable fluctuation of muscle tone, the goal of physical therapy is to increase function as much as possible and prevent injuries. Some treatment ideas have been suggested that make use of the structures and neurophysiological principles described here. Later chapters in this text explain more fully how physical agents may be used to manage some of the problems presented when muscle tone is abnormal. The reader is referred to the Evolve website at http://evolve.elsevier.com/Cameron for study questions pertinent to this chapter.

References

1. Keshner EA: Reevaluating the theoretical model underlying the neurodevelopmental theory: a literature review, *Phys Ther* 61:1035-1040, 1981.
2. Brooks VB: Motor control: how posture and movements are governed, *Phys Ther* 63:664-673, 1983.
3. Lance JW: The control of muscle tone, reflexes, and movement: Robert Wartenberg lecture, *Neurology* 30:1303-1313, 1980.
4. Sahrmann SA, Norton BJ: The relationship of voluntary movement to spasticity in the upper motor neuron syndrome, *Ann Neurol* 2:460-465, 1977.
5. Bobath B: *Adult Hemiplegia: Evaluation and Treatment,* ed 2, London, 1978, Heinemann.
6. Teasell R: Musculoskeletal complications of hemiplegia following stroke, *Semin Arthritis Rheum* 20(6):385-395, 1991.
7. Dietz V, Quintern J, Berger W: Electrophysiological studies of gait in spasticity and rigidity: evidence that altered mechanical properties of muscle contribute to hypertonia, *Brain* 104:431-449, 1981.
8. Claypool DW, Duane DD, Ilstrup DM et al: Epidemiology and outcome of cervical dystonia (spasmodic torticollis) in Rochester, Minnesota, *Movement Disorders* 10(5):608-614, 1995.
9. Giuliani C: Dorsal rhizotomy for children with cerebral palsy: support for concepts of motor control, *Phys Ther* 71:248-259, 1991.
10. Boiteau M, Malouin F, Richards CL: Use of a hand-held dynamometer and a Kin-Com^R dynamometer for evaluating spastic hypertonia in children: a reliability study, *Phys Ther* 75:796-802, 1995.
11. Wolf SL, Catlin PA, Blanton S et al: Overcoming limitations in elbow movement in the presence of antagonist hyperactivity, *Phys Ther* 74:826-835, 1994.
12. Basmajian JV, De Luca CJ: *Muscles Alive: Their Functions Revealed by Electromyography,* ed 5, Baltimore, 1985, Williams & Wilkins.
13. Bajd T, Vodovnik L: Pendulum testing of spasticity, *J Biomed Eng* 6:9-16, 1984.
14. Bohannon RW: Variability and reliability of the pendulum test for spasticity using a Cybex II Isokinetic Dynamometer, *Phys Ther* 67:659-661, 1987.
15. O'Sullivan SB: Assessment of motor function. In O'Sullivan SB, Schmitz TJ, eds: *Physical Rehabilitation: Assessment and Treatment,* ed 4, Philadelphia, 2001, FA Davis.
16. Bates B: *A Guide to Physical Examination,* ed 4, Philadelphia, 1987, JB Lippincott.
17. Ashworth B: Preliminary trial of carisoprodol in multiple sclerosis, *Practitioner* 192:540-542, 1964
18. Bohannon RW, Smith MB: Interrater reliability of a modified Ashworth scale of muscle spasticity, *Phys Ther* 67:206-207, 1987.
19. Bohannon RW, Andrews AW: Influence of head-neck rotation on static elbow flexion force of paretic side in patients with hemiparesis, *Phys Ther* 69:135-137, 1989.
20. DeLong MR: The basal ganglia. In Kandel ER, Schwartz JH, Jessell TM, eds: *Principles of Neural Science,* ed 4, New York, 2000, McGraw-Hill.
21. Jessell TM: Reactions of neurons to injury. In Kandel ER, Schwartz JH, Jessell TM, eds: *Principles of Neural Science,* ed 3, New York, 1991, Elsevier.
22. Koester J, Siegelbaum SA: Local signaling: passive membrane properties of the neuron. In Kandel ER, Schwartz JH, Jessell TM, eds: *Principles of Neural Science,* ed 4, New York, 2000, McGraw-Hill.
23. Rothwell J: *Control of Human Voluntary Movement,* ed 2, New York, 1994, Chapman and Hall.
24. De Jesus P, Housmanowa-Petrusewicz I, Barchi R: The effect of cold on nerve conduction of human slow and fast nerve fibers, *Neurology* 23:1182-1189, 1973.
25. Dewhurst DJ: Neuromuscular control system, *IEEE Trans Bio-Med Eng* 14:167-171, 1967.
26. Rowland LP: Diseases of the motor unit. In Kandel ER, Schwartz JH, Jessell TM, eds: *Principles of Neural Science,* ed 4, New York, 2000, McGraw-Hill.
27. Nashner LM: Adapting reflexes controlling the human posture, *Exp Brain Res* 26:59-72, 1976.
28. Vallbo AB: Afferent discharge from human muscle spindles in non-contracting muscles: steady state impulse frequency as a function of joint angle, *Acta Physiol Scand* 90:303-318, 1974a.
29. Vallbo AB: Human muscle spindle discharge during isometric voluntary contractions: amplitude relations between spindle frequency and torque, *Acta Physiol Scand* 90:319-336, 1974b.
30. Matthews PBC: *Mammalian Muscle Receptors and Their Central Actions,* London, 1972, Arnold.
31. Houk J, Henneman E: Responses of golgi tendon organs to active contractions of the soleus muscle of the cat, *J Neurophysiol* 30:466-481, 1967.
32. Jami L: Golgi tendon organs in mammalian skeletal muscle: functional properties and central actions, *Physiol Rev* 72:623-666, 1992.
33. O'Sullivan SB: Strategies to improve motor control and motor learning. In O'Sullivan SB, Schmitz TJ, eds: *Physical Rehabilitation: Assessment and Treatment,* ed 4, Philadelphia, 2001, FA Davis.
34. Gracies JM, Meunier S, Pierrot-Deseilligny E, et al: Patterns of propriospinal-like excitation to different

species of human upper limb motor neurons, *J Physiol* 434:151-167, 1990.

35. Knott M, Voss DE: *Proprioceptive Neuromuscular Facilitation: Patterns and Techniques,* ed 2, New York, 1968, Harper & Row.

36. Brunnstrom S: *Movement Therapy in Hemiplegia: A Neurophysiological Approach,* Hagerstown, MD, 1970, Harper & Row.

37. Sawner KA, LaVigne JM: *Brunnstrom's Movement Therapy in Hemiplegia: A Neurophysiological Approach,* ed 2, Philadelphia, 1992, JB Lippincott.

38. Nagi S: Disability concepts revisited. In Pope AM, Tarlov AR, eds: *Disability in America: Toward a National Agenda for Prevention,* Washington, DC, 1991, National Academy Press.

39. Schenkman M, Butler RB: A model for multisystem evaluation, interpretation, and treatment of individuals with neurologic dysfunction, *Phys Ther* 69:538-547, 1989.

40. McDonald-Williams MF: Exercise and postpolio syndrome, *Neurol Rep* 20(2):37-44, 1996.

41. Stockert BW: Peripheral neuropathies. In Umphred DA, ed: *Neurological Rehabilitation,* ed 3, St Louis, 1995, Mosby.

42. Bassile CC: Guillain-Barre syndrome and exercise guidelines, *Neurol Rep* 20(2):31-36, 1996.

43. Morris DM: Aquatic neurorehabilitation, *Neurol Rep* 19(3):22-28, 1995.

44. Barnard P, Dill H, Eldredge P et al: Reduction of hypertonicity by early casting in a comatose head-injured individual, *Phys Ther* 64:1540-1542, 1984.

45. Duncan PW, Badke MB: Therapeutic strategies for rehabilitation of motor deficits. In Duncan PW, Badke MB, eds: *Stroke Rehabilitation: The Recovery of Motor Control,* Chicago, 1987, Year Book Medical Publishers.

46. Lehmkuhl LD, Krawczyk L: Physical therapy management of the minimally-responsive patient following traumatic brain injury: coma stimulation, *Neurol Rep* 17(1):10-17, 1993.

47. Gowland C, deBruin H, Basmajian JV et al: Agonist and antagonist activity during voluntary upper-limb movement in patients with stroke, *Phys Ther* 72:624-633, 1992.

48. Knutsson E, Martensson A: Dynamic motor capacity in spastic paresis and its relation to prime mover dysfunc-

tion, spastic reflexes and antagonist co-activation, *Scand J Rehab Med* 12:93-106, 1980.

49. Campbell SK, Almeida GL, Penn RD et al: The effects of intrathecally administered baclofen on function in patients with spasticity, *Phys Ther* 75:352-362, 1995.

50. Somers MF: *Spinal Cord Injury: Functional Rehabilitation,* Norwalk, CT, 1992, Appleton & Lange.

51. Schmitz TJ: Traumatic spinal cord injury. In O'Sullivan SB, Schmitz TJ, eds: *Physical Rehabilitation: Assessment and Treatment,* ed 3, Philadelphia, 1994, FA Davis.

52. Ostrosky KM: Facilitation vs. motor control, *Clin Management* 10(3):34-40, 1990.

53. Duncan PW, Badke MB: Determinants of abnormal motor control. In Duncan PW, Badke MB, eds: *Stroke Rehabilitation: The Recovery of Motor Control,* Chicago, 1987, Year Book Medical Publishers.

54. Horak FB: Assumptions underlying motor control for neurologic rehabilitation. In *Proceedings of the II Step Conference: Contemporary Management of Motor Control Problems,* Alexandria, VA, 1991, Foundation for Physical Therapy.

55. Rosner LJ, Ross S: *Multiple Sclerosis,* New York, 1987, Prentice Hall Press.

56. Bobath B: *Abnormal Postural Reflex Activity Caused by Brain Lesions,* ed 2, London, 1971, Heinemann.

57. Giorgetti MM: Serial and inhibitory casting: implications for acute care physical therapy management, *Neurol Rep* 17(1):18-21, 1993.

58. McClure PW, Blackburn LG, Dusold C: The use of splints in the treatment of joint stiffness: biologic rationale and an algorithm for making clinical decisions, *Phys Ther* 74:1101-1107, 1994.

59. Cutson TM, Laub KC, Schenkman M: Pharmacological and nonpharmacological interventions in the treatment of Parkinson's disease, *Phys Ther* 75:363-373, 1995.

60. Stockmeyer SA: An interpretation of the approach of Rood to the treatment of neuromuscular dysfunction, *Am J Phys Med* 46(1):900-956, 1967.

61. Maitland GD: *Vertebral Manipulation,* ed 6, London, 2000, Butterworth-Heinemann.

62. Grieve GP: *Common Vertebral Joint Problems,* ed 2, Edinburgh, 1988, Churchill Livingstone.

63. Saunders HD, Saunders R: *Evaluation, Treatment and Prevention of Musculoskeletal Disorders,* ed 3, vol 1: *Spine,* Bloomington, MN, 1993, Educational Opportunities.

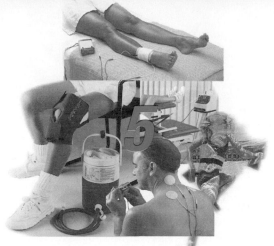

Motion Restrictions

Linda G. Monroe, MPT, OCS

SUMMARY OF INFORMATION COVERED

OBJECTIVES

Upon completion of this chapter, the reader will be able to:

1. Define different types of motion.
2. Describe different patterns of motion restrictions.
3. Identify tissues that can restrict motion.
4. Discuss pathologies that can contribute to motion restrictions.
5. Select and apply appropriate tools and methods to quantify and qualify motion restrictions.
6. Select and apply appropriate methods to determine the structures and pathologies contributing to motion restrictions.
7. When presented with a clinical case involving a motion restriction, evaluate the clinical findings, propose treatment goals, and identify possible interventions.

INTRODUCTION

This chapter discusses motion between body segments and the factors that can restrict such motion. The amount of motion that occurs when one segment of the body moves in relation to an adjacent segment is known as *range of motion (ROM)*.[1] When a segment of the body moves through its available ROM, all tissues in that region, including the bones, joint capsule, ligaments, tendons, intraarticular structures, muscles, nerves, fascia, and skin, may be affected. When all of these tissues function normally, full, normal ROM can be achieved; however, dysfunction of any of these tissues may contribute to a restriction of the available ROM. Many patients in rehabilitation seek medical treatment with an impairment of restricted ROM. To restore motion most effectively, the therapist must understand both the factors that influence normal motion and the factors that may contribute to motion restrictions.[2]

The impairment of restricted motion may contribute directly or indirectly to patient functional limitation and disability.[3-6] For example, restricted shoulder ROM may stop an individual from raising the arm above shoulder height and may prevent him or her from performing a job that involves overhead lifting. This impairment may also contribute indirectly to further pathology by causing impingement of the rotator cuff tendons, resulting in pain, weakness, and additional limitation of lifting capacity.

In the absence of pathology, ROM is generally limited by the lengthening or approximation of anatomical structures.[7] The integrity and flexibility of the soft tissues surrounding a joint, and the shape and relationship of the articular structures, affect the amount of motion that can occur. When a joint is at midrange, it can generally be moved with the application of a small force. This is because the collagen fibers in the connective tissue surrounding the joint are in a relaxed state, loosely oriented in various directions, and only sparsely cross-linked with other fibers, allowing them to distend readily. As the joint approaches terminal motion, the collagen fibers begin to align in the direction of the stress and start to straighten. Motion ceases at the normal terminal range when the fibers have achieved their maximum alignment or when soft or bony tissues approximate. For example, ankle dorsiflexion normally ceases when the fibers of the calf muscles have achieved maximum alignment and the muscles are fully extended, whereas elbow flexion normally ceases when the soft tissues of the anterior arm approximate with the soft tissues of the anterior forearm, and elbow extension ceases when the olecranon process of the ulna approximates with the olecranon fossa of the humerus (Fig. 5-1).

The normal ROM for all human joints has been measured and documented; however, these measures vary with the individual's age, sex, and health status.[8-10] Range of motion generally decreases with age and is greater in women than in men, although these differences vary with different motions and joints and are not consistent for all individuals.[11-19] Because of this variability, normal ROM is generally determined by comparison with the motion of the contralateral limb, if available, rather than by comparison with normative data. A motion is considered to be restricted when it is less than that available for the same segment on the contralateral side of the same individual. When a normal contralateral side is not available—as occurs, for example, with the spine—motion is considered to be restricted when it is less than normal for the individual's age and sex.

TYPES OF MOTION

Active and Passive Motion

The motion of body segments can be classified as either *active* or *passive*. Active motion is the movement produced by contraction of the muscles crossing a joint. Assessment of active ROM can provide information about an individual's functional abilities. Active motion may be restricted by muscle weakness, abnormal muscle tone, pain originating from the musculotendinous unit or other local structures, an inability or unwillingness of the subject to follow directions, or as the result of restrictions in passive ROM.[20]

Passive motion is movement produced entirely by an external force without voluntary muscle contraction by the subject. The external force may be produced by gravity, a machine, another individual, or another part of the subject's own body.[1] Passive motion may be restricted by shortening of the soft tissues, edema, adhesion, mechanical block, spinal disc herniation, or adverse neural tension.

Normal passive ROM is greater than normal active ROM when motion is limited by the distention or approximation of soft tissue, but both types of motion are equal when motion is limited by approximation of bone. For example, a few degrees of passive

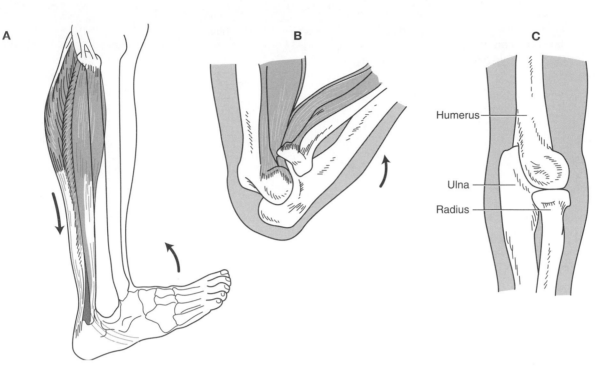

Figure 5-1. A, Ankle dorsiflexion limited by soft tissue distension. **B,** Elbow flexion limited by soft tissue approximation. **C,** Elbow extension limited by bone approximation.

ankle dorsiflexion motion are available beyond the limit of active motion because the limiting tissues are elastic and may be extended by an external force that is greater than that of the active muscles when at terminal active ROM. A few degrees of additional passive elbow flexion are available beyond the limit of active range because the limiting tissues are compressible by an external force greater than that of the active muscles in that position and because the approximating muscles may be less bulky when relaxed. This additional passive ROM may protect joint structures by absorbing external forces during activities, particularly those performed at or close to the end of active range.

Physiological and Accessory Motion

Physiological motion is the motion of one segment of the body relative to another segment. For example, physiological knee extension is the straightening of the knee that occurs when the leg moves away from the thigh. Accessory motion is the motion that occurs between the joint surfaces during normal physiological motion.[21,42,43] For example, anterior gliding of the

tibia on the femur is the accessory motion that occurs during physiological knee extension (Fig. 5-2). Accessory motions may be intraarticular, as in the prior example of anterior tibial gliding during knee extension, or extraarticular, as with the upward rotation of the scapula during physiological shoulder flexion (Fig. 5-3). Accessory motions cannot be performed actively in isolation from their associated physiological movement; however, they may be performed passively in isolation from their associated physiological movement.

Normal accessory motion is required for normal active and passive joint motion to occur. The direction of normal accessory motion depends on the shape of the articular surfaces and the direction of physiological motion. Concave joint surfaces require accessory gliding to be available in the direction of the associated physiological motion of the segment, whereas convex joint surfaces require accessory gliding to be available in the opposite direction of the associated physiological motion of the segment.[21] For example, the tibial plateau, which has a concave surface at the knee, glides anteriorly during knee extension when the tibia is moving anteriorly, and the

Figure 5-2. Accessory anterior gliding of the tibia on the femur during physiological knee extension.

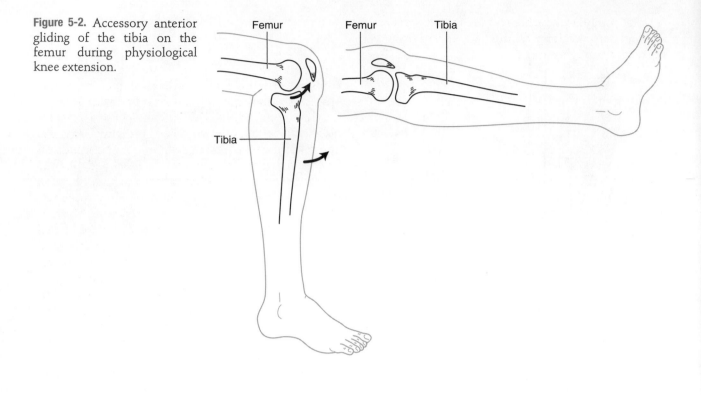

Figure 5-3. Extraarticular accessory motion, which is the upward rotation of the scapula that accompanies shoulder flexion.

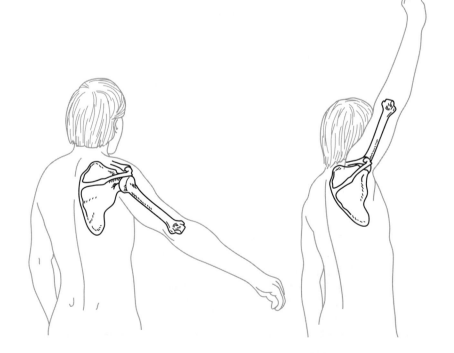

femoral condyles, which have convex surfaces at the knee, glide posteriorly during knee extension when the femur is moving anteriorly.

PATTERNS OF MOTION RESTRICTION

Capsular and Noncapsular Patterns of Motion Restriction

The restriction of motion at a joint can be classified as having either a *capsular* or a *noncapsular* pattern. A capsular pattern of restriction is the specific combination of motion loss that is caused by shortening of the joint capsule surrounding a joint. Each synovial joint has a unique capsular pattern of restriction. Capsular patterns generally include restrictions of motion in multiple directions. For example, the capsular pattern for the glenohumeral joint involves restriction of external rotation, abduction, internal rotation, and flexion to progressively smaller degrees. Capsular patterns of restriction may be caused by the effusion, fibrosis, or inflammation commonly associated with degenerative joint disease, arthritis, immobilization, and acute trauma.

A noncapsular pattern of restriction is a combination of motion loss that does not follow the capsular pattern. A noncapsular pattern of motion loss may be caused by ligamentous adhesion, an internal derangement, or an extraarticular lesion. Ligamentous adhesion will limit motion in the directions that stretch the adhered ligament. For example, an adhesion of the talofibular ligament after an ankle sprain will restrict ankle inversion because this motion places the adhered ligament on stretch; however, this adhesion will not alter the motion of the ankle in other directions. Internal derangement, the displacement of loose fragments within a joint, will generally limit motion only in the direction that compresses the fragment. For example, a cartilage fragment in the knee will generally limit knee extension but will not limit knee flexion. Extraarticular lesions, such as muscle adhesions, hematomas, cysts, or inflamed bursae, may limit motion in the direction of either stretch or compression, depending on the nature of the lesion. For example, adhesion of the quadriceps muscle to the shaft of the femur will limit stretching of the muscle, while a popliteal cyst will limit compression of the popliteal area. Both of these lesions will restrict motion in the noncapsular pattern of restricted knee flexion, with full, painless knee extension.

TISSUES THAT CAN RESTRICT MOTION

Contractile and Noncontractile Tissues

Any of the musculoskeletal tissues in the area of a motion restriction may contribute to that restriction. These tissues are most readily classified as *contractile* or *noncontractile* (Table 5-1). Contractile tissue is composed of the musculotendinous unit, which includes the muscle, the musculotendinous junction, the tendon, and the tendon's interface with bone. Skeletal muscle is considered to be contractile because it can contract by forming cross-bridges of the myosin proteins with the actin proteins within its fibers.[24] Tendons and their attachments to bone are considered contractile because contracting muscles apply tension directly to these structures. When a muscle contracts, it applies tension to its tendons, causing the bones to which it is attached and the surrounding tissues to move through the available active ROM. When all the components of the musculotendinous unit and the noncontractile tissues are functioning normally, the available active ROM will be within normal limits for the age and sex of the subject. Injury or dysfunction of contractile tissue generally results in a restriction of active ROM in the direction of movement produced by contraction of the musculotendinous unit. Dysfunction of contractile tissue may also result in pain or weakness on resisted testing of the musculotendinous unit. For example, a tear in the anterior tibialis muscle or tendon can restrict active dorsiflexion at the ankle and reduce the force generated by resisted testing of ankle dorsiflexion, but this lesion is not

TABLE 5-1	Contractile and Noncontractile Sources of Motion Restrictions	
Contractile tissue	**Noncontractile tissue**
Muscle	Skin
Musculotendinous junction	Ligament
Tendon	Bursa
Tendinous interface with bone	Capsule Articular cartilage
	Intervertebral disc
	Peripheral nerve
	Dura mater

likely to alter passive plantar flexion, dorsiflexion, ROM, or active plantar flexion strength.

All tissues that are not components of the musculotendinous unit are considered noncontractile. Noncontractile tissues include skin, fascia, scar tissue, ligament, bursa, capsule, articular cartilage, bone, intervertebral disc, nerve, and dura mater. When the noncontractile tissues in an area are functioning normally, the passive ROM of the segments in that area will be within normal limits. Injury or dysfunction of noncontractile tissue can cause a restriction of the passive ROM of the joints in the area of the tissue in question and may also contribute to restriction of active ROM.[25] The direction, degree, and nature of the motion restriction depends on the type of noncontractile tissue involved, the type of tissue dysfunction, and the severity of involvement. For example, adhesive capsulitis of the shoulder, which involves shortening of the glenohumeral joint capsule and elimination of the inferior axillary fold, will restrict both passive and active shoulder ROM in a capsular pattern[26-31] (Fig. 5-4).

PATHOLOGIES THAT CAN CAUSE MOTION RESTRICTIONS

Contracture

Motion may be restricted if any of the soft tissue structures in an area have become shortened. Such soft tissue shortening, known as a *contracture,* may occur in contractile or noncontractile tissues.[32,33] A contracture may be caused by immobilization resulting from external splinting provided by a cast or splint, for example. Contractures are also caused by imbalance of muscle power resulting from weakness, as could be caused by poliomyelitis or from spasticity from central, nervous system (CNS) damage, for example.[33,34] It has been proposed that immobilization results in contracture because it allows anomalous cross-links to form between collagen fibers and it causes fluid to be lost from fibrous connective tissue, including tendon, capsule, ligament, and fascia.[34-36] Anomalous cross-links can develop when tissues remain stationary because, in the absence of normal stress and motion, fibers remain in contact with each other for prolonged periods and start to adhere at their points of interception. These cross-links may prevent normal alignment of the collagen fibers when motion is attempted. They also increase the stress required to stretch the tissue, limit tissue extension, and result in contracture (Fig. 5-5). Fluid loss can also impair normal fiber gliding, causing collagen fibrils to have closer contact and limiting tissue extension.[32]

The risk of contracture formation in response to immobilization is increased when the tissue has been injured because scar tissue, which is formed during the proliferation phase of healing, tends to have poor fiber alignment and a high degree of cross-linking between

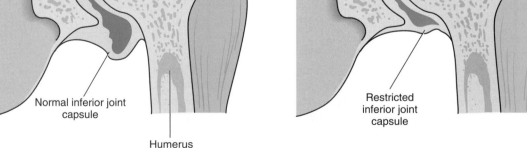

Figure 5-4. Joint capsule shortening and adhesion restricting shoulder range of motion.

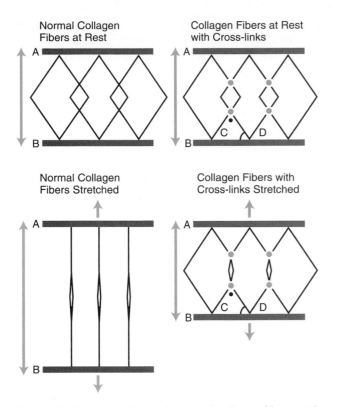

Figure 5-5. Normal collagen fibers and collagen fibers with cross-links. (From Woo SL, Matthews JV, Akeson WH et al: Connective tissue response to immobility. Correlative study of biomechanical measurements of normal and immobilized rabbit knees, *Arthritis and Rheumatism,* May-June 18(3):262, 1975. This material is used by permission of Wiley-Liss, Inc., a subsidiary of John Wiley & Sons, Inc.)

its fibers. Restriction of motion after an injury may be further aggravated if a concurrent problem, such as sepsis or ongoing trauma, amplifies the inflammatory response and causes excessive scarring.[33]

A persistent shortening of a muscle that is resistant to stretch is known as a *muscle contracture.* A muscle contracture can be caused by prolonged muscle spasm, guarding, muscle imbalance, muscle disease, or ischemic muscle necrosis, and by immobilization.[33] A muscle contracture may limit both active and passive motion of the joint(s) that the muscle crosses and can also cause deformity of the joint(s) normally controlled by the muscle.

Edema

Normally, a joint capsule contains fluid but is not fully distended. This allows the capsule to fold or distend when the joint moves, altering its size and shape as required for movement through full ROM. If excessive fluid forms inside a joint capsule, a condition known as *intraarticular edema,* the joint capsule becomes more distended, limiting its folding and further distention and potentially restricting both passive and active joint motion in a capsular pattern. For example, intraarticular edema in the knee will produce the capsular pattern of knee flexion being more limited than knee extension.

Accumulation of fluid outside of the joint, a condition known as *extraarticular edema,* may also restrict active and passive motion by causing soft tissue approximation to occur earlier in the range. Extraarticular edema generally restricts motion in a noncapsular pattern. For example, edema in the calf muscle may restrict knee flexion ROM while having no effect on knee extension ROM.

Adhesion

Adhesion is the abnormal joining of parts to each other.[37] Adhesion may occur between different types of tissue for various reasons and frequently causes restriction of motion. During the healing process, scar tissue can adhere to surrounding structures, and fibrofatty tissue may proliferate inside joints and adhere between intraarticular structures as it matures into scar tissue.[38] Prolonged joint immobilization, even in the absence of local injury, can also cause the synovial membrane surrounding the joint to adhere to the cartilage inside the joint. Adhesions can affect both the quality and the quantity of joint motion. For example, with adhesive capsulitis, not only does the joint capsule shorten, it also adheres to the synovial membrane. This limits motion and reduces, or even obliterates, the space between the cartilage and the synovial membrane, thus blocking normal synovial fluid nutrition and causing articular cartilage degeneration that can alter the quality of joint motion.[33]

Mechanical Block

Motion can be mechanically blocked by bone or fragments of articular cartilage, or by tears in intraarticular discs or menisci. Degenerative joint disease or malunion of bony segments following fracture healing frequently results in a bony block that restricts joint motion in one or more directions (Fig. 5-6). This is because these pathologies cause bone to

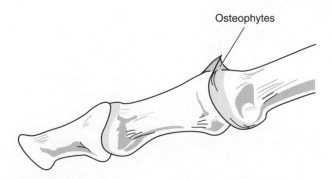

Osteophytes

Figure 5-6. Osteophytes blocking metatarsophalangeal extension.

hypertrophy in or around the joints. Loose bodies or fragments of articular cartilage, caused by avascular necrosis or trauma, can also alter the mechanics of the joint, causing "locking" in various positions, pain, and other dysfunctions.[33] Tears in intraarticular fibrocartilaginous discs and menisci caused by high-force traumatic injury or by repetitive low-force strain generally block motion in one direction only.

Spinal Disc Herniation

Spinal disc herniation may result in direct blockage of spinal motion if a portion of the discal material becomes trapped in a facet joint or if the disc compresses a spinal nerve root where it passes through the vertebral foramen. Other pathologies associated with spinal disc herniation, including inflammation, hypertrophic changes, decreased disc height, and pain, may further limit spinal motion. Inflammation about the spinal facet joint or herniated segment can limit motion by narrowing the vertebral foramen and compressing the nerve root. Hypertrophic changes at the vertebral margins and facet joints, as well as decreased disc height, also narrow the vertebral foramen, making the nerve root more vulnerable to compression. Pain may limit motion by causing involuntary muscle spasms or by causing the individual to restrict movements voluntarily.

Adverse Neural Tension

Under normal circumstances, the nervous system, including the spinal cord and the peripheral nerves, must adapt to both mechanical and physiological stresses.[39] For example, during forward flexion of the trunk, the nervous system must adapt to the increased length of the spinal column without interruption of transmission.[40] Adverse neural tension is the presence of abnormal responses produced from peripheral nervous system structures when their ROM and stretch capabilities are tested.[41] Adverse neural tension may result from major or minor nerve injury or may be caused indirectly by extraneural adhesions that result in tethering of the nerve to surrounding structures. Nerve injury may be the result of trauma due to friction, compression, or stretch. It may also be caused by disease, ischemia, inflammation, or a disruption in the axonal transport system.[42] Ischemia can be caused by pressure from extravascular fluid, blood, disc material, or soft tissues with decreased mobility.

Adverse neural tension is most commonly due to restriction of nerve motion. A number of structural features predispose nerve motion to restriction. Nerve motion is commonly restricted where nerves pass through tunnels, as, for example, where the median nerve passes through the carpal tunnel or where the spinal nerves pass through the intervertebral foramina. Peripheral nerve motion is also likely to be restricted at points where the nerves branch; for example, where the ulnar nerve splits at the hook of the hammate or where the sciatic nerve splits into the peroneal and tibial nerves in the thigh. Places where the system is relatively fixed are also points of vulnerability; for example, at the dura mater at L4 or where the common peroneal nerve passes the head of the fibula. The system is also relatively fixed where nerves are close to unyielding interfaces; for example, where the cords of the brachial plexus pass over the first rib or the greater occipital nerve passes through the fascia in the posterior skull.[41]

Weakness

When muscles are too weak to generate the force required to move a segment of the body through its normal ROM, active ROM will be restricted. Muscle weakness may be the result of contractile tissue changes such as atrophy or injury, poor transmission along the motor nerves, or poor synaptic transmission at the neuromuscular junction.

Other Factors

Motion restrictions may also be caused by many other factors, including pain, psychological factors, and tone. Pain may restrict active or passive motion, depending on whether contractile or noncontractile structures are the source of the pain. Psychological factors such as fear, poor motivation, or poor comprehension are most likely to cause restriction of only active ROM. Tone abnormalities, particularly hypotonia or flaccidity, may also impair the control of active muscle contractions and may thus limit active ROM.

ASSESSMENT OF MOTION RESTRICTIONS

When a patient seeks medical treatment for complaints of limited motion, an examination of the mobility of all the structures in the area of the restriction, including the joints, muscles, intra- and extraarticular structures, and nerves, should be made. Evaluation of all these findings is required to determine the pathophysiology underlying the motion restriction, identify the tissues limiting motion, and assess the severity and irritability of the dysfunction.[43] This complete examination and evaluation will direct treatment to the appropriate structure(s) and will facilitate selection of the optimal intervention to meet goals. Ongoing assessment of outcomes is required to modify treatment appropriately in response to changes in the dysfunction. This will accelerate and optimize progress toward the treatment goals.[22,23,42] A variety of tools and methods are available for quantitative and qualitative assessment of motion and motion restrictions.

Quantitative Measures

Goniometers, tape measures, and various types of inclinometers are commonly used in the clinical setting for quantitative assessment of ROM. These tools provide objective and moderately reliable measures of ROM, and are practical and convenient for clinical use. Radiographs, photographs, electrogoniometers, flexometers, and plumb lines may be used to increase the accuracy and reliability of ROM measurement. These additional tools are often used for research purposes but are not available in most clinical settings. The different tools provide different information about the available or demonstrated ROM. Most tools, including goniometers, inclinometers, and electrogoniometers, provide measures of the angle, or change in angle, between body segments, whereas other tools, such as the tape measure, provide measures of the change in length of body segments.[44]

Qualitative Measures

Qualitative assessment techniques such as soft tissue palpation, accessory motion testing, and end-feel provide valuable information about motion restrictions that can help to guide treatment. Soft tissue palpation may be used to assess the mobility of skin or scar tissue, local tenderness, the presence of muscle spasm, skin temperature, and the quality of edema. It is also used to identify bony landmarks before quantitative measurement of ROM.

Test Methods and Rationale

Active, resisted, passive, and accessory motion, and neural tension testing can be used to determine which tissues are restricting motion and the nature of the pathologies contributing to a motion restriction.

Active range of motion

Active ROM is tested by asking the subject to move the desired segment to its limit in a given direction. The subject is asked to report any symptoms or sensations, such as pain or tingling, experienced during this activity. The maximum motion is measured, and the quality or coordination of the motion and any associated symptoms are noted. Testing of active ROM yields information regarding the subject's ability and willingness to move functionally and is generally most useful for assessing the integrity of contractile structures.

The following questions should be noted when testing active ROM:
1. Is the ROM symmetrical, normal, restricted, or excessive?
2. What is the quality of the available motion?
3. Are any signs or symptoms associated with the motion?

Resisted muscle testing

Resisted muscle testing is performed by having the subject contract his or her muscle against a resistance strong enough to prevent movement.[45,46] Resisted muscle tests provide information about the ability of a muscle to produce force. This information may help determine whether contractile or noncontractile tissues are the source of a motion restriction since muscle weakness is commonly the cause of a loss of active ROM.[47]

Cyriax[25] has identified four possible responses to resisted muscle testing and has proposed interpretations for each of these responses (Table 5-2).

TABLE 5-2	Cyriax's Interpretation of Resisted Muscle Tests

Finding	Interpretation
1. Strong and painless	No apparent pathology of contractile or nervous tissue
2. Strong and painful	Minor lesion of musculotendinous unit
3. Weak and painless	Complete rupture of the musculotendinous unit Neurological lesion
4. Weak and painful	Partial disruption of the musculotendinous unit Inhibition by pain due to pathology such as inflammation, fracture, or neoplasm Concurrent neurological deficit

From Cyriax J: *Textbook of Orthopedic Medicine,* ed 6, Baltimore, 1975, Williams & Wilkins.

When the force is strong and there is no pain with testing, this indicates no pathology of contractile or nervous tissues. When the force is strong but pain is produced with testing, this usually indicates a minor structural lesion of the musculotendinous unit. When the force is weak and there is no pain with testing, this indicates a complete rupture of the musculotendinous unit or a neurological deficit. When the force is weak but pain is produced with testing, this indicates a minor structural lesion of the musculotendinous unit with a concurrent neurological deficit or inhibition of contraction resulting from pain caused by pathology such as inflammation, fracture, or neoplasm.

Passive range of motion

Passive ROM is assessed by the tester moving the segment to its limit in a given direction. During passive ROM testing, the quantity of available motion is measured, and the quality of motion and symptoms associated with motion and the end-feel are noted. End-feel is the quality of the resistance at the limit of passive motion felt by the clinician. An end-feel may be normal (physiological) or abnormal (pathological). A normal end-feel exists when passive ROM is full and the normal anatomy of the joint stops movement. Certain end-feels are normal for some joints but may be pathological at other joints or at abnormal points in the range. Other end-feels are abnormal if felt at any point in the motion of any joint. Normal and abnormal end-feels for most joints are listed in Table 5-3.[20,42,47] Passive ROM is normally limited by stretching of soft tissues or by the opposition of soft tissues or bone and may be restricted as a result of soft tissue contracture, mechanical block, or edema. The amount of passive motion available and the quality of the end-feel can assist in the determination of the structures at fault and the nature of the pathologies contributing to the motion restriction.[47]

Combining the findings of active range of motion assessment, resisted muscle testing, and passive range of motion

Combining the findings of active ROM, resisted muscle testing, and passive ROM can assist in differentiating between restrictions of motion caused by contractile and noncontractile structures. For example, if active elbow flexion is restricted, the elbow flexors are weak and passive elbow flexion range is normal, then the structures limiting motion are most likely to be contractile. In contrast, if both active and passive elbow flexion ROM are restricted and the strength of the elbow flexors is normal, then noncontractile tissues are probably involved. Other combinations of abnormality may indicate muscle substitution during active ROM testing, psychological factors limiting motion, the use of poor testing technique, or pain inhibiting muscle contraction (Table 5-4). To definitely implicate a particular pathology or a particular structure, the findings of these noninvasive tests may need to be correlated with the findings of other diagnostic

TABLE 5-3 **Descriptions and Examples of Different Types of End-Feels**

Type	Description	Examples	Comments
Hard	Abrupt halt to movement when two hard surfaces meet	Normal: elbow extension Abnormal: result of malunion fracture or heterotopic ossification	May be normal or abnormal
Firm	Leathery, firm resistance when range is limited by joint capsule	Normal: shoulder rotation Abnormal: result of adhesive capsulitis	May be normal or abnormal
Soft	Gradual onset of resistance when soft tissue approximates or when range is limited by length of muscle	Approximation: knee flexion Muscle length: cervical side bending	May be normal or abnormal, depending on tissue bulk and muscle length
Empty	Movement stopped by subject prior to tester's feeling resistance	Passive shoulder abduction stopped by subject due to pain	Always abnormal
Spasm	Movement stopped abruptly by reflex muscle contraction	Passive ankle dorsiflexion in subject with spasticity due to upper motor neuron lesion Active trunk flexion in subject with acute low back injury	Always abnormal
Springy block	Rebound felt and seen at end of range	Caused by loose body or displaced meniscus	Always abnormal
Boggy	Resistance by fluid	Knee joint effusion	Always abnormal
Extended	No resistance felt within the normal range expected for the particular joint	Joint instability or hypermobility	Always abnormal

From Cote L, Crutcher MD: The basal ganglia. In Kandel ER, Schwartz JH, Jessell TM, eds: *Principles of Neural Science*, ed 3, New York, 1991, Elsevier.

TABLE 5-4 **Combining the Findings of Active Range of Motion, Resisted Muscle Testing, and Passive Range of Motion Assessment**

Active range of motion	Resisted testing	Passive range of motion	Interpretation
Normal	Normal	Normal	No pathology restricting motion
Normal	Normal	Abnormal	Pathology beyond terminal active range of motion Poor testing technique for passive range of motion
Normal	Abnormal	Abnormal	Poor testing technique for passive range of motion Strength at least 3/5 but less than 5/5
Normal	Abnormal	Normal	Strength at least 3/5 but less than 5/5
Abnormal	Normal	Abnormal	Noncontractile tissue restricting motion
Abnormal	Abnormal	Normal	Contractile tissue injury restricting motion
Abnormal	Normal	Normal	Poor testing techniques for active range of motion or psychological factors limiting active range of motion
Abnormal	Abnormal	Abnormal	Contractile and noncontractile tissues restricting motion

procedures such as radiographic imaging, diagnostic injection, arthroscopic exploration, and blood tests.

Passive accessory motion

Passive accessory motion is tested using joint mobilization treatment techniques.[5,13] The clinician can use these treatment techniques to assess the motion of joint surfaces and the extensibility of major ligaments and portions of the joint capsule. During accessory motion testing the clinician notes qualitatively if the motion felt is greater than, less than, or similar to the normal accessory motion expected for that joint in that plane in the particular individual and if pain is produced with testing.[22,48-50] Accessory motion testing may provide information about joint mechanics not available from other tests. For example, a reduction of accessory gliding of the glenohumeral joint when passive shoulder flexion is normal may indicate that glenohumeral joint motion is restricted, and the motion of the scapulothoracic joint is excessive.

Muscle length

Muscle length is tested by passively positioning muscle attachments as far apart as possible to elongate the muscle in the direction opposite to its action.[45] The testing of muscle length by this technique will produce valid results only if pathology of the noncontractile structures or muscle tone does not limit joint motion. When testing the length of muscles that cross only one joint, the passive ROM available at that joint will indicate the length of the muscle. For example, the length of the soleus muscle can be assessed by measurement of passive dorsiflexion ROM at the ankle. To test the length of a muscle that crosses two or more joints, the muscle must first be elongated across one of the joints and then that joint must be held in that position while the muscle is elongated as far as possible across the other joint that it crosses.[45] The passive ROM available at the second joint will indicate the length of the muscle. For example, the length of the gastrocnemius muscle can be tested by first elongating it across the knee, by placing the knee in full extension, and then measuring the amount of passive dorsiflexion available at the ankle. It is essential that multijoint muscles be fully extended across one joint before measurement

at the other joint to obtain a valid test of muscle length.

Adverse neural tension

Adverse neural tension is usually tested by passively placing neural structures in their position of maximum length. Evaluation is based on comparison with the contralateral side, comparison with norms, and assessment of the symptoms produced in the position of maximum length.

Adverse neural tension tests include the passive straight leg raise (PSLR, Lasegue's sign), prone knee bend, passive neck flexion, and upper limb tension tests. The PSLR is the most commonly used neural tension test and is intended to test for adverse neural tension in the sciatic nerve.

Because adverse neural tension tests may also provoke symptoms in the presence of pathologies associated with the muscles or joints, it is recommended that maneuvers that apply tension to the nervous system but do not additionally stress the muscles or joints be used to differentiate the source of symptoms with this type of test. For example, the PSLR test can provoke symptoms in the presence of pathologies associated with the hamstring muscles or the sacroiliac, iliofemoral, or lumbar spinal facet joints. Therefore at the onset of symptoms with this test, additional tension can be applied to the nervous system by passively dorsiflexing the ankle to increase the tension on the sciatic nerve distally or by passively flexing the neck to tighten the dura proximally. If these maneuvers increase the patient's symptoms, adverse neural tension rather than joint or muscle pathology is probably the cause of symptoms.[41]

Contraindications and Precautions to Range of Motion Techniques

Range of motion techniques are contraindicated when motion of a part may disrupt the healing process. However, some controlled motion within the range, speed, and tolerance of the patient may be beneficial during the acute recovery stage or immediately following acute tears, fractures, and surgery. Limited, controlled motion is recommended to reduce the severity of adhesion, contracture, decreased circulation, and loss of strength associated with complete immobilization.[33,47]

Contraindications

Active and passive assessment techniques are contraindicated:

1. In the region of a dislocation or an unhealed fracture.
2. Immediately following surgical procedures to tendons, ligaments, muscle, joint capsule, or skin.

Precautions

Caution should be observed when performing active or passive ROM techniques when motion to the part might aggravate the condition. This may occur:

1. When there is an infection or an inflammatory process in or around the joint.
2. In patients taking pain medication who may not be able to respond appropriately.
3. In the presence of osteoporosis or any condition that causes bone fragility.
4. With hypermobile joints or joints prone to subluxation.
5. In painful conditions where the techniques might reinforce the severity of the symptoms.
6. In patients with hemophilia.
7. In the region of a hematoma.
8. If bony ankylosis is suspected.
9. Immediately after an injury where there has been a disruption of soft tissue.
10. In the presence of myositis ossificans.

In addition, neural tension testing should be performed with caution in the presence of inflammatory conditions; spinal cord symptoms; tumors; signs of nerve root compression; unrelenting night pain; neurological symptoms such as weakness, reflex changes, or loss of sensation; recent paresthesia or anesthesia; and reflex sympathetic dystrophy.[39,41,42] Detailed contraindications and precautions for each specific neural tension test are provided in other texts devoted to the assessment and treatment of adverse neural tension.[41]

TREATMENT APPROACHES FOR MOTION RESTRICTIONS

Stretching

Currently, most noninvasive interventions for reestablishing soft tissue ROM involve stretching. Clinical

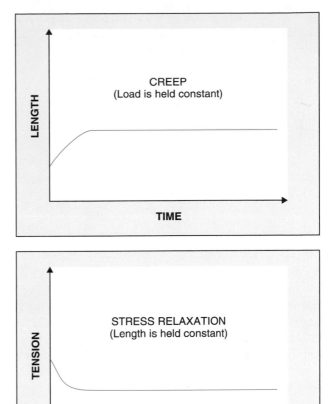

Figure 5-7. The relationships of time, tension, and length during creep and stress relaxation.

and experimental evidence demonstrates that stretching can increase motion; however, the results may not be consistent and the recommended protocols vary.[51] When a stretch is applied to connective tissues, within the elastic limit, over time the tissues may demonstrate creep, stress relaxation, and plastic deformation.[52] Creep is transient lengthening or deformation with the application of a fixed load. Stress relaxation is a decrease in the amount of force required over time to hold a given length (Fig. 5-7). Creep and stress relaxation can occur in soft tissue in a short time and are thought to be dependent on the viscous components of the tissue.[53-55] Plastic

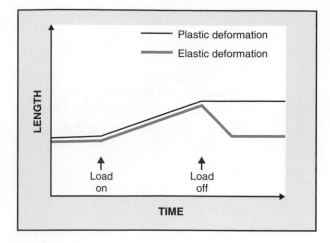

Figure 5-8. Plastic deformation versus elastic deformation.

applied for a prolonged time to cause plastic deformation. The length of time necessary to determine that no further ROM gains are possible is not known and is probably dependent on the specific pathology or pathologies causing the restriction and its duration. In addition to time, the force direction and speed of the stretch must be controlled to produce optimal lengthening of the appropriate structures without damaging tissue or causing hypermobility.

Many stretching techniques to increase soft tissue length have been described. The most common types of stretching are passive stretching, proprioceptive neuromuscular facilitation (PNF), and ballistic stretching (Table 5-5). To perform a passive stretch, the limb is held passively in a position in which the subject feels a mild stretch. The force of gravity on the involved body part, the force of other limbs, or another individual can apply passive stretch. External devices such as progressive end range splints, serial casts, or dynamic splints may also be used to stretch tissue passively. Although optimal parameters for passively stretching normal and

deformation is the elongation produced under loading that remains after the load is removed (Fig. 5-8). After plastic deformation, tissue will have a permanent increase in length. A controlled stretch must be

---

TABLE **5-5** **Types of Stretching**

Method	Description	Examples	Comments
1. Passive	Limb held passively in a position in which the subject feels a mild stretch	Manual passive stretching Progressive end range splinting Dynamic splinting	Pain perception is a factor[*] Results in no motor learning Optimal parameters have not been established[†‡]
2. Proprioceptive neuromuscular facilitation[‡]	Active muscle contraction followed by muscle relaxation in conjunction with passive stretch	Contract-relax Hold-relax Subject resists and aids	Requires the assistance of an individual proficient in the technique May result in motor learning
3. Ballistic	Active, quick, short-amplitude movements at the end of the subject's available range of motion	Active stretching with "bounce" at end of range	Not generally used or recommended because this may increase tissue tightness by activating the stretch reflex in normal and spastic muscles

[*]Magnusson SP, Simonsen EB, Aagaard P, et al: A mechanism for altered flexibility in human skeletal muscle, *J Physiol* 497(1):291-298, 1996.
[†]Zito M, Driver D, Parker C et al: Lasting effects of one bout of two 15-second passive stretches on ankle dorsiflexion range of motion, *JOSPT* 26:214-221, 1997.
[‡]Bandy WD, Irion JM, Briggler M: The effect of time and frequency of static stretching on flexibility of the hamstring muscles, *Phys Ther* 77:1090-1096, 1997.

pathological tissues have not been established, it is generally recommended that low-load, prolonged forces be applied to minimize the risk of adverse effects.

Manipulation of a joint while the subject is anesthetized also involves passive stretching of the soft tissues to increase ROM. Manipulation under anesthesia can produce a rapid increase in ROM because high forces that would otherwise be painful or cause muscles to spasm may be applied. These high forces may cause greater increases in soft tissue length and may tear adhesions to increase motion; however, the risk of damaging structures or exacerbating inflammation may be greater with such techniques than with stretching while the subject is fully conscious.

Proprioceptive neuromuscular facilitation techniques for muscle stretching inhibit contraction of the muscle being stretched and facilitate contraction of its opponent.[56] This is achieved by having the subject actively contract and then voluntarily relax the muscles to be stretched before the application of the stretching force. PNF techniques have the advantage over other stretching techniques of including a motor learning component from the repeated active muscle contractions; however, their use is frequently limited by the requirement that a skilled individual help the patient perform the technique.

Ballistic stretching is a technique in which the subject performs short, bouncing movements at the end of the available range. Although some people attempt to stretch in this manner, ballistic stretching is not generally used or recommended, because it may increase tissue tightness by activating the stretch reflex.[57]

Motion

The formation of contractures is a time-related process that may be inhibited by motion.[35] Motion can inhibit contracture formation by physically disrupting the adhesions between gross structures and/or by limiting intermolecular cross-linking. Active or passive motion also stretches tissues, promotes their lubrication, and may also alter their metabolic activity.[34] Because active ROM may be

contraindicated during early stages of healing, particularly when contractile tissue is damaged, passive motion may be used to limit contracture formation at this stage. For example, continuous passive motion (CPM) can be used to prevent motion loss after joint trauma or surgery. In addition to inhibiting the formation of contractures and adhesions, CPM has been shown to accelerate healing, improve the orientation of collagen fibers, and inhibit edema formation.[58-61]

Surgery

Although the noninvasive approaches of stretching and motion frequently resolve or prevent motion restrictions, in some cases these approaches are not effective and surgery may be required to optimize motion. Surgery will be necessary if motion is restricted by a mechanical block, particularly if the mechanical block is bony. In such cases, the surgical procedure removes some or all of the tissue blocking motion. Surgery may also be required if stretching techniques cannot lengthen a contracture adequately or if the functional length of a tendon is decreased due to hypertonicity. For example, Z-plasty procedures are frequently performed to lengthen the Achilles tendon in children with limited dorsiflexion caused by congenital plantar flexion contractures or by hypertonicity of the plantar flexor muscles. Z-plasty is generally preformed when it can be expected to permit a more functional gait than is achieved with noninvasive techniques alone.[9] Surgical procedures to increase ROM are also frequently performed in adults. For example, surgical release may be performed to restore motion limited by a Dupuytren's contracture, and tenotomy may be performed when tendon length limits motion. Surgery may also be performed to release adhesions and lengthen scars that have formed after prolonged immobilization. For example, patients with extensive burns who have received limited medical intervention frequently develop contractures that cannot be stretched sufficiently to allow full function and therefore require surgical release. Surgery is more commonly required to release adhesions that form after injury if scarring is exaggerated by prolonged inflammation or infection.

THE ROLE OF PHYSICAL AGENTS IN THE TREATMENT OF MOTION RESTRICTIONS

Although physical agents alone are generally not sufficient to reverse or prevent motion restrictions, they may be used as adjuncts to the treatment of such impairments. Physical agents combined with other appropriate treatment can enhance the functional recovery associated with regaining normal motion. Physical agents are generally used as components of the treatment of motion restrictions because they can increase soft tissue extensibility, control inflammation, control pain, and facilitate motion.

Increase Soft Tissue Extensibility

Physical agents that increase tissue temperature may be used as components of the treatment of motion restriction because they can increase soft tissue extensibility, thereby decreasing the force required to increase tissue length and decreasing the risk of injury during the stretching procedure.[62-64] Applying physical agents to soft tissue before prolonged stretching can alter the viscoelasticity of the fibers, allowing plastic deformation to occur.[65,66] To achieve the maximum benefit from the use of physical agents that increase soft tissue extensibility, agents that increase superficial tissue temperature, such as those described in Chapter 6, should be used before stretching superficial tissues, whereas agents that increase deep tissue temperature, such as ultrasound and diathermy, should be used before stretching deep soft tissues.

Control Inflammation and Adhesion Formation

A number of physical agents, particularly cryotherapy and certain types of electrical currents, are thought to control inflammation and its associated signs and symptoms after tissue injury.[67,68] Controlling inflammation may help to prevent the development of motion restrictions by limiting the formation of edema during the acute inflammatory stage and thereby limiting the degree of immobilization. Controlling the severity and duration of inflammation also limits the duration and extent of the proliferative response and may thus limit the formation of adhesions during tissue healing.

Control Pain During Stretching

Many physical agents, including thermotherapy, cryotherapy, and electrical currents, can help to control pain. This effect may assist in the treatment of motion restrictions because, if pain is well controlled, tissues may be stretched for a longer period, which may increase tissue length more effectively. If pain is controlled, motion may also be initiated sooner after injury, limiting the loss of motion caused by immobilization.

Facilitate Motion

Some physical agents facilitate motion and thus assist in the treatment of motion restrictions. Electrical stimulation of the motor nerves of innervated muscles or direct electrical stimulation of denervated muscle can make muscles contract. These muscle contractions may complement motion produced by normal physiological contractions or substitute for such contractions if the subject does not or cannot move independently. Water may also facilitate motion since it provides buoyancy to an immersed body to assist with motion against gravity. The buoyancy of water may prove particularly beneficial in assisting patients with active ROM restrictions caused by contractile tissue weakness.

▶ *Clinical Case Studies* ◀

The following case studies summarize the concepts of motion restrictions discussed in this chapter. Based on the scenario presented, an evaluation of the clinical findings and goals of treatment are proposed. These are followed by a discussion of the factors to be considered in treatment selection.

Case 1

TR is a 45-year-old male who has been referred to physical therapy with a diagnosis of a right L5, S1 radiculopathy. He complains of constant mild to moderately severe right low back pain that radiates to his right buttock and lateral thigh after sitting for more than 20 minutes and that is relieved to some degree by walking or lying down. He reports no numbness, tingling, or weakness of the lower extremities. The pain started about 6 weeks ago, the morning after TR spent a day stacking firewood, at which time he woke up with severe low back and right lower extremity pain down to his lateral calf. He also had difficulty standing up straight. He has had similar problems in the past; however, they have always fully resolved after a couple of days of bed rest and a few aspirins. TR first saw his doctor regarding his present problem 5 weeks ago, and at that time he was prescribed a nonsteroidal antiinflammatory drug and a muscle relaxant and was told to take it easy. His symptoms improved to their current level over the following 2 weeks but have not changed since that time. He has also not been able to return to his job as a telephone installer since the onset of symptoms 6 weeks ago. An MRI scan last week showed a mild posterolateral disc bulge at L5-S1 on the right. The patient has had no prior physical therapy for his back problem. The objective exam is significant for a 50% restriction of lumbar active ROM in forward bending and right side bending, both of which cause increased right low back and lower extremity pain. Left side bending decreases the patient's pain. Passive straight leg raising is 35% (on the right, limited by right lower extremity pain), and 60% (on the left, limited by hamstring tightness). Palpation reveals stiffness and tenderness to right unilateral posterior-anterior pressure at L5-S1 and no notable areas of hypermobility. All other tests, including lower extremity sensation, strength, and reflexes, are within normal limits.

EVALUATION OF THE CLINICAL FINDINGS

This patient presents with the impairments of restricted lumbar forward-bending and right side-bending motion, pain, restricted lumbar nerve root mobility on the right, as indicated by the restricted passive straight leg raising test, and bulging of the L5-S1 disc. These impairments have resulted in a limitation of sitting tolerance and an inability to return to work.

PREFERRED PRACTICE PATTERN

Impaired Joint Mobility, Motor Function, Muscle Performance, Range of Motion, and Reflex Integrity Associated With Spinal Disorders, (4F)

PLAN OF CARE

The anticipated goals of treatment at this time are to reduce pain and increase sitting tolerance sufficiently for the patient to be able to return to limited duty work. The long-term goals of treatment are to fully alleviate pain, return lumbar range of motion to normal, increase passive straight leg raising and sitting tolerance to within normal limits, and have the patient return to his full work duties.

ASSESSMENT REGARDING SELECTION OF THE OPTIMAL TREATMENT

The optimal treatment for this patient would separate the disc spaces and/or reduce disc protrusion, thus decreasing compression on the nerve root and allowing improved, pain free motion. Therefore the intervention of choice at this time is traction. The appropriate type of traction and the parameters of treatment are discussed in Chapter 10.

Case 2

MP is a 40-year-old female diagnosed with adhesive capsulitis of the left shoulder. She reports that her shoulder first began to hurt about 6 months ago without any apparent cause. Although the pain has almost completely resolved since that time, her shoulder has also gradually become more stiff, preventing her from reaching up to brush her hair and from reaching behind herself to zip up her skirts. The objective evaluation is significant for restricted ROM of the left shoulder as follows:

Active Range of Motion	Right	Left
Flexion	170°	100°
Abduction	170°	80°
Hand behind back	Central thoracolumbar junction	Left sacroiliac joint

Continued

▶ *Clinical Case Studies—cont'd* ◀

Passive Range of Motion	Right	Left
Internal rotation	90°	50°
External rotation	80°	10°

Glenohumeral passive inferior and posterior glide are both restricted on the left. MP has had no prior treatment for this problem.

EVALUATION OF THE CLINICAL FINDINGS

This patient presents impairments of restricted active and passive motion of her left shoulder in a capsular pattern, reducing her ability to perform activities of daily living, including grooming and dressing. This patient's signs and symptoms and their duration indicate that the problem has probably progressed to the remodeling stage of healing, with some possibility of chronic inflammation. MP does not report significant pain at this time. No tone abnormalities are noted.

This patient's signs and symptoms are consistent with the diagnosis of adhesive capsulitis, which occurs most often in the shoulder.[30,69,70] The onset of this problem is frequently reported to be insidious, although it may be associated with other pathology such as local trauma, tendinitis, cerebrovascular accident, or surgery of the neck and thorax.[27,29,30,69] Predisposing factors include female gender, history of diabetes, immobilization, and age over 40 years.[29,30,71]

PREFERRED PRACTICE PATTERN

Impaired Joint Mobility, Motor Function, Muscle Performance, and Range of Motion Associated With Connective Tissue Dysfunction, (4D)

PLAN OF CARE

The anticipated goals of treatment at this time are to restore normal active and passive motion of the left shoulder and to give MP the ability to perform all activities of daily living in the manner she used previously, using both upper extremities. Since her shoulder ROM is probably restricted by soft tissue shortening, intervention should be directed at increasing the extensibility and length of the shortened tissues, particularly the anterior inferior capsule of the glenohumeral joint. Other appropriate goals for this late stage of healing are to control scar tissue formation and to ensure adequate circulation. Although no strength abnormalities were noted on this initial evaluation, the patient's strength should be reevaluated as she regains ROM since she may have strength deficits at these end ranges due to disuse. Should strength deficits become apparent, an additional goal of treatment would be to restore normal strength to the left shoulder muscles.

ASSESSMENT REGARDING SELECTION OF THE OPTIMAL TREATMENT

Although there is disagreement concerning the optimal intervention for adhesive capsulitis, it has been suggested that treatments that increase the extensibility and length of the restricted soft tissues around the glenohumeral joint and decrease local inflammation facilitate the resolution of this problem.[30,72,73] As is explained in greater detail in Section 2 of this book, a number of physical agents that provide localized deep heating may increase the extensibility of the tissues, whereas other physical agents, such as ice or low-dose ultrasound, may facilitate resolution of the inflammation. Thermotherapy could be used in conjunction with stretching and range-of-motion activities to lengthen the shortened tissues. Joint mobilization and later strengthening may also be necessary to regain full function of the shoulder.

Preferred Physical Therapist PatternsSM [4D and 4F] are copyright 2002 American Physical therapy Association. All rights reserved.

CHAPTER REVIEW

The musculoskeletal and neural structures of the body are normally able to move. Active movement occurs when muscles contract, and passive movement occurs when the body is acted on by an outside force. Physiological joint motion is the motion of one segment of the body relative to another, while accessory motion is the motion that occurs between the joint surfaces during normal physiological motion.

The amount of motion normally available depends on the joint being considered and may also vary with the subject's age, sex, and health status; however, motion may be restricted by a variety of pathologies including contractures, edema, adhesions, mechanical blocks, spinal disc herniation, adverse neural tension, and weakness. Motion will be restricted in a capsular pattern if the capsule surrounding a joint is affected and otherwise can be restricted in a noncapsular pattern. Various tests and measures may be used to determine the degree of motion restriction, the tissue involved, and the nature of the pathology contributing to a motion restriction. Motion restrictions may be treated conservatively by stretching and motion or, in some cases, may require invasive surgery. Physical agents may serve as adjuncts to these interventions by increasing soft tissue extensibility before stretching, controlling inflammation and adhesion formation during tissue healing, controlling pain during stretching or motion, or causing or assisting with motion. The reader is referred to the Evolve website at http://evolve.elsevier.com/Cameron for study questions pertinent to this chapter.

References

1. Kisner C, Colby LA: *Therapeutic Exercise: Foundations and Techniques,* ed 3, Philadelphia, 1996, FA Davis.
2. Cummings GS: Comparison of muscle to other soft tissue in limiting elbow extension, *J Orthop Sports Phys Ther* 5(4):170-174, 1984.
3. Sojberg JO: The stiff elbow, *Acta Orthop Scand* 67:626-631, 1996.
4. Cooper JE, Shwedyk E, Quanbury AO et al: Elbow joint restriction: Effect on upper limb motion during performance of three feeding activities, *Arch Phys Med Rehabil* 74:805-809, 1993.
5. Badley EM, Wagstaff S, Wood PH: Measures of functional ability (disability) in arthritis in relation to impairment of joint motion, *Ann Rheum Dis* 43:563-569, 1984.
6. Godges JJ, MacRae PG, Engelke KA: Effects of exercise on hip range of motion, trunk muscle performance and gait economy, *Phys Ther* 73:468-477, 1993.
7. Nordin M, Frankel VH: *Basic Biomechanics of the Musculoskeletal System,* ed 2, Philadelphia, 1989, Lea & Febiger.
8. American Academy of Orthopaedic Surgeons: *Joint Motion: Methods of Measuring and Recording,* Edinburgh, Scotland, 1965, Churchill Livingstone.
9. Shinaburger NI: Limited joint mobility in adults with diabetes mellitus, *Phys Ther* 67:215-218, 1987.
10. Libby AK, Sherry DD, Dudgeon BJ: Shoulder limitation in juvenile rheumatoid arthritis, *Arch Phys Med Rehabil* 72:382-384, 1991.
11. Roach KE, Miles TP: Normal hip and knee active range of motion: the relationship to age, *Phys Ther* 71:656-665, 1991.
12. Filbert I, Fuhri JR, New MD: Elbow, forearm, and wrist passive range of motion in persons aged sixty and older, *Phys Occup Ther Geriatr* 10:17-32, 1992.
13. Sullivan MS, Dickinsin CE, Troup JD: The influence of age and gender on lumbar spine sagittal plane range of motion, *Spine* 19:682-686, 1994.
14. Holmes A, Wang C, Han ZH et al: The range and nature of flexion-extension motion in the cervical spine, *Spine* 19:2505-2510, 1994.
15. Kuhlman KA: Cervical range of motion in the elderly, *Arch Phys Med Rehabil* 74:1071-1079, 1993.
16. Einkauf DK, Gohdes ML, Jensen GM et al: Changes in spinal mobility with increasing age in women, *Phys Ther* 67:370-375, 1987.
17. Lind B, Sihlbom H, Nordwall A et al: Normal range of motion of the cervical spine, *Arch Phys Med Rehabil* 70:692-695, 1989.
18. Desrosiers J, Hebert R, Bravo , et al: Shoulder range of motion of healthy elderly people: a normative study, *Phys Occup Ther Geriatr* 13:101-114, 1995.
19. Fiebert IM, Downed PA, Brown J: Active shoulder range of motion in persons aged 60 years and older, *Phys Occup Ther Geriatr* 13:115-128, 1995.
20. Kessler RM, Hertling D: *Management of Common Musculoskeletal Disorders, Physical Therapy Principles and Methods,* Philadelphia, 1983, Harper & Row.
21. Kaltenborn FM: *Mobilization of the Extremity Joints: Examination and Basic Treatment Techniques,* ed 3, Oslo, Norway, 1980, Olaf Norlis Bokhandel.
22. Maitland GD: *Vertebral Manipulation,* ed 5, London, 1986, Butterworths.
23. Saunders HD, Saunders R: *Evaluation, Treatment and Prevention of Musculoskeletal Disorders: Spine,* ed 3, Chaska, MN, 1995, Saunders Group.
24. Guyton AC: *Textbook of Medical Physiology,* Philadelphia, 1981, WB Saunders.
25. Cyriax J: *Textbook of Orthopaedic Medicine,* ed 6, Baltimore, 1975, Williams & Wilkins.
26. Neviaser RJ, Neviaser TJ: The frozen shoulder: Diagnosis and management, *Clin Orthop* 223:59-64, 1987.
27. Andrews AW, Bohannon RW: Decreased shoulder range of motion on paretic side after stroke, *Phys Ther* 66:768-772, 1989.
28. Rizk TE, Pinals RS: Frozen shoulder, *Semin Arthritis Rheum* 11:440-452, 1982.
29. Bunker TD, Anthony PP: The pathology of frozen shoulder: a Dupuytren-like disease, *J Bone Joint Surg Br* 77:677-683, 1995.
30. Parker RD, Froimson AI, Winsberg DD et al: Frozen shoulder. Part 1: chronology, pathogenesis, clinical picture, and treatment, *Orthopedics* 12:869-873, 1989.
31. Grubbs N: Frozen shoulder syndrome: a review of literature, *J Orthop Sports Phys Ther* 18:479-487, 1993.
32. Akeson WH, Amiel D, Woo SL-Y: Immobility effects on synovial joints, the pathomechanics of joint contracture, *Biorheology* 17:95-110, 1980.

33. Salter RB: *Textbook of Disorders and Injuries of the Musculoskeletal System,* ed 2, Baltimore, 1983, Williams & Wilkins.

34. Frank C, Akeson WH, Woo SL-Y, et al: Physiology and therapeutic value of passive joint motion, *Clin Orthop* 185:113-125, 1984.

35. Woo SL, Matthews JV, Akeson WH et al: Connective tissue response to immobility. Correlative study of biomechanical and biochemical measurements of normal and immobilized rabbit knees, *Arthritis Rheum* 18:257-264, 1975.

36. Akeson WH, Amiel D, Abel MF et al: Effects of immobilization on joints, *Clin Orthop* 219:28-37, 1987.

37. *Dorland's Illustrated Medical Dictionary*, ed 29, Philadelphia, 2000, WB Saunders.

38. Enneking WF: The intraarticular effects of immobilization on the human knee, *J Bone Joint Surg* 54A:973, 1972.

39. Slater H, Butler DS: The dynamic central nervous system. In *Grieve's Modern Manual* ed 2, New York, 1994, Churchill Livingstone.

40. Oliver J, Middleditch A: *Functional Anatomy of the Spine*, London, 1991, Butterworth-Heinemann.

41. Butler DS: *Mobilization of the Nervous System*, Edinburgh, 1991, Churchill Livingstone.

42. Tomberlin JP, Saunders HD: *Evaluation, Treatment and Prevention of Musculoskeletal Disorders: Extremities,* ed 3, Chaska, MN, 1994, Saunders Group.

43. Greenman PE: *Principles of Manual Medicine,* ed 2, Baltimore, 1996, Williams & Wilkins.

44. Norkin CC, White DJ: *Measurement of Joint Motion: A Guide to Goniometry,* Philadelphia, 1985, FA Davis.

45. Kendall FP, McCreary EK: *Muscles: Testing and Function,* ed 3, Baltimore, 1983, Williams & Wilkins.

46. Daniels L, Worthingham C: *Muscle Testing: Techniques of Manual Examination*, ed 4, Philadelphia, 1980, WB Saunders.

47. Clarkson HM, Gilewich GB: *Musculoskeletal Assessment: Joint Range of Motion and Manual Muscle Strength,* Baltimore, 1989, Williams & Wilkins.

48. Riddle DL: Measurement of accessory motion: critical issues and related concepts, *Phys Ther* 72:865-874, 1992.

49. Mints N, Dvir Z: Wrist complex mobility: a study of passive flexion and extension and accessory movements, *Physiother Canada* 40:282-285, 1988.

50. Binkley J, Stratford PW, Gill C: Interrater reliability of lumbar accessory motion mobility testing, *Phys Ther* 75:786-795, 1995.

51. Bonutti PM, Windau JE: Static progressive stretch to reestablish elbow range of motion, *Clin Orthop* 303:128-134, 1994.

52. Taylor DC, Dalton JD, Seaber AV et al: Viscoelastic properties of muscle-tendon units: the biomechanics of stretching, *Am J Sports Med* 18:300, 1900.

53. Fung YC: Biomechanics: Mechanical Properties of Living Tissues, ed 2. New York: Springer-Verlag; 1993.

54. McClure PW, Blackburn LG, Dusold C: The use of splints in the treatment of stiffness: biologic rationale and an algorithm for making clinical decisions, *Phys Ther* 74:1101-1107, 1994.

55. Norkin CC, Levangie PK: *Joint Structure and Function: A Comprehensive Analysis,* ed 2, Philadelphia, 1990, FA Davis.

56. Voss DE, Ionta MK, Myers BJ: *Proprioceptive Neuromuscular Facilitation,* ed 3, Philadelphia, 1985, Harper & Row.

57. Lamontagne A, Maloun F, Richards CL: Viscoelastic behavior of plantar flexor muscle-tendon unit at rest, *J Orthop Sports Phys Ther* 26:244-252, 1997.

58. Salter RB, Simmonds DF, Malcolm BW et al: The biological effect of continuous passive motion on the healing of full thickness defects in articular cartilage: an experimental investigation in the rabbit, *J Bone Joint Surg* 62A:1232-1251, 1980.

59. Salter RB, Bell RS, Keeley FW: The protective effect of continuous passive motion on living articular cartilage in acute septic arthritis: an experimental investigation in the rabbit, *Clin Orthop* 159:223-247, 1981.

60. Frank C, Akeson W, Woo S et al: Physiology and therapeutic value of passive joint motion, *Clin Orthop* 185:113-125, 1984.

61. Covey MH, Dutcher K, Marvin JA et al: Efficacy of continuous passive motion (CPM) devices with hand burns, *J Burn Care Rehabil* 9:397-400, 1988.

62. Lentell G, Hetherington T, Eagan J et al: The use of thermal agents to influence the effectiveness of low load prolonged stretch, *J Orthop Sport Phys Ther* 16(5):200-207, 1992.

63. Warren C, Lehmann J, Koblanski J: Elongation of rat tail tendon: effect of load and temperature, *Arch Phys Med Rehabil* 52:465-474, 484, 1971.

64. Warren C, Lehmann J, Koblanski J: Heat and stretch procedures: an evaluation using rat tail tendon, *Arch Phys Med Rehabil* 57:122-126, 1976.

65. Gersten JW: Effect of ultrasound on tendon extensibility, *Am J Phys Med* 34:362-369, 1955.

66. Lehmann J, Masock A, Warren C et al: Effect of therapeutic temperatures on tendon extensibility, *Arch Phys Med Rehabil* 51:481-487, 1970.

67. Hocutt JE, Jaffe R, Ryplander CR: Cryotherapy in ankle sprains, *Am J Sports Med* 10:316-319, 1982.

68. Cote DJ, Prentice WE, Hooker DN et al: Comparison of three treatment procedures for minimizing ankle sprain swelling, *Phys Ther* 68(7):1072-1076, 1988.

69. Patten C, Hillel AD: The 11th nerve syndrome, *Arch Otolaryngol Head Neck Surg* 119:215-220, 1993.

70. Emig EW, Schweitzer ME, Karasic D et al: Adhesive capsulitis of the shoulder: MR diagnosis, *Am J Roentgenol* 164(6):1457-1459, 1995.

71. Kozin F: Two unique shoulders: adhesive capsulitis and sympathetic dystrophy syndrome of motion, *Postgrad Med* 73:207-216, 1983.

72. Rizk TE, Morris L, Gavant ML: Treatment of adhesive capsulitis (frozen shoulder) with arthrographic capsular distension and rupture, *Arch Phys Med Rehabil* 75: 803-807, 1994.

73. Rizk TE, Pinals RS, Talaiver AS: Corticosteroid injections in adhesive capsulitis: investigation of their value and site, *Arch Phys Med Rehabil* 72:20-22, 1991.

Section Two

The Physical Agents

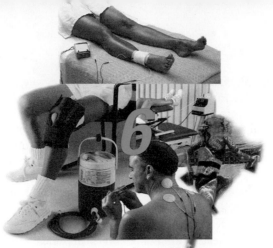

Thermal Agents: Cold and Heat

SUMMARY OF INFORMATION COVERED

Physical Principles of Thermal Energy
Specific Heat
Modes of Heat Transfer
Cold—Cryotherapy
Effects of Cold
Uses of Cryotherapy
Contraindications and Precautions for Cryotherapy
Adverse Effects of Cryotherapy
Application Techniques
Clinical Case Studies
Heat—Thermotherapy
Effects of Heat

Uses of Superficial Heat
Contraindications and Precautions for
    Thermotherapy
Adverse Effects of Thermotherapy
Application Techniques
Other Means of Applying Thermotherapy
Clinical Case Studies
**Choosing Between Cryotherapy and
    Thermotherapy**
Chapter Review

OBJECTIVES

Upon completion of this chapter, the reader will be able to:

1. Identify the physical properties of, and the physiological responses to, thermal agents.
2. Analyze the physiological responses to thermal agents necessary to promote particular treatment goals.
3. Assess the indications, contraindications, and precautions for the use of thermal agents with respect to different patient management situations.
4. Evaluate different types of thermal agents with respect to their potential to produce

desired physical and physiological effects.
5. Choose and use the most appropriate thermal agent to obtain desired treatment goals.
6. Presented with a clinical case, evaluate the clinical findings, propose goals of treatment, assess whether a superficial thermal agent would be the best treatment, and, if so, formulate an effective treatment plan, including the most appropriate thermal agent, for achieving the goals of treatment.

This chapter discusses the basic physical principles and physiological effects of transferring heat to or from patients by using thermal agents. The clinical applications of cold and superficial heating agents are also addressed. Superficial heating agents are those that primarily increase the temperature of the skin and superficial subcutaneous tissues. In contrast, deep heating agents also increase the temperature of deeper tissues, including large muscles and periarticular structures, and generally reach to a depth of about 5 cm. The clinical applications of deep-heating agents are not covered in this chapter but are discussed in Chapters 7 and 12.

The therapeutic application of thermal agents results in the transfer of heat to or from a patient's body and between the various component tissues and fluids of the body. Heat transfer may occur by conduction, convection, conversion, radiation, or evaporation. Heating agents transfer heat to the body, whereas cooling agents transfer heat away from the body. Thermoregulation by the body also uses the above processes to maintain core body temperature and to maintain equilibrium between internal metabolic heat production and heat loss or gain at the skin surface. The following section of this chapter discusses the physical principles of heat transfer to or from the body and within the body. This section is followed by discussions of the physiological effects of cooling and heating and directions for the clinical application of superficial cooling and heating modalities.

PHYSICAL PRINCIPLES OF THERMAL ENERGY

SPECIFIC HEAT

Specific heat is the amount of energy required to raise the temperature of a given weight of a material by a given number of degrees. Different materials used as thermal agents and different body tissues have different specific heats (Table 6-1). For example, skin has higher specific heat than fat or bone, and water has a higher specific heat than air. Materials with a high specific heat require more energy to achieve the same temperature increase than materials with a low specific heat. Materials with a high specific heat also hold more energy than materials with a low specific heat when both are at the same temperature. Thermal agents with a high specific heat, such as water, are therefore applied at lower temperatures than air-based thermal agents, such as Fluidotherapy, to transfer the same amount of heat to a patient. The specific heat of a material is generally expressed in joules per gram per degrees Celsius.

MODES OF HEAT TRANSFER

Different physical agents transfer heat by different modes. These include conduction, convection, conversion, radiation, and evaporation, as discussed in detail in the following sections.

Conduction: Heat Transfer by Direct Contact Such as Hot Packs and Cold Packs

Heating by conduction is the result of energy exchange by direct collision between the molecules of two materials at different temperatures. Heat is conducted from the material at the higher temperature to the material at the lower temperature as the faster moving molecules in the warmer material collide with the molecules in the cooler material and cause them to accelerate. Heat transfer continues until the temperature and the speed of molecular movement of both materials become equal. Heat may be transferred to or from a patient by conduction. If the physical agent used has a higher temperature than the patient's skin, for example, a hot pack or warm paraffin, heat will be transferred from the agent to the patient, and the temperature of the superficial tissues in contact with the heating agent will rise. If the physical agent used is colder than the patient's skin, for

TABLE 6-1 Specific Heat of Various Materials	
Material	**Specific heat in J/g/ °C**
Water	4.19
Air	1.01
Average for human body	3.56
Skin	3.77
Muscle	3.75
Fat	2.30
Bone	1.59

example, an ice pack, heat will be transferred from the patient to the agent, and the temperature of the superficial tissues in contact with the cooling agent will fall.

Heat can also be transferred from one area of the body to another by conduction. For example, when one area of the body is heated by an external thermal agent, the tissues adjacent to and in contact with that area will increase in temperature due to heating by conduction.

Heat transfer by conduction occurs only between materials of different temperatures that are in direct contact with each other. If there is any air between a conductive thermal agent and the patient, the heat is first conducted from the thermal agent to the air and then from the air to the patient.

Rate of heat transfer by conduction

The rate at which heat is transferred by conduction between two materials depends on the temperature difference between the materials, their thermal conductivity, and their area of contact, and is expressed by the following formula.

$$\text{Rate of heat transfer} = \frac{\text{area of contact} \times \text{thermal conductivity} \times \text{temperature difference}}{\text{tissue thickness}}$$

The thermal conductivity of a material describes the rate at which it transfers heat by conduction and is generally expressed in $(\text{cal/sec})/(\text{cm}^2 \times {}^\circ\text{C/cm})$ (Table 6-2). Note that this is not the same as a material's specific heat.

A number of guidelines can be derived from the preceding formula.

TABLE 6-2 Thermal Conductivity of Various Materials

Material	Thermal conductivity (cal/sec)/ (cm² × °C/cm)
Silver	1.01
Aluminum	0.50
Ice	0.005
Water at 20 °C	0.0014
Bone	0.0011
Muscle	0.0011
Fat	0.0005
Air at 0 °C	0.000057

Guidelines for heat transfer by conduction

1. The greater the temperature difference between a heating or cooling agent and the body part it is applied to, the faster the rate of heat transfer. For example, the higher the temperature of a hot pack, the more rapidly the temperature of the area of the patient's skin in contact with the hot pack will increase. Generally, the temperatures of conductive physical agents are selected to achieve a fast but safe rate of temperature change. If a heating agent is only a few degrees warmer than the patient, heating will take too long; by contrast, if the temperature difference is large, heat transfer could be so rapid as to quickly burn the patient.

2. Materials with high thermal conductivity transfer heat more rapidly than those with low thermal conductivity. Metals have high thermal conductivity, whereas water has moderate thermal conductivity and air has low thermal conductivity.

Heating and cooling agents are generally composed of materials with moderate thermal conductivity to provide a safe and effective rate of heat transfer. Materials with low thermal conductivity can be used as insulators to limit the rate of heat transfer. For example, some types of hot packs are kept hot by soaking in and absorbing water that is kept at approximately 70 °C (175 °F). The high temperature, high specific heat, and moderate thermal conductivity of the water allow efficient heat transfer; however, if the pack is applied directly to a patient's skin, the patient will probably soon feel uncomfortably hot and could easily be burned. Therefore towels or terrycloth hot pack covers that trap air, which has low thermal conductivity, are placed between the pack and the patient to limit the rate of heat transfer. In general, six to eight layers of toweling are placed between a hot pack and a patient; however, if the patient gets too hot, additional layers of toweling can be added to further limit the rate of heat conduction.

Note that newer towels and covers are generally thicker and therefore act as more effective insulators than older ones. Since subcutaneous fat has low thermal conductivity, it also acts as an insulator, limiting the conduction of heat to or from the deeper tissues.

Because metal has high thermal conductivity, metal jewelry should be removed from any area that will be in contact with a conductive thermal agent. If metal jewelry is not removed, heat will rapidly transfer to the metal, with the potential to burn the skin that is in contact with it.

Because ice has higher thermal conductivity than water, it causes more rapid cooling than water even at the same temperature. The thermal conductivities of different commercially available cold packs vary, some being higher than water or ice and others being lower. Therefore, when changing the brand or type of cold pack used, one should not assume that the new pack can be applied in the same manner, for the same amount of time, or with the same number of layers of insulating material as the old pack.

3. The larger the area of contact between a thermal agent and the patient, the greater the total heat transfer. For example, when a hot pack is applied to the entire back, or when a patient is immersed up to the neck in a whirlpool or a Hubbard tank, the total amount of heat transferred will be greater than if a hot pack is applied only to a small area overlying the calf.

4. The rate of temperature rise decreases in proportion to tissue thickness. When a thermal agent is in contact with a patient's skin, the skin temperature increases the most and deeper tissues are progressively less affected. The deeper the tissue, the less its temperature will change. Therefore conductive thermal agents are well-suited to heating or cooling superficial tissues but should not be used when the goal is to change the temperature of deeper tissues.

Convection: Heat Transfer by Circulation of a Medium of a Different Temperature Such as Fluidotherapy, Whirlpool, Blood Circulation

Heat transfer by convection occurs as the result of direct contact between a circulating medium and another material of a different temperature. This is in contrast to heating by conduction, in which there is constant contact between a stationary thermal agent and the patient. During heating or cooling by convection the thermal agent is in motion, so new parts of the agent at the initial treatment temperature keep coming into contact with the patient's body part. As a result, heat transfer by convection transfers more heat in the same period of time than heat transfer by conduction when the same material at the same initial temperature is used. For example, immersion in a whirlpool will heat a patient's skin more rapidly than immersion in a bowl of water of the same temperature, and the faster the water moves, the more rapid the rate of heat transfer will be.

Blood circulating in the body also transfers heat by convection to reduce local changes in tissue temperature. For example, when a thermal agent is applied to an area of the body and produces a local change in tissue temperature, the circulation constantly moves the heated blood out of the area and moves cooler blood into the area to return the local tissue temperature to a normal level. This local cooling by convection reduces the impact of superficial heating agents on the local tissue temperature. Vasodilation increases the rate of circulation, increasing the rate at which the tissue temperature returns to normal.[1] Thus, the vasodilation that occurs in response to heat protects the tissues by reducing the risk of burning.

Conversion: Conversion from One Type of Energy to Another Such as Ultrasound Diathermy, and Metabolism

Heat transfer by conversion involves the conversion of a nonthermal form of energy, such as mechanical, electrical, or chemical energy, into heat. For example, ultrasound, which is a mechanical form of energy, is converted into heat when applied at a sufficient intensity to a tissue that absorbs ultrasound waves. Ultrasound causes vibration of molecules in the tissue, which generates friction between the molecules, resulting in an increase in tissue temperature. When diathermy, an electromagnetic form of energy, is applied to the body, it causes rotation of polar molecules, which also results in friction between the molecules and an increase in tissue temperature. Some types of cold packs cool by converting heat into chemical energy. Striking these chemical cold packs initiates a chemical reaction that extracts heat from the pack, causing it to become cold. Thermal energy is converted into chemical energy to drive this reaction.

Unlike heating by conduction or convection, heating by conversion is not affected by the temperature of the thermal agent. When transferring heat by conversion, the rate of heat transfer depends on the power of the energy source. The power of ultrasound and diathermy is usually measured in watts, which is the amount of energy in joules output per second. The amount of energy output by a chemical reaction depends on the reacting chemicals and is usually measured in joules. The rate of tissue temperature increase also depends on the size of the area being treated, the size of the applicator, efficiency of transmission from the applicator to the patient, and the type of tissue being treated. Different types of tissues absorb different forms of energy to different extents and therefore heat differently.[2]

Heat transfer by conversion does not require direct contact between the thermal agent and the body; however, it does require any intervening material to be a good transmitter of that type of energy. For example, a transmission gel, lotion, or water must be used between an ultrasound transducer and the patient to transmit the ultrasound because air, which might otherwise come between the transducer and the patient, transmits ultrasound poorly.

Physical agents that heat by conversion may also have other nonthermal physiological effects. For example, although the mechanical energy of ultrasound and the electrical energy of diathermy can produce heat by conversion, they are also thought to have direct mechanical or electrical effects on tissue. A full discussion of absorption and the thermal and nonthermal effects of ultrasound and diathermy can be found in Chapters 7 and 12, respectively.

Radiation: Exchange of Energy Directly without an Intervening Medium Such as Infrared Lamp

Heating by radiation involves the direct transfer of energy from a material with a higher temperature to one with a lower temperature without the need for an intervening medium or contact. This is in contrast to heat transfer by conversion, in which the medium and the patient may be at the same temperature. It is also different from heat transfer by conduction or convection, which both require the thermal agent to be in contact with the tissue being heated. The rate of temperature increase caused by radiation depends on the intensity of the radiation, the relative sizes of the radiation source and the area being treated, the distance of the source from the treatment area, and the angle of the radiation to the tissue.

Evaporation: Absorption of Energy as the Result of Conversion of a Material from a Liquid to a Vapor State Such as Vapocoolant Sprays

Sweating

A material must absorb energy to evaporate and thus change form from a liquid to a gas or vapor. This energy is absorbed in the form of heat, either from the material itself or from an adjoining material, resulting in a decrease in temperature. For example, when a vapocoolant spray is heated by the warm skin of the body, it changes from its liquid form to a vapor at its specific evaporation temperature. During this process, the spray absorbs heat and thus cools the skin. Another example is the evaporation of sweat, which also acts to cool the body. The temperature of evaporation for sweat is a few degrees higher than the normal skin temperature; therefore, if the skin temperature increases from exercise or an external source and the humidity of the environment is low enough, the sweat produced in response to the increased temperature will evaporate, reducing the local body temperature. If the ambient humidity is high, evaporation will be impaired. Sweating is a homeostatic mechanism that serves to cool the body when it is overheated to help return body temperature toward the normal range.

COLD—CRYOTHERAPY

Cryotherapy, the therapeutic use of cold, has clinical applications both in rehabilitation and other areas of medicine. The primary use of cryotherapy outside of rehabilitation is for the destruction of malignant and nonmalignant tissue growths, for which very low temperatures are used and the cooling is generally applied directly to the tissue being treated. In rehabilitation, mild cooling is used to control inflammation, pain, and edema; to reduce spasticity; to control symptoms of multiple sclerosis; and to facilitate movement (Fig. 6-1). This type of cryotherapy is applied to the skin but can decrease tissue temperature deep to the area of application, including intraarticular areas.[3] Cryotherapy exerts its therapeutic

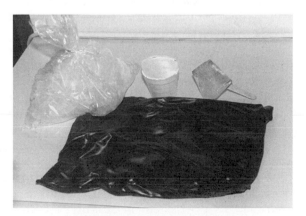

Figure 6-1. Cryotherapy agents.

effects by influencing hemodynamic, neuromuscular, and metabolic processes, the mechanisms of which are explained in detail in the following sections.

EFFECTS OF COLD

Hemodynamic effects
Initial decrease in blood flow
Later increase in blood flow

Neuromuscular effects
Decreased nerve conduction velocity
Increased pain threshold
Altered muscle strength
Decreased spasticity
Facilitation of muscle contraction

Metabolic effects
Decreased metabolic rate

Hemodynamic Effects

Initial decrease in blood flow

Generally, if cold is applied to the skin, it causes an immediate constriction of the cutaneous vessels and a reduction in blood flow. This vasoconstriction persists as long as the duration of the cold application is limited to less than 15 to 20 minutes.[4] Studies show that repeating ice application after an initial 20-minute application for 2 repetitions of 10 minutes off and 10 minutes on lowers blood flow significantly more than a single 20-minute ice application.[5] The vasoconstriction and reduction in blood flow produced by cryotherapy is most pronounced in the area where the cold is applied because this is where the tissue temperature decrease is greatest.

Cold causes cutaneous vasoconstriction by both direct and indirect mechanisms (Fig. 6-2). Activation of the cutaneous cold receptors by cold directly stimulates the smooth muscles of the blood vessel walls to contract. Cooling of the tissue also decreases the production and release of vasodilator mediators, such as histamine and prostaglandins, resulting in reduced vasodilation. Decreasing the tissue temperature also causes a reflex activation of sympathetic adrenergic neurons, resulting in cutaneous vasoconstriction both in the area that is cooled and, to a lesser extent, in areas distant from the site of cold application.[6] Cold is also thought to reduce

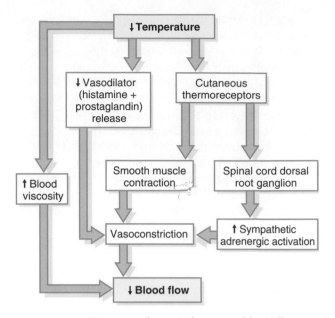

Figure 6-2. How cryotherapy decreases blood flow.

the circulatory rate by increasing blood viscosity, thereby increasing the resistance to flow.

It is thought that the body reduces blood flow in response to a decrease in tissue temperature to protect other areas from excessive decreases in temperature and stabilize core body temperature. The less blood that flows through an area being cooled, the smaller the amount of blood that is cooled and thus the less other areas in the circulatory system are affected. Reducing circulation results in a greater decrease in the temperature of the area to which a cooling agent is applied because warmer blood is not being brought into the area to raise its temperature by convection, and less of a decrease in temperature in other areas of the body because little of the cold blood is circulated to these areas.

Later increase in blood flow

The immediate vasoconstriction response to cold is a consistent and well-documented phenomenon; however, when cold is applied for longer periods of time or when the tissue temperature reaches less than 10 °C (50 °F), vasodilation may occur. This phenomenon is known as *cold-induced vasodilation (CIVD)* and was first reported by Lewis in 1930.[7] His findings were replicated in a number of later studies;[8-10] however, vasodilation has not been found to be a consistent response to prolonged cold application.[4,11]

Lewis reported that when an individual's fingers were immersed in an ice bath, their temperature initially decreased; however, after 15 minutes, their temperature cyclically increased and decreased (Fig. 6-3). Lewis correlated this temperature cycling with alternating vasoconstriction and vasodilation and called this the *hunting response*. It is proposed that the hunting response is mediated by an axon reflex in response to the pain of prolonged cold or very low temperatures, or that it is caused by inhibition of contraction of the smooth muscles of the blood vessel walls by extreme cold.[12] Maintained vasodilation, without cycling, has also been observed with cooling human forearms at 1 °C (35 °F) for 15 minutes. [8]

Cold-induced vasodilation is most likely to occur in the distal extremities, such as the fingers or toes, with applications of cold for more than 15 minutes at temperatures below 1 °C. Although the amount of vasodilation is usually small, in clinical situations where vasodilation should be avoided, it is generally recommended that cold application be limited to 15 minutes or less, particularly when treating the distal extremities. When vasodilation is the intended goal of treatment, cryotherapy is also not recommended because it does not consistently have this effect.

Although the increase in skin redness seen with the application of cold may appear to be a sign of CIVD, it is actually thought to be primarily the result of an increase in the oxyhemoglobin concentration of the blood due to the decrease in oxygen-hemoglobin dissociation that occurs at lower temperatures[13] (Fig. 6-4). Since cooling decreases oxygen-hemoglobin dissociation, making less oxygen available to the tissues, cold-induced vasodilation is not considered to be an effective means of increasing oxygen delivery to an area.

Neuromuscular Effects

Cold has a variety of effects on neuromuscular function, including decreasing nerve conduction velocity, elevating the pain threshold, altering muscle force generation, decreasing spasticity, and facilitating muscle contraction.

Decreased nerve conduction velocity

When nerve temperature is decreased, nerve conduction velocity decreases in proportion to the degree and duration of the temperature change.[14] Decreased nerve conduction velocity has been documented in response to the application of a superficial cooling agent to the skin for 5 minutes or longer.[15] The decrease in nerve conduction velocity that occurs with 5 minutes of cooling fully reverses within 15 minutes in individuals with normal circulation. However, after 20 minutes of cooling, nerve conduction velocity may take 30 minutes or longer to recover due to the greater reduction in temperature caused by the longer duration of cooling.[16]

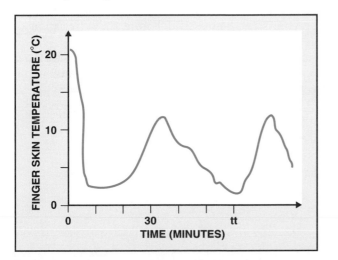

Figure 6-3. Hunting response, cold-induced vasodilation of finger immersed in ice water, measured by skin temperature change. (From Lewis T: Observations upon the reactions of the vessels of the human skin to cold, *Heart* 15:177-208, 1930.)

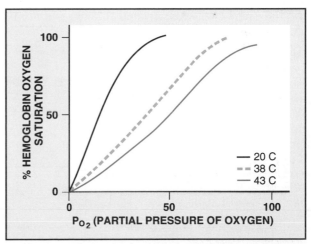

Figure 6-4. Effect of temperature on oxygen-hemoglobin dissociation curve. (From Barcroft J, King W: The effect of temperature on the dissociation curve of blood, *J Physiol* 39:374-384, 1909.)

Cold can decrease the conduction velocity of both sensory and motor nerves. It has the greatest effect on conduction by myelinated and small fibers and the least effect on conduction by unmyelinated and large fibers.[16] A-delta fibers, which are small-diameter, myelinated, pain-transmitting fibers, demonstrate the greatest decrease in conduction velocity in response to cooling. Reversible total nerve conduction block can also occur with the application of ice over superficially located major nerve branches such as the peroneal nerve at the lateral aspect of the knee.[17]

Increased pain threshold

The application of cryotherapy can increase the pain threshold and decrease the sensation of pain. The proposed mechanisms for these effects include counter-irritation via the gate control mechanism and the reduction of muscle spasm, sensory nerve conduction velocity, or postinjury edema.[18]

Stimulation of the cutaneous cold receptors by cold may provide sufficient sensory input to block the transmission of painful stimuli fully or partially along the spinal cord to the cerebral cortex, increasing pain threshold or decreasing pain sensation. Such gating of the sensation of pain can also reduce muscle spasms by interrupting the pain-spasm-pain cycle, as described in Chapter 3. Cryotherapy may also reduce the pain associated with an acute injury by reducing the rate of blood flow in an area and decreasing the rate of reactions related to acute inflammation, thus controlling post-injury edema formation.[19] Reducing edema can alleviate pain that results from compression of nerves or other pressure-sensitive structures.

Altered muscle strength

Depending on the duration of treatment and the timing of measurement, cryotherapy has been associated with both increases and decreases in muscle strength. Isometric muscle strength has been found to increase directly after the application of ice massage for 5 minutes or less; however, the duration of this effect has not been documented.[20] The proposed mechanisms for this response to brief cooling include facilitation of motor nerve excitability and an increased psychological motivation to perform. In contrast, after cooling for 30 minutes or longer, isometric muscle strength has been found to decrease initially and then to increase an hour later, to reach greater than precooling strength for the following 3 hours or longer[21-23] (Fig. 6-5). The proposed mechanisms for the reduced strength after prolonged cooling include reduction of blood flow to the muscles, slowed motor nerve conduction, increased muscle viscosity, and increased joint or soft tissue stiffness.

It is important to be aware of these changes in muscle strength in response to the application of cryotherapy since they can obscure accurate, objective assessment of muscle strength and patient progress. It is therefore recommended that muscle strength be consistently measured before the application of

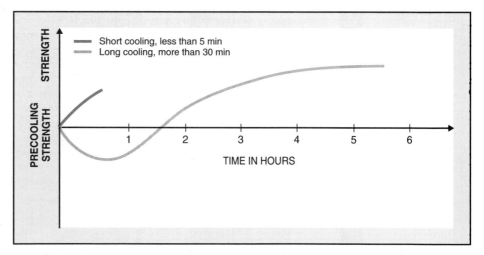

Figure 6-5. Effects of cold on strength of muscle contraction. (Data from Oliver RA, Johnson DJ, Wheelhouse WW et al: Isometric muscle contraction response during recovery from reduced intramuscular temperature, *Arch Phys Med Rehabil* 60:126-129, 1979; Johnson J, Leider FE: Influence of cold bath on maximum handgrip strength, *Percept Mot Skills* 44:323-325, 1977; Davies CTM, Young K: Effect of temperature on the contractile properties and muscle power of triceps surae in humans, *J Appl Physiol* 55:191-195, 1983.)

cryotherapy and that pre-cooling strength not be compared with postcooling strength when trying to assess patient progress.

Decreased spasticity

When applied appropriately, cryotherapy can temporarily decrease spasticity. Two mechanisms are proposed to act sequentially to produce this effect: first, a decrease in gamma motor neuron activity and, later, a decrease in afferent spindle and Golgi tendon organ activity. A decrease in the amplitude of the Achilles tendon reflex and integrated electromyography (EMG) activity have been observed within a few seconds of the application of cold to the skin.[24,25] These changes are thought to be related to a decrease in the activity of the gamma motor neurons as a reflex reaction to stimulation of the cutaneous cold receptors. This fast response must be related to stimulation of cutaneous structures sincethe temperature of the muscles cannot decrease after such a brief period of cooling.

After more prolonged cooling, lasting for 10 to 30 minutes, a temporary decrease or elimination of spasticity and clonus, depression of the Achilles tendon reflex, and a reduction in resistance to passive motion have also been observed in some patients with spasticity.[25-29] These changes are thought to be caused by a decrease in the discharge from the afferent spindles and Golgi tendon organs as a result of decreased muscle temperature.[30] These later effects generally persist for 1 to 1.5 hours and can therefore be taken advantage of in treatment by applying cryotherapy to hypertonic areas for up to 30 minutes before other interventions, to reduce spasticity during functional or therapeutic activities.

Facilitation of muscle contraction

The stimulus of a brief application of cryotherapy is thought to facilitate alpha motor neuron activity to produce a contraction in a muscle that is flaccid due to upper motor neuron dysfunction.[25] This effect is observed in response to a few seconds of cooling and also lasts for only a short time. With more prolonged cooling of even a few minutes, a decrease in gamma motor neuron activity reduces the force of muscle contraction. This brief facilitation effect of cryotherapy is occasionally used clinically when trying to stimulate the production of appropriate motor patterns in patients with upper motor neuron lesions.

Metabolic Effects

Decreased metabolic rate

Cold decreases the rate of all metabolic reactions, including those involved in inflammation and healing. Thus cryotherapy can be used to control acute inflammation, because it is not recommended when healing is delayed because it may further impair recovery. The activity of cartilage-degrading enzymes, including collagenase, elastase, hyaluronidase, and protease, is inhibited by decreases in joint temperature, almost ceasing at joint temperatures of 30 °C (86 °F) or lower.[31] Thus cryotherapy is recommended as a treatment for the prevention or reduction of collagen destruction in inflammatory joint diseases such as osteoarthritis and rheumatoid arthritis.

USES OF CRYOTHERAPY

> **Inflammation control**
> **Edema control**
> **Pain control**
> **Modification of spasticity**
> **Symptom management in multiple sclerosis**
> **Facilitation**
> **Cryokinetics and cryostretch**

Inflammation Control

Cryotherapy can be used to control acute inflammation and thereby accelerate recovery from injury or trauma.[32] Decreasing tissue temperature slows the rate of the chemical reactions that occur during the acute inflammatory response and also reduces the heat, redness, edema, pain, and loss of function associated with this phase of tissue healing. Cryotherapy directly reduces the heat associated with inflammation by decreasing the temperature of the area to which it is applied. The decrease in blood flow caused by vasoconstriction and increased blood viscosity, and the decrease in capillary permeability associated with cryotherapy, impede the movement of fluid from the capillaries to the interstitial tissue, thereby controlling bleeding and fluid loss after acute trauma. These effects reduce the redness and edema associated with inflammation. As described in more detail below, cryotherapy is thought to control pain by decreasing the activity of the A-delta pain fibers and by gating at the spinal cord level. Controlling the edema and pain associated with inflammation limits the loss of function associated with this phase of tissue healing.

It is recommended that cryotherapy be applied immediately following an injury and throughout the acute inflammatory phase. Immediate application helps to control bleeding and edema; therefore, the sooner the treatment is applied, the greater and more immediate the potential benefit.[33] Clinically, local skin temperature can be used to estimate the stage of healing and thus to determine if cryotherapy is indicated. If the temperature of an area is elevated, the area is probably still inflamed and cryotherapy is likely to be beneficial. Once the local temperature returns to normal, the acute inflammation has probably resolved and therefore cryotherapy should be discontinued. Acute inflammation usually resolves within 48 to 72 hours of acute trauma but may be prolonged with severe trauma, inflammatory diseases such as rheumatoid arthritis, or with chronic recurrent injuries. If the temperature of an area remains elevated for longer than appropriate for the patient's condition, the possibility of an infection should be considered and the patient should be referred to a physician for further evaluation. Cryotherapy should be discontinued when acute inflammation has resolved to avoid slowing chemical reactions or impairing circulation during the later stages of healing when these effects of cryotherapy can impede recovery.

The prophylactic use of cryotherapy after exercise has also been shown to reduce the severity of delayed-onset muscle soreness (DOMS).[34] DOMS is thought to be the result of inflammation from muscle and connective tissue damage caused by exercise.[35,36] Clinically, the prophylactic use of cryotherapy after aggressive joint or soft tissue mobilization, or after light activity in an area with a preexisting inflammation, can effectively decrease postactivity soreness.

Although cryotherapy can help to control inflammation and its associated signs and symptoms, the cause of the inflammation must also be addressed directly to prevent recurrence. For example, if inflammation is caused by overuse of a tendon, the patient's use of that tendon must be modified if recurrence of symptoms is to be avoided.

When cryotherapy is applied with the goal of controlling inflammation, the treatment time is generally limited to 15 minutes or less because longer application has been associated with vasodilation and increased circulation.[7-10] However, since reflex vasodilation in response to cold has not been shown to occur outside of the distal extremities, longer treatment durations may be used for areas other than the distal extremities.[4,11] To limit the probability of excessive decreases in tissue temperature and cold-induced injury, cryotherapy applications should be at least 1 hour apart so that the tissue temperature can return to normal between treatments.

Edema Control

Cryotherapy can be used to control the formation of edema, particularly when the edema is associated with acute inflammation.[37] During acute inflammation, edema is caused by extravasation of fluid into the interstitium caused by increased intravascular fluid pressure and increased vascular permeability. Cryotherapy reduces the intravascular fluid pressure by reducing blood flow into the area via vasoconstriction and increased blood viscosity. Cryotherapy also controls increases in capillary permeability by reducing the release of vasoactive substances, such as histamine.

To minimize edema formation, cryotherapy should be applied as soon as possible after an acute trauma. The formation of edema associated with inflammation will be most effectively controlled if the cryotherapy is applied in conjunction with compression and elevation of the affected area.[38,39] Compression can easily be applied with an elastic wrap (Fig. 6-6), and elevation should be above the level of the heart. Compression and elevation reduce edema by driving extravascular fluid out of the swollen area into the venous and lymphatic drainage systems. The combined treatment of rest, ice, compression, and elevation is frequently referred to by the acronym *RICE*.

Cryotherapy is not effective in controlling the formation of edema caused by immobility and poor circulation. In such cases, increased rather than decreased venous or lymphatic circulation is required to move fluid out of the affected area. This is best accomplished with compression, elevation, heat, exercise, and massage.[40] The mechanisms of action of this combination of treatments are discussed in detail in Chapter 11 in the section on compression.

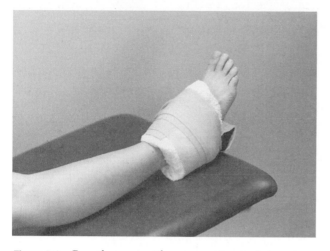

Figure 6-6. Cryotherapy with compression and elevation.

Pain Control

The decrease in tissue temperature produced by cryotherapy may directly or indirectly reduce the sensation of pain. Cryotherapy directly and rapidly modifies the sensation of pain by gating pain transmission with activity of the cutaneous thermal receptors. This immediate analgesic effect of cold is exploited when vapocoolant sprays or ice massage are used to cool the skin before stretching the muscles below. The reduced sensation of pain allows the stretch to be more forceful and thus potentially more effective.

Applying cryotherapy for 10 to 15 minutes or longer can control pain for 1 or more hours. This prolonged effect is thought to be the result of blocking conduction by deep pain-transmitting A-delta fibers, and by gating of pain transmission by the cutaneous thermal receptors.[16] The effect is thought to be prolonged because the temperature of the area remains lower than normal for 1 or 2 hours after removal of the cooling modality. Rewarming of the area is slow because cold-induced vasoconstriction limits the flow of warm blood into the area, and subcutaneous fat insulates the deeper tissues from rewarming by conduction from the ambient air.

The reduction of pain by cryotherapy can also interrupt the pain-spasm-pain cycle, resulting in reduced muscle spasm and prolonged alleviation of pain even after the temperature of the treated area has returned to normal. Cryotherapy can also reduce pain indirectly by alleviating the underlying cause of this symptom, such as inflammation or edema.

Modification of Spasticity

Cryotherapy can be used to temporarily reduce spasticity in patients with upper motor neuron dysfunctions. As explained above, brief applications of cold, lasting for about 5 minutes, cause an almost immediate decrease in deep tendon reflexes. Longer applications, for 10 to 30 minutes, also decrease or eliminate clonus and decrease the resistance of muscles to passive stretch.[24] Because longer applications of cryotherapy control more of the signs of spasticity, cryotherapy should be applied for up to 30 minutes when this is the treatment goal. The decrease in spasticity produced by prolonged cooling generally lasts for 1 hour or longer after the treatment, which is sufficient to allow for a variety of therapeutic interventions, including active exercise, stretching, functional activities, or hygiene.

Symptom Management in Multiple Sclerosis

The symptoms of some patients with multiple sclerosis are aggravated by generalized heating, such as occurs in warm environments or with activity. This group of patients can respond well to generalized cooling, with improvements in electrophysiological measures and in clinical symptoms and function.[41] Cooling with a vest has been shown to improve fatigue, muscle strength, and postural stability in a group of patients with heat-sensitive multiple sclerosis when compared with a sham noncooling vest.[42]

Facilitation

The rapid application of ice as a stimulus to elicit desired motor patterns, known as *quick icing,* is a technique developed by Rood. Although this technique may be used effectively in the rehabilitation of patients with flaccidity resulting from upper motor neuron dysfunction, it tends to have unreliable results and is therefore not commonly used.[43] The results of quick icing are unreliable because the initial phasic withdrawal pattern stimulated in the agonist muscles may lower the resting potential of the antagonists, so that a second stimulus elicits activity in the antagonist muscles rather than in the agonists.[44] This produces motion first in the desired direction, followed by a rebound movement in the opposite direction. It has also been proposed that icing may adversely impact motor control caused by dysynchronization of the cortex as a result of increased sympathetic tone.[45]

Cryokinetics and Cryostretch

Cryokinetics is a technique that combines the use of cold and exercise in the treatment of pathology or disease.[46] This technique involves applying a cooling agent to the point of numbness shortly after any injury to reduce the sensation of pain and thus allow the patient to exercise and work toward regaining range of motion (ROM) as early as possible in the recovery process.[47] This approach is most commonly used in the rehabilitation of athletes. Cold is applied first for up to 20 minutes, or until the patient reports numbing of the area; then the patient performs strengthening and stretching exercises for 3 to 5 minutes until sensation returns.[48] The cooling agent is then reapplied until analgesia is regained. This sequence of cooling, exercise, and recooling is repeated approximately five times. Because the numbness produced by the cryotherapy masks the pain related to the injury, to avoid further trauma and tissue damage it is essential that, before applying this technique, the exact nature of the injury is known and the therapist is certain that it is safe to exercise the area involved.

Cryostretch is the application of a cooling agent before stretching. The purpose of this sequence of treatments is to reduce muscle spasm and thus allow greater range-of-motion increases with stretching.[49]

CONTRAINDICATIONS AND PRECAUTIONS FOR CRYOTHERAPY

Although cryotherapy is a relatively safe treatment modality, its use is contraindicated in some circumstances and it should be applied with caution in others. Cryotherapy may be applied by a qualified clinician or by a properly instructed patient. Rehabilitation clinicians may use all forms of cryotherapy that are noninvasive and do not destroy tissue. Patients may use cold packs or ice packs, ice massage, or contrast baths to treat themselves.

If the patient's condition is worsening or is not improving within the period of two or three treatments, the treatment approach should be reevaluated and changed or the patient should be referred to a physician for further evaluation even when cryotherapy is not contraindicated.

CONTRAINDICATIONS
for the Application of Cryotherapy

- Cold hypersensitivity
- Cold intolerance
- Cryoglobulinemia
- Paroxysmal cold cryoglobinuria
- Raynaud's disease or phenomenon
- Over a regenerating peripheral nerve
- Over an area with circulatory compromise or peripheral vascular disease

....

The use of cryotherapy is contraindicated . . .

. . . **in patients with cold hypersensitivity, cold intolerance, cryoglobulinemia, paroxysmal cold hemoglobinuria, Raynaud's disease, or Raynaud's phenomenon**[50]

Cold Hypersensitivity (Cold-induced Urticaria). Some individuals have a familial or acquired hypersensitivity to cold that causes them to develop a vascular skin reaction in response to cold exposure.[51] This reaction is marked by the transient appearance of smooth, slightly elevated patches, which are redder or more pale than the surrounding skin and are often attended by severe itching. This response is

known as *cold hypersensitivity* or *cold-induced urticaria*. These symptoms can occur only in the area of cold application or all over the body.

Cold Intolerance. Cold intolerance, in the form of severe pain, numbness, and color changes in response to cold, can occur in patients with some types of rheumatic diseases or following severe accidental or surgical trauma to the digits.

Cryoglobulinemia. Cryoglobulinemia is an uncommon disorder characterized by the aggregation of serum proteins in the distal circulation when the distal extremities are cooled. These aggregated proteins form a precipitate or gel that can impair circulation, causing local ischemia and then gangrene. This disorder may be idiopathic or may be associated with multiple myeloma, systemic lupus erythematosus, rheumatoid arthritis, or other hyperglobulinemic states. Therefore the therapist should check with the referring physician before applying cryotherapy to the distal extremities of any patient with these predisposing disorders.

Paroxysmal Cold Hemoglobinuria. Paroxysmal cold hemoglobinuria is the release of hemoglobin into the urine from lysed red blood cells in response to local or general exposure to cold.

Raynaud's Disease and Phenomenon. Raynaud's disease is the primary or idiopathic form of paroxysmal digital cyanosis. Raynaud's phenomenon, which is more common, is paroxysmal digital cyanosis due to some other regional or systemic disorder. Both conditions are characterized by sudden pallor and cyanosis followed by redness of the skin of the digits precipitated by cold or emotional upset and relieved by warmth. These disorders occur primarily in young women. In Raynaud's disease the symptoms are bilateral and symmetric even when cold is applied to only one area, whereas in Raynaud's phenomenon, the symptoms generally occur only in the cooled extremity. Raynaud's phenomenon may be associated with thoracic outlet syndrome, carpal tunnel syndrome, or trauma.

ASK THE PATIENT:

- Do you have any unusual responses to cold? If the patient answers "yes" to this question, ask for further details. Include the following questions:
- Do you develop a rash when cold? (A sign of cold hypersensitivity)
- Do you have severe pain, numbness, and color changes in your fingers when exposed to cold? (Signs of Raynaud's disease/phenomenon)
- Do you get blood in your urine after being cold? (A sign of paroxysmal cold hemoglobinuria)

If the responses indicate that the patient may have cold hypersensitivity, cold intolerance, cryoglobulinemia, paroxysmal cold hemoglobinuria, Raynaud's disease, or Raynaud's phenomenon, cryotherapy should not be applied.

. . . over regenerating peripheral nerves

Cryotherapy should not be applied directly over a regenerating peripheral nerve because local vasoconstriction or altered nerve conduction may delay nerve regeneration.

ASK THE PATIENT:

- Do you have any nerve damage in this area?
- Do you have any numbness or tingling in this limb? If so, where?

ASSESS:

- Test sensation
  In the presence of sensory impairment or other signs of nerve dysfunction, cryotherapy should not be applied directly over the affected nerve.

. . . over an area with circulatory compromise or peripheral vascular disease

Cryotherapy should not be applied over an area with impaired circulation because it may aggravate the condition by causing vasoconstriction and increasing blood viscosity. Circulatory impairment may be the result of peripheral vascular disease, trauma to the vessels, or early healing, and is often associated with edema. When edema is present, it is important that its cause be determined, since edema due to inflammation can benefit from cryotherapy, while edema due to impaired circulation may be increased. These causes of edema can be distinguished by observation of local skin coloration and temperature. Edema due to inflammation is characterized by warmth and redness, whereas edema due to poor circulation is characterized by coolness and pallor.

ASK THE PATIENT:

- Do you have poor circulation in this limb?

ASSESS:

- Skin temperature and color.
  If the patient has signs of impaired circulation, such as pallor and coolness of the skin in the area being considered for treatment, cryotherapy should not be applied.

PRECAUTIONS
for the Application of Cryotherapy

- Over the superficial main branch of a nerve
- Over an open wound

- Hypertension
- In patients with poor sensation or poor mentation
- Very young and very old patients

Apply cryotherapy with caution . . .

. . . over a superficial main branch of a nerve

Applying cold directly over the superficial main branch of a nerve, such as the peroneal nerve at the lateral knee or the radial nerve at the posterolateral elbow, may cause a nerve conduction block.[14,17,52,53] Therefore when applying cryotherapy to such an area, one should monitor for signs of changes in nerve conduction, such as distal numbness or tingling, and discontinue cryotherapy if these occur.

. . . over an open wound

Cryotherapy should not be applied directly over any deep open wound because it can delay wound healing by reducing circulation and metabolic rate.[54] Cryotherapy may be applied in areas of superficial skin damage; however, it is important to realize that this can reduce the efficacy and safety of the treatment because when there is superficial skin damage, the cutaneous thermal receptors may also be damaged or absent. These receptors play a part in activating the vasoconstriction, pain control, and spasticity reduction produced by cryotherapy; therefore, these responses are likely to be less pronounced when cryotherapy is applied to areas with superficial skin damage. Caution should also be used if cryotherapy is applied to such areas because the absence of skin reduces the insulating protection of the subcutaneous layers and increases the risk of excessive cooling to these tissues.

ASSESS:

- Inspect the skin closely for deep wounds, cuts, or abrasions. Do not apply cryotherapy in the area of a deep wound, and use less intense cooling if cuts or abrasions are present.

. . . when treating patients with hypertension

Since cold can cause transient increases in systolic or diastolic blood pressure, patients with hypertension should be carefully monitored during the application of cryotherapy.[55] Treatment should be discontinued if blood pressure increases beyond safe levels during treatment. Guidelines for safe blood pressures for individual patients should be obtained from the physician.

. . . when treating patients with poor sensation or mentation

Although adverse effects with cryotherapy are rare, if the patient cannot sense or report discomfort or other abnormal responses, the clinician should monitor the patient's response directly. Check for adverse responses to cold such as wheals or abnormal changes in color or strength, both in the area of cold application and generally.

. . . when treating very young and very old patients

Caution should be used when applying cryotherapy to the very young or the very old because these individuals frequently have impaired thermal regulation and a limited ability to communicate.

ADVERSE EFFECTS OF CRYOTHERAPY

Tissue death
Frostbite
Nerve damage
Unwanted vasodilation

A variety of adverse effects have been reported when cold is applied incorrectly or when contraindicated. The most severe adverse effect from the improper application of cryotherapy is tissue death caused by prolonged vasoconstriction, ischemia, and thromboses in the smaller vessels. Tissue death may also result from freezing of the tissue. Tissue damage can occur when the tissue temperature reaches 15 °C (59 °F); however, freezing (frostbite) does not occur until the skin temperature drops to between – 4° and –10 °C (39° to 14 °F) or lower. Excessive exposure to cold may also cause temporary or permanent nerve damage, resulting in pain, numbness, tingling, hyperhidrosis, or nerve conduction abnormalities.[56] To avoid soft tissue or nerve damage, the duration of cold application should be limited to under 45 minutes, and the tissue temperature should be maintained above 15 °C (59 °F).

Because the prolonged application of cryotherapy to the distal extremities may cause reflex vasodilation and increased blood flow, cryotherapy should be applied for only 10 to 15 minutes when the goal of treatment is vasoconstriction.

APPLICATION TECHNIQUES

Cryotherapy may be applied using a variety of materials, including cold or ice packs, ice cups, controlled cold compression units, vapocoolant sprays, frozen towels, ice water, cold whirlpools, and contrast baths. The following section gives details on application techniques for these different cooling agents and the decisions to be made when selecting a specific agent and an application technique.

APPLICATION TECHNIQUE
Cryotherapy

1. Evaluate the patient and set the goals of treatment.
2. Determine if cryotherapy is the most appropriate treatment.
3. Determine that cryotherapy is not contraindicated for this patient or condition.

    Inspect the area to be treated for open wounds and rashes and assess sensation. Check the patient's chart for any record of previous adverse responses to cold and for any diseases that would predispose the patient to an adverse response. Ask the appropriate questions of the patient as described in the preceding sections on contraindications and precautions.
4. Select the appropriate cooling agent according to the body part to be treated and the desired response.

    Select an agent that provides the desired intensity of cold treatment, best fits the location and size of the area to be treated, is easily applied for the desired duration and in the desired position, is readily available, and is reasonably priced. An agent that conforms to the contours of the area being treated should be used to maintain good contact with the patient's skin. With agents that cool by conduction or convection, such as cold packs or a cold whirlpool, good contact must be maintained between the agent and the patient's body at all times to maximize the rate of cooling. For brief cooling the best choice is an agent that is quick to apply and remove. Any of the cooling agents described as follows may be available for use in a clinical setting, and the patient can readily use ice packs, ice cups, and cold packs at home. Ice packs and ice massage are the least expensive means of

providing cryotherapy, whereas controlled cold compression units are the most expensive.
5. Explain to the patient the procedure and reason for applying cryotherapy and the sensations the patient can expect to feel.

    During the application of cryotherapy by any means the patient will usually experience the following sequence of sensations: intense cold followed by burning, then aching, and finally analgesia and numbness. These sensations are thought to correspond to increasing stimulation of the thermal receptors and pain receptors followed by blocking of sensory nerve conduction as the tissue temperature decreases.

SEQUENCE OF SENSATIONS IN RESPONSE TO CRYOTHERAPY
- Intense cold
- Burning
- Aching
- Analgesia and numbness
6. Apply the appropriate cooling agent.
    Select from the following list:
    Cold packs or ice packs
    Ice cups for ice massage
    Controlled cold compression units
    Vapocoolant sprays or brief icing
    Frozen towels
    Ice water immersion
    Cold whirlpool
    Contrast bath

    } See application methods for each cooling agent on the following pages.

Continued

APPLICATION TECHNIQUE—cont'd
Cryotherapy

7. Assess the outcome of treatment.

   After completing cryotherapy with any of the preceding agents, reassess the patient, checking particularly for progress toward the set goals of treatment and for any adverse effects of the treat-

ment. Remeasure quantifiable subjective conditions and objective limitations, and reassess the impairments and disabilities.

8. Document the treatment.

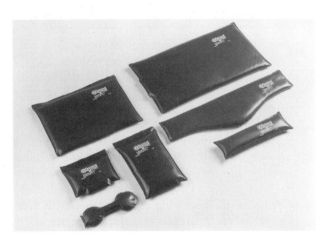

Figure 6-7. Cold packs. (Courtesy Chattanooga Group, Inc., Hixson, TN.)

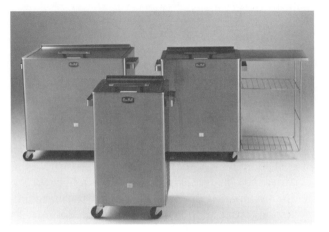

Figure 6-8. Cooling units for cold packs. (Courtesy Chattanooga Group, Inc., Hixson, TN.)

Cold Packs or Ice Packs

Cold packs are usually filled with a gel composed of silica or a mixture of saline and gelatin and are usually covered with vinyl (Fig. 6-7). The gel is formulated to be semisolid at between 0° and 5 °C (32° to 41 °F) for the pack to conform to the body contours when it is within this temperature range. The temperature of a cold pack is maintained by storing it in a specialized cooling unit (Fig. 6-8) or in a freezer at –5 °C (23 °F). Cold packs should be cooled for at least 30 minutes between uses and for 2 hours or longer before initial use. Patients can use plastic bags of frozen vegetables at home as a substitute for cold packs, or they can make their own cold packs from plastic bags filled with a 4:1 ratio mixture of water and rubbing alcohol

cooled in a home freezer. The addition of alcohol to the water decreases the freezing temperature of the mixture so that it is semisolid and flexible at –5 °C (23 °F).

Ice packs are made of crushed ice placed in a plastic bag. Ice packs provide more aggressive cooling than cold packs at the same temperature because ice has a higher specific heat than most gels and because ice absorbs a large amount of energy when it melts and changes from a solid to a liquid. [57] Both cold packs and ice packs are applied in a similar manner, as described below; however, more insulation should be used when applying an ice pack because it provides more aggressive cooling.

APPLICATION TECHNIQUE
Cold Pack/Ice Pack

Equipment Required

Cold Packs
- Cold packs in a variety of sizes and shapes appropriate for different areas of the body
- Freezer or specialized cooling unit
- Towels or pillow cases for hygiene and/or insulation

Ice Packs
- Plastic bags
- Ice chips
- Ice chip machine or freezer
- Towels or pillow cases for hygiene and/or insulation

PROCEDURE

1. Remove all jewelry and clothing from the area to be treated and inspect the area.
2. Wrap the cold pack or ice pack in a towel. Use a damp towel if a maximal rate of tissue cooling is desired. It is recommended that warm water be used to dampen the towel to allow the patient to gradually become accustomed to the cold sensation. A thin, dry towel can be used if slower, less intense cooling is desired. A damp towel is generally appropriate for a cold pack, whereas a dry towel should be used for an ice pack since ice provides more intense cooling.
3. Position the patient comfortably, elevating the area to be treated if edema is present.
4. Place the wrapped pack on the area to be treated and secure it well. Packs can be secured with elastic bandages or towels to ensure good contact with the patient's skin (Fig. 6-9).

5. Leave the pack in place for 10 to 15 minutes to control pain, inflammation, or edema.[58] A recent systematic review of the research on cryotherapy found that a 10-minute application time is most effective for reducing the pain and swelling associated with soft tissue injury and minimizing the risk of side effects and possible further injury.[59]

   When cold is applied over bandages or a cast, the application time should be increased to allow the cold to penetrate through these insulating layers to the skin.[60] In this circumstance, the cold pack should be replaced with a newly frozen pack if the original pack melts during the course of treatment.

   If cryotherapy is being used to control spasticity, the pack should be left in place for up to 30 minutes. With these longer applications, check every 10 to 15 minutes for any signs of adverse effects.
6. Provide the patient with a bell or other means to call for assistance.
7. When the treatment is completed, remove the pack and inspect the treatment area for any signs of adverse effects such as wheals or a rash. It is normal for the skin to be red or dark pink after icing.
8. Cold or ice pack application can be repeated every 1 to 2 hours to control pain and inflammation.[61]

ADVANTAGES
- Easy to use
- Inexpensive materials and equipment
- Short use of clinician's time
- Low level of skill required for application
- Covers moderate to large areas
- Can be applied to an elevated limb

DISADVANTAGES
- Pack must be removed to visualize the treatment area during treatment
- Patient may not tolerate weight of the pack

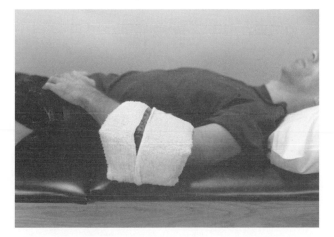

Figure 6-9. Application of a cold pack.

Continued

APPLICATION TECHNIQUE—cont'd
Cold Pack/Ice Pack

- Pack may not be able to maintain good contact on small or contoured areas
- Long duration of treatment compared to massage with an ice cup

ICE PACK VERSUS COLD PACK
- Ice pack provides more intense cooling
- Ice pack is less expensive
- Cold pack is quicker to apply

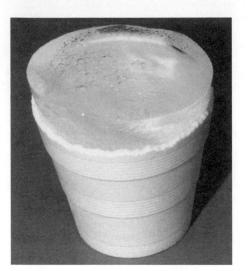

Figure 6-10. Ice cup.

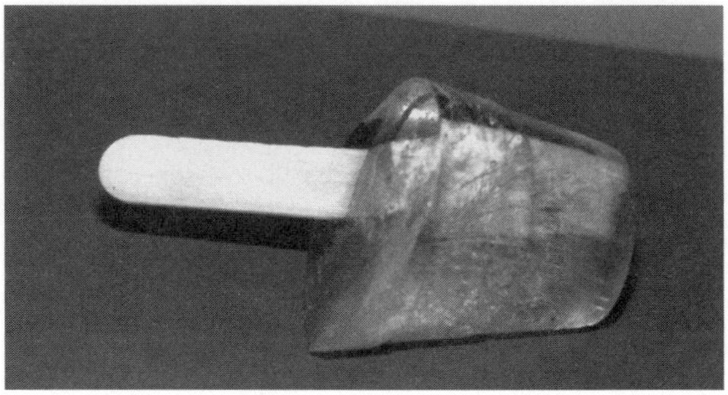

Figure 6-11. Water popsicle.

Ice Massage

Ice cups (Fig. 6-10) or frozen water popsicles[62] (Fig. 6-11) can be used to apply ice massage. Frozen ice cups are made by freezing small paper or Styrofoam cups of water. To use these, the therapist holds on to the bottom of the cup and gradually peels back the edge to expose the surface of the ice and puts it in direct contact with the patient's skin. Water popsicles are made by placing a stick or tongue depressor into the water cup before freezing. When frozen, the ice can be completely removed from the cup and the stick used as a handle for applying the ice. Patients can easily make ice cups or popsicles for home use.

APPLICATION TECHNIQUE
Ice Massage

Equipment Required
- Small paper or Styrofoam cups
- Freezer

- Tongue depressors or popsicle sticks (optional)
- Towels to absorb water

PROCEDURE

1. Remove all jewelry and clothing from the area to be treated and inspect the area.
2. Place towels around the treatment area to absorb any dripping water and to wipe away water on the skin during treatment.
3. Rub the ice over the treatment area using small, overlapping circles (Fig. 6-12). Wipe away any water as it melts on the skin.
4. Continue ice massage application for 5 to 10 minutes or until the patient experiences analgesia at the site of application.
5. When the treatment is completed, inspect the treatment area for any signs of adverse effects such as wheals or a rash. It is normal for the skin to be red or dark pink after the application of ice massage. Ice massage may be applied in the above manner for the local control of pain, inflammation, or edema. Ice massage can also be used as a stimulus for facilitating the production of desired motor patterns in patients with impaired motor control. When applied for this purpose, the ice is either rubbed with pressure for 3 to 5 seconds or quickly stroked over the muscle bellies to be facilitated. This technique is known as *quick icing*.

ADVANTAGES

- Treatment area can be observed during application

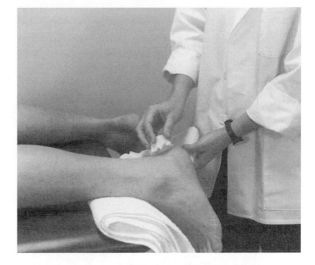

Figure 6-12. Application of ice massage.

- Can be used for small and irregular areas
- Short duration of treatment
- Inexpensive
- Can be applied to an elevated limb

DISADVANTAGES

- Too time-consuming for large areas
- Requires active participation by the clinician or patient throughout application

Controlled Cold Compression Unit

Controlled cold compression units alternately pump cold water and air into a sleeve that is wrapped around a patient's limb (Fig. 6-13 *A,B*). The temperature of the water can be set at between 10° and 25 °C (50° to 77 °F) to provide cooling. Compression is applied by intermittent inflation of the sleeve with air. Controlled cold compression units are most commonly used directly after surgery for the control of postoperative inflammation and edema; however, they may also be used to control inflammation and related edema in other circumstances. When applied postoperatively, the sleeve is put on the patient's affected limb immediately after completion of the surgery while the patient is in the recovery room, and the unit is sent home with the patient so that it can be used for a few days or weeks after surgery. The application of cold with compression in this manner has been shown to be more effective than ice or compression alone in controlling swelling, pain, and blood loss after surgery and in assisting the patient in regaining ROM.[63,64]

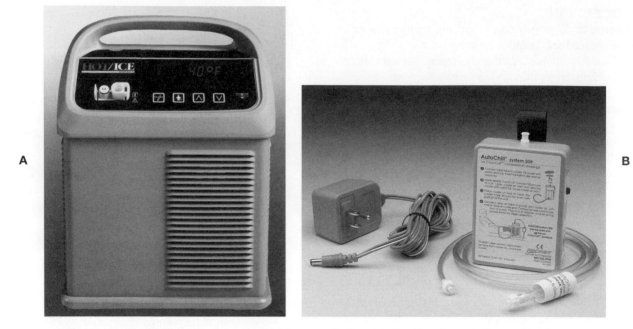

Figure 6-13. **A,** Controlled cold compression unit. (Courtesy InCare Medical Products, Libertyville, IL). **B,** AutoChill® System 20B. (Courtesy AIRCAST® Inc., Summit, NJ.)

APPLICATION TECHNIQUE
Controlled Cold Compression

Equipment Required
• Controlled cold compression unit
• Sleeves appropriate for area(s) to be treated
• Stockinette for hygiene

PROCEDURE

1. Remove all jewelry and clothing from the area to be treated and inspect the area.
2. Cover the limb with a stockinette before applying the sleeve.
3. Wrap the sleeve around the area to be treated (Fig. 6-14).
4. Elevate the area to be treated.
5. Set the temperature at 10° to 15 °C (50° to 59 °F).
6. Cooling can be applied continuously or intermittently. For intermittent treatment, apply cooling for 15 minutes every 2 hours.
7. Cycling intermittent compression may be applied at all times when the area is elevated.
8. When the treatment is completed, remove the sleeve and inspect the treatment area.

ADVANTAGES

• Allows simultaneous application of cold and compression
• Temperature and compression force are easily and accurately controlled
• Can be applied to large joints

DISADVANTAGES

• Treatment site cannot be visualized during treatment
• Expensive
• Usable only for extremities
• Cannot be used for trunk or digits

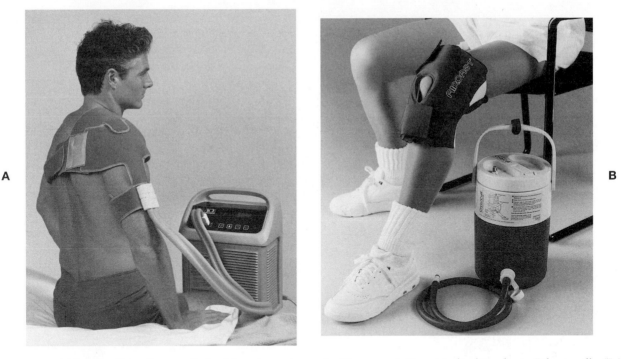

Figure 6-14. **A,** Application of controlled cold compression unit. (Courtesy InCare Medical Products, Libertyville, IL.); and, **B,** Knee Cryo/Cuff®. (Courtesy AIRCAST® Inc., Summit, NJ.)

Vapocoolant Sprays and Brief Icing

The vapocoolant sprays ethyl chloride and Fluori-Methane have been used for many years to achieve brief and rapid cutaneous cooling (Fig. 6-15). These products cool by evaporation. Ethyl chloride was first used for this purpose; however, since it is volatile, flammable, and capable of causing excessive temperature decreases,[65] Fluori-Methane, which also effectively cools the skin but is nonflammable and causes less reduction in temperature, was introduced.[66] However, Fluori-Methane is a volatile chlorofluorocarbon that can damage the ozone layer; therefore, its use is not permitted by a number of facilities, although it has been granted a nonessential class I product exemption from the Environmental Protection Agency (EPA) to permit its use in a clinical setting.[67] Due to these limitations of vapocoolant spray products, many clinicians apply brief ice massage, using ice cups or popsicles, when rapid cutaneous cooling is desired.

Rapid cutaneous cooling is generally used as a component of the treatment of trigger points. For this application, the vapocoolant spray or brief icing is applied in parallel strokes along the skin overlying the muscles with trigger points immediately before stretching these muscles[68] (Figs. 6-16 and 6-17). This type of treatment is frequently applied directly after trigger point injection. The purpose of the rapid cooling is to provide a counterirritant stimulus to the cutaneous thermal afferents overlying the muscles to cause a reflex reduction in motor neuron activity and thus a reduction in the resistance to stretch.[69] This technique was developed by Janet Travell, who describes this combination with the phrase "Stretch is the action; spray is the distraction."[70] The "distraction" of rapid cutaneous cooling is intended to promote greater elongation of the muscle with passive stretching. The combination of spraying with vapocoolant spray followed by stretching is known as *"spray and stretch."*

Other Means of Applying Cryotherapy

Cryotherapy may also be applied using frozen wet towels, a bucket of ice or cold water, a cold whirlpool, or a contrast bath. Frozen wet towels are rarely used because they are inconvenient and messy. The use of cold water, cold whirlpools, and contrast baths is discussed in detail in Chapter 9 of this book.

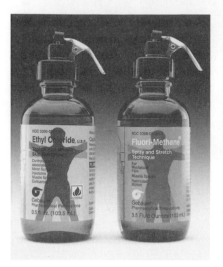

Figure 6-15. Vapocoolant sprays: ethyl chloride and Fluori-Methane. (Courtesy Gebauer Company, Cleveland, OH.)

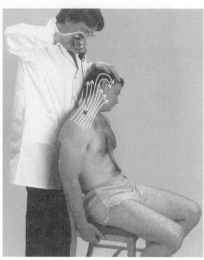

Figure 6-16. Application of vapocoolant spray. (Courtesy Gebauer Company, Cleveland, OH.)

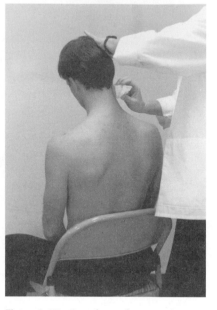

Figure 6-17. Quick stroking with ice cup.

APPLICATION TECHNIQUE
Vapocoolant Sprays and Brief Icing[71]

PROCEDURE

1. Identify trigger points and their related tight muscles.
2. Position the patient comfortably, with all limbs and the back well supported and the area to be treated exposed and accessible. Inspect the area to be treated. If using ethyl chloride spray, protect the surrounding areas of skin with petrolatum to avoid excessive cooling. Because Fluori-Methane produces less intense cooling than ethyl chloride, the surrounding areas of skin do not need protection when Fluori-Methane is being used.
3. Apply two to five parallel sweeps of the spray or brief ice massage at a speed of approximately 10 cm per second along the direction of the muscle fibers. When using a spray, hold the bottle about 45 cm from the skin and angled so that the spray hits the skin at an angle of about 30 degrees. If applying the spray near or around the patient's head, try to minimize the patient's inhalation of the spray, particularly with ethyl chloride, since this substance can produce general anesthetic effects.
4. During the cooling, maintain gentle, smooth, steady tension on the muscle to take up any slack that may develop.
5. Immediately after the cooling, have the patient take a deep breath and then perform a gentle passive stretch while exhaling. Contraction/relaxation techniques may also be used to enhance the ROM increases obtained with this procedure.
6. Following this procedure, the skin should be rewarmed with moist heat, and then the muscles should be moved through their full active ROM.

ADVANTAGES
- Brief duration of cooling
- Very localized area of application

DISADVANTAGES
- Fluori-Methane spray damages the ozone layer

- Limited to use for brief, localized, superficial application of cold before stretching
- Possible narcotic or general anesthetic effect if ethyl chloride is inhaled

Documentation

Document the area of the body treated, the type of cooling agent used, the treatment duration, patient positioning, and the response to treatment. Documentation is typically written in the SOAP note (Subjective, Objective, Assessment, Plan) format. The following examples only summarize the modality component of treatment and are not intended to represent a comprehensive plan of care.

Examples

When applying an ice pack (IP) to the left knee (L knee) for 15 minutes (15 °C) to control postoperative swelling, document:

S: Pt c/o L knee pain and swelling that increases with walking.

O: IP L anterior knee × 15', L LE elevated

A: Midpatellar girth decreased from 16 ½ to 15, gait improved from "step to" to "step through" ascending stairs.

P: Instruct pt. in home program of IP to L anterior knee, 15', with L LE elevated, 3X each day until next treatment session.

When applying ice massage (IM) to the area of the right (R) lateral epicondyle to treat epicondylitis, document:

S: Pt c/o pain in R lateral elbow at 8/10

O: IM R lat elbow × 5'

A: Pain decreased from 8/10 to 6/10. Elbow ROM improved – full extension after treatment.

P: Continue IM at end of treatment sessions until goal of pain-free elbow function is achieved.

▶ Clinical Case Studies ◀

The following case studies summarize the concepts of cryotherapy discussed in this chapter. Based on the scenario presented, an evaluation of the clinical findings and goals of treatment are proposed. These are followed by a discussion of the factors to be considered in the selection of cryotherapy as the indicated treatment modality and in the selection of the ideal cryotherapy agent to promote progress toward the set goals.

Case 1

TF is a 20-year-old male accountant. He injured his right knee 4 months ago while playing football and was treated conservatively with nonsteroidal antiinflammatory drugs (NSAIDs) and physical therapy for 8 weeks, with moderate improvement in symptoms; however, he was not able to return to sports due to continued complaints of medial knee pain. A magnetic resonance imaging (MRI) scan 3 weeks ago revealed a tear of the medial meniscus, and the patient underwent arthroscopic partial medial meniscectomy of his right knee 4 days ago. He has been referred to physical therapy with an order to evaluate and treat. TF complains of pain in his knee that has decreased in intensity from 9/10 to 7/10 since the surgery but that increases with weight bearing on the right lower extremity. He also complains of knee stiffness. The objective exam reveals moderate warmth of the skin of the right knee, particularly at the anteromedial aspect, and ROM restricted to –10 degrees of extension and 85 degrees of flexion. The patient is ambulating without any assistive device but with a decreased stance phase on the right lower extremity and with his right knee held stiffly in approximately 30 degrees of flexion throughout the gait cycle. Knee girth at the midpatellar level is 17 inches on the right and 15 ½ inches on the left.

EVALUATION OF THE CLINICAL FINDINGS

This patient presents with the impairments of pain, loss of motion, and increased girth of the right knee, resulting in the disabilities of limited ambulation and sports activity. He is independent in his home environment without the use of adaptive equipment.

Continued

◗ *Clinical Case Studies—cont'd* ◖

PREFERRED PRACTICE PATTERN

Impaired Joint Mobility, Motor Function, Muscle Performance, and Range of Motion Associated With Bony or Soft Tissue Surgery, (4I)

PLAN OF CARE

The goals of treatment at this time are to control pain and edema, accelerate resolution of the acute inflammation phase of healing, and accelerate the recovery of ROM and function.

ASSESSMENT REGARDING THE APPROPRIATENESS OF CRYOTHERAPY AS THE OPTIMAL TREATMENT

Cryotherapy is an indicated treatment for the control of pain, edema, and inflammation. It can control the formation of edema, and compression and elevation can reduce edema already present in the patient's knee. The application of cryotherapy early during the recovery from articular surgery has also been associated with an acceleration of functional recovery.[72] Since the peroneal nerve is superficial at the lateral knee, the patient should be monitored for signs of nerve conduction block, such as tingling or numbness in his lateral leg, during treatment. The presence of any contraindications to the application of cryotherapy, such as Raynaud's syndrome, should also be ruled out before the application of cryotherapy. Cryotherapy also should not be applied if infection is suspected. Although this patient does have signs of inflammation, including heat, redness, pain, swelling, and loss of function, the fact that his signs and symptoms have decreased since surgery indicates an appropriate course of recovery and the probable absence of infection. A progressive increase in the signs and symptoms of inflammation or complaints of fever and general malaise would suggest the presence of infection, requiring physician evaluation before the initiation of rehabilitation.

PROPOSED TREATMENT PLAN AND RATIONALE

To obtain maximum cooling of the knee, cryotherapy should be applied to all the skin surfaces surrounding the knee joint. A cold pack, ice pack, or controlled cold compression unit could adequately cover this area. In choosing among these agents, one should consider the convenience and ease of application of a cold pack, the low expense and ready availability of an ice pack, and the additional benefits (although greater cost) of intermittent compression provided by a controlled cold compression unit. Ice massage would not be an appropriate treatment because it would take too long to apply to such a large area. Immersion in ice or cold water would also not be appropriate since this would require the swollen knee to be in a dependent position, potentially aggravating the edema, and would require the additional discomfort of immersing the entire distal lower extremity in cold water.

Whether using a cold pack, ice pack, or controlled cold compression unit, cryotherapy should generally be applied for approximately 15 minutes to ensure adequate cooling of the tissues and minimizing the probability of excessive cooling or reactive vasodilation. This treatment should be reapplied by the patient at home every 2 to 3 hours while signs of inflammation are still present (Fig. 6-18).

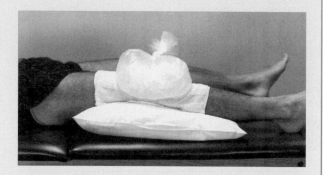

Figure 6-18. Application of ice pack to right knee.

Case 2

SG is a 40-year-old female office worker. She has been referred to therapy with a diagnosis of lateral epicondylitis and an order to evaluate and treat. SG complains of constant moderate to severe pain at her right lateral elbow that prevents her from playing tennis. The pain started about 1 month ago, the morning after she spent a whole day pulling weeds, and remained unchanged in severity or frequency until 3 days ago. She reports a slight decrease in pain severity over the last 3 days, which she associates with starting to take an NSAID prescribed by her physician. She has had similar symptoms previously, after gardening or playing tennis, but these have always resolved within a couple of days without any medical intervention. Objective examination reveals tenderness and mild swelling at the right lateral epicondyle and pain without weakness with resisted wrist extension. All other tests, including upper extremity sensation, ROM, and strength, are within normal limits.

EVALUATION OF THE CLINICAL FINDINGS

This patient presents with the impairments of pain, tenderness, and swelling of the right elbow resulting in an inability to participate in her normal sports activity of tennis.

PREFERRED PRACTICE PATTERN

Impaired Joint Mobility, Motor Function, Muscle Performance, and Range of Motion Associated With Localized Inflammation, (4E)

PLAN OF CARE

The goals of treatment at this time are to resolve the inflammation and control pain. The anticipated long-term goals of treatment include the patient's return to playing tennis and prevention of recurrences of this problem.

ASSESSMENT REGARDING THE APPROPRIATENESS OF CRYOTHERAPY AS THE OPTIMAL TREATMENT

Cryotherapy is an indicated treatment for inflammation and pain, and can also be used prophylactically after exercise to prevent the onset of inflammation and soreness. The advantages of cryotherapy over other treatments indicated for these applications, such as ultrasound or electrical stimulation, are that it is quick, easy, and inexpensive to apply, and the patient can apply it at home. Cryotherapy alone may not resolve the present symptoms and may therefore need to be applied in conjunction with other physical agents, activity modification, manual therapy techniques, and/or exercises to achieve the proposed goals of treatment. Since the radial nerve is superficial at the lateral elbow, the patient should be monitored for signs of nerve conduction blockage during treatment, such as tingling or numbness in her dorsal arm. The presence of any contraindications to the application of cryotherapy, such as Raynaud's syndrome, should be ruled out before the application of cryotherapy.

PROPOSED TREATMENT PLAN AND RATIONALE

Ice massage, an ice pack, or a cold pack can be used to provide cryotherapy to the area of the lateral epicondyle (Fig. 6-19). Since ice massage has the advantages of taking little time to apply to this small area while allowing visualization of the treatment area and assessment of signs and symptoms throughout the treatment, this would be the most appropriate agent to use for this patient, although an ice pack or cold pack could also be used. An ice pack or cold pack would be more appropriate if the symptomatic area was larger; for example, if the area extended into the dorsal forearm. Cryotherapy should be applied until the treatment area is numb,

which usually takes 5 to 10 minutes when using ice massage or about 15 minutes when using an ice pack or a cold pack. Treatment should be discontinued sooner if numbness extends into the hand in the distribution of the radial nerve. Cryotherapy treatments should continue to be applied until the signs and symptoms of inflammation have resolved. Treatments should be discontinued thereafter since the vasoconstriction produced by cryotherapy may retard the later stages of tissue healing. The patient should also be instructed to apply cryotherapy prophylactically after activities that have previously resulted in elbow pain, such as tennis or gardening, to reduce the risk of a recurrence of her present symptoms.

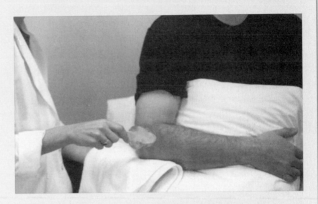

Figure 6-19. Application of ice massage to elbow.

Case 3

FB is a 60-year-old male truck driver. He has been referred to physical therapy with a diagnosis of osteoarthritis of the left knee and an order to evaluate and treat. He reports that he has had arthritis in this knee for the last 5 years and that he recently started performing exercises that have increased the strength, stability, and endurance of his legs but cause knee pain and thigh muscle soreness the next day. His goals in therapy are to control this postexercise discomfort to allow continuation of his exercise program. He performed his exercises yesterday, and today the objective evaluation reveals a mild increase in the temperature of the left knee and tenderness of the anterior thigh. Knee girth and ROM are equal bilaterally.

EVALUATION OF THE CLINICAL FINDINGS

This patient presents with the impairments of intermittent left knee and thigh pain resulting in the disability of restricted exercise activity.

PREFERRED PRACTICE PATTERN

Impaired Joint Mobility, Motor Function, Muscle Performance, and Range of Motion Associated With Localized Inflammation, (4E)

Continued

▶ *Clinical Case Studies—cont'd* ◀

PLAN OF CARE

The goals of treatment at this time are to eliminate postexercise thigh muscle and knee joint soreness.

ASSESSMENT REGARDING THE APPROPRIATENESS OF CRYOTHERAPY AS THE OPTIMAL TREATMENT

Cryotherapy is an indicated treatment for delayed-onset muscle soreness and joint inflammation; however, the patient's exercise program should also be evaluated and modified as appropriate to reduce his discomfort after exercising. The presence of any contraindications to the application of cryotherapy, such as Raynaud's syndrome, should be ruled out before the application of cryotherapy.

PROPOSED TREATMENT PLAN AND RATIONALE

As in Case 1, the application of cryotherapy for 15 minutes with an ice pack or cold pack would be appropriate for treatment of this patient's knee. The additional expense of a controlled cold compression unit is not justified in this case since there is no edema and therefore compression is not needed. The patient should apply the pack immediately after completing his exercise program. Since the peroneal nerve is superficial at the lateral knee, the patient should be monitored for signs of nerve conduction blockage, such as tingling or numbness in his lateral leg, during treatment.

HEAT—THERMOTHERAPY

The therapeutic application of heat is known as *thermotherapy*. Thermotherapy is used clinically outside of rehabilitation primarily to destroy malignant tissue growth or to treat cold-related injuries. Within rehabilitation, thermotherapy is used primarily to control pain, increase soft tissue extensibility, increase circulation, and accelerate healing. Heat has these therapeutic effects due to its influence on hemodynamic, neuromuscular, and metabolic processes, the mechanisms of which are explained in detail following.

EFFECTS OF HEAT

Hemodynamic effects
Vasodilation

Neuromuscular effects
Changes in nerve conduction velocity and firing rate
Increased pain threshold
Changes in muscle strength

Metabolic effects
Increased metabolic rate

Altered tissue extensibility
Increased collagen extensibility

Hemodynamic Effects

Vasodilation

Heat causes vasodilation and thus an increase in the rate of blood flow.[73] When heat is applied to one area of the body, there is vasodilation where the heat is applied, and to a lesser degree, systemically, in areas distant from the site of heat application. Superficial heating agents produce more pronounced vasodilation in the local cutaneous blood vessels, where they cause the greatest change in temperature, and less pronounced dilation in the deeper vessels that run through muscles, where they cause little if any change in temperature. Thermotherapy applied to the whole body can also cause generalized vasodilation and may improve vascular endothelial function in the setting of cardiac risk factors.[74]

Thermotherapy may cause vasodilation by a variety of mechanisms, including direct reflex activation of the smooth muscles of the blood vessels by the cutaneous thermoreceptors, indirect activation of local spinal cord reflexes by the cutaneous thermoreceptors, or by increasing the local release of chemical mediators of inflammation.[75,76] (Fig. 6-20). A recent study demonstrated that at least two independent mechanisms contribute to the rise in skin blood flow during local heating: a fast-responding vasodilator system mediated by the axon reflexes and a more

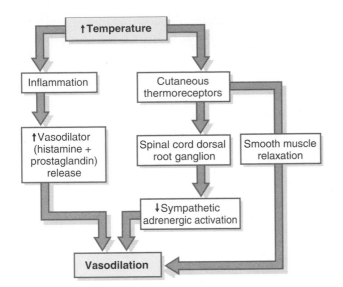

Figure 6-20. How heat causes vasodilation.

slowly responding vasodilator system that relies on local production of nitrous oxide.[77]

Superficial heating agents stimulate increased activity of the cutaneous thermoreceptors. It is proposed that transmission from the cutaneous thermoreceptors via their axons directly to nearby cutaneous blood vessels causes the release of bradykinin and nitrous oxide. Bradykinin and nitrous oxide act as vasoactive mediators stimulating relaxation of the smooth muscles of the vessel walls to cause vasodilation.[76-78] This vasodilation occurs locally, in the area where the heat is applied.

Cutaneous thermoreceptors also project via the dorsal root ganglion to synapse with interneurons in the dorsal horn of the gray matter of the spinal cord. These interneurons synapse with sympathetic neurons in the lateral gray horn of the thoracolumbar segments of the spinal cord to inhibit their firing and thus decrease sympathetic output.[79] This decrease in sympathetic activity causes a reduction in smooth muscle contraction, resulting in vasodilation both at the site of heat application and in the cutaneous vessels of the distal extremities.[80] This distant vasodilative effect of thermotherapy may be used to increase cutaneous blood flow to an area where it is difficult or unsafe to apply a heating agent directly.[81] For example, if a patient has an ulcer on his leg as the result of arterial insufficiency in the extremity, thermotherapy may be applied to his lower back to increase the circulation to his lower extremity and thereby facilitate wound healing. This would be most appropriate if the ulcer was bandaged or did not tolerate pressure, or if the area lacked sufficient circulation or sensation to tolerate the direct application of heat.

Because blood flow in the skeletal muscles is primarily influenced by metabolic factors rather than by changes in sympathetic activity, and superficial heating agents do not increase the temperature to the depth of most muscles, skeletal muscle blood flow is much less affected by superficial heating modalities than is skin blood flow.[82,83] The use of exercise or deep heating modalities, such as ultrasound or diathermy, or a combination of these interventions, is therefore recommended when the goal of treatment is to increase skeletal muscle blood flow.

Cutaneous vasodilation, and the resulting increase in blood flow that occurs in response to increased tissue temperature, acts to protect the body from excessive heating and tissue damage. The increased rate of blood flow increases the rate at which an area is cooled by convection. Thus when an area is heated with a thermal agent, it is simultaneously cooled by circulating blood, and as the temperature of the area increases, the rates of circulation and cooling both increase to reduce the impact of the thermal agent on tissue temperature thereby reducing the risk of burning.

Neuromuscular Effects

Changes in nerve conduction velocity and firing rate

Increased temperature has long been known to increase nerve conduction velocity and decrease the conduction latency of both sensory and motor nerves.[84,85] Nerve conduction velocity has been reported to increase by approximately 2 meters/second for every 1 °C (1.8 °F) increase in temperature. Although the clinical implications of these effects are not well understood, they may contribute to the reduced pain perception or improved circulation that occurs in response to increasing tissue temperature.

Nerve firing rate (frequency) has also been found to change in response to changes in temperature. Elevation of muscle temperature to 42 °C (108 °F) has been shown to result in a decreased firing rate of type II muscle spindle efferents and gamma efferents and an increased firing rate of type Ib fibers from Golgi tendon organs.[86,87] These changes in nerve firing rates are thought to contribute to a reduction in the firing rate of alpha motor neurons and thus to a reduction in muscle spasm.[88] The decrease in gamma neuron activity causes the stretch on the muscle spindles to decrease, reducing afferent firing from the spindles.[89] The decreased spindle afferent activity results in decreased alpha motor neuron activity and thus in relaxation of muscle contraction.

Increased pain threshold

Several studies demonstrate that the application of local heat can increase pain threshold.[90,91] The proposed mechanisms of this effect include a direct and immediate reduction of pain by activation of the spinal gating mechanism and an indirect, later, and more prolonged reduction of pain by reduction of ischemia and muscle spasm or facilitation of tissue healing. Heat increases the activity of the cutaneous thermoreceptors, which can have an immediate inhibitory gating effect on the transmission of the sensation of pain at the spinal cord level. Stimulation of the thermoreceptors can also result in vasodilation, as described above, causing an increase in blood flow and thus potentially reducing pain caused by ischemia. Ischemia may also be decreased as a result of reduction of spasm in muscles that compress blood vessels. The vasodilation produced by thermotherapy may also accelerate the recovery of the local pain threshold to a normal level by speeding tissue healing.

Changes in muscle strength

Muscle strength and endurance have been found to decrease during the initial 30 minutes after the application of deep or superficial heating agents.[92-94] It is proposed that this initial decrease in muscle strength is the result of changes in the firing rates of type II muscle spindle efferent, gamma efferent, and type Ib fibers from Golgi tendon organs caused by heating of the motor nerves. In turn, this decreases the firing rate of alpha motor neurons. Beyond 30 minutes after the application of heat, and for the next 2 hours, muscle strength gradually recovers and then increases to above pretreatment levels. This delayed increase in strength is thought to result in augmentation of the individual's pain threshold.

Although changes in muscle strength produced by heating are not generally used to modify a rehabilitation program, it is important to be aware of them when assessing muscle strength as a measure of patient progress. Since comparing preheating strength with postheating strength from the same session or another session can provide misleading information, it is recommended that muscle strength and endurance always be measured before applying a heating modality.

Metabolic Effects

Increased metabolic rate

Heat increases the rate of endothermic chemical reactions, including the rate of enzymatic biological reactions. Increased enzymatic activity has been observed in tissues at 39° to 43 °C (102° to 109 °F), with the reaction rate increasing by approximately 13% for every 10 °C (18 °F) increase in temperature and doubling for every 10 °C (18 °F) increase in temperature.[32] Enzymatic and metabolic activity rates continue to increase up to a temperature of 45 °C (113 °F). Beyond this temperature, the protein constituents of enzymes begin to denature and enzyme activity rates decrease, ceasing completely at about 50 °C (122 °F).[95]

Any increase in enzymatic activity will result in an increase in the rate of cellular biochemical reactions. This can increase oxygen uptake and accelerate healing but may also increase the rate of destructive processes. For example, heat may accelerate the healing of a chronic wound; however, it has also been shown to increase the activity of collagenase and may thus accelerate the destruction of articular cartilage in patients with rheumatoid arthritis.[31] Therefore thermotherapy should be used with caution in patients with acute inflammatory disorders.

Increasing tissue temperature also shifts the oxygen-hemoglobin dissociation curve to the right, making more oxygen available for tissue repair (see Fig. 6-4). It has been shown that hemoglobin releases twice as much oxygen at 41 °C (106 °F) as it does at 36° C (97 °F).[96] In conjunction with the increased rate of blood flow stimulated by increased temperature and the increased enzymatic reaction rate, this increased oxygen availability may contribute to acceleration of tissue healing by thermotherapy.

Altered Tissue Extensibility

Increased collagen extensibility

Increasing the temperature of soft tissue increases its extensibility.[97] When soft tissue is heated before stretching, it maintains a greater increase in length after the stretching force is applied, less force is required to achieve the increase in length, and the risk of tissue tearing is reduced.[98,99] If heat is applied to collagenous soft tissue such as tendon, ligament, scar tissue, or joint capsule before prolonged stretching, plastic deformation, whereby the tissue increases in length and maintains most of the increase after cooling, can be achieved.[100,101] In contrast, if collagenous tissue is stretched without prior heating, elastic deformation, whereby the tissue increases in length while the force is applied but loses most of the increase when the force is removed, generally occurs. The maintained elongation of collagenous tissue that occurs after heating and stretching is caused by changes in the organization of the collagen fibers and to changes of the viscoelasticity of the fibers themselves rather than to increases in the number of fibers.

For heat to increase the extensibility of soft tissue, the appropriate temperature range and structures must be reached. A maximum increase in residual length is achieved when the tissue temperature is maintained at 40° to 45 °C (104° to 113 °F) for 5 to 10 minutes.[86,101] The superficial heating agents described in the following sections can cause this level of temperature increase in superficial structures, such as cutaneous scar tissue or superficial tendons. However, to adequately heat deeper structures, such as the joint capsules of large joints or deep tendons, deep-heating agents such as ultrasound or diathermy must be used.

USES OF SUPERFICIAL HEAT

> **Pain control**
> **Increased ROM and decreased joint stiffness**
> **Accelerated healing**
> **Infrared radiation for psoriasis and dermal ulcers**

Pain Control

Thermotherapy can be used clinically to control pain. This therapeutic effect may be caused by gating of pain transmission by activation of cutaneous thermoreceptors or may indirectly be the result of improved healing, decreased muscle spasm, or reduced ischemia.[102] Increasing skin temperature may also reduce the sensation of pain by altering nerve conduction and/or transmission.[103] For example, it is likely that the analgesia produced in the sensory distribution of the ulnar nerve (the volar and medial forearm), when infrared radiation is applied over the ulnar nerve at the elbow, is caused by altered nerve conduction.[90] The indirect effects of thermotherapy on tissue healing and ischemia are primarily attributable to vasodilation and increased blood flow. It has also been proposed that the psychological experience of heat as comfortable and relaxing may influence the patient's perception of pain.

Although thermotherapy may reduce pain of any etiology, it is not recommended as a treatment for pain caused by acute inflammation because an increase in tissue temperature may aggravate other signs and symptoms of inflammation including heat, redness, and edema.[104]

Increased Range of Motion and Decrease Joint Stiffness

Thermotherapy can be used clinically to increase joint ROM and decrease joint stiffness. Both of these effects are thought to be the result of the increase in soft tissue extensibility that occurs with increasing soft tissue temperature. Increasing soft tissue extensibility contributes to increasing joint ROM because it results in greater increases in soft tissue length and less injury when a passive stretch is applied. A maximum increase in length, with the lowest risk of injury, is obtained if the tissue temperature is maintained at 40° to 45 °C (104° to 113 °F) for 5 to 10 minutes and if a low-load, prolonged stretch is applied during the heating period and while the tissue is cooling[86,101] (Fig. 6-21). Therefore it is recommended that stretching be performed during and/or immediately after the application of thermotherapy, since if the tissues are allowed to cool before being stretched, the effects of the prior heating on tissue extensibility will be lost.

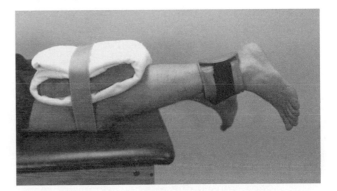

Figure 6-21. Low-load prolonged stretch with heat.

Thermotherapy can decrease joint stiffness, a quality related to the amount of force and the time required to move a joint; as joint stiffness decreases, less force and time are required to produce joint motion.[105-107] For example, increasing tissue temperature by placing the hands in a warm water bath or warm paraffin, or heating the surface with an infrared lamp, have all been shown to decrease finger joint stiffness.[108] The proposed mechanisms of this effect are increased extensibility and viscoelasticity of the periarticular structures, including the joint capsule and surrounding ligaments.

When using a heating agent to increase soft tissue extensibility before stretching, an agent that can reach the shortened tissue must be used. Thus superficial agents such as hot packs, paraffin, or infrared lamps are appropriate for use before stretching skin, superficial muscle, joints, or fascia, whereas deep heating agents such as ultrasound or diathermy should be used before stretching deeper joint capsules, muscles, or tendons.

Accelerated Healing

Thermotherapy can accelerate tissue healing by increasing circulation and enzymatic activity rate and by increasing the availability of oxygen to the tissues. Increasing the rate of circulation accelerates the delivery of blood to the tissues, bringing in oxygen and other nutrients and removing waste products. The application of any physical agent that increases circulation can be beneficial during the proliferative or remodeling stages of healing or when chronic inflammation is present. However, since increasing circulation can increase edema, the application of thermotherapy during the acute inflammation phase can prolong this phase and delay healing and is therefore not recommended.

By increasing the enzymatic activity rate, thermotherapy also increases the rate of metabolic reactions, thus allowing the processes of inflammation and healing to proceed more rapidly. Increasing the temperature of the blood also increases the dissociation of oxygen from hemoglobin, making more oxygen available for the processes of tissue repair.

Because superficial heating agents increase the temperature of only the superficial few millimeters of tissue, they are most likely to accelerate the healing of only superficial structures, such as the skin, or deeper tissue layers exposed due to skin ulceration. Deeper effects may also occur as the result of consensual vasodilation in areas distant from or deep to the area of increased temperature.

Infrared Radiation for Psoriasis

Although the ultraviolet (UV) frequency range of electromagnetic radiation is used most commonly in the treatment of psoriasis, the infrared (IR) range is also used occasionally for this application.[109,110] The increased temperature of the upper epidermis and dermis in the region of psoriatic plaques produced by IR radiation has been proposed as the mechanism for the reduction in psoriatic plaques that occurs in some individuals exposed to IR radiation.[110]

Infrared Radiation for Dermal Ulcers

Infrared radiation has been used for the treatment of dermal ulcers. The purpose of such treatment was to improve healing by increasing circulation, retarding bacterial growth, and dehydrating the wound site.[111] However, because current research indicates that wound healing is optimized with a moist rather than a dry environment, the application of IR radiation to open wounds is no longer recommended.[112]

CONTRAINDICATIONS AND PRECAUTIONS FOR THERMOTHERAPY

Although thermotherapy is a relatively safe treatment modality, its use is contraindicated in some circumstances, and it should be applied with caution in others. Thermotherapy may be applied by a qualified clinician or by a properly instructed patient. Clinicians may use all forms of thermotherapy, and patients may be instructed to use hot packs, paraffin, or IR lamps at home to treat themselves. When patients are taught to use these modalities at home, they should be instructed how to use the modality, including the location it should be applied to, the temperature to be used, safety precautions, and the duration and frequency of treatment. Patients must also be taught how to identify possible adverse effects and must be told to discontinue treatment should any of these occur.

Even when thermotherapy is not contraindicated, as with all treatments, if the patient's condition is worsening or not improving after two to three treatments, the treatment approach should be reevaluated or the patient should be referred to a physician for reevaluation.

CONTRAINDICATIONS
for the Use of Thermotherapy

- Acute injury or inflammation
- Recent or potential hemorrhage
- Thrombophlebitis

- Impaired sensation
- Impaired mentation
- Malignancy
- Infrared irradiation of the eyes[113]

The use of thermotherapy is contraindicated . . .

. . . in the area of an acute injury or acute inflammation

Do not apply heat to the area of an acute injury or acute inflammation because increasing tissue temperature can increase edema and bleeding as a result of vasodilation and increased blood flow.[114] This may aggravate the injury, increase pain, and/or delay recovery.

ASK THE PATIENT:
- When did this injury occur?
  Do not apply heat within the first 48 to 72 hours after an injury.

ASSESS:
- Skin temperature and color and local edema
  Elevation of skin temperature, rubor, and local edema demonstrate the presence of acute inflammation and indicate that heat should not be applied to the area.

. . . over an area of recent or potential hemorrhage

Heat causes vasodilation and an increased rate of blood flow. Because vasodilation may cause reopening of a vascular lesion, increasing the rate of blood flow in an area of recent hemorrhage can restart or worsen the bleeding. In addition, increasing blood flow in an area of potential hemorrhage can cause hemorrhage to start. Therefore it is recommended that heat not be applied to areas of recent or potential hemorrhage.

ASK THE PATIENT:
- When did this injury occur?
- Did you have any bruising or bleeding?

ASSESS:
- Visually inspect for ecchymosis

Do not apply thermotherapy if the patient reports bruising or bleeding in the previous 48 to 72 hours or if recently formed red, purple, or blue ecchymosis is present.

. . . in areas with thrombophlebitis

The vasodilation and increased rate of circulation caused by increased tissue temperature may cause a thrombus or a blood clot to become dislodged from the area being treated and to be moved to the vessels of vital organs, resulting in morbidity or even death.

ASK THE PATIENT:
- Do you have a blood clot in this area?

ASSESS:
- Check for calf swelling and tenderness (Homan's sign) before applying heat to the leg. Do not apply thermotherapy if the patient says that there is a blood clot in the area. Do not apply thermotherapy to the leg if there is tenderness and swelling of the calf until the presence of a thrombus in the lower extremity has been ruled out.

. . . over areas with impaired sensation or to patients with impaired mentation

A patient's sensation and a report of heat or pain are used as the primary indicators of the maximum safe temperature for thermotherapy; therefore, a patient who cannot feel or report the sensation of heat can easily be burned before the clinician realizes that there is a problem. Therefore heat should not be applied to areas where sensation is impaired or to patients who may have any other difficulty letting the therapist know when they are too hot.

ASK THE PATIENT:
- Do you have normal feeling in this area?

Continued

CONTRAINDICATIONS—cont'd

ASSESS:

- Sensation in the area

Test tubes containing hot and cold water can be used to test thermal sensation. If sensation is impaired only in the treatment area, heat may be applied proximally to increase peripheral circulation via the spinal cord reflex, as described above. Note that sensation in the distal extremities is frequently impaired in patients with neuropathy due to diabetes mellitus.

- Alertness and orientation

Do not apply thermotherapy if the patient is unresponsive or confused.

. . . over or near malignant tissue

Thermotherapy may increase the growth rate or rate of metastasis of malignant tissue, either by increasing circulation to the area and/or by increasing metabolic rate.

ASK THE PATIENT:

Because a patient may not know that he or she has cancer, or may be uncomfortable discussing this diagnosis directly, the therapist should first check the chart for a diagnosis of cancer. Then ask the patient:

- Are you under the care of a physician for any major medical problem? If so, what is the problem?
- Have you experienced any recent unexplained weight loss or gain?
- Do you have constant pain that does not change?

If the patient has experienced recent unexplained changes in body weight or has constant pain that does not change, defer thermotherapy until a physician has performed a follow-up evaluation to rule out malignancy. If the patient is known to have cancer, ask:

- Do you know if you have a tumor in this area?

Thermotherapy should generally not be applied in the area of a known or possible malignancy; however, such treatment may be given, with informed consent, to provide relief of pain for the terminally ill patient.

Infrared irradiation of the eyes

IR irradiation of the eyes should be avoided because such treatment may cause optical damage. To avoid irradiation of the eyes, IR opaque goggles should be worn by the patient throughout treatment using an IR lamp, and by the therapist when near the lamp, as occurs when setting up the treatment.

PRECAUTIONS
for the Use of Thermotherapy

- Pregnancy
- Impaired circulation
- Poor thermal regulation
- Edema
- Cardiac insufficiency
- Metal in the area
- Over an open wound
- Over areas where topical counterirritants have recently been applied

Use heat with caution . . .

. . . during pregnancy

A fetus may be damaged by maternal hyperthermia; however, since this is unlikely to occur with superficial heating of the limbs, thermotherapy may be applied to such areas, but full body heating, as occurs with immersion of most of the body in a whirlpool, should be avoided during pregnancy.

Although maternal hyperthermia has not been demonstrated with application of hot packs to the low back or abdomen, such application is also generally not recommended.

ASK THE PATIENT:

- Are you pregnant?
- Do you think you may be pregnant?
- Are you trying to get pregnant?

If the patient is or may be pregnant, do not apply heat to the abdomen or low back and do not immerse the patient in a warm or hot whirlpool.

...over areas with poor circulation or in patients with poor thermal regulation

Areas with poor circulation and patients with poor thermal regulation may not vasodilate to a normal degree in response to an increase in tissue temperature and therefore may not have a sufficient increase in blood flow when tissue temperature increases to protect the tissues from burning. In general, poor thermal regulation is encountered in the elderly and very young.

ASSESS:
- Check skin temperature and quality and nail quality, and look for tissue swelling or ulceration. Decreased skin temperature, thin skin, poor nails, tissue swelling, and ulceration are all signs of impaired circulation.

  Use milder superficial heat in areas with poor circulation or in elderly or very young patients. Apply heat at a lower temperature or with more insulation, and check these patients frequently for any discomfort or signs of burning.

...in areas with edema

The application of thermotherapy to a dependent extremity has been shown to increase edema.[104] This effect is thought to be the result of the vasodilation and enhanced circulation that occur with raised tissue temperature and the increase in inflammation caused by increased metabolic rate.

ASSESS:
- Measure limb girth in the area to be treated and compare this with the contralateral side.
- Palpate for pitting or brawny edema. Check for other signs of inflammation, including heat, redness, and pain.

  Do not apply heat with the area in a dependent position if edema is present. Heat may be applied with caution with the area elevated if edema is present and is thought to be a result of impaired venous circulation.

...with patients with cardiac insufficiency

Heat can cause both local and generalized vasodilation, which can contribute to increased cardiac demand. Because this may not be well tolerated by patients with cardiac insufficiency, such patients should be monitored closely if heat is applied, particularly if the heat is applied to a large area.

ASK THE PATIENT:
- Do you have any problems with your heart?

ASSESS:
- In patients with heart problems, check heart rate and blood pressure before, during, and after treatment. A slight decrease in blood pressure and an increase in heart rate are normal consensual responses to the application of heat. Discontinue heat treatment in a patient with cardiac insufficiency if the patient's heart rate falls or the patient complains of feeling faint.

...in areas with metal

Metal has a higher thermal conductivity and higher specific heat than body tissue and therefore may become very hot with the application of conductive heating modalities. For this reason, jewelry should be removed before the application of superficial heating modalities, and caution should be applied when there is metal, such as staples or bullet fragments, in the superficial tissues of the area being treated.

ASK THE PATIENT:
- Do you have any metal in you in this area, such as staples or bullet fragments?
- Please remove your jewelry in the area to be heated.

  If there is metal present that cannot easily be removed, apply heat with caution. Use milder heat, at a lower temperature or intensity, or with more insulation, and check the area frequently during treatment for any signs of burning.

ASSESS:
- Inspect skin for scars that may cover metal.

...over any open wound

Do not use paraffin over an open wound because it may contaminate the wound and is difficult to remove. All other forms of thermotherapy should be applied over open wounds with caution because the loss of epidermis reduces the insulation of the subcutaneous tissues. If forms of thermotherapy other than paraffin are used in the area of an open wound, they should be applied at a lower temperature or intensity,

Continued

PRECAUTIONS—cont'd

or with more insulation than would be used when treating areas with intact skin. One should also check frequently during treatment for any signs of burning. When applying a heating agent with the goal of increasing circulation and accelerating the healing of an open wound, hydrotherapy with clean, warm water may be applied directly to the wound, or other superficial heating agents may be applied close to, but not directly over, the wound to provide a therapeutic effect while reducing the risk of cross-contamination and burns.

. . . over areas where topical counterirritants have recently been applied

Topical counterirritants are ointments or creams that cause a sensation of heat when applied to the skin. Such preparations generally contain substances such as menthol that stimulate the sensation of heat by

causing a mild inflammatory reaction in the skin. These preparations also cause local superficial vasodilation. If a thermal agent is applied to an area that is already vasodilated as the result of application of a topical counterirritant, the vessels in the area may not be able to vasodilate further to dissipate the heat from the thermal agent, and a burn may result.

ASK THE PATIENT:
- Have you applied any cream or ointment to this area today?
- If so, what type?

If the patient has recently applied a topical counterirritant to an area, do not apply a superficial heating agent. Tell the patient not to use this type of preparation before future treatment sessions and not to apply a superficial heating agent at home after using this type of preparation.

ADVERSE EFFECTS OF THERMOTHERAPY

Burns
Fainting
Bleeding
Skin and eye damage from IR irradiation

Burns

Excessive heating can cause protein denaturation and cell death. These effects may occur when heat is applied for too long, when the heating agent is too hot, or if heat is applied to a patient who does not have the appropriate protective vasodilation response to increased tissue temperature. The effects of heat on cell viability are exploited in the medical treatment of malignancies, where heat is applied with the goal of killing the malignant cells; however, in application of heat in rehabilitation, cell death is to be avoided. Because protein begins to denature at 45 °C (113 °F), and cell death has been observed when cells were maintained at 43 °C (109 °F) for 60 minutes or at 46 °C (115 °F) for only 7½ minutes, when applying heat in rehabilitation, the duration and tissue temperature should be kept below these levels.[115,116]

Overheating and tissue damage can be avoided by using superficial heating agents that get cooler during their application, by limiting the initial temperature of the agent, and/or by using insulation between the agent and the patient's skin. For example, hot packs that are warmed in hot water before being placed on the patient start to cool as soon as they are removed from the hot water and applied, and are therefore unlikely to cause burns. In contrast, superficial heating agents such as plug-in electric hot packs or IR lamps that do not cool with use are more likely to cause burns. The higher the temperature of a conductive superficial heating agent, the greater the rate of heat transfer to the patient and thus the greater the risk of burns; therefore it is important not to overheat a conductive superficial heating agent and to always use adequate insulation.

To avoid burns, heating agents should be applied in the manner recommended below. They should not be applied for longer periods or at higher temperatures, and the treatment time and temperature of the heating agent should be reduced if the patient has impaired circulation. Heating agents should not be applied where contraindicated, and all patients should be provided with a means of calling for assistance, such as a bell, if the clinician or another staff member is not in the immediate treatment area. During the treatment, check to be sure that the patient has not fallen asleep, and instruct the patient to use a timer that rings loudly at the end of the treatment time if the patient uses a superficial heating agent at home.

A superficial heating agent used at home should be the type that cools over time, such as a microwavable hot pack or a hot water bottle. If an electric heating pad is used by a patient at home, it should be the type that requires the patient to hold down a switch at all times for it to stay on. This safety feature ensures that the heating pad will turn off if the patient falls asleep and stops holding down the switch.

It is recommended that the patient's skin be inspected for burns before initiating treatment since a patient may have been burned previously. The skin should also be inspected during and after thermotherapy. A recent superficial burn will appear red and may have blistering. As the burn heals, the skin will appear pale and scarred.

Fainting

Occasionally, a patient may feel faint when heat is applied. Fainting, a sudden, transient loss of consciousness, is generally due to inadequate cerebral blood flow and is most commonly caused by peripheral vasodilation and decreased blood pressure, generally in association with a decreased heart rate.[117] Heating an area of the body generally causes vasodilation locally and, to a lesser extent, in areas distant from the site of application. This distant, or consensual, response can result in a sufficient decrease in cerebral blood flow to cause a patient to faint during the application of thermotherapy. If a patient feels faint while heat is being applied, lowering the head and raising the feet will bring more blood to the brain to help the patient recover. Heating as small an area as clinically beneficial, and removing excessive heavy clothing that insulates the whole body, may also help to limit this consensual decrease in blood pressure and thus reduce the probability of fainting.

Patients may also feel faint when getting up after thermotherapy. This is due to the additive hypotensive effects of postural (orthostatic) hypotension and the hypotensive effect of the heat, as described above. Keeping the patient's head elevated with a pillow during the heat application can help to decrease post-treatment postural hypotension by reducing the extent of positional change at the completion of the treatment. It is also recommended that the patient remain in the position used during the treatment for a few minutes after the thermal agent is removed to allow blood pressure to normalize before rising.

Bleeding

The vasodilation and increased blood flow caused by increasing tissue temperature may cause or aggravate bleeding in areas of acute trauma or in patients with hemophilia. The vasodilation may also cause reopening of any recent vascular lesion.

Skin and Eye Damage from Infrared Irradiation

Infrared radiation can produce adverse effects that are not produced by other superficial thermal agents. These include permanent damage to the eyes and permanent changes in skin pigmentation. Injury to the eyes, including corneal burning and retinal and lenticular damage, is considered to be the most likely and most severe hazard of IR radiation application.[113] Prolonged exposure to IR radiation may also cause epidermal hyperplasia.[118]

APPLICATION TECHNIQUE
Superficial Thermotherapy

1. Evaluate the patient problem and set the goals of treatment.
2. Determine if thermotherapy is the most appropriate treatment.
3. Determine that thermotherapy is not contraindicated for this patient or this condition.

   Inspect the treatment area for open wounds and rashes and assess sensation. Check the patient's chart for any record of previous adverse responses to heat or for any disease that may predispose the patient to an adverse response. Ask the appropriate questions of the patient, as described in the preceding sections on contraindications and precautions.
4. Select the appropriate superficial heating agent according to the body part to be treated and the desired response.

Continued

APPLICATION TECHNIQUE—cont'd
Superficial Thermotherapy

When applying superficial heat, select an agent that best fits the location and size of the area to be treated, is easily applied in the desired position, allows the desired amount of motion during application, is available, and is reasonably priced. Choose an agent that will conform to the area being treated so that it maintains good contact with the body. If edema is present, an agent that can be applied with the area elevated should be used. When applying thermotherapy with the goal of increasing ROM, it can be beneficial to allow active or passive motion while the treatment is being applied. Any of the heating agents described below can be applied in the clinic; only hot packs and paraffin may be applied by patients at home.

5. Explain to the patient the procedure and the reason for applying thermotherapy, and describe the sensations the patient can expect to feel.

   During the application of thermotherapy the patient should feel a sensation of mild warmth. Depending on the agent and the amount of insulation, the warmth may not be felt for the first few minutes of treatment. The patient should not feel excessively hot or feel any sensation of increased pain or burning. If the patient reports any of these sensations, discontinue the treatment or reduce the intensity of the heat.

6. Apply the appropriate superficial heating agent.

   Select from the following list:
   Hot packs
   Paraffin
   Fluidotherapy   See applications for
   IR lamp   each superficial heating
   Whirlpool or   agent on the following
      contrast bath   pages.

7. Inspect the treated area and assess the outcome of treatment.

   After completing thermotherapy with any of the above agents, reassess the patient, checking particularly for progress toward the set goals of treatment and for any adverse effects of the treatment. Remeasure quantifiable subjective complaints and objective impairments and disabilities.

8. Document the treatment.

APPLICATION TECHNIQUES

Hot Packs

Commercially available hot packs are usually made of bentonite, a hydrophilic silicate gel, covered with canvas. Bentonite is used for this application because it can hold a large quantity of water for the efficient delivery of heat. Hot packs are made in various sizes and shapes designed to fit different areas of the body (Fig. 6-22). They are stored in hot water kept at about 70° to 75 °C (158° to 167 °F) inside a purpose-designed, thermostatically controlled water cabinet (Fig. 6-23) that stays on at all times. This type of hot pack initially takes 2 hours to heat and 30 minutes to reheat between each use.

Electric, plug-in heating pads are not recommended for clinical use because they do not cool during application and therefore may more easily burn a patient. If patients are using a plug-in electric heating pad at home, advise them to use a pad that requires the "on" switch to be held down for the pad to heat, to use only the medium or low settings, to limit application at the medium setting to 20 minutes, and to discontinue use if any sensation of pain, overheating, or burning occurs. Patients should also be advised to inspect their skin for any signs of burns directly after the use of a hot pack and for the following 24 hours.

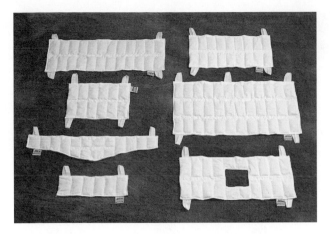

Figure 6-22. Hot packs of various shapes and sizes. (Courtesy Chattanooga Group, Inc., Hixson, TN.)

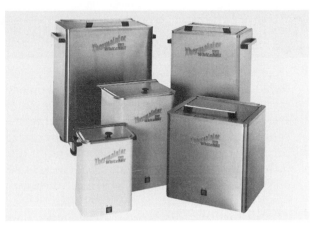

Figure 6-23. Thermostatically controlled hot pack containers. (Courtesy Whitehall Manufacturing, City of Industry, CA.)

APPLICATION TECHNIQUE
Hot Pack

Equipment Required
- Hot packs in a variety of sizes and shapes appropriate for different areas of the body
- Specialized heating unit
- Towels
- Hot pack covers (optional)
- Timer
- Bell

PROCEDURE

1. Remove clothing and jewelry from the area to be treated and inspect the area.
2. Wrap the hot pack in six to eight layers of dry towels. Hot pack covers, which come in various sizes to match the hot packs, can substitute for two to three layers of towels (Fig. 6-24). More layers should be used if the towels or hot pack covers are old and have become thin or if the patient complains of feeling too warm during treatment. The towels can be preheated to achieve more uniform heating throughout the treatment period. More layers of towels should be used if the body part is on top of the hot pack than if the hot pack is placed over the body part because when the body part is on top of the pack the towels are compressed, reducing insulation of the body, and the underlying table provides more insulation to the pack, causing it to cool more slowly.[119] If the patient complains of not feeling enough heat, fewer layers of towels may be used for the next treatment session; however, towels should not be removed during heating with hot packs because

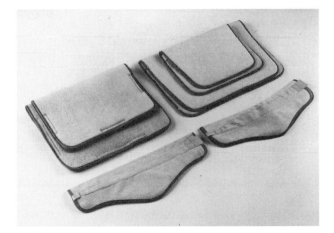

Figure 6-24. Hot pack covers of various shapes and sizes. (Courtesy Chattanooga Group, Inc., Hixson, TN.)

the increased skin temperature may decrease the patient's thermal sensitivity and the ability to judge the tissue's heat tolerance accurately and safely.

3. Apply the wrapped hot pack to the treatment area and secure it well (Fig. 6-25).

Continued

APPLICATION TECHNIQUE—cont'd
Superfical Thermotherapy

4. Provide the patient with a bell or other means to call for assistance while the hot pack is on and instruct the patient to call immediately if he or she experiences any increase in discomfort. If the patient feels too hot, extra towels should be placed between the hot pack and the patient. If the patient does not feel hot enough, fewer layers of towels should be used at the next treatment session.

5. After 5 minutes, check the patient's report and inspect the area being treated for excessive redness, blistering, or other signs of burning. Discontinue thermotherapy in the presence of signs of burning. If there are any signs of burning, brief application of a cold pack or an ice pack is recommended to curtail the inflammatory response.

6. After 20 minutes, remove the hot pack and inspect the treatment area. It is normal for the area to appear slightly red and to feel warm to the touch.

ADVANTAGES
- Easy to use
- Inexpensive materials (packs and towels)
- Short use of clinician's time
- Low level of skill needed for application
- Can be used to cover moderate to large areas
- Safe, as packs start cooling on removal from the water cabinet
- Readily available for patient purchase and home use

DISADVANTAGES
- Hot pack must be moved to observe the treatment area during treatment

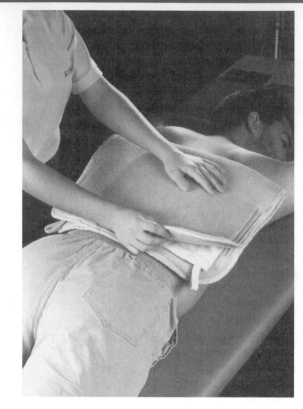

Figure 6-25. Application of a hot pack. (Courtesy Whitehall Manufacturing, City of Industry, CA.)

- Patient may not tolerate the weight of the hot pack
- Pack may not be able to maintain good contact with small or contoured areas
- Active motion not practical during treatment
- Moderately expensive equipment (heated water cabinet)

Paraffin

Warm, melted paraffin can be used for thermotherapy. For this application, the paraffin is mixed with mineral oil in a 6:1 or 7:1 ratio of paraffin to oil to reduce the melting temperature of the paraffin from 54 °C (129 °F) to between 45° and 50 °C (113° to 122 °F). Paraffin can safely be applied directly to the skin at this temperature because of its low specific heat and thermal conductivity. For this application, the paraffin is heated and stored in a thermostatically controlled container. Such containers are available in small portable sizes for home or clinic use and in larger sizes designed primarily for clinic use (Fig. 6-26 *A,B*). Paraffin is usually used for heating the distal extremities because it can maintain good contact with these irregularly contoured areas. Paraffin may also be applied to more proximal areas such as the elbows and knees, or even the low back, by using the paint method described following.

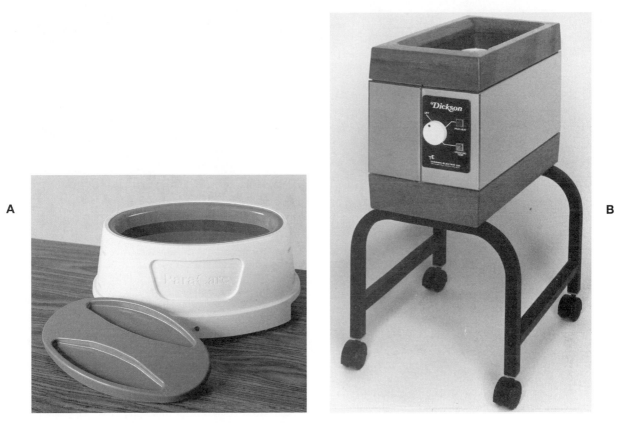

Figure 6-26. Thermostatically controlled paraffin baths. **A,** Small size for home or clinic use. (Courtesy Chattanooga Group, Inc., Hixson, TN). **B,** Large size for clinic use. (Courtesy Thermo-Electric, Imperial, PA.)

APPLICATION TECHNIQUE
Paraffin

Equipment Required
- Paraffin
- Mineral oil (or commercially available premixed paraffin intended for this application)
- Thermostatically controlled container
- Plastic bags or paper
- Towels

PROCEDURE

There are three different methods by which paraffin is commonly applied: dip-wrap, dip-immersion, and paint. The dip-wrap and dip-immersion methods can only be used for treating the distal extremities. The paint method can be used for any area of the body. For all three methods, do the following:

1. Remove all jewelry from the area to be treated and inspect the area.
2. Thoroughly wash and dry the area to be treated to minimize contamination of the paraffin.

For the Dip-wrap Method (for the wrist and hand):

3. With fingers apart, dip the hand into the paraffin as far as possible and remove (Fig. 6-27).

   Advise the patient to avoid moving the fingers during the treatment because this will crack the paraffin coating. Also, advise the patient to avoid touching the sides or bottom of the tank because these may be hotter than the paraffin.
4. Wait briefly for the layer of paraffin to harden and become opaque.

Continued

APPLICATION TECHNIQUE—cont'd
Paraffin

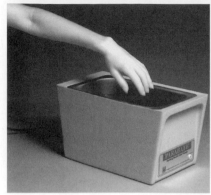 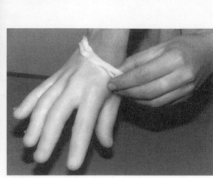 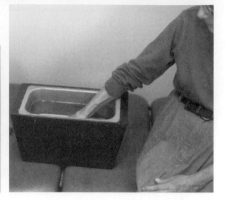

Figure 6-27. Application of paraffin by the dip-wrap method. (Courtesy The Hygenic Corporation, Akron, OH.)

Figure 6-28. Removing paraffin from a patient's hand.

Figure 6-29. Application of paraffin by the dip-immersion method.

5. Redip the hand, keeping the fingers apart. Repeat steps 3 through 5 six to ten times.
6. Wrap the patient's hand in a plastic bag, wax paper, or treatment table paper and then in a towel. The plastic bag or paper prevents the towel from sticking to the paraffin, and the towel acts as insulation to slow the cooling of the paraffin. Caution the patient not to move the hand during dipping or during the rest period because this may crack the coating of paraffin, allowing air to penetrate and the paraffin to cool more rapidly.
7. Elevate the extremity.
8. Leave the paraffin in place for 10 to 15 minutes or until it cools.
9. When the treatment is completed, peel the paraffin off the hand and either replace the paraffin in the container to melt or discard it (Fig. 6-28).

For the Dip-immersion Method:

3. With fingers apart, dip the hand into the paraffin and remove.
4. Wait 5 to 15 seconds for the layer of paraffin to harden and become opaque.
5. Redip the hand, keeping the fingers apart.
6. Allow the hand to remain in the paraffin for up to 20 minutes and then remove it (Fig. 6-29).
   The temperature of the paraffin should be at the lower end of the range for this method of application because the hand cools less during treat-

ment than with the dip-wrap method. The heater should be turned off during the treatment so that the sides and bottom of the tank do not become too hot.

For the Paint Method:

3. Paint a layer of paraffin onto the treatment area with a brush.
4. Wait for the layer of paraffin to become opaque.
5. Paint on another layer of paraffin no larger than the first layer. Repeat steps 3 through 5 six to ten times.
6. Cover the area with plastic or paper and then with toweling. As with the dip-immersion method, the plastic or paper is used to prevent the towel from sticking to the paraffin and the towel acts as insulation to slow down the cooling of the paraffin. Caution the patient not to move the area during treatment as this may crack the coating of paraffin, allowing air to penetrate and the treatment area to cool more rapidly.
7. Leave the paraffin in place for 20 minutes or until it cools.
8. When the treatment is completed, peel off the paraffin and either replace it in the container to melt or discard it.

For All Methods:

When the treatment is complete, inspect the treatment area for any signs of adverse effects and document the treatment.

Paraffin may be sterilized by heating it to 80 °C (176 °F) and then allowing it to cool overnight. Its temperature should be allowed to return to between 45° and 50 °C (113° to 122 °F) before it is used again for treatment.

ADVANTAGES
- Maintains good contact with highly contoured areas
- Easy to use
- Inexpensive
- Body part can be elevated if using the dip-wrap method

- Oil lubricates and conditions the skin
- Can be used by patient at home

DISADVANTAGES
- Messy and time-consuming to apply
- Cannot be used over an open skin lesion as it may contaminate the lesion
- Risk of cross-contamination if the paraffin is reused
- Part in dependent position for dip-immersion method

Fluidotherapy

Fluidotherapy is a dry heating agent that transfers heat by convection.[120] It consists of a cabinet containing finely ground cellulose particles made from corn cobs (Fig. 6-30). Heated air is circulated through the particles, suspending and moving them so that they act like a liquid. The patient extends a body part into the cabinet, where it floats, as if in water. There are also portals in the cabinet that allow the therapist to access the patient's body part while it is being heated. Fluidotherapy units come in a variety of sizes suitable for treating different body parts. Both the temperature and the amount of particle agitation can be controlled by the clinician.

APPLICATION TECHNIQUE
Fluidotherapy

Equipment Required
- Fluidotherapy unit of appropriate size and shape for areas to be treated

PROCEDURE
1. Remove all jewelry and clothing from the area to be treated and inspect the area.
2. Cover any open wounds with a plastic barrier to prevent the cellulose particles from becoming lodged in the wound.
3. Extend the body part to be treated through the portal of the unit (Fig. 6-31).
4. Secure the sleeve to prevent particles from escaping from the cabinet.
5. Set the temperature at 38° to 48 °C (100° to 118 °F).
6. Adjust the degree of agitation to achieve patient comfort.
7. The patient may move or exercise during the treatment.
8. Treat for 20 minutes.

ADVANTAGES
- Patient can move during the treatment to work on gaining active ROM
- Minimal pressure applied to the area being treated
- Temperature well-controlled and constant throughout treatment
- Easy to administer

DISADVANTAGES
- Expensive equipment
- Limb must be in dependent position in some units, increasing the risk of edema formation
- The constant heat source may result in overheating
- If the corn cob particles spill onto a smooth floor, they will make the floor slippery

Continued

APPLICATION TECHNIQUE—cont'd
Fluidotherapy

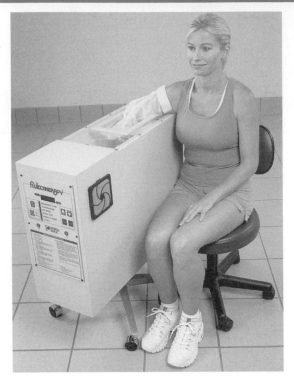

Figure 6-30. Fluidotherapy controls. (Courtesy Chattanooga Group, Inc., Hixson, TN.)

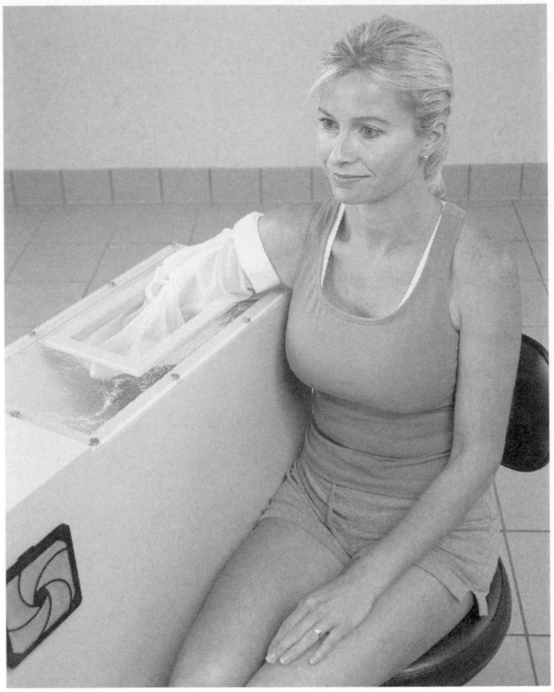

Figure 6-31. Application of Fluidotherapy. (Courtesy Chattanooga Group, Inc., Hixson, TN.)

Infrared Lamps

Infrared lamps emit electromagnetic radiation within the frequency range that gives rise to heat when absorbed by matter (Fig. 6-32). Infrared radiation has a wavelength of 770 nm to 1 mm (10^6 nm), lying between visible light and microwaves on the electromagnetic spectrum (see Fig. 12-1) and is emitted by many sources that emit visible light or UV radiation, such as the sun. Infrared radiation is divided into three bands with different wavelength ranges: IR-A, with wavelengths of 770 to 1400 nm; IR-B, with wavelengths of 1400 to 3000 nm; and IR-C, with wavelengths of 3000 to 10^6 nm. The IR sources used in rehabilitation include sunlight, IR lamps, and low intensity lasers. Infrared lamps that emit IR radiation in both the luminous (visible) and nonluminous (invisible) ranges were available for clinical use in the past; however, only those emitting luminous IR-A radiation are currently being manufactured. The lamps

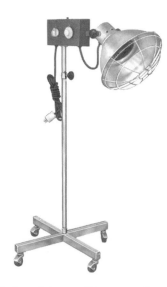

Figure 6-32. Infrared lamp. (Courtesy Brandt Industries, Inc., Bronx, NY.)

available at this time generally emit IR radiation with wavelengths of between 780 and 1500 nm with a peak intensity at 1000 nm.

The tissue temperature increase produced by IR radiation is directly proportional to the amount of radiation that penetrates the tissue. This is related to the power and wavelength of the radiation, the distance of the radiation source from the tissue, the angle of incidence of the radiation to the tissue, and the absorption coefficient of the tissue. Higher power IR will deliver more radiation to the skin. Most lamps deliver IR radiation with power in the range of 50 to 1500 watts. The wavelength of IR radiation used clinically, which is between 780 and 1500 nm, is absorbed within the first 1 to 3 mm of human tissue. It has been shown that at least 50% of IR radiation of 1200 nm wavelength penetrates beyond 0.8 mm and is therefore able to pass through the skin to interact with subcutaneous capillaries and cutaneous nerve endings.[121] Human skin allows maximum penetration of radiation with a wavelength of 1200 nm while being virtually opaque to IR radiation with a wavelength of 2000 nm or greater.[113]

The amount of energy reaching the patient from an IR radiation source is also related to the distance between the source and the tissue. As the distance of the source from the target increases, the intensity of radiation reaching the target changes in proportion to the inverse square of the distance. For example, if the source is moved from a position 5 cm from the target to a position 10 cm from the target, increasing by a factor of 2, the intensity of radiation reaching the target will fall to one-fourth of its prior level. The amount of energy reaching the target is also related to the angle of incidence of the radiation. As the angle of incidence of the radiation changes, the intensity of the energy reaching the target changes in proportion to the cosine of the angle of incidence of the radiation. For example, if the angle of incidence changes from 0 degrees (i.e.,

perpendicular to the surface of the skin), with a cosine of 1, to 45 degrees, with a cosine of $\sqrt{2}/2$, the intensity of radiation will fall by a factor of $\sqrt{2}/2$. Thus, the intensity reaching the skin is greatest when the radiation source is close to the patient's skin and the radiation beam is perpendicular to the skin surface, and, as the distance or the angle of incidence increases, the intensity of the radiation reaching the skin will diminish.

Infrared radiation is absorbed most by tissues with high IR absorption coefficients. Because IR absorption coefficients are primarily affected by skin color, with darker skins absorbing more radiation than lighter skins, with the same radiation and lamp positioning, dark skin will absorb more IR radiation and therefore increase more in temperature than light skin.

A number of authors have provided formulae for calculating the exact amount of heat being delivered to a patient by IR radiation,[109,122] or methodologies for measuring the exact tissue temperature increase;[110] however, in clinical practice, the sensory report of the patient is usually used to gauge the skin temperature. The amount of heat transfer is adjusted by changing the power output of the lamp and/or the distance of the lamp from the patient so that the patient feels a comfortable level of warmth.

Although the clinical use of IR lamps for heating superficial tissues was popular during the 1940s and 1950s, this practice has waned in recent years. Its fall in popularity appears to be the result of changes in practice style preferences and limitations in the quantity of published research data rather than because of any evidence of excessive adverse effects or lack of therapeutic efficacy. Most of the current use and recent literature regarding clinical applications of IR radiation relate to high-intensity IR lasers intended to produce local burning and photocoagulation rather than to the lower-intensity lamps intended for gentle heating during rehabilitation.

APPLICATION TECHNIQUE
Infrared Lamp

Equipment Required
- IR lamp
- IR opaque goggles
- Tape measure to measure distance of treatment area from IR source
- Towels

Continued

APPLICATION TECHNIQUE—cont'd
Infrared Lamp

PROCEDURE

1. Remove clothing and jewelry from the area to be treated and inspect the area. Drape the patient for modesty, leaving the area to be treated uncovered.
2. Put IR opaque goggles on the patient and the therapist if there is a possibility of IR irradiation of the eyes.
3. Allow the IR lamp to warm up for 5 to 10 minutes so it will reach a stable level of output.[109]
4. Position the patient with the surface of the area to be treated perpendicular to the IR beam and about 45 to 60 cm away from the source. Remember that the intensity of the IR radiation reaching the skin decreases, with an inverse square relationship, as the distance from the source increases, and in proportion to the cosine of the angle of incidence of the beam. Adjust the distance from the source and wattage of the lamp output so that the patient feels a comfortable level of warmth. Measure and record the distance of the lamp from the target tissue.
5. Provide the patient with a means to call for assistance, and instruct the patient to call if discomfort occurs.
6. Instruct the patient to avoid moving closer to or farther from the lamp and to avoid touching the lamp since movement toward or away from the lamp will alter the amount of energy reaching the patient.
7. Set the lamp to treat for 15 to 30 minutes. Generally, treatment times of about 15 minutes are used for subacute conditions and up to 30 minutes for chronic conditions. Most lamps have a timer that automatically shuts off the lamp when the treatment time has elapsed.
8. Monitor the patient's response during treatment. It may be necessary to move the lamp farther away if the patient becomes too warm. Be cautious in moving the lamp closer if the patient reports not feeling warm enough as the patient may have accommodated to the sensation and may not judge the heat level accurately once warm.
9. When the treatment is completed, turn off the lamp and dry any perspiration from the treated area.

ADVANTAGES

- Does not require contact of the medium with the patient. This reduces the risk of infection and the possible discomfort of the weight of a hot pack. It also avoids the problem of poor contact when treating highly contoured areas.
- The area being treated can be observed throughout the treatment.

DISADVANTAGES

- Infrared radiation is not easily localized to a specific treatment area.
- It is difficult to ensure consistent heating in all treatment areas because the amount of heat transfer is affected by the distance of the skin from the radiation source and the angle of the beam with the skin, both of which vary with tissue contours and may be inconsistent between treatment sessions.

OTHER MEANS OF APPLYING THERMOTHERAPY

Superficial heat may also be applied by immersion in a warm whirlpool or a contrast bath, as described in detail in Chapter 9.

Documentation

Document the area of the body treated, the type of heating agent used, the treatment duration, and the response to treatment. Also document treatment parameters such as the temperature or power of the agent, the number and type of insulation layers used, the distance of the agent from the patient, and the patient's position or activity if these can be varied with the agent used. Documentation is typically written in the SOAP note format. The following examples only summarize the modality component of treatment and are not intended to represent a comprehensive plan of care.

Examples

When applying a hot pack to the low back, document:

S: Pt c/o low back pain at level 7/10

O: HP low back, 20', pt prone, six layers of towels

A: Pain decreased from 7/10 to 4/10. Sitting tolerance increased from 30' to 60'.
P: Continue use of HP as above before stretching and the ex program

When applying paraffin to the right hand, document:

S: Pt c/o R hand stiffness especially with finger extension
O: Paraffin R hand, 50 °C, 10', dip-wrap, seven dips
A: Decreased joint stiffness. Proximal interphalangeal extension increased 10–20 degrees after active and passive stretching. Able to tie shoe laces without assistance.
P: Continue use of paraffin as above to R hand before stretching and mobilization

When applying Fluidotherapy to the left leg, ankle, and foot, document:

S: Pt c/o L ankle stiffness
O: Fluidotherapy L LE, 42 °C, 20'. Ankle AROM during heating
A: Ankle DF increased from neutral to 5 degrees
P: Discontinue fluidotherapy. Progress to active and passive ROM and gait activities in weight bearing position

When applying IR radiation to the right forearm, document:

S: Pt c/o R forearm pain with writing
O: IR R forearm, IR-A 1000 nm, 100 W at 50 cm for 20 minutes.
A: Mild sensation of warmth at forearm; pain with writing decreased 50%
P: Continue IR as above 2× per week

▶ Clinical Case Studies ◀

The following case studies summarize the concepts of superficial heat discussed in this chapter. Based on the scenarios presented, an evaluation of the clinical findings and goals of treatment are proposed. These are followed by a discussion of the factors to be considered in the selection of superficial thermotherapy as the indicated treatment modality and in the selection of the ideal thermotherapy agent to promote progress toward the set goals.

Case 1

MP is a 75-year-old female who has been referred for therapy with a diagnosis of osteoarthritis of the hands and an order to evaluate and treat with a focus on developing a home program. MP complains of stiffness and aching in all her finger joints, causing difficulties in gripping cooking utensils and performing other houschold tasks and pain with writing. She reports that these symptoms have gradually worsened over the last 10 years and have become much more severe in the last month since she stopped taking ibuprofen due to gastric side effects. The objective exam reveals stiffness and restricted flexion ROM of the proximal interphalangeals to approximately 90 degrees, and mild ulnar drift at the carpometacarpal joints bilaterally. The joints are not warm or edematous, and sensation is intact in both hands.

EVALUATION OF THE CLINICAL FINDINGS

This patient presents with the impairments of restricted finger ROM, stiffness and swelling of the finger joints, and abnormal ulnar drift of the carpometacarpal joints of the hands. These impairments have resulted in difficulties with the functional activities of cooking, household tasks, and writing.

PREFERRED PRACTICE PATTERN

Impaired Joint Mobility, Motor Function, Muscle Performance, and Range of Motion Associated With Connective Tissue Dysfunction, (4D)

PLAN OF CARE

The goals of treatment at this time are to increase joint ROM, reduce joint stiffness, control pain, and increase the patient's ability to grip cooking utensils, perform household tasks, and write. Given the chronic, progressive nature of osteoarthritis, the treatment should focus on maintaining the patient's status, optimizing her function, and slowing progression of her disabilities if possible.

ASSESSMENT REGARDING THE APPROPRIATENESS OF THERMOTHERAPY AS THE OPTIMAL TREATMENT

Superficial heating agents can increase the extensibility of superficial soft tissue and are therefore indicated for the treatment of joint stiffness and restricted ROM. Superficial heating agents can also reduce joint-related pain. Reducing these impairments may also help decrease this patient's disability. Thermotherapy is not contraindicated for this patient at this time because, although she has a diagnosis of osteoarthritis, which is an inflammatory disease, her hands do not show signs of acute inflammation such as increased temperature or edema of the finger joints. Her

Continued

▶ *Clinical Case Studies—cont'd* ◀

hands also have intact sensation. Caution should be used, however, since at the age of 75 years she may have impaired circulation or impaired thermal regulation. Therefore the intensity of the thermal agent should be at the lower end of the range typically used.

PROPOSED TREATMENT PLAN AND RATIONALE

It is proposed that superficial heat be applied to the wrists, hands, and fingers of both hands. Paraffin, Fluidotherapy, or water are appropriate treatments for these areas; however, a hot pack is not appropriate because it would not provide good contact with these highly contoured areas. Paraffin has the additional advantage of allowing elevation while heat is being applied, thus reducing the risk of edema formation. It is also inexpensive and safe enough to be used at home; however, it has the disadvantage of not allowing motion during application. Therefore for optimal benefit, if paraffin is used to treat this patient, she should perform active ROM exercises directly after removing the paraffin from her hands. Fluidotherapy and water have the advantage of allowing motion during their application; however, Fluidotherapy is generally too expensive and cumbersome for use at home or in many clinics, and water immersion may result in edema formation because the patient's hands must be in a dependent position while being heated. Given these advantages and disadvantages, warm water soaks together with exercise would be most appropriate if the patient does not develop edema with this treatment, and paraffin followed by exercise would be most appropriate if the patient develops edema with soaking in warm water. If paraffin is used, it should be applied using the dip-wrap method rather than the dip-immersion method since the former allows elevation of the hand and results in less intense and prolonged heating. Therefore it is less likely to result in edema formation and is safer for the older patient who may have impaired circulation and/or thermal regulation.

Case 2

KB is a 45-year-old male patient with mild low back pain. Two months ago, he fell 10 feet from a ladder and sustained severe soft tissue bruising; however, there was no evidence of a fracture or disc damage with this trauma. KB was referred for physical therapy 1 month ago with the diagnosis of a lumbar strain and with an order to optimize function with the goal of the patient returning to work. KB is currently participating in an active exercise program to work on spinal flexibility and stabilization, but he often feels stiff when starting to exercise and has

not returned to his job as a carpenter because of low back pain that is aggravated by forward bending and low back stiffness that is most intense during the first few hours of the day. KB reports that his pain is also aggravated by lying supine for more than 5 minutes and is alleviated to some degree by taking a hot shower. He had been making good progress, with increasing lumbar ROM, strength, and endurance, until the last 2 weeks, when his progress reached a plateau. The objective exam reveals spasms of the lumbar paravertebral muscles, a 50% restriction of active forward-bending ROM, and a 30% restriction of side bending bilaterally, with a complaint of pulling of the low back at the end of the range. Other objective measures, including active backward bending, passive joint mobility, sensation, and lower extremity strength, are within normal limits.

EVALUATION OF THE CLINICAL FINDINGS

This patient presents with impairments of restricted trunk forward- and side-bending ROM, paravertebral muscle spasms, and low back pain. He also has not returned to work since his injury.

PREFERRED PRACTICE PATTERN

Impaired Joint Mobility, Motor Function, Muscle Performance, Range of Motion, and Reflex Integrity Associated With Spinal Disorders, (4F)

PLAN OF CARE

The goals of treatment at this time are to decrease low back pain and stiffness, to increase lumbar forward-bending and side-bending ROM, and to have the patient return to work.

ASSESSMENT REGARDING THE APPROPRIATENESS OF THERMOTHERAPY AS THE OPTIMAL TREATMENT

It is important to realize that 2 months after a soft tissue injury, a patient's rehabilitation program should generally focus on active participation in a program of stretching and strengthening; however, the application of a physical agent before active exercise may be indicated to improve performance and accelerate progress. Thermotherapy may be indicated for this patient since it can reduce pain, stiffness, and soft tissue shortening and because this patient has reported that a hot shower, which provides superficial heating, helps to alleviate his symptoms. There are also no contraindications to the use of thermotherapy for this patient.

PROPOSED TREATMENT PLAN AND RATIONALE

A deep or superficial heating agent would be appropriate for providing thermotherapy to this patient. A deep heating agent would be ideal since it could directly increase the temperature of both the superficial tissues and the muscles of the low back; however, a superficial heating agent would generally be used because diathermy, which can provide deep heating to large areas, is not available in most clinical settings (see Chapter 12) and ultrasound can only provide deep heating to small areas (see Chapter 7). Superficial heating could be provided to the low back using an IR lamp or a hot pack. A hot pack is most likely to be used since IR lamps are also not available in most clinical settings. There are no contraindications to the use of thermotherapy for this patient.

A hot pack could be applied with the patient in a prone, side-lying, or sitting position; however, supine positioning should be avoided since he reports that this aggravates his pain. More insulating towels may be needed in the sitting position than in the prone or side-lying position due to compression of the towels and the insulating effect of the back of the chair. Treatment with any superficial heating agent would generally be applied for 20 to 30 minutes. Also, to optimize the benefit of increased soft tissue extensibility, active or passive stretching should be performed immediately following the application of the thermal agent.

Case 3

BD is a 72 year old female with a 10-year history of non–insulin-dependent diabetes mellitus and a full-thickness ulcer on her lateral right ankle caused by arterial insufficiency. The ulcer has been present for 6 months and has been treated only with dressing changes. BD has poor arterial circulation in her distal lower extremities, but her physician has determined that she is not a candidate for lower extremity bypass surgery. Sensation is impaired distal to the patient's knees and is intact proximal to the knees. The patient is alert and oriented. She lives alone at home and is independent in all activities of daily living; however, her walking is limited to approximately 500 feet because of calf pain. BD has been referred to physical therapy for evaluation and treatment of her ulcer.

EVALUATION OF CLINICAL FINDINGS

This patient presents with the impairments of loss of skin and underlying soft tissue on her right lateral ankle and reduced sensation in both lower extremities. Her ambulation tolerance is limited, and she is required to change the dressing on her wound two or three times per week.

PREFERRED PRACTICE PATTERN

Impaired Integumentary Integrity Associated With Full-Thickness Skin Involvement and Scar Formation, (7D)

PLAN OF CARE

The goals of treatment at this time are to decrease the wound area, achieve wound closure, and eliminate the high infection risk associated with open wounds and the need for dressing changes.

ASSESSMENT REGARDING THE APPROPRIATENESS OF THERMOTHERAPY AS THE OPTIMAL TREATMENT

Thermotherapy may be indicated to achieve the proposed goals of treatment because it can improve circulation and thus facilitate tissue healing. Superficial heating agents can increase circulation both in the area to which the heat is applied and distally. Increasing tissue temperature can also increase oxygen-hemoglobin dissociation, increasing the availability of oxygen for tissue healing. Because the application of thermotherapy directly to the distal lower extremities of this patient is contraindicated due to her impaired sensation in these areas, proximal application of thermotherapy to the patient's low back or thighs may be used to increase the circulation to her distal lower extremities without excessive risk.

PROPOSED TREATMENT PLAN AND RATIONALE

Thermotherapy using a deep or superficial heating agent would be appropriate for this patient. As with Case 2, deep heating would be ideal since this would affect both deep and superficial tissue temperatures; however, a superficial heating agent is more likely to be used because of greater availability. A hot pack or an IR lamp could be used to heat this patient's low back or thighs and should be applied for about 20 minutes.

TABLE 6-3	Effects of Cryotherapy and Thermotherapy	
Effect	**Cryotherapy**	**Thermotherapy**
Pain	–	–
Muscle spasm	–	–
Blood flow	–	+
Edema formation	–	+
Nerve conduction velocity	–	+
Metabolic rate	–	+
Collagen extensibility	–	+
Joint stiffness	+	–
Spasticity	–	0

– = decreases; + = increases; 0 = no effect.

CHOOSING BETWEEN CRYOTHERAPY AND THERMOTHERAPY

Because some of the effects and clinical indications for the use of cryotherapy and thermotherapy are the same and others are different, there are some situations in which either may be used and others in which only one or the other would be appropriate. Table 6-3 provides a summary of the effects of cryotherapy and thermotherapy to assist the clinician in choosing between these treatment options.

Chapter Review

Thermal agents transfer heat to or from patients by conduction, convection, conversion, or radiation. Cryotherapy is the transfer of heat from a patient by use of a cooling agent, and thermotherapy is the transfer of heat to a patient by use of a heating agent. Cryotherapy has been shown to decrease blood flow, decrease nerve conduction velocity, increase pain threshold, alter muscle strength, decrease enzymatic activity rate, temporarily decrease spasticity, and facilitate muscle contraction. These effects of cryotherapy are used clinically to control inflammation, pain, edema, and muscle spasm; to reduce spasticity temporarily; and to facilitate muscle contraction. Thermotherapy has been shown to increase

blood flow, increase nerve conduction velocity, increase pain threshold, alter muscle strength, and increase enzymatic activity rate. These effects of thermotherapy are used clinically to control pain, increase soft tissue extensibility, and accelerate healing. Thermal agents should not be applied in situations in which they may aggravate an existing pathology, such as a malignancy, or may cause damage, such as frostbite or burns. The reader is referred to the Evolve website at http://evolve.elsevier.com/Cameron for study questions pertinent to this chapter.

References

1. Darlas Y, Solassol A, Clouard R et al: Ultrasonotherapie: calcul del thermogenese, *Ann Readapt Med Phys* 32: 181-192, 1989.
2. Coakley WT: Biophysical effects of ultrasound at therapeutic intensities, *Physiotherapy* 64(4):166-168, 1978.
3. Martin SS, Spindler KP, Tarter JW et al: Cryotherapy: an effective modality for decreasing intraarticular temperature after knee arthroscopy, *Am J Sports Med* May-Jun;29(3):288-291, 2000.

4. Weston M, Taber C, Casagranda L et al: Changes in local blood volume during cold gel pack application to traumatized ankles, *J Orthop Sport Phys Ther* 19(4):197-199, 1994.

5. Karunakara RG, Lephart SM, Pincivero DM: Changes in forearm blood flow during single and intermittent cold application, *J Orthop Sports Phys Ther* Mar; 29(3):177-180, 1999.

6. Wolf SL: Contralateral upper extremity cooling from a specific cold stimulus, *Phys Ther* 51:158-165, 1971.

7. Lewis T: Observations upon the reactions of the vessels of the human skin to cold, *Heart* 15:177-208, 1930.

8. Clark RS, Hellon RF, Lind AR: Vascular reactions of the human forearm to cold, *Clin Sci* 17(1):165-179, 1958.

9. Fox R, Wyatt H: Cold-induced vasodilation in various areas of the body surface in man, *J Physiol* 162(1): 289-297, 1962.

10. Keating WR: The effect of general chilling on the vasodilation response to cold, *J Physiol* 139(3):497-507, 1957.

11. Taber C, Countryman K, Fahrenbruch J et al: Measurement of reactive vasodilation during cold gel pack application to nontraumatized ankles, *Phys Ther* 72(4):294-299, 1992.

12. Keating WR: *Survival in Cold Water,* Oxford, 1978, Blackwell.

13. Comroe JH Jr: *The Lung: Clinical Physiology and Pulmonary Function Tests,* ed 2, Chicago, 1962, Year Book Medical Publishers.

14. Lee JM, Warren MP, Mason SM: Effects of ice on nerve conduction velocity, *Physiotherapy* 64:2-6, 1978.

15. Zankel HT: Effect of physical agents on motor conduction velocity of the ulnar nerve, *Arch Phys Med Rehabil* 47:787-792, 1966.

16. Douglas WW, Malcolm JL: The effect of localized cooling on cat nerves, *J Physiol* 130:53-54, 1955.

17. Bassett FH, Kirkpatrick JS, Engelhardt DL et al: Cryotherapy induced nerve injury, *Am J Sport Med* 22:516-528, 1992.

18. Ernst E, Fialka V: Ice freezes pain? A review of the clinical effectiveness of analgesic cold therapy, *J Pain Symptom Mgmt* 9(1):56-59, 1994.

19. McMaster WC, Liddie S: Cryotherapy influence on posttraumatic limb edema, *Clin Orthop Relat Res* 150: 283-287, 1980.

20. McGown HL: Effects of cold application on maximal isometric contraction, *Phys Ther* 47:185-192, 1967.

21. Oliver RA, Johnson DJ, Wheelhouse WW et al: Isometric muscle contraction response during recovery from reduced intramuscular temperature, *Arch Phys Med Rehabil* 60:126-129, 1979.

22. Johnson J, Leider FE: Influence of cold bath on maximum handgrip strength, *Percept Mot Skills* 44:323-325, 1977.

23. Davies CTM, Young K: Effect of temperature on the contractile properties and muscle power of triceps surae in humans, *J Appl Physiol* 55:191-195, 1983.

24. Knuttsson E, Mattsson E: Effects of local cooling on monosynaptic reflexes in man, *Scand J Rehabil Med* 52:166-168, 1969.

25. Knuttsson E: Topical cryotherapy in spasticity, *Scand J Rehabil Med* 2:159-162, 1970.

26. Hartvikksen K: Ice therapy in spasticity, *Acta Neurol Scand* 38:79-83, 1962.

27. Miglietta O: Electromyographic characteristics of clonus and influence of cold, *Arch Phys Med Rehabil* 45:502-503, 1964.

28. Miglietta O: Action of cold on spasticity, *Am J Phys Med* 52:198-205, 1973.

29. Price R, Lehmann JF, Boswell-Bassette S et al: Influence of cryotherapy on spasticity at the human ankle, *Arch Phys Med Rehabil* 74:300-304, 1993.

30. Wolf SL, Letbetter WD: Effect of skin cooling on spontaneous EMG activity in triceps surae of the decerebrate cat, *Brain Res* 91:151-155, 1975.

31. Harris ED, McCroskery PA: The influence of temperature and fibril stability on degradation of cartilage collagen by rheumatoid synovial collagenase, *N Engl J Med* 290:1-6, 1974.

32. Hocutt JE, Jaffe R, Ryplander CR et al: Cryotherapy in ankle sprains, *Am J Sports Med* 10(5):316-319, 1982.

33. Ohkoshi Y, Ohkoshi M, Nagasaki S: The effect of cryotherapy on intraarticular temperature and postoperative care after anterior cruciate ligament reconstruction, *Am J Sports Med* May-Jun;27(3):357-362, 1999.

34. Meeusen R, Lievens P: The use of cryotherapy in sport injuries, *Sports Med* 3:398-414, 1986.

35. Friden J, Sjostrom M, Ekblom B: A morphological study of delayed onset muscle soreness, *Experientia* 37:506-507, 1981.

36. Jones D, Newhan D, Round J et al: Experimental human muscle damage: morphological changes in relation to other indices of damage, *J Physiol* 375:435-448, 1986.

37. Cote DJ, Prentice WE, Hooker DN et al: Comparison of three treatment procedures for minimizing ankle sprain swelling, *Phys Ther* 68(7):1072-1076, 1988.

38. Wilkerson GB: Treatment of inversion ankle sprain through synchronous application of focal compression and cold, *Athl Train* 26:220-225, 1991.

39. Quillen WS, Roullier LH: Initial management of acute ankle sprains with rapid pulsed pneumatic compression and cold, *J Orthop Sports Phys Ther* 4:39-43, 1982.

40. Boris M, Wiedorf S, Lasinski B et al: Lymphedema reduction by noninvasive complex lymphedema therapy, *Oncology* 8(9):95-106, 1994.

41. Beenakker EA, Oparina TI, Hartgring A et al: Cooling garment treatment in MS: clinical improvement and decrease in leukocyte NO production, *Neurology* Sep 11;57(5):892-894, 2001.

42. Capello E, Gardella M, Leandri M et al: Lowering body temperature with a cooling suit as symptomatic treatment for thermosensitive multiple sclerosis patients, *Ital J Neurol Sci* Nov;16(8):533-539, 1995.

43. Umphred DA: *Neurological Rehabilitation,* St. Louis, 1985, Mosby.

44. Selbach H: The principles of relaxation oscillation as a special instance of the law of initial value in cybernetic functions, *Ann NY Acad Sci* 98:1221-1228, 1962.

45. Gelhorn E: *Principles of Autonomic-Somatic Integration: Physiological Basis and Psychological and Clinical Implications,* Minneapolis, 1967, University of Minnesota Press.

46. Knight KL: *Cryotherapy: Theory, Technique, Physiology,* Chattanooga, Tenn, 1985, Chattanooga Corp.

47. Hayden CA: Cryokinetics in an early treatment program, *J Am Phys Ther Assoc* 44:990, 1964.

48. Bugaj R: The cooling, analgesic, and rewarming effects of ice massage on localized skin, *Phys Ther* 55(1):11-19, 1975.

49. Prentice WE: An electromyographic analysis of the effectiveness of heat or cold and stretching for inducing relaxation in injured muscle, *J Orthop Sports Phys Ther* 3:133-137, 1982.

50. Tierney LM, McPhee SJ, Papadakis MA et al: *Current Medical Diagnosis and Treatment.* Norwalk, CT, 1998, Appleton & Lange.

51. Day MJ: Hypersensitive response to ice massage: report of a case, *Phys Ther* 54:592-593, 1974.

52. Parker JT, Small NC, Davis DG: Cold-induced nerve palsy, *Athl Train* 18:76-77, 1983.

53. Green GA, Zachazewski JE, Jordan SE: Peroneal nerve palsy induced by cryotherapy, *Physician Sport Med* 17(9):63-70, 1989.

54. Lundgren C, Murren A, Zederfeldt B: Effect of cold vasoconstriction on wound healing in the rabbit, *Acta Chir Scand* 118:1, 1959.

55. Boyer JT, Fraser JRE, Doyle AE: The hemodynamic effects of cold immersion, *Clin Sci* 19:539-543, 1980.

56. Covington DB, Bassett FH: When cryotherapy injures, *Physician Sport Med* 21(3):78-93, 1993.

57. Knight KL: *Cryotherapy in Sport Injury Management,* Champaign, IL, 1995, Human Kinetics.

58. Benson TB, Copp EP: The effects of therapeutic forms of heat and ice on the pain threshold of the normal shoulder, *Rheumatol Rehabil* 13:101-104, 1974.

59. MacAuley DC: Ice therapy: how good is the evidence? *Int J Sports Med* Jul;22(5):379-384, 2001.

60. Metzman L, Gamble JG, Rinsky LA: Effectiveness of ice packs in reducing skin temperature under casts, *Clin Orthop* Sep;(330):217-221, 1996.

61. Farry PJ, Prentice NG: Ice treatment of injured ligaments: an experimental model, *NZ Med J* 9:12-14, 1980.

62. Krumhansl BR: Ice lollies for ice massage, *Phys Ther* 49(10):1098, 1969.

63. Schroder D, Passler HH: Combination of cold and compression after knee surgery:a prospective randomized study, *Knee Surg Sports Traumatol Arthrosc* 2(3):158-165, 1994.

64. Webb JM, Williams D, Ivory JP et al: The use of cold compression dressings after total knee replacement: a randomized controlled trial, *Orthopedics* Jan;21(1): 59-61, 1998.

65. Travel J: Temporomandibular joint pain referred from muscles of the head and neck, *J Prosthetic Dent* 10(4): 745-763, 1960.

66. Rubin D: Myofascial trigger point syndromes: an approach to management, *Arch Phys Med Rehabil* 62:107-110, 1981.

67. *Fluorimethane technical specifications,* Cleveland, OH, 1996, Gebauer Co.

68. Travell JG, Simons DG: *Myofascial Pain and Dysfunction: The Trigger Point Manual,* Baltimore, 1983, Williams & Wilkins.

69. Travell JG: Myofascial trigger points: clinical view. In Bonica JJ, Albe-Fessard D, eds: *Advances in Pain Research and Therapy,* New York, 1976, Raven Press.

70. Simons DG, Travell JG: Myofascial origins of low back pain. 1: Principles of diagnosis and treatment, *Postgrad Med* 73(2):70-77, 1983.

71. Simons DG: Myofascial pain syndrome due to trigger points, *Int Rehabil Med Assoc* Monogr 1, 1987.

72. Scarcella JB, Cohn BT: The effect of cold therapy on the postoperative course of total hip and total knee arthroplasty patients, *Am J Orthop* 24(11):847-852, 1955.

73. Bickford RH, Duff RS: Influence of ultrasonic irradiation on temperature and blood flow in human skeletal muscle, *Circ Res* 1:534-538, 1953.

74. Imamura M, Biro S, Kihara T et al: Repeated thermal therapy improves impaired vascular endothelial function in patients with coronary risk factors, *J Am Coll Cardiol* Oct;38(4):1083-1088, 2001.

75. Crockford GW, Hellon RF, Parkhouse J: Thermal vasomotor response in human skin mediated by local mechanisms, *J Physiol* 161:10-15, 1962.

76. Kellogg DL Jr, Liu Y, Kosiba IF et al: Role of nitric oxide in the vascular effects of local warming of the skin in humans, *J Appl Physiol* Apr;86(4):1185-1190, 1999.

77. Minson CT, Berry LT, Joyner MJ: Nitric oxide and neurally mediated regulation of skin blood flow during local heating, *J Appl Physiol* Oct;91(4):1619-1626, 2001.

78. Fox HH, Hilton SM: Bradykinin formation in human skin as a factor in heat vasodilation, *J Physiol* 142:219, 1958.

79. Guyton AC: *Textbook of Medical Physiology,* ed 8, Philadelphia, 1991, WB Saunders.

80. Abramson DI: Indirect vasodilation in thermotherapy, *Arch Phys Med Rehabil* 46:412-415, 1965.

81. Wessman MS, Kottke FJ: The effect of indirect heating on peripheral blood flow, pulse rate, blood pressure and temperature, *Arch Phys Med Rehabil* 48:567-576, 1967.

82. Wyper DJ, McNiven DR: Effects of some physiotherapeutic agents on skeletal muscle blood flow, *Physiotherapy* 62:83-85, 1976.

83. Crockford GW, Hellon RF: Vascular responses in human skin to infra-red radiation, *J Physiol* 149: 424-426, 1959.

84. Currier DP, Kramer JF: Sensory nerve conduction: heating effects of ultrasound and infrared radiation, *Physiother Canada* 34:241-246, 1982.

85. Halle JS, Scoville CR, Greathouse DG: Ultrasound effect on the conduction latency of the superficial radial nerve in man, *Phys Ther* 61:345-350, 1981.

86. Lehmann JF, DeLateur BJ: Therapeutic heat. In Lehmann JF, ed: *Therapeutic Heat and Cold,* ed 4, Baltimore, 1990, Williams & Wilkins.

87. Rennie GA, Michlovitz SL: Biophysical principles of heating and superficial heating agents. In Michlovitz SL, ed: *Thermal Agents in Rehabilitation*, Philadelphia, 1996, FA Davis.

88. Fountain FP, Gersten JW, Senger O: Decrease in muscle spasm produced by ultrasound, hot packs and IR, *Arch Phys Med Rehabil* 41:293-299, 1960.

89. Fischer M, Schafer SS: Temperature effects on the discharge frequency of primary and secondary endings of isolated cat muscle spindles recorded under a ramp-and-hold stretch, *Brain Res* 840(1-2):1-15, 1999.

90. Lehmann JF, Brunner GD, Stow RW: Pain threshold measurements after therapeutic application of ultrasound, microwaves and infrared, *Arch Phys Med Rehabil* 39:560-565, 1958.

91. Benson TB, Copp EP: The effects of therapeutic forms of heat and ice on the pain threshold of the normal shoulder, *Rheumatol Rehabil* 13:101-104, 1974.

92. Chastain PB: The effect of deep heat on isometric strength, *Phys Ther* 58:543-546, 1978.

93. Wickstrom R, Polk C: Effect of whirlpool on the strength and endurance of the quadriceps muscle in trained male adolescents, *Am J Phys Med* 40:91-95, 1961.

94. Edwards R, Harris R, Hultman E et al: Energy metabolism during isometric exercise at different temperatures of m. quadriceps femoris in man, *Acta Physiol Scand* 80:17-18, 1970.

95. Miller MW, Ziskin MC: Biological consequences of hyperthermia, *Ultrasound Med Biol* 15(8):707-722, 1989.

96. Barcroft J, King W: The effect of temperature on the dissociation curve of blood, *J Physiol* 39:374-384, 1909.

97. Lentell G, Hetherington T, Eagan J et al: The use of thermal agents to influence the effectiveness of low-load prolonged stretch, *J Orthop Sport Phys Ther* 16(5): 200-207, 1992.

98. Warren C, Lehmann J, Koblanski J: Elongation of rat tail tendon: effect of load and temperature, *Arch Phys Med Rehabil* 52:465-474, 484, 1971.

99. Warren C, Lehmann J, Koblanski J: Heat and stretch procedures: an evaluation using rat tail tendon, *Arch Phys Med Rehabil* 57:122-126, 1976.

100. Gersten JW: Effect of ultrasound on tendon extensibility, *Am J Phys Med* 34:362-369, 1955.

101. Lehmann J, Masock A, Warren C et al: Effect of therapeutic temperatures on tendon extensibility, *Arch Phys Med Rehabil* 51:481-487, 1970.

102. Kramer JF: Ultrasound: evaluation of its mechanical and thermal effects, *Arch Phys Med Rehabil* 65:223-227, 1984.

103. Steilan J, Habot B: Improvement of pain and disability in elderly patients with degenerative osteoarthritis of the knee treated with narrow band light therapy, *J Am Geriatr Soc* 40(1):23-26, 1992.

104. Magness J, Garrett T, Erickson D: Swelling of the upper extremity during whirlpool baths, *Arch Phys Med Rehabil* 51:297-299, 1970.

105. Wright V, Johns R: Physical factors concerned with the stiffness of normal and diseased joints, *Johns Hopkins Hosp Bull* 106:215-229, 1960.

106. Kik JA, Kersley GD: Heat and cold in the physical treatment of rheumatoid arthritis of the knee, *Ann Phys Med* 9:270-274, 1968.

107. Blacklung L, Tiselius P: Objective measurement of joint stiffness in rheumatoid arthritis, *Acta Rheum Scand* 13:275, 1967.

108. Johns R, Wright V: Relative importance of various tissues in joint stiffness, *J Appl Physiol* 17:824-828, 1962.

109. Orenberg EK, Noodleman FR, Koperski JA et al: Comparison of heat delivery systems for hyperthermia treatment of psoriasis, *Int J Hypertherm* 2(3): 231-241, 1986.

110. Westerhof W, Siddiqui AH, Cormane RH et al: Infrared hyperthermia and psoriasis, *Arch Dermatol Res* 279:209-210, 1987.

111. Hyland DB, Kirkland VJ: Infra red therapy for skin ulcers, *Am J Nurs* 80(10):1800-1801, 1980.

112. Cummings J: Role of light in wound healing. In Kloth L, McCulloch JM, Feedar JA, eds: *Wound Healing: Alternatives in Management,* Philadelphia, 1990, FA Davis.

113. Moss C, Ellis R, Murray W et al: *Infrared Radiation, Nonionising Radiation Protection,* ed 2, WHO Regional Publications, European Series, 25. Geneva, 1989, World Health Organization.

114. Schmidt KL: Heat, cold and inflammation, *Rheumatology* 38:391-404, 1979.

115. Sapareto SA, Dewey WC: Thermal dose determination in cancer therapy, *Int J Radiol Oncol Biol Phys* 10:787-800, 1984.

116. Hornback NB: *Hyperthermia and Cancer,* Boca Raton, FL, 1984, CRC Press.

117. Ganong WF: *Review of Medical Physiology,* ed 13, Norwalk, CT, 1987, Appleton & Lange.

118. Kligman LH: Intensification of ultraviolet-induced dermal damage by infra-red radiation, *Arch Dermatol Res* 272:229-238, 1982.

119. Enwemeka CS, Booth CK, Fisher SL et al: Decay time of temperature of hot packs in two application positions, *Phys Ther* 76(5):S96, 1996.

120. Borrell RM, Henley ES, Purvis H et al: Fluidotherapy: evaluation of a new heat modality, *Arch Phys Med Rehabil* 58:69-71, 1977.

121. Hardy JD: Spectral transmittance and reflectance of excised human skin, *J Appl Physiol* 9:257-264, 1956.

122. Selkins KM, Emery AF: Thermal science for physical medicine. In Lehmann JF, ed: *Therapeutic Heat and Cold,* ed 3, Baltimore, 1982, Williams & Wilkins.

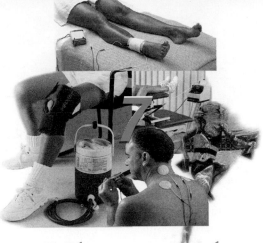

Ultrasound

OBJECTIVES

Upon completion of this chapter, the reader will be able to:

1. Recognize and distinguish the terminology used to describe therapeutic ultrasound.
2. Analyze the physiological responses to ultrasound necessary to promote particular treatment goals.
3. Identify the physical properties of, and the physiological responses to, therapeutic ultrasound.
4. Evaluate the indications, contraindications, and precautions for the use of therapeutic ultrasound with respect to different patient management situations.
5. Design appropriate methods for selecting therapeutic ultrasound treatment parameters to produce desired physical and physiological effects.
6. Choose and use the most appropriate therapeutic ultrasound device and treatment parameters to obtain the desired treatment goals.
7. Evaluate different therapeutic ultrasound devices with respect to their potential for treating different patient problems.
8. Presented with a clinical case, evaluate the clinical findings, propose goals of treatment, assess whether therapeutic ultrasound would be the best treatment, and, if so, formulate an effective treatment plan, including the appropriate treatment parameters, for achieving the goals of treatment.

HISTORY

Methods to generate and detect ultrasound first became available in the United States in the 19th century; however, the first large-scale application of ultrasound was for SONAR (Sound Navigation and Ranging) during World War II. For this application, a short pulse of ultrasound is sent from a submarine through the water, and a detector is used to pick up the echo of the signal. Because the time required for the echo to reach the detector is proportional to the distance of the detector from a reflecting surface, the duration of this period can be used to calculate the distance to objects under the water, such as other submarines or rocks. This pulse-echo technology has since been adapted for medical imaging applications, for "viewing" a fetus or other internal masses. Early SONAR devices used high-intensity ultrasound for ease of detection; however, it was found that these devices can heat and thus damage underwater life. Although this fact limited the intensity of ultrasound appropriate for SONAR, it led to the development of clinical ultrasound devices specifically intended for heating of biological tissue. Ultrasound was found to heat tissue with a high collagen content, such as tendons, ligaments, or fascia and, for the past 50 years or more, has been widely used in the clinical setting for this purpose. More recently, ultrasound has also been found to have nonthermal effects and, over the past 20 years, therapeutic applications of these effects have been developed. Low-intensity pulsed ultrasound, which produces only nonthermal effects, has been shown to facilitate tissue healing, modify inflammation, and enhance transdermal drug delivery.

What Is Ultrasound?

Ultrasound is a type of sound, and all forms of sound consist of waves that transmit energy by alternately compressing and rarefying material (Fig. 7-1). Ultrasound is defined as sound with a frequency of greater than 20,000 cycles per second (Hertz, Hz). This definition is based on the limits of normal human hearing. Humans can hear sound with a frequency of 16 to 20,000 Hz; sound with a frequency greater than this is known as *ultrasound*. Generally, therapeutic ultrasound has a frequency of between 0.7 and 3.3 megahertz (MHz) in order to maximize energy absorption at a depth of 2 to 5 cm of soft tissue.

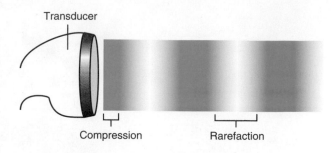

Figure 7-1. Ultrasound compression-rarefaction wave.

Audible sound and ultrasound have many similar properties. For example, as ultrasound travels through material, it gradually decreases in intensity due to attenuation in the same way that the sound we hear becomes quieter as we move farther from its source (Fig. 7-2). Ultrasound waves cause a slight circular motion of material as they are transmitted, but they do not carry the material along with the wave. Similarly, when someone speaks, the audible sound waves of the voice reach across the room, but the air in front of the speaker's mouth is agitated only slightly, not moved across the room.

Ultrasound has a variety of physical effects that can be classified as *thermal* or *nonthermal*. Its ability to increase tissue temperature is its thermal effect, and its ability to cause acoustic streaming, microstreaming, and cavitation, which may alter cell membrane permeability, are its nonthermal effects. This chapter describes the physical properties of ultrasound and its effects on the body in order to derive guidelines for the optimal clinical application of therapeutic ultrasound.

The following section lists and defines the terms used specifically to describe therapeutic ultrasound and its effects. Terms used to describe ultrasound and other physical agents are defined in the glossary at the end of this book.

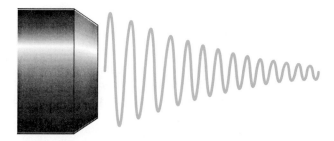

Figure 7-2. Decreasing ultrasound intensity as the wave travels through tissue.

TERMINOLOGY

Transducer (sound head): A crystal that converts electrical energy into sound (Fig. 7-3). This term is also used to describe the part of an ultrasound unit that contains the crystal.

Power: The amount of acoustic energy per unit time. This is usually expressed in Watts (W).

Intensity: The power per unit area of the sound head. This is usually expressed in Watts/centimeter squared (W/cm^2). The World Health

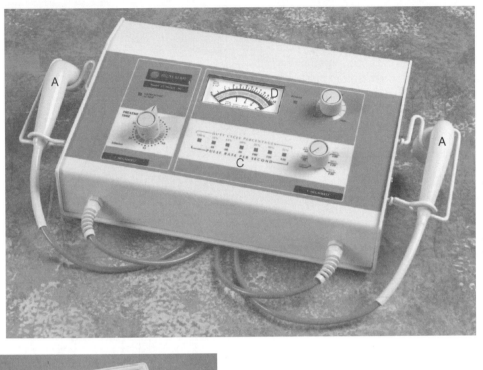

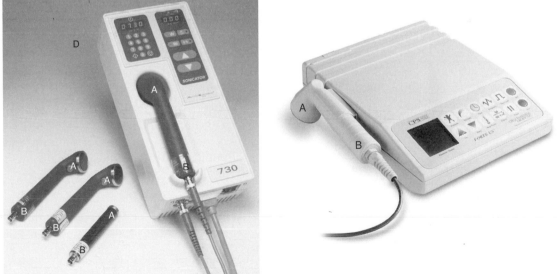

Figure 7-3. Ultrasound units: **A**, transducer; **B**, frequency indicator; **C**, pulse duty cycle indicator; and **D**, power/intensity indicator. (*Part one* courtesy Rich-Mar, Inola, OK; *Part Two* courtesy Mettler Electronics, Anaheim, CA; *Part Three* courtesy Chattanooga Group, Hixson, TN.)

Organization limits the average intensity output by therapeutic ultrasound units to 3 W/cm^2.[1]

Spatial Average Intensity: The average intensity of the ultrasound output over the area of the transducer.

Spatial Peak Intensity: The peak intensity of the ultrasound output over the area of the transducer. The intensity is usually greatest in the center of the beam and lowest at the edges of the beam.

Beam Nonuniformity Ratio (BNR): The ratio of the spatial peak intensity to the spatial average intensity (Fig. 7-4). For most units this is usually between 5:1 and 6:1, although it can be as low as 2:1.

EXAMPLES

Using a transducer with a maximum BNR of 5:1, when the spatial average intensity is set at 1 W/cm^2, the spatial peak intensity within the field could be as high as 5 W/cm^2.

Using a transducer with a maximum BNR of 6:1, when the spatial average intensity is set at 1.5 W/cm^2, the spatial peak intensity within the field could be as high as 9 W/cm^2.

The FDA requires that the maximum BNR for an ultrasound transducer be specified on the device.

Continuous Ultrasound: Continuous delivery of ultrasound throughout the treatment period (Fig. 7-5).

Pulsed Ultrasound: Delivery of ultrasound during only a portion of the treatment period. Delivery of ultrasound is pulsed on and off throughout the

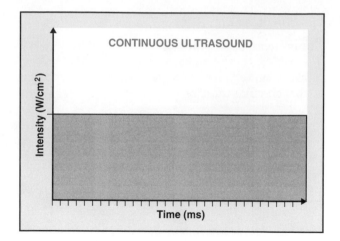

Figure 7-5. Continuous ultrasound.

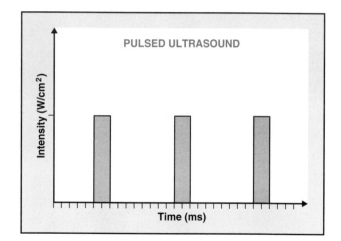

Figure 7-6. Pulsed ultrasound.

treatment period. Pulsing the ultrasound minimizes its thermal effects (Fig. 7-6).

Duty Cycle: The proportion of the total treatment time that the ultrasound is on. This can be expressed either as a percentage or a ratio.

EXAMPLES

20% or 1:5 duty cycle, is on 20% of the time and off 80% of the time. This is generally delivered 2 ms on, 8 ms off (Fig. 7-7).

100% duty cycle is on 100% of the time and is the same as continuous ultrasound.

Spatial Average Temporal Peak (SATP) Intensity: The spatial average intensity of the ultrasound during the on time of the pulse (Fig. 7-8). Therapeutic

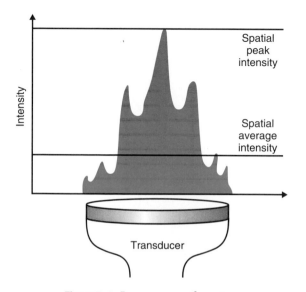

Figure 7-4. Beam nonuniformity.

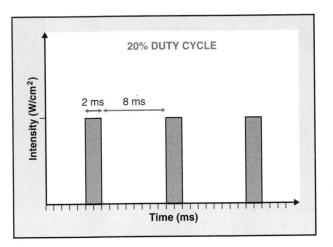

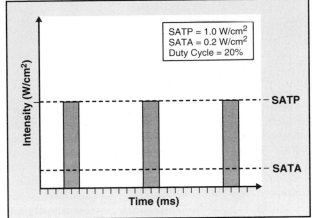

Figure 7-8. SATP and SATA intensity.

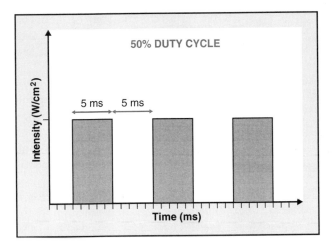

Figure 7-7. Duty cycles: 20% and 50%.

Note that SATA is equal to SATP for continuous ultrasound.

EXAMPLE
1 W/cm² SATP at 100% duty cycle =
$$1 \times 1 = 1 \text{ W/cm}^2 \text{ SATA}$$

Frequency: The number of compression-rarefaction cycles per unit of time, usually expressed in *cycles per second* (Hertz, Hz) (Fig. 7-9). Increasing the frequency of ultrasound causes a decrease in its depth of penetration and concentration of the ultrasound energy in the superficial tissues (Fig. 7-10).

Effective Radiating Area (ERA): The area of the transducer from which the ultrasound energy radiates (Fig. 7-11). Because the crystal does not vibrate uniformly, the ERA is always smaller than the area of the treatment head.

ultrasound units display the SATP intensity and the duty cycle. In this chapter, all intensities are expressed as *SATP*, followed by the duty cycle, unless stated otherwise.

Spatial Average Temporal Average (SATA) Intensity: The spatial average intensity of the ultrasound averaged over both the on time and the off time of the pulse.
SATP × duty cycle = SATA

EXAMPLE
1 W/cm² SATP at 20% duty cycle =
$$1 \times 0.2 = 0.2 \text{ W/cm}^2 \text{ SATA}$$

This is a measure of the amount of energy delivered to the tissue. SATA units are frequently used in the nonclinical literature on ultrasound.

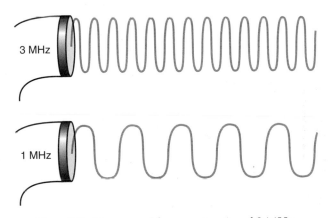

Figure 7-9. Ultrasound frequencies: 1 and 3 MHz.

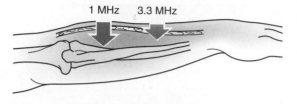

Figure 7-10. Frequency controls the depth of penetration of ultrasound; 1 MHz ultrasound penetrates approximately 3 times as far as 3.3 MHz ultrasound. (Courtesy Mettler Electronics, Anaheim, CA.)

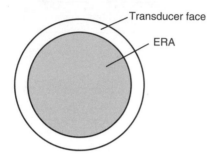

Figure 7-11. Effective radiating area.

Near Field/Far Field: The ultrasound beam delivered from a transducer initially converges and then diverges (Fig. 7-12). The near field, also known as the Fresnel zone, is the convergent region, and the far field, also known as the Fraunhofer zone, is the divergent region. In the near field there is interference of the ultrasound beam, causing variations in ultrasound intensity. In the far field there is little interference, resulting in a more uniform distribution of ultrasound intensity. The length of the near field is dependent on the ultrasound frequency and the ERA of the transducer and can be calculated from the following formula (Table 7-1):

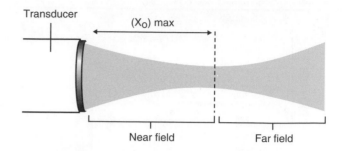

Figure 7-12. Longitudinal cross-section of an ultrasound beam.

$$\text{Length of near field} = \frac{\text{Radius of transducer}^2}{\text{Wavelength of ultrasound}}$$

In most human tissue the majority of the ultrasound intensity is attenuated within the first 2 to 5 cm of tissue depth, which, for transducers of most frequencies and sizes, lies within the near field.

Absorption: Conversion of the mechanical energy of ultrasound into heat. The amount of absorption that occurs in a tissue type at a specific frequency is expressed by its absorption coefficient. The absorption coefficient is determined by measuring the rate of temperature rise in a homogeneous tissue model exposed to an ultrasound field of known intensity. Absorption coefficients are tissue and frequency specific. They are highest for tissues with the highest collagen content and increase in proportion to the ultrasound frequency (Table 7-2).

Reflection: The redirection of an incident beam away from a reflecting surface at an angle equal and opposite to the angle of incidence (Fig. 7-13). Ultrasound is reflected at tissue interfaces, with most reflection occurring where there is the greatest difference between the acoustic impedance of

TABLE 7-1	Length of the Near Field for Different Frequencies of Ultrasound and Different Areas (ERA) of Ultrasound Transducers	
Ultrasound frequency (MHz)	**ERA (cm^2)**	**Length of near field (cm)**
1	5	11
3	5	33
1	1	2.1
3	1	6.3

TABLE 7-2	Absorption Coefficients in Decibels/cm at 1 and 3 MHz	
Tissue	**1 MHz**	**3 MHz**
Blood	0.028	0.084
Fat	0.14	0.42
Nerve	0.2	0.6
Muscle (parallel)	0.28	0.84
Muscle (perpendicular)	0.76	2.28
Blood vessels	0.4	1.2
Skin	0.62	1.86
Tendon	1.12	3.36
Cartilage	1.16	3.48
Bone	3.22	

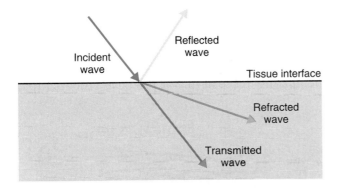

Figure 7-13. Ultrasound reflection and refraction.

adjacent tissues. In the body, most reflection, about 35%, occurs at soft tissue-bone interfaces. There is 100% reflection of ultrasound at the air-skin interface and only 0.1% reflection at the transmission medium–skin interface. There is no reflection at the transmission medium–sound head interface. A transmission medium that eliminates the air between the sound head and the body is used in order to avoid an air-skin interface with high reflection.

Refraction: The redirection of a wave at an interface (see Fig. 7-13). When refraction occurs, the ultrasound wave enters the tissue at one angle and continues through the tissue at a different angle.

Attenuation: A measure of the decrease in ultrasound intensity as the ultrasound wave travels through tissue. Attenuation is the result of absorption, reflection, and refraction, with absorption accounting for about one-half of attenuation. Attenuation coefficients are tissue and frequency specific. They are higher for tissues with a higher collagen content and increase in proportion to the frequency of the ultrasound (Table 7-3).

Half Depth: The depth of tissue at which the ultrasound intensity is half its initial intensity (Table 7-4).

Standing Wave: Intensity maxima and minima at fixed positions one-half wavelength apart. Standing waves occur when the ultrasound transducer and a reflecting surface are an exact multiple of wavelengths apart, allowing the reflected wave to

TABLE 7-3	Attenuation of 1 MHz Ultrasound	
Tissue	**Attenuation (dB/cm)**	**%/cm**
Blood	0.12	3
Fat	0.61	13
Nerve	0.88	–
Muscle	1.2	24
Blood vessels	1.7	32
Skin	2.7	39
Tendon	4.9	59
Cartilage	5.0	68
Bone	13.9	96

TABLE 7-4	Half Depths in mm at 1 and 3 MHz	
Tissue	**1 MHz**	**3 MHz**
Water	11,500	3833
Fat	50	16.5
Muscle (parallel)	24.6	8
Muscle (perpendicular)	9	3
Skin	11.1	4
Tendon	6.2	2
Cartilage	6	2
Bone	2.1	–

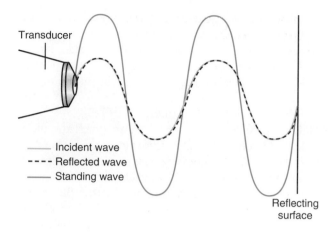

Figure 7-14. Formation of standing waves.

superimpose on the incident wave entering the tissue (Fig. 7-14). Standing waves can be avoided by moving the sound head throughout the treatment.

Cavitation: The formation, growth, and pulsation of gas- or vapor-filled bubbles caused by ultrasound. During the compression phase of an ultrasound wave, bubbles present in the tissue are made smaller, and during the rarefaction phase they expand. Cavitation may be stable or unstable (transient). With stable cavitation, the bubbles oscillate in size throughout many cycles but do not

burst. With unstable cavitation, the bubbles grow over a number of cycles and then suddenly implode (Fig. 7-15). This implosion produces large, brief, local pressure and temperature increases and causes free radical formation. Stable cavitation has been proposed as a mechanism for the nonthermal therapeutic effects of ultrasound, while unstable cavitation is thought not to occur at the intensities of ultrasound used therapeutically.[2]

Microstreaming: Microscale eddying that takes place near any small, vibrating object. Microstreaming occurs around the gas bubbles set into oscillation by cavitation.[3]

Acoustic Streaming: The steady, circular flow of cellular fluids induced by ultrasound. This flow is larger in scale than with microstreaming and is thought to alter cellular activity by transporting material from one part of the ultrasound field to another.[3]

Phonophoresis: The application of ultrasound with a topical drug in order to facilitate transdermal drug delivery (Fig. 7-16).

In summary, ultrasound is a high-frequency sound wave that can be described by its intensity, frequency, duty cycle, ERA, and BNR. It enters the body and is attenuated in the tissue by absorption, reflection, and refraction. Attenuation is greatest in tissues with a high collagen content and with the use of high ultra-

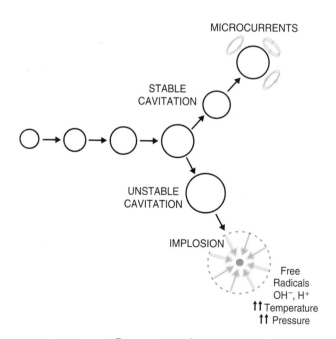

Figure 7-15. Cavitation and microstreaming.

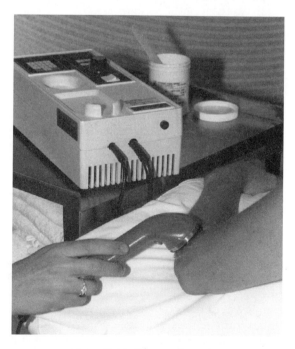

Figure 7-16. Phonophoresis.

sound frequencies. Ultrasound can generate heat, its thermal effect, and has the mechanical effects of cavitation, microstreaming, and acoustic streaming. Both the thermal and mechanical effects can be used to accelerate the achievement of treatment goals when ultrasound is applied to the appropriate pathology at the appropriate time.

GENERATION OF ULTRASOUND

Ultrasound is generated by applying a high-frequency alternating electrical current to the crystal in the transducer of an ultrasound unit. The crystal is made of a material with piezoelectric properties causing it to respond to the alternating current by expanding and contracting at the same frequency at which the current changes polarity. When the crystal expands it compresses the material in front of it, and when it contracts it rarefies the material in front of it. This alternating compression-rarefaction is the ultrasound wave (Fig. 7-17).

The property of piezoelectricity, the ability to generate electricity in response to a mechanical force or to change shape in response to an electrical current, was first discovered by Paul-Jacques and Pierre Currie in the 1880s. A variety of materials are piezoelectric, including bone, natural quartz and synthetic plumbium zirconium titanate (PZT), and barium titanate. At this time, ultrasound transducers are usually made of PZT because this is the least costly and most efficient piezoelectric material readily available.

In order to obtain a pure single frequency of ultrasound from a piezoelectric crystal, a single frequency of alternating current must be applied to it and the crystal must be of the appropriate thickness to resonate with this frequency. Resonance occurs when the ultrasound frequency and the crystal thickness conform to the following formula:

$$f = \frac{c}{2t}$$

where f is frequency, c is the speed of sound in the material, and t is the thickness of the crystal. Thus thinner, more fragile crystals are generally used to generate higher frequencies of ultrasound. These crystals should be handled with care.

Multifrequency transducers use a single crystal of a thickness optimized for only one of the frequencies. The crystal is made to vibrate at other frequencies by application of those frequencies of alternating electrical currents; however, this is associated with decreased efficiency, variability in the output frequency, reduction of the ERA, and increased BNR.[4] Recently, composite materials have been developed to deliver multiple frequencies of ultrasound more accurately and efficiently.[5]

Pulsed ultrasound is produced when the high-frequency alternating electrical current is delivered to the transducer for only a limited proportion of the treatment time, as determined by the selected duty cycle.

EFFECTS OF ULTRASOUND

Ultrasound has a variety of biophysical effects. It can increase the temperature of deep and superficial tissues and has a range of nonthermal effects. Traditionally, these effects have been considered separately, although the reader should be aware that to some degree both occur with all applications of ultrasound. Continuous ultrasound has the most effect on tissue temperature; however, nonthermal effects can also occur with the use of continuous ultrasound. Additionally, although pulsed ultrasound produces minimal sustained changes in tissue temperature, it probably does have a small brief heating effect during the on time of a pulse. Although a number of studies have demonstrated the biophysical effects of ultrasound, the degree to which the findings can be extrapolated from the experimental conditions to specific clinical applications is still uncertain and requires further study.[6]

THERMAL EFFECTS

Tissues Affected

The earliest studies demonstrating that ultrasound can increase tissue temperature were published by

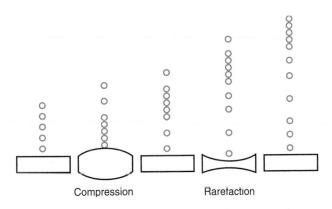

Compression   Rarefaction

Figure 7-17. Ultrasound production by piezoelectric crystal.

Harvey in 1930.[7] The thermal effects of ultrasound, including acceleration of metabolic rate, reduction or control of pain and muscle spasm, alteration of nerve conduction velocity, increased circulation, and increased soft tissue extensibility, are the same as those obtained with other heating modalities, as described in Chapter 6, except that the structures heated are different.[8-10] Ultrasound reaches more deeply and heats smaller areas than most superficial heating agents. Ultrasound also heats tissues with high ultrasound absorption coefficients more than those with low absorption coefficients. Tissues with high absorption coefficients are generally those with a high collagen content, while tissues with low absorption coefficients generally have a high water content. Thus, ultrasound is particularly well-suited to heating tendons, ligaments, joint capsules, and fascia while not overheating the overlying fat. Ultrasound is generally not the ideal physical agent for heating muscle tissue because muscle has a relatively low absorption coefficient; also, most muscles are much larger than the available ultrasound transducers.

Factors Affecting the Amount of Temperature Increase

The increase in tissue temperature produced by the absorption of ultrasound varies according to the tissue to which the ultrasound is applied, as well as with the frequency, intensity, and duration of the ultrasound. The heating rate is proportional to the tissue's absorption coefficient at the applied ultrasound frequency.[11] Tissue absorption coefficients increase with increased collagen content and in proportion to the ultrasound frequency. Thus, higher temperatures are achieved in tissues with a high collagen content and with the application of higher-frequency ultrasound. When the absorption coefficient is high, the temperature increase is distributed in a smaller volume of more superficial tissue than when the absorption coefficient is low, since changing the absorption coefficient alters the heat distribution but does not change the total amount of heat being delivered (Fig. 7-18). To increase the total amount of heat being delivered to the tissue, the duration of ultrasound application or the average ultrasound intensity must be increased. One MHz frequency ultrasound can be used to heat tissues up to 5 cm deep, whereas 3 MHz frequency should be used when the goal is to heat tissues only 1 to 2 cm deep. Note that with 3 MHz ultra-

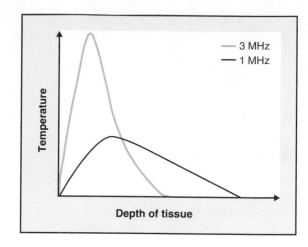

Figure 7-18. Temperature distribution for 1 and 3 MHz ultrasound at the same intensity.

sound, although the maximum temperature achieved is higher, the depth of penetration is lower. Although theoretical models predict that 3 MHz ultrasound will increase tissue temperature 3 times more than 1 MHz ultrasound, an in vivo study in which ultrasound was applied to human calf muscle found an almost fourfold greater temperature increase with 3 MHz ultrasound than with 1 MHz ultrasound applied at 0.5 to 2.0 W/cm^2; therefore, clinically, an intensity 3 to 4 times lower should be used when applying 3 MHz ultrasound than when applying 1 MHz ultrasound.[12]

During ultrasound application, tissue temperature change is also affected by factors other than ultrasound absorption. Blood circulating through the tissue will cool the tissues while conduction from one warmed area of tissue to another and reflection of ultrasound waves in regions of soft tissue–bone interfaces will heat the tissues.[13]

On average, soft tissue temperature has been shown to increase by 0.2° C per minute *in vivo* with ultrasound delivered at 1 W/cm^2 at 1 MHz.[12,14] Nonuniformity of the intensity of ultrasound output, the variety of tissue types with different absorption coefficients in a clinical treatment area, and reflection at tissue boundaries, cause the temperature increase within the ultrasound field not to be uniform. The the highest temperature is generally produced at soft tissue–bone interfaces where reflection is greatest. Moving the sound head throughout the application helps to equalize the heat distribution and minimize the incidence of excessively hot or cold areas.

The number of unknown variables, including the thickness of each tissue layer, the amount of circulation, and the distance to reflecting soft tissue-bone interfaces, makes it difficult to predict accurately the temperature increase that will be produced clinically when ultrasound is applied to a patient. Thus, initial treatment parameters are set according to theoretical and research predictions; however, the patient's report of warmth is used to determine the final ultrasound intensity. If the ultrasound intensity is too high, the patient will complain of a deep ache from overheating of the periosteum. If this occurs, the ultrasound intensity must be reduced in order to avoid burning the tissue. If the ultrasound intensity is too low, the patient will not feel any increase in temperature. More specific guidelines for selection of the optimal ultrasound treatment parameters for tissue heating are given below in the section on application technique. Because the patient's report is used to determine the maximum safe ultrasound intensity, it is recommended that thermal-level ultrasound not be applied to patients who are unable to feel or report discomfort caused by overheating.

Applying Other Physical Agents in Conjunction with Ultrasound

Various physical agents can be applied together with, prior to, or after the application of ultrasound. Applying a hot pack prior to ultrasound treatment has been shown to increase the temperature of only the superficial 1 to 2 mm of skin and subcutaneous tissue while not affecting the temperature of deeper tissue layers.[15] Similarly, using a warm conduction medium will not affect the heating of deep tissues. Applying ultrasound in cold water cools the superficial skin by conduction and convection, thereby reducing the increase in superficial tissue temperature produced by ultrasound. Applying ice prior to the application of ultrasound has also been shown to reduce the temperature increase produced by ultrasound in the deeper tissues.[16] Ice, or any other thermal agent, should be applied with caution prior to the application of ultrasound since the loss of sensation that may be caused by these agents can reduce the accuracy of the patient's feedback regarding deep tissue temperature. Although many clinicians apply ultrasound in conjunction with electrical stimulation, with the goal of combining the benefits of both modalities, there is no published research at this time evaluating the efficacy of this combination of interventions. In general, one should analyze the effects of each physical agent independently when considering applying a combination of agents either concurrently or in sequence.

NONTHERMAL EFFECTS

Ultrasound has a variety of effects on biological processes that are thought to be unrelated to any increase in tissue temperature. These effects are the result of the mechanical events produced by ultrasound, including cavitation, microstreaming, and acoustic streaming. When ultrasound is delivered in a pulsed mode, with a 20% or lower duty cycle, the heat generated during the on time of the cycle is dispersed during the off time, resulting in no measurable net increase in temperature. Thus, pulsed ultrasound with a 20% duty cycle has generally been used to apply and study the nonthermal effects of ultrasound. Some recent studies have also used low intensities of continuous ultrasound to study these effects.[17]

Ultrasound with a low average intensity has been shown to increase intracellular calcium,[18] increase skin and cell membrane permeability,[19] increase mast cell degranulation, increase chemotactic factor and histamine release,[20] increase macrophage responsiveness,[21] and increase the rate of protein synthesis by fibroblasts.[22] These effects have been demonstrated using ultrasound at intensities and duty cycles that did not produce any measurable increase in temperature and are therefore considered to be nonthermal effects. They have been attributed to cavitation, acoustic streaming, and microstreaming.[21,23] Because these cellular-level processes are essential components of tissue healing, the changes in these processes produced by ultrasound are thought to underlie the enhanced healing observed to occur in response to the application of ultrasound to a variety of pathologies. For example, increasing intracellular calcium can alter the enzymatic activity of cells and stimulate their synthesis and secretion of proteins because calcium ions act as chemical signals (second messengers) to cells. The greatest changes in intracellular calcium levels have been reported to occur in response to 20% pulsed ultrasound at intensities of 0.5 to 0.75 W/cm^2.[18] The fact that ultrasound can affect macrophage responsiveness explains, in part, why ultrasound is particularly effective during the inflammatory phase of repair, when the macrophage is the dominant cell type. It is interesting to note that pulsed ultrasound has been shown to have a significantly greater effect on membrane permeability than continuous ultrasound delivered at the same SATA intensity.[19]

CLINICAL APPLICATIONS OF ULTRASOUND

Soft tissue shortening
Pain control
Dermal ulcers
Surgical skin incisions
Tendon injuries
Resorption of calcium deposits
Bone fractures
Carpal tunnel syndrome
Phonophoresis
Plantar warts
Herpes zoster infection

Ultrasound is commonly used as a component of the treatment of a wide variety of pathologies. These applications take advantage of both the thermal and nonthermal effects of ultrasound. The thermal effects are used primarily prior to stretching shortened soft tissue and for the reduction of pain. The nonthermal effects are used primarily for altering membrane permeability in order to accelerate tissue healing. Although much of the research on the nonthermal effects of ultrasound has been done using in vitro models, ultrasound at nonthermal levels has been shown to facilitate the healing of dermal ulcers, surgical skin incisions, tendon injuries, and bone fractures in both humans and animals. Ultrasound has also been shown to enhance transdermal drug penetration, probably via both thermal and nonthermal mechanisms. This mode of transdermal drug delivery is known as *phonophoresis*. Ultrasound has also been found to assist in the resorption of calcium deposits, in the removal of plantar warts, and in the recovery from herpes zoster virus infection. The mechanism of these effects is uncertain.

A summary of the research on the use of ultrasound for these applications follows. Gaps in current research do not allow one to conclude with certainty that ultrasound can consistently produce the clinical effects described. Although there is evidence to support these recommended clinical applications, recent systematic reviews of the randomized controlled studies of the clinical effects of ultrasound found that there were insufficient studies to clearly demonstrate that ultrasound is more effective than placebo.[24,25]

Many studies were limited by poor design and by the fact that the ultrasound doses varied considerably without any rationale. Further well-controlled studies using appropriate ultrasound doses are needed to determine with greater certainty the clinical efficacy of therapeutic ultrasound and the optimal treatment parameters to use.

Soft Tissue Shortening

Soft tissue shortening can be the result of immobilization, inactivity, or scarring, and can cause joint range-of-motion (ROM) restrictions, pain, and functional limitations. Shortening of the joint capsule, surrounding tendons, or ligaments is frequently responsible for such adverse consequences, and stretching of these tissues can help them regain their normal length and thereby reverse the adverse consequences of soft tissue shortening. Increasing the temperature of soft tissue temporarily increases its extensibility, increasing the length gained for the same force of stretch while also reducing the risk of tissue damage.[26,27] The increase in soft tissue length is also maintained more effectively if the stretching force is applied while the tissue temperature is elevated. This increased ease of stretching is thought to be the result of altered viscoelasticity of collagen and alteration of the collagen matrix.

Because ultrasound can penetrate to the depth of most joint capsules, tendons, and ligaments, and since these tissues have high ultrasound absorption coefficients, ultrasound can be an effective physical agent for heating these tissues prior to stretching. The deep heating produced by 1 MHz continuous ultrasound at 1.0 to 2.5 W/cm^2 has been shown to be more effective at increasing hip joint ROM than the superficial heating produced by infrared radiation when applied in conjunction with exercise.[28] One MHz continuous ultrasound at 1.5 W/cm^2 applied to the triceps surae combined with static dorsiflexion stretching has also been shown to be more effective than static stretching alone at increasing dorsiflexion ROM.[29] The increased ROM observed in both of these studies was attributed to increased extensibility of the soft tissues due to heating by ultrasound.

The studies cited above indicate that continuous ultrasound of sufficient intensity and duration to increase tissue temperature may increase soft tissue extensibility, thereby combatting soft tissue shortening and increasing joint ROM when applied in conjunction with stretching. The treatment parameters found to be effective for this application are 1 or 3 MHz frequency, depending on the tissue depth, at 1.0 to 2.5 W/cm² intensity, applied for 5 to 10 minutes. For optimal effect, it is recommended that stretching be applied during heating by ultrasound and maintained for 5 to 10 minutes after ultrasound application while the tissue is cooling (Fig. 7-19).

Pain Control

Ultrasound may control pain by altering its transmission or perception or by modifying the underlying condition causing the pain. These effects may be the result of stimulation of the cutaneous thermal receptors or increased soft tissue extensibility due to increased tissue temperature, the result of changes in nerve conduction due to increased tissue temperature or the nonthermal effects of ultrasound, or the result of modulation of inflammation due to the nonthermal effects of ultrasound.

Studies have shown that ultrasound can be more effective in controlling pain than placebo ultrasound or treatment with other thermal agents, and that the addition of ultrasound to an exercise program can further improve pain relief.[30-32] Continuous ultrasound at 0.5 to 2.0 W/cm² intensity and 1.5 MHz frequency has also been reported to be more effective than superficial heating with paraffin or infrared or deep heating with shortwave diathermy for relieving the pain from soft tissue injuries when applied within 48

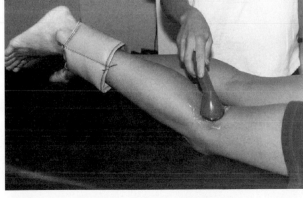

Figure 7-19. Ultrasound being applied to the posterior knee in conjunction with an extension stretching force.

hours of injury.[30] Persons treated with ultrasound had less pain, tenderness on pressure, erythema, restricted ROM, and swelling than those treated with the other thermal agents. Also, more subjects in the ultrasound-treated group were symptom free 2 weeks after injury than subjects who received the other treatments. Given the wide range of possible diagnoses treated in this study and the wide range of ultrasound doses used, the mechanism of the observed effects is uncertain. Ultrasound may have improved circulation or accelerated the processes of inflammation and healing of the involved tissues.

Continuous ultrasound applied 3 times a week for 4 weeks at 1.0 to 2.0 W/cm² for 10 minutes to the low backs of patients with recent onset of pain due to prolapsed discs and nerve root compression between L4 and S2 has also been shown to result in significantly faster relief of pain and return of ROM than placebo ultrasound or no treatment.[22] The authors discuss the concern that ultrasound at the intensity used may aggravate an acute disc rupture and state that this did not occur because so little ultrasound was able to reach the disc through the overlying bone.

Continuous ultrasound applied at 1.5 W/cm² for 3 to 5 minutes for 10 treatments over a 3-week period followed by exercise has been found to be more effective than exercise alone in relieving pain and increasing ROM in patients with shoulder pain.[22] Also, at the 3-month follow-up, significantly more patients who received ultrasound treatment reported no pain than those who received exercise alone. The short duration of ultrasound used in this study may have produced a slight increase in tissue temperature, which may have resulted in increased patient comfort or increased soft tissue extensibility, allowing greater gains in ROM with exercise and better resolution of the underlying pathology.

The studies cited above indicate that continuous ultrasound may be effective for reducing pain. The treatment parameters found to be effective for this application are 1 or 3 MHz frequency, depending on the tissue depth, and 0.5 to 3.0 W/cm² intensity, for 3 to 10 minutes.

Dermal Ulcers

Some studies have shown that ultrasound accelerates the healing of vascular and pressure ulcers; however, others have failed to demonstrate any beneficial effects with this application, and recent systematic reviews of the randomized controlled trials on the treatment of venous ulcers and pressure ulcers with therapeutic ultrasound concluded that there is no good evidence of a benefit of ultrasound therapy in these types of dermal ulcers.[33,34]

Dyson and Suckling found that the addition of ultrasound treatment to conventional wound care procedures resulted in significantly greater reduction in the area of lower extremity varicose ulcers.[35] Ultrasound was applied pulsed at 20% duty cycle, at 1.0 W/cm^2 intensity, 3 MHz frequency, for 5 to 10 minutes to the intact skin around the border of 13 lower extremity varicose ulcers 3 times a week for 4 weeks. Sham ultrasound was applied, in a double-blind manner, to 12 other ulcers to serve as a control. At 28 days the treated ulcers were approximately 30% reduced in size, whereas the sham-treated ulcers were not significantly smaller than their initial size. Using a similar procedure, McDiarmid and colleagues found that infected pressure ulcers healed significantly more quickly with the application of ultrasound than with sham treatment, whereas clean sores did not.[36] The ultrasound was applied pulsed at a 20% duty cycle, 0.8 W/cm^2 intensity, 3 MHz frequency, for 5 to 10 minutes 3 times a week.

In contrast, three more recent studies have failed to demonstrate improved healing of venous ulcers with ultrasound.[37-39] One MHz ultrasound was used in the first two of these studies, and it is possible that this lower frequency may have altered the efficacy of the treatment. In the third study, 3 MHz pulsed ultrasound was used; however, 0.1% chlorhexidine, a cytotoxic agent, was used to cleanse some of the wounds. The addition of this cleanser to the treatment may have obscured the benefits of the ultrasound.

The studies cited above indicate that pulsed ultrasound may be effective in facilitating wound healing. The treatment parameters found to be effective for this application are 20% duty cycle, 0.8 to 1.0 W/cm^2 intensity, 3 MHz frequency for 5 to 10 minutes. Ultrasound can be applied to a dermal ulcer either by applying transmission gel to the intact skin around the wound perimeter and treating only over this area (Fig. 7-20), or the wound can be treated directly by covering it with an ultrasound coupling sheet (Fig. 7-21) or by placing it and the ultrasound transducer in water (Fig. 7-22).

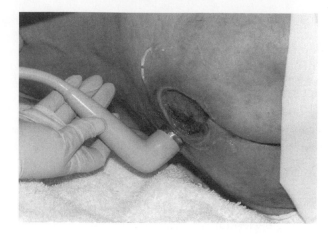

Figure 7-20. Ultrasound treatment of a wound: peri-wound application technique.

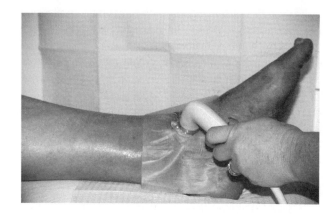

Figure 7-21. Ultrasound being used to treat a venous stasis ulcer. (Courtesy Jim Staicer, Beverly Manor Convalescent Hospital, Fresno, CA.)

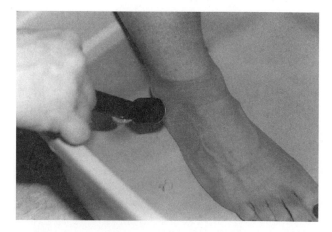

Figure 7-22. Ultrasound treatment of a wound: underwater application technique.

Surgical Skin Incisions

The effect of ultrasound on the healing of surgical skin incisions has been studied in both animal and human subjects. Ultrasound applied at 0.5 W/cm^2, pulsed 20%, for 5 minutes daily to full-thickness skin lesions in adult rats has been shown to accelerate the evolution of angiogenesis, a vital component of early wound healing.[40] Angiogenesis is the development of new blood vessels at an injury site that serves to reestablish circulation and thus limit ischemic necrosis and facilitate repair. It is proposed that ultrasound may accelerate the development of angiogenesis by altering cell membrane permeability, particularly to calcium ions, and by stimulating angiogenic factor synthesis and release by macrophages.[32]

Byl and associates reported that low-dose and high-dose ultrasound can increase the breaking strength of incisional wounds in pigs when applied for 1 week and that low-dose ultrasound increases wound breaking strength only in the second week.[41,42] The low dose was 0.5 W/cm^2, pulsed 20%, 1 MHz and the high dose was 1.5 W/cm^2, continuous, 1 MHz. Both were applied for 5 minutes daily, starting 1 day after the incision.

Ultrasound has also been reported to be beneficial in the treatment of gynecological surgical wounds and episiotomies in humans.[43,44] Ultrasound applied on the first and second postoperative days at 0.5 W/cm^2, 20% duty cycle, 1 MHz for 3 minutes has been reported to reduce pain and accelerate hematoma resolution after these procedures. Treatment with ultrasound has also been found to relieve the pain from episiotomy scars when applied months or years after the procedure. Fieldhouse reported successful treatment of painful, thickened scars with ultrasound at 0.5 to 0.8 W/cm^2, for 5 minutes, 3 times a week for 6 to 16 weeks, at 15 months to 4 years after episiotomy.[44] Earlier intervention was recommended for earlier relief of symptoms.

The preceding studies indicate that ultrasound can accelerate the healing of surgical incisions, relieve the pain associated with these procedures, and facilitate development of stronger repair tissue. The treatment parameters found to be most effective were 0.5 to 0.8 W/cm^2 intensity, pulsed 20% for 3 to 5 minutes, 3 to 5 times a week.

Tendon Injuries

Ultrasound has been reported to assist in the healing of tendons after surgical incision and repair. Although some studies with both animal and human subjects have reported treatment success, others have failed to support these findings.

Binder and colleagues reported significantly enhanced recovery in patients with lateral epicondylitis treated with ultrasound compared with those treated with sham ultrasound.[45] The ultrasound was applied pulsed with a 20% duty cycle, 1.0 to 2.0 W/cm^2 intensity, 1 MHz frequency, for 5 to 10 minutes for 12 treatments over a 4- to 6-week period. In addition, Ebenbichler and co-workers reported greater resolution of calcium deposits, greater decreases in pain, and greater improvements in the quality of life in patients with calcific tendinitis of the shoulder treated with ultrasound compared with those treated with sham ultrasound.[46] For this study, ultrasound was applied for 24 15-minute sessions with a frequency of 0.89 MHz and an intensity, 2.5 W/cm^2 pulsed mode 1:4 (sic.). In contrast to the positive findings of these studies, Lundeberg and colleagues reported no significant difference in the healing of lateral epicondylitis between ultrasound-treated groups and sham ultrasound-treated groups using either continuous or pulsed ultrasound.[47,48] Downing and Weinstein also failed to demonstrate any benefit of continuous ultrasound at 10% lower intensity than patient discomfort in the treatment of subacromial symptoms.[49]

The differences in outcome between the above studies may be due to the use of different treatment parameters and the application of treatment at different stages of healing. Because applying ultrasound with parameters that would increase tissue temperature may aggravate acute inflammation, and because, conversely, pulsed ultrasound may be ineffective in the chronic, late stage of recovery if the tissue requires heating to promote more effective stretching or increased circulation, applying ultrasound with the same parameters to all patients may obscure any treatment effect.

It is recommended that ultrasound be applied in a pulsed mode at a low intensity during the acute phase of tendon inflammation in order to minimize the risk of aggravating the condition and to accelerate recovery, and that continuous ultrasound at a high enough intensity to increase tissue temperature be applied in combination with stretching to assist in the resolution of chronic tendinitis if the problem is accompanied by soft tissue shortening due to scarring.

Studies on the effect of ultrasound on the healing of tendons after surgical incision and repair have yielded more consistently positive results, although one study has reported tendon weakening after 6 weeks of ultrasound treatment. Ultrasound at 0.5 or 1.0 W/cm^2, continuous, 1 MHz applied daily for the first 9 postoperative days has been shown to enhance the breaking strength of cut and sutured Achilles tendons in rabbits.[50,51] The strength of the ultrasound-treated tendons was greater than that of sham-treated controls, and the strength of those treated with 0.5 W/cm^2 intensity ultrasound was greater than that of those treated at 1.0 W/cm^2. Similar benefits have been reported from the application of 1.5 W/cm^2, continuous, 1 MHz ultrasound for 3 to 4 minutes starting 1 day postoperatively to repaired Achilles tendons in rats.[52,53] Treatment was applied daily for the first 8 days and every other day thereafter for up to 3 weeks.

In contrast to the above findings, Roberts and colleagues reported reduced strength and healing in surgically repaired flexor profundus tendons in 7 rabbits after treatment with pulsed ultrasound at 0.8 W/cm^2, 1 MHz, for 5 minutes daily for 6 weeks.[54] The results of this study have been called into question because the strength of the tendons in both the treated and untreated groups was more than 10 times lower than has been reported in other studies for normal flexor tendon healing in rabbits.[55] Although immobilization was attempted throughout the post-injury period, technical difficulties in maintaining cast fixation, and thus apposition of the tendon ends, may have resulted in gap formation and thus poor strength in all subjects. The small sample size and poor reporting of the data also call into question the validity of this study. Adverse effects of ultrasound on tendon healing have not been reported in other research.

Overall, research supports the early use of ultrasound for facilitation of tendon healing after rupture and repair. The ultrasound doses found to be effective for this application are 0.5 to 1.5 W/cm^2 intensity, continuous, 1 or 3 MHz frequency for 3 to 5 minutes. Although high-intensity ultrasound has been found to promote tendon healing, the lower end of the range is recommended in order to minimize the risk of any potentially adverse effect from heating acutely inflamed tissue postoperatively.

Resorption of Calcium Deposits

Ultrasound may facilitate the resorption of calcium deposits. Two published case studies and a randomized control trial have reported functional recovery, pain resolution, and elimination of a calcific deposit in the shoulder following application of ultrasound; however, the mechanisms of this effect are unknown.[46,56,57] Although the mechanism underlying calcific deposits resorption is not known, the decrease in pain and improvements in function may be due to the reduction in inflammation produced by ultrasound.

Bone Fractures

Although prior reports have recommended that ultrasound not be applied over unhealed fractures, because they have failed to provide data to support this recommendation and because recent studies have demonstrated that low-dose ultrasound can reduce the fracture healing time in animals and humans, the use of low-dose ultrasound to accelerate fracture healing is now recommended.[58,59] The stimulation of bone growth by physical means has been investigated for many years. At the beginning of the 18th century, it was observed that small direct currents acting at the periosteum induced bone formation, and in 1957 Fukada and Yasuda proposed that the piezoelectricity of bone was the mechanism behind this observed phenomenon.[60] In 1983 Duarte proposed that ultrasound may be a safe, noninvasive, and effective means to stimulate bone growth, also theoretically linked to the piezoelectric property of bone.[61] He applied very low-intensity ultrasound, delivered pulsed with a 0.05% duty cycle at approximately 10 W/cm^2 SATP intensity, at either 4.93 or 1.65 MHz frequency to 23 rabbit fibulae that were osteomized and 22 femurs with drilled holes. Treatment was applied for 15 minutes per day, starting 1 day postoperatively, for 4 to 18 days. All animals received bilateral osteotomies and were treated with ultrasound unilaterally so that the contralateral extremity could serve as a control. The treated bones were found to develop callus and trabeculae more rapidly than the untreated bones (Fig. 7-23).

A similar study with a larger sample size (139) has also reported acceleration of bone healing with ultrasound.[62] The ultrasound was delivered pulsed with a 20% duty cycle, 0.15 W/cm^2 SATP intensity, 1.5 MHz frequency. Treatment was applied for 20 minutes daily, starting 1 day postoperatively, for 14 to 28 days. Biomechanical healing was accelerated by a factor of 1.7, with treated fractures being as strong as intact bone in 17 days compared with 28 days for the control fractures.

Two double-blind, placebo-controlled studies have also demonstrated acceleration of fracture healing in

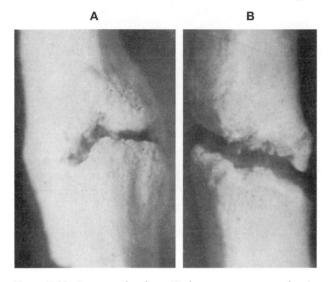

A   **B**

Figure 7-23. Fracture healing 17 days postoperatively, **A,** with and, **B,** without ultrasound application. (Used with permission. From Duarte LR: The stimulation of bone growth by ultrasound. *Arch Orthop Trauma Surg* 101:153-159, 1983.)

human subjects with the application of ultrasound. Both used the ultrasound signal and treatment durations described directly above. One study reported accelerated healing of Colles' and tibial diaphyseal fractures by a factor of 1.5 (as demonstrated by radiography),[63] and the other reported acceleration of tibial fracture healing by a factor of 1.3 for clinical healing and a factor of 1.6 for overall clinical and radiographic healing.[64]

A device specifically designed for the application of ultrasound for fracture healing was approved by the FDA in 1994 for home use. It has unadjustable, preset treatment parameters of 20% duty cycle pulsed, 0.15 W/cm^2 SATP intensity, 1.5 MHz frequency and a treatment duration of 20 minutes (Fig. 7-24). This device is available by prescription only.

Current research supports the use of very low-dose ultrasound for facilitation of fracture healing. The parameters found to be effective are 0.15 W/cm^2 intensity, 20% duty cycle, 1.5 MHz frequency for 15 to 20 minutes daily.

Carpal Tunnel Syndrome

Continuous ultrasound has generally not been recommended for the treatment of carpal tunnel syndrome because of the risk of adversely impacting nerve conduction velocity by overheating.[65,66] However, a recent study found that pulsed ultrasound produced

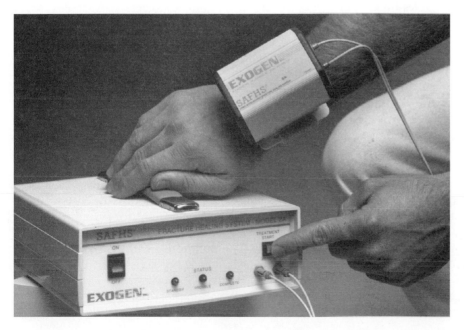

Figure 7-24. Ultrasound device for home use for fracture healing. (Courtesy Exogen, Piscataway, NJ.)

significantly greater improvement in subjective complaints (*p* <0.001, paired *t* test), hand grip and finger pinch strength, and electroneurographic variables (motor distal latency *p* <0.001, paired *t* test; sensory antidromic nerve conduction velocity *p* <0.001, paired *t* test) than sham ultrasound treatment.[67] These benefits were sustained at 6 months' follow up. The ultrasound was applied for 20 sessions at 1 MHz frequency, 1.0 W /cm², pulsed mode 1:4, for 15 minutes per session. The proposed mechanisms for these benefits are the anti-inflammatory and tissue stimulating effects of ultrasound.

Phonophoresis

Phonophoresis is the application of ultrasound in conjunction with a topical drug preparation as the ultrasound conduction medium. The ultrasound is intended to enhance delivery of the drug through the skin, thereby delivering the drug for local or systemic effects. Transcutaneous drug delivery has a number of advantages over oral drug administration. It provides a higher initial drug concentration at the delivery site,[68] avoids gastric irritation, and avoids first-pass metabolism by the liver. Transcutaneous delivery also avoids the pain, trauma, and infection risk associated with injection and allows delivery to a larger area than is readily achieved by injection.

The first report of the use of ultrasound to enhance drug delivery across the skin was published in 1954.[69] This was followed by a series of studies by Griffin and colleagues evaluating the location and depth of hydrocortisone delivery and the effects of varying ultrasound parameters on hydrocortisone phonophoresis.[70-73] The authors of these initial studies proposed that ultrasound enhanced drug delivery by exerting pressure on the drug to drive it through the skin. However, because ultrasound exerts only a few grams of force, it is now thought that ultrasound increases transdermal drug penetration by increasing the permeability of the stratum corneum through cavitation.[74] This theory is supported by the observation that ultrasound can enhance drug penetration even when the ultrasound is applied before the drug is put on the skin.[75]

The stratum corneum is the superficial cornified layer of the skin that acts as a protective barrier, preventing foreign materials from entering the body through the skin (Fig. 7-25). Ultrasound may change stratum corneum permeability by both thermal and

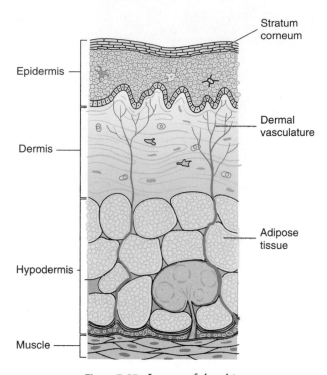

Figure 7-25. Layers of the skin.

nonthermal mechanisms. It has been proposed that ultrasound alters the skin porous pathways by enlarging the skin effective pore radii and by creating more pores or making the pores less tortuous.[76] Drug diffusion across the stratum corneum depends on both diffusion and partition coefficients. A recent study demonstrated ultrasound enhancement of diffusion coefficients of a variety of solutes by up to 15-fold. Ultrasound, however, did not significantly enhance partition coefficients.[77]

When the permeability of the stratum corneum is increased, a drug will diffuse across it due to the difference in concentration on either side of the skin. Once a drug diffuses across the stratum corneum, it is initially more concentrated at the delivery site and is then distributed throughout the body by the vascular circulation; therefore, therapists should be aware that drugs delivered by phonophoresis do become systemic and the contraindications for systemic delivery of these drugs also apply to this mode of delivery. Because six phonophoresis treatments with the corticosteroid dexamethasone have been shown not to cause an increase in urinary free cortisol, which is a measure of adrenal suppression, a course of six treatments is considered safe for patients who do not have other contraindications for corticosteroid treatment.[78] It is recommended that a drug not be delivered by phonophoresis if the patient is already receiving a drug of the same type by another route of administration since this increases the risk of adverse effects. For example, if a patient with rheumatoid arthritis or asthma is taking corticosteroids by mouth, hydrocortisone or dexamethasone should not be given by phonophoresis.

Phonophoresis has been studied for its efficacy in local and systemic drug delivery. In rehabilitation, phonophoresis is studied and used primarily for local delivery of corticosteroid and nonsteroidal anti-inflammatory drugs for treatment of tissue inflammation, such as tendinitis or bursitis; however, there is also a medical interest in transcutaneous systemic delivery of substances such as insulin that cannot be delivered effectively by mouth.

A brief review of the research on phonophoresis follows. For a more complete review of the principles and research of phonophoresis, please consult the recently published literature review by Byl.[79] Griffin and colleagues found that, with the application of hydrocortisone phonophoresis to pigs, more hydrocortisone was deposited in nerve than in muscle.[70] They also reported that the highest ultrasound frequency they used, 3.6 MHz, was most effective and that a low intensity (0.1 W/cm^2) for a long duration (51 minutes) or a high intensity (3.0 W/cm^2) for a short duration (5 minutes) resulted in the most hydrocortisone delivery.[71-73]

In comparing the efficacy of different drug concentrations used for phonophoresis, Kleinkort and Wood found that 10% hydrocortisone was more effective than 1% hydrocortisone in relieving pain associated with tendinitis or bursitis.[80] However, a comparison of the ability of different media customarily used for phonophoresis to transmit ultrasound found that the hydrocortisone preparations most commonly used for this application do not transmit ultrasound effectively.[81] This calls into question the mechanism of hydrocortisone phonophoresis since, when a poorly transmitting medium is used, very little ultrasound is able to reach the tissue. The energy is absorbed by the medium or reflected back to the transducer, causing heating of the transducer. It has been proposed that the enhanced hydrocortisone penetration reported by Griffin and colleagues may have been caused by heating of the skin by conduction from the warm sound head rather than being a direct effect of the ultrasound.[81]

More recent studies, using media that transmit ultrasound effectively, have demonstrated enhanced transdermal penetration of drugs other than hydrocortisone using phonophoresis. For example, ultrasound has been shown to increase transdermal penetration of mannitol and inulin in rats and guinea pigs, increasing the output of radiolabeled mannitol and inulin in the urine of the ultrasound-treated animals by 5- to 20-fold for 1 to 2 hours after treatment compared with controls.[82] Urinary output was used as a measure of the systemic uptake of these drugs.

An in vitro comparison of the penetration of ibuprofen through human skin with ultrasound or with equal heating using a conductive heater has demonstrated that the enhancement of transdermal drug penetration by ultrasound was not only the result of the thermal effects of ultrasound.[83] Drug penetration was increased with the application of both conductive heating and ultrasound; however, the increase produced by ultrasound was significantly greater than that produced by conductive heating alone.

The research at this time supports the use of ultrasound for facilitation of transdermal drug penetration. The treatment parameters most likely to be effective are 3 MHz frequency, to optimize ultrasound absorption by the skin; pulsed 20% duty cycle, to avoid heating of any inflammatory condition; at 0.5 to 0.75 W/cm^2 intensity, for 5 to 10 minutes. The drug preparation used should also transmit ultrasound effectively.

Plantar Warts and Herpes Zoster

Plantar warts and herpes zoster are both viral cutaneous lesions. Studies have shown that ultrasound may facilitate healing of these lesions; however, this application of ultrasound is not widely used by rehabilitation professionals in the United States at this time.

Plantar warts are skin lesions containing thrombosed capillaries in a soft, whitish core covered by hyperkeratotic epithelial tissue. They usually occur on the plantar surface of the feet of children or young adults. They resemble plantar corns or calluses and are tender on pressure. Like other warts, they are probably viral in origin. Plantar warts are prone to spreading and recurrence but also frequently resolve spontaneously without treatment. A wide range of treatments, including surgical excision and cryosurgery, can effectively eradicate plantar warts; however, most treatments are painful and result in scar formation. Ultrasound has been proposed as a painless, relatively safe method of treatment of these lesions and has been used for this application for the past 30 years; however, studies regarding this use of ultrasound have had varying results. Although all studies report success rates exceeding 50%, the only published double-blind, controlled study showed little clinically significant difference in the healing time between ultrasound and sham-treated groups.[84,85] The studies reporting treatment success with ultrasound used the treatment parameters of 0.6 to 0.8 W/cm^2 intensity, continuous application, for 7 to 15 minutes with 2 to 15 treatments.

Ultrasound has been reported to be effective in the treatment of pain resulting from acute herpes zoster.[86,87] The treatment parameters used were 1 MHz frequency, 25% pulsed duty cycle, applied for 1 minute per ERA of the transducer at 0.8 W/cm^2 intensity adjacent to the vertebral column and at 0.5 W/cm^2 intensity around the periphery of the vesicles. More than 80% of the patients treated with ultrasound in this manner were pain free at the conclusion of treatment and on long-term follow-up compared with 46% of the placebo-treated patients. The authors propose that ultrasound may have had a viricidal effect in these patients.

CONTRAINDICATIONS AND PRECAUTIONS FOR ULTRASOUND

Although ultrasound is a relatively safe treatment modality, it must be applied with care to avoid harming the patient. Ultrasound may not be used by patients to treat themselves. It must be used by, or under the supervision of, a licensed practitioner.

Even when ultrasound is not contraindicated, if the patient's condition is worsening or not improving within 2 to 3 treatments, reevaluate the treatment approach and consider changing the treatment or referring the patient to a physician for reevaluation.

CONTRAINDICATIONS
for the Use of Ultrasound

- Malignant tumor
- Pregnancy
- Central nervous system tissue
- Joint cement
- Plastic components
- Pacemaker
- Thrombophlebitis
- Eyes
- Reproductive organs

The use of ultrasound is contraindicated . . .

. . . over a limb or body part with a malignant tumor

Although there are no research data concerning the effects of applying therapeutic ultrasound to malignant tumors in humans, the application of continuous ultrasound at 1.0 W/cm^2, 1 MHz, for 5 minutes for 10 treatments over a period of 2 weeks to mice with malignant subcutaneous tumors has been shown to produce significantly larger and heavier tumors compared to those of untreated controls.[88] The treated mice also developed more lymph node metastases. Because this study indicates that therapeutic ultrasound may increase the rate of tumor growth or metastasis, it is recommended that therapeutic ultrasound not be applied to malignant tumors in humans. Caution should also be used when treating a patient who has a history of a malignant tumor or tumors, since it can be difficult to ascertain whether any small tumors remain. It is therefore recommended that the therapist consult with the referring physician before applying ultrasound to a patient with a history of malignancy within the last 5 years.

One should note that ultrasound is used as a component of the treatment of certain types of malignant tumors; however, the devices used for this application allow a number of ultrasound beams to be directed at the tumor in order to achieve a temperature within the range of 42° to 43°C.[89-91] Some malignant tumors decrease in size or are eradicated when heated to within this narrow range, while healthy tissue is left undamaged. Because the therapeutic ultrasound devices generally available to physical therapists do not allow such precise determination and control of tissue temperature, and because primary treatment of malignancy is outside the scope of practice of rehabilitation professionals, therapeutic ultrasound devices intended for rehabilitation applications should not be used for treatment of malignancy.

ASK THE PATIENT:

- Have you ever had cancer? Do you have cancer now?
- Do you have fevers, chills, sweats, or night pain?
- Do you have pain at rest?
- Have you had recent unexplained weight loss?

If the patient has cancer at this time, ultrasound should not be used. If the patient has a history of cancer or signs of cancer such as fevers, chills, sweats, night pain, pain at rest, or recent unexplained weight loss, the therapist should consult with the referring physician in order to rule out the presence of malignancy before applying ultrasound.

. . . over the abdomen, low back, or pelvis of a patient who is, or may be, pregnant

Maternal hyperthermia has been associated with fetal abnormalities, including growth retardation, microphthalmia, exencephaly, microencephaly, neural tube defects, and myelodysplasia.[92,93] There is also a published report documenting a case of sacral agenesis, microcephaly, and developmental delay in a child whose mother was treated 18 times with low-intensity pulsed ultrasound for a left psoas bursitis between days 6 and 29 of gestation.[94] It is therefore recommended that therapeutic ultrasound not be applied at any level in areas where it may reach a developing fetus.

The diagnostic ultrasound frequently used during pregnancy to assess the position and development of the fetus and placenta has been shown to be safe and without adverse consequences for the fetus or the mother.[95,96]

ASK THE PATIENT:

- Are you pregnant, might you be pregnant, or are you trying to become pregnant?

The patient may not know if she is pregnant, particularly in the first few days or weeks after conception; however, since damage may occur during early development, ultrasound should not be applied in any area where the beam may reach the fetus of a patient who is or might be pregnant.

. . . over central nervous system tissue

There is concern that ultrasound may damage CNS tissue. However, because CNS tissue is usually covered by bone, both in the spinal cord and in the brain, this is rarely a problem. The spinal cord may be exposed if the patient has had a laminectomy above the L2 level. In such cases, ultrasound should not be applied over or near the area of the laminectomy.

. . . over methylmethacrylate cement or plastic

Methylmethacrylate cement and plastic are materials used for fixation or as components of prosthetic joints. Because these materials are rapidly heated by ultrasound,[97] it is generally recommended that ultrasound not be applied over a cemented prosthesis or in areas where plastic components are used. Although very little ultrasound is able to reach to the depth of most prosthetic joints, it is still recommended that the clinician err on the side of caution and not use this modality in areas where plastic or cement may be present. Ultrasound may be used over areas with metal implants such as screws, plates, or all-metal joint replacements since metal is not rapidly heated by ultrasound, and ultrasound has been shown not to loosen screws or plates.[98]

ASK THE PATIENT:

- Do you have a joint replacement in this area?
- Was cement used to hold it in place?
- Does it have plastic components?

If the patient has a joint replacement, ultrasound should not be applied in the area of the prosthesis until the therapist has determined that neither cement nor plastic was used.

. . . over a pacemaker

Because ultrasound may heat a pacemaker or interfere with its electrical circuitry, ultrasound should not be applied in the area of a pacemaker. Ultrasound may be applied to other areas in patients with pacemakers.

Continued

CONTRAINDICATIONS—cont'd

ASK THE PATIENT:
• Do you have a pacemaker?

. . . over an area of thrombophlebitis

Because ultrasound may dislodge or cause partial disintegration of a thrombus, which could then result in obstruction of the circulation to vital organs, ultrasound should not be applied over or near an area where a thrombus is or may be present.

ASK THE PATIENT:
• Do you have a blood clot in this area?

. . . over the eyes

It is recommended that ultrasound not be applied over the eyes because cavitation in the ocular fluid may damage the eyes.

. . . over the male or female reproductive organs

Because ultrasound at the levels used for rehabilitation may affect gamete development, it is recommended that it not be applied in the areas of the male or female reproductive organs.

PRECAUTIONS
for the Application of Ultrasound

• Acute inflammation
• Epiphyseal plates

• Fractures
• Breast implants

Ultrasound at sufficient intensity to produce heat should be used with caution . . .

. . . in areas of acute inflammation

Because heat can exacerbate acute inflammation, causing increased bleeding, pain, and swelling, impairing healing and delaying functional recovery, ultrasound at sufficient intensity to produce heat should be applied with caution in areas of acute inflammation.

. . . over growing epiphyseal plates

The literature regarding the application of ultrasound over epiphyseal plates is controversial. Although one study reported that ultrasound applied at greater than 3.0 W/cm^2 may damage epiphyseal plates,[99] Lehmann states that it is safe to apply ultrasound over epiphyseal plates as long as there is no pain.[8] Also, a recent study reported no change in bone growth in skeletally immature rats with ultrasound applied at the low levels used for fracture healing.[100] At this time, it is recommended that high-dose ultrasound not be applied over growing epiphyseal plates.

Because the age of epiphyseal closure varies, radiographic evaluation rather than age should be used to determine if epiphyseal closure is complete.

. . . over a fracture

Although low-dose ultrasound has been shown to accelerate fracture healing, the application of high-intensity ultrasound over a fracture generally causes pain. There is also concern that high-level ultrasound may impair fracture healing. Therefore only low-dose ultrasound, as described in the section above on fracture healing, should be applied over the area of a fracture.

. . . over breast implants

Because heat may increase the pressure inside a breast implant and cause it to rupture, high-dose ultrasound should not be applied over breast implants.

ADVERSE EFFECTS OF ULTRASOUND

In general, ultrasound has rarely been reported to produce adverse effects.[101] However, a variety of adverse effects can occur if ultrasound is applied incorrectly or when contraindicated. The most common adverse effect is a burn, which may occur when high-intensity, continuous ultrasound is applied, particularly if a stationary application technique is used. The risk of burns is further increased in areas with impaired circulation or sensation and with superficial bone. To minimize the risk of burning a patient, always move the ultrasound head and do not apply thermal-level ultrasound to areas with impaired circulation or sensation. Reduce the ultrasound intensity in areas with superficial bone or if the patient complains of any increase in discomfort with the application of ultrasound.

Ultrasound standing waves can cause blood cell stasis due to collections of gas bubbles and plasma at antinodes and collection of cells at nodes[102,103] (Fig. 7-26). This is accompanied by damage to the endothelial lining of the blood vessels. These effects have been demonstrated with ultrasound of 1 to 5 MHz frequency with intensity as low as 0.5 W/cm^2 and with as short an exposure as 0.1 second. Although the stasis is reversed when ultrasound application stops,

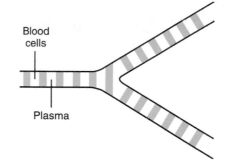

Figure 7-26. Banding of blood cells and plasma due to standing waves.

the endothelial damage remains. Therefore in order to prevent the adverse effects of standing waves, it is recommended that the ultrasound transducer be moved throughout treatment application.

APPLICATION TECHNIQUE

This section provides guidelines for the sequence of procedures required for the safe and effective application of therapeutic ultrasound.

APPLICATION TECHNIQUE
Ultrasound

1. Evaluate the patient's clinical findings and set the goals of treatment.
2. Determine if ultrasound is the most appropriate treatment.
3. Determine that ultrasound is not contraindicated for the patient or the condition. Check with the patient and check the patient's chart for contraindications or precautions regarding the application of ultrasound.
4. Apply an ultrasound transmission medium to the area to be treated.
   Apply enough medium to eliminate any air between the sound head and the treatment area. Select a medium that transmits ultrasound well, does not stain, is not allergenic, is not rapidly absorbed by the skin, and is inexpensive. Gels or lotions meeting these criteria have been specifically formulated for use with ultrasound.
   OR

For the application of ultrasound under water, place the area to be treated in a container of water (see Fig. 7-22).

5. Select a sound head with an ERA approximately half the size of the treatment area.
6. Select the optimal treatment parameters including ultrasound frequency, intensity, duty cycle, and duration; the appropriate size of the treatment area; and the appropriate number and frequency of treatments. Specific recommendations for different clinical applications are given above in the sections concerning the specific clinical conditions. General guidelines for treatment parameters follow.

FREQUENCY

Select the frequency according to the depth of tissue to be treated. Use 1 MHz for tissue up to 5 cm deep and 3 MHz for tissue 1 to 2 cm deep. The depth of

Continued

APPLICATION TECHNIQUE—cont'd
Ultrasound

penetration is lower in tissues with a high collagen content and in areas of increased reflection.

DUTY CYCLE

Select the duty cycle according to the treatment goal. When the goal is to increase tissue temperature, a 100% (continuous) duty cycle should be used.[3] When applying ultrasound where only the nonthermal effects without tissue heating are desired, pulsed ultrasound with a 20% or lower duty cycle should be used. Although the nonthermal effects of ultrasound are produced by continuous ultrasound, it is thought that they are not optimized with application at this level.[14] Almost all published studies on the effects of pulsed ultrasound have used a duty cycle of 20%.

INTENSITY

Select intensity according to the treatment goal. When the goal is to increase tissue temperature, the patient should feel some warmth within 2 to 3 minutes of initiating ultrasound application and should not feel increased discomfort at any time during the treatment. When using 1 MHz frequency ultrasound, an intensity of 1.5 to 2.0 W/cm^2 will generally produce this effect. When using 3 MHz frequency, an intensity of about 0.5 W/cm^2 is generally sufficient. A lower intensity is effective at the higher frequency because the energy is absorbed in a smaller, more superficial volume of tissue, resulting in a greater temperature increase with the same ultrasound intensity. Adjust the intensity up or down from these levels according to the patient's report. Increase the intensity if there is no sensation of warmth within 2 to 3 minutes and decrease the intensity immediately if there is any complaint of discomfort. If there is superficial bone in the treatment area, a slightly lower intensity will be sufficient to produce comfortable heating because the ultrasound reflected by the bone will cause a greater increase in temperature.

When applying ultrasound for nonthermal effects, successful treatment outcomes have been documented for most applications using an intensity of 0.5 to 1.0 W/cm^2 SATP (0.1 to 0.2 W/cm^2 SATA), with as low as 0.15 W/cm^2 SATP (0.03 W/cm^2 SATA) being sufficient for facilitation of bone healing.

DURATION

Select the treatment duration according to the treatment goal, the size of the area to be treated, and the ERA of the sound head. For most thermal or nonthermal applications, ultrasound should be applied for 5 to 10 minutes for each treatment area that is twice the ERA of the transducer. For example, when treating an area 20 cm^2 with a sound head that has an ERA of 10 cm^2, the treatment duration should be 5 to 10 minutes. When treating an area of 40 cm^2 with the same 10 cm^2, the treatment duration should be extended to between 10 and 20 minutes.

When the goal of treatment is to increase tissue temperature, the treatment duration should also be adjusted according to the frequency and intensity of the ultrasound. For example, if the goal is to increase tissue temperature by 3°C, and thus reach the minimal therapeutic level of 40°C, if 1 MHz ultrasound at an intensity of 1.5 W/cm^2 is applied to an area twice the ERA of the transducer, the treatment duration must be at least 9 minutes, whereas if the intensity is increased to 2 W/cm^2, the treatment duration need be only 8 minutes.[8] If 3 MHz ultrasound is used at an intensity of 0.5 W/cm^2, the treatment duration must be at least 10 minutes to achieve the same temperature level.

In general, treatment duration should be increased when lower intensities or lower frequencies of ultrasound are used, when treating areas larger than twice the ERA of the transducer, or when higher tissue temperatures are desired. Treatment duration should be decreased when higher intensities or frequencies of ultrasound are used, when treating areas smaller than twice the ERA of the transducer, or when lower tissue temperatures are desired.

When ultrasound is used to facilitate bone healing, longer treatment times of 15 to 20 minutes are recommended.

AREA TO BE TREATED

The size of area that can be treated with ultrasound depends on the ERA of the transducer and the duration of treatment. As explained in the previous discussion of duration of treatment, a treatment area equal to twice the ERA of the sound head can be treated in 5 to 10 minutes. Smaller areas can be treated in proportionately shorter times; however, it is impractical to treat areas less than $1^1/_2$ times the ERA of the sound head and still keep the sound head moving within the area. Larger areas can be treated in proportionately longer times; however, ultrasound should not be used to treat areas larger than four times the ERA of the transducer, such as the whole low back, because this requires excessively long treatment durations and, when heating is desired, results in some areas being heated while other previously heated areas are already cooling (Figs. 7-27 and 7-28).

NUMBER AND FREQUENCY OF TREATMENTS

The recommended number of treatments depends on the goals of treatment and the patient's response. If the patient is making progress at an appropriate rate toward the established goals for this treatment, the treatment should be continued. If the patient is not progressing appropriately, the treatment should be modified, either by changing the ultrasound parameters or by selecting a different intervention. In most cases, an effect should be detectable within 1 to 3 treatments. For problems in which progress is commonly slow, such as chronic wounds, or in which progress is hard to detect, such as with fractures, treatment may need to be continued for a longer period. The frequency of treatments depends on the level of ultrasound being used and the stage of healing. Thermal-level ultrasound is usually applied only during the subacute or chronic phase of healing, when treatment 3 times a week is recommended; ultrasound at nonthermal levels may be applied at earlier stages, when treatment may be as frequent as daily. These frequencies of treatment are based on current clinical standards of practice since there are no published studies at this time comparing the efficacy of different treatment frequencies.

SEQUENCE OF TREATMENT

In most cases, ultrasound may be applied before or after other treatment interventions; however, when using ultrasound to heat tissue, it should not be applied after any intervention that may impair sensation, such as ice. Also, when thermal-level ultrasound is used to increase collagen extensibility in order to maximize the increase in length produced with stretching, the ultrasound must be applied directly before, and if possible during, the application of the stretching force. Do not wait or apply another treatment between applying the ultrasound and stretching since the tissue starts to cool as soon as the ultrasound application ends.

7. Prior to treatment of any area with a risk of cross-infection, swab the sound head with 0.5% alcoholic chlorhexidine, or use the antimicrobial approved for this use in the facility.[43]
8. Place the sound head on the treatment area.
9. Turn on the ultrasound machine.
10. Move the sound head within the treatment area. The sound head is moved in order to optimize the uniformity of ultrasound intensity delivered to the tissues and to minimize the risk of standing wave formation.[45]

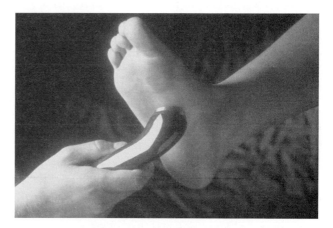

Figure 7-27. Ultrasound application to the foot. (Courtesy Mettler Electronics, Anaheim, CA.)

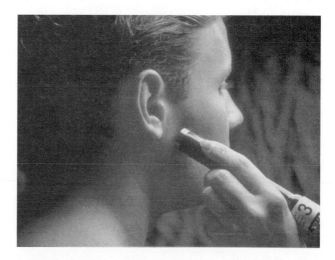

Figure 7-28. Ultrasound application to the temporomandibular joint (TMJ) area. (Courtesy Mettler Electronics, Anaheim, CA.)

Continued

APPLICATION TECHNIQUE—cont'd
Ultrasound

Move the sound head at approximately 4 cm/second, quickly enough to maintain motion and slowly enough to maintain contact with the skin. If the sound head is kept stationary or moved too slowly, the area of tissue under the center of the transducer, where the intensity is greatest, will receive much more ultrasound than the areas under the edges of the transducer. With continuous ultrasound this can result in overheating and burning of the tissues at the center of the field, and with pulsed ultrasound this can reduce the efficacy of the treatment. A stationary sound head should not be used when applying either continuous or pulsed ultrasound. If the sound head is moved too quickly, the therapist may not be able to maintain good contact of the sound head with the skin, and thus the ultrasound will not be able to enter the tissue.

Move the sound head in a manner that causes the center of the head to change position so that all parts of the treatment area receive similar exposure. Strokes overlapping by half the ERA of the sound head are recommended (Fig. 7-29). Keep within the predetermined treatment area of one and a half to four times the ERA only.

Keep the surface of the sound head in constant parallel contact with the skin in order to ensure

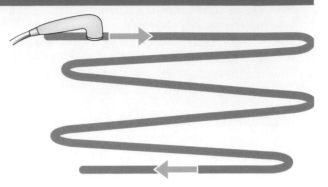

Figure 7-29. Stroking technique for ultrasound application.

that the ultrasound is transmitted to the tissues. Poor contact will impede the transmission of ultrasound because much of it will be absorbed by intervening air or reflected at the air-tissue interface. In order to promote more effective treatment, some clinical ultrasound units are equipped with a transmission sensor that gives a signal when contact is poor.

11. When the treatment is completed, remove the conduction medium from the sound head and the patient and reassess for any changes in status.

12. Document the treatment.

Documentation

Document the area of the body treated, the ultrasound frequency, intensity, and duty cycle, the treatment duration, if the treatment was delivered under water, and the patient's response to the treatment. Documentation is typically written in the SOAP note format. The following examples only summarize the modality component of treatment and are not intended to represent a comprehensive plan of care.

Examples

1. When applying ultrasound (US) to the left lateral knee (L lat knee) over the lateral collateral ligament (LCL), to facilitate tissue healing, document:

S: Pt reports his c/o L lateral knee pain with turning has decreased from frequent to occasional since last week following therapy treatment

O: US L lat. knee, LCL, 0.5 W/cm², pulsed 20%, 3 MHz, 5 min.

A: Pain at L lateral knee with turning to L decreasing in frequency

P: Reassess pain level next treatment, if pain resolved then discontinue US

2. When applying ultrasound to the right inferior anterior shoulder capsule, document:

S: Pt notes slowly improving R shoulder ROM and is now able to use R UE when combing her hair

O: US R inf ant shoulder, 2.0 W/cm², continuous, 1 MHz, 5 min, followed by jt mob inf glide grade IV

A: Shoulder abduction increased from 120° to 130°

P: Continue US as above followed by mobilization and ROM to R shoulder

▶ *Clinical Case Studies* ◀

The following case studies summarize the concepts of applying therapeutic ultrasound as discussed in this chapter. Based on the scenarios presented, an evaluation of the clinical findings and goals of treatment are proposed. These are followed by a discussion of factors to be considered in the selection of ultrasound as the indicated treatment modality and in selection of the ideal treatment parameters to promote progress toward the goals (Fig. 7-30).

Case 1

TR is a 60-year-old male, 3 months post-open reduction and internal fixation of a right hip fracture, with placement of a plate and screws. He has been referred to physical therapy for gait training with the restriction of limiting weight bearing to his tolerance. TR complains of intermittent dull pain in the right anterior groin that is aggravated by standing or walking without an assistive device and by lying prone. His pain is eased when he sits or lies on his side. Since the hip fracture he has walked only up to approximately 50 feet, maintaining partial weight bearing on his right lower extremity by using bilateral crutches and by flexing his right hip and knee throughout the gait cycle. He has not been able to return to work due to his restricted ambulation. Prior to the hip fracture, TR walked

2 miles a day at his job without an assistive device and without pain. The objective exam reveals decreased hip passive ROM into extension and abduction, with tightness of the anteromedial hip capsule and guarding and spasms of the hip adductor and flexor muscles. All other objective measures are within normal limits.

EVALUATION OF THE CLINICAL FINDINGS

This patient presents with the impairments of intermittent dull pain in the right anteromedial hip and shortening of the right anteromedial hip capsule, resulting in the disabilities of limited ambulation and inability to work.

PREFERRED PRACTICE PATTERN

Impaired Joint Mobility, Muscle Performance, and Range of Motion Associated With Bony or Soft Tissue Surgery, (4I)

PLAN OF CARE

Goals of treatment include resolution of pain in the right anteromedial hip, normalization of the length of the anteromedial hip capsule, a return to 2 miles of ambulation per day without an assistive device, and full return to work.

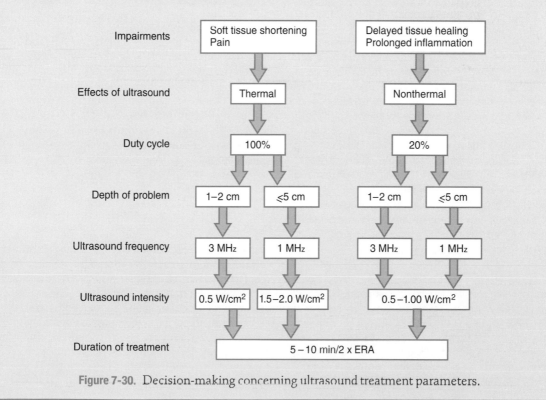

Figure 7-30. Decision-making concerning ultrasound treatment parameters.

Continued

◗ *Clinical Case Studies—cont'd* ◖

ASSESSMENT REGARDING THE APPROPRIATENESS OF THERAPEUTIC ULTRASOUND AS THE OPTIMAL TREATMENT

Therapeutic ultrasound is an indicated treatment for pain and for shortened deep soft tissue with a high collagen content. A superficial heating agent would not be appropriate since the heat will not penetrate to the hip capsule, and diathermy would not be appropriate since the presence of metal contraindicates diathermy application. Therapeutic ultrasound can reach deep tissues and is not contraindicated in the presence of metal plates and screws. The presence of malignancy should be ruled out, and the patient's sensation in the anterior hip should be assessed prior to initiating treatment. Ultrasound should not be used if the hip fracture was associated with a malignancy. Thermal-level ultrasound should not be used if sensation in the treatment area is not intact.

PROPOSED TREATMENT PLAN AND RATIONALE

It is proposed that ultrasound be applied over the area of greatest soft tissue shortening, the right anterior groin. A frequency of 1 MHz in order to reach the depth of the hip joint capsule, a continuous duty cycle in order to increase tissue temperature and thereby increase soft tissue extensibility, and an intensity of 1.5 to 2.0 W/cm^2, adjusting as necessary so that the patient feels a sensation of mild warmth after 2 to 3 minutes of ultrasound application in order to produce an adequate increase in the temperature of the hip capsule are recommended. Since the treatment area will probably be in the range of 20 cm^2, a large sound head with an ERA of 10 cm^2 should be used. Given this relationship of sound head ERA to treatment area, ultrasound should be applied for approximately 10 minutes in order to raise the temperature of the hip capsule to within the therapeutic range of 40° to 45°C. It is essential that the shortened soft tissues be stretched immediately following the ultrasound application and ideally during the ultrasound application as well. Treatment would generally be applied 2 or 3 times per week, consistent with present practice patterns, and should be continued as long as progress is being made toward the treatment goals.

Case 2

BJ is an 18-year-old female college student. She sustained a complete rupture of her left Achilles tendon 6 weeks ago while playing basketball, and the tendon was surgically repaired 2 weeks later. She has been referred for physical therapy in order to attain a pain-free return to sports as rapidly as possible. She complains of mild discomfort at the surgical incision site that increases with walking. Her leg was in a cast, and BJ ambulated without weight bearing on the left, using bilateral axillary crutches, for 4 weeks postoperatively. The cast was removed yesterday and she has been instructed to walk, bearing weight as tolerated, wearing a heeled "boot." She has been instructed to avoid running or jumping for 6 more weeks. The objective exam reveals restricted dorsiflexion ROM of –15°, mild swelling, tenderness, and redness in the area of the surgical repair, and atrophy of the calf muscles on the left. All other objective measures are within normal limits.

EVALUATION OF THE CLINICAL FINDINGS

This patient presents with the impairments of restricted dorsiflexion ROM, mild swelling, tenderness and redness in the area of the surgical repair indicating continued inflammation, and atrophy of the calf muscles. She also has the disabilities of limited ambulation and of being unable to participate in sporting activities at this time.

PREFERRED PRACTICE PATTERN

Impaired Joint Mobility, Motor Function, Muscle Performance, and Range of Motion Associated With Bony or Soft Tissue Surgery, (4I)

PLAN OF CARE

The goals of treatment are to resolve the inflammation, thereby limiting excessive scar formation, and to promote maximal strengthening of the repaired tendon in the shortest period of time. At this initial stage of treatment, the problems of restricted ankle ROM and calf atrophy would generally not be addressed directly due to the fragile status of the repair. As the inflammation resolves, these problems would be addressed, with proposed goals of achieving normal ROM, strength, and muscle mass.

ASSESSMENT REGARDING THE APPROPRIATENESS OF THERAPEUTIC ULTRASOUND AS THE OPTIMAL TREATMENT

Therapeutic ultrasound may be used at this time for facilitation of tendon repair in order to promote the development of greater strength in the repaired tendon. Therapeutic ultrasound may also promote completion of the inflammation stage of tissue healing and progression to the proliferation and remodeling stages. As the signs of inflammation resolve, ultrasound may be used to increase the temperature of the tendon in order to facilitate stretching and recovery of normal ankle ROM; however, ultrasound will not promote the recovery of muscle mass or strength.

Since ultrasound should be used with caution over unclosed epiphyseal plates, and since this patient is of an age where epiphyseal closure may or may not be complete, radiographic studies of skeletal maturity should be performed prior to applying ultrasound. If the studies indicate that the epiphyseal plates are closed, ultrasound may be applied in the usual manner. If they indicate that the epiphyseal plates are not closed, thermal-level ultrasound should not be used; however, most authors agree that low-level, pulsed ultrasound may be used.

PROPOSED TREATMENT PLAN AND RATIONALE

It is proposed that ultrasound be applied over the area of the tendon repair. Select a frequency of 3 MHz in order to maximize absorption in the Achilles tendon, which is a superficial structure. For the initial treatment, select a 20% pulsed duty cycle in order to avoid increasing the tissue temperature, thereby potentially aggravating the inflammatory reaction, and select an intensity of 0.5 W/cm^2, consistent with the studies demonstrating improved tendon repair with ultrasound. When the signs of inflammation have resolved and the goal of treatment with ultrasound is to increase dorsiflexion ROM, the duty cycle should be increased to 100%, and the intensity may be increased to between 0.5 and 0.75 W/cm^2 in order to heat the tendon prior to stretching. Since the treatment area will probably be in the range of 5 cm^2, a small sound head with an ERA of 2 to 3 cm^2 should be used. Given this relationship of sound head ERA to treatment area, ultrasound should be applied for 5 to 10 minutes. Treatment would generally be applied 3 to 5 times per week, depending on the availability of resources and the importance of a rapid functional recovery. In studies demonstrating enhanced tendon healing with the application of therapeutic ultrasound, the ultrasound was applied daily; however, treatment 3 times per week is more consistent with present practice patterns. Due to the contouring of this area and its accessibility, treatment may be applied under water.

Case 3

JG is an 80-year-old female with a 10 cm^2 stage IV infected pressure ulcer over her left greater trochanter. She is bedridden, minimally responsive, and completely dependent on others for feeding and bed mobility as the result of three strokes over the past 5 years. She developed the present ulcer 6 months ago after suffering a loss of appetite due to an upper respiratory infection. JG is turned every 2 hours, avoiding left side lying, has been placed on systemic antibiotics, and is receiving conventional wound care; however, her wound has not improved in the last month. She has been referred to physical therapy with the hope that the addition of other interventions may promote tissue healing.

EVALUATION OF THE CLINICAL FINDINGS

This patient presents with the impairments of soft tissue ulceration and delayed tissue healing. Her impairment of reduced strength and her disability of limited mobility have contributed to the development of the pressure ulcer, placing her at risk for systemic infection.

PREFERRED PRACTICE PATTERN

Impaired Integumentary Integrity Associated With Skin Involvement Extending Into Fascia, Muscle, or Bone and Scar Formation, (7E)

PLAN OF CARE

The goals of treatment at this time include resolution of wound infection, decrease in wound size, wound closure, and prevention of reulceration.

ASSESSMENT REGARDING THE APPROPRIATENESS OF THERAPEUTIC ULTRASOUND AS THE OPTIMAL TREATMENT

Therapeutic ultrasound has been shown in some studies to facilitate the healing of chronic wounds, including those with infection. Since conventional modes of treatment have failed to promote any improvement in wound status over the last month, it is appropriate to consider the addition of adjunctive treatments such as ultrasound to the treatment regimen at this time. The use of ultrasound is not contraindicated in this patient, although thermal-level ultrasound should not be used since the patient is minimally responsive and would therefore not be able to report excessive heating by the ultrasound.

PROPOSED TREATMENT PLAN AND RATIONALE

In most studies demonstrating improved healing with the application of ultrasound to chronic wounds, ultrasound was applied to the periwound area alone; therefore, it is recommended that treatment of this patient should focus on the area of intact periwound skin using a gel conduction medium. Select a frequency of 3 MHz in accordance with research findings regarding the use of ultrasound for wound healing and in order to maximize absorption in the superficial tissues surrounding the wound. Select a 20% pulsed duty cycle in order to produce the nonthermal effects of ultrasound while avoiding increasing tissue temperature. Select an intensity of 0.5 to 1.0 W/cm^2, consistent with the studies demonstrating improved wound healing with ultrasound. Because the treatment area is in the range

Continued

> ▶ *Clinical Case Studies—cont'd* ◀

of 10 cm², a medium-sized sound head with an ERA of approximately 5 cm² should be used. Given this relationship of sound head ERA to treatment area, ultrasound should be applied for 5 to 10 minutes, and the treatment should be provided 3 to 5 times per week, depending on the availability of resources. Treatment with ultrasound should be continued until the wound closes or progress plateaus. One can expect approximately a 30% reduction in wound size per month. It is important to note that standard wound care procedures should be continued when ultrasound is added to the treatment regimen for a chronic wound.

Chapter Review

Ultrasound is sound with a frequency greater than that audible by the human ear. It is a mechanical compression-rarefaction wave that travels through tissue, producing both thermal and nonthermal effects. The thermal effects of ultrasound increase the temperature of deep tissue with a high collagen content, and thus increase the tissue's extensibility or control pain. The nonthermal effects of ultrasound can alter cell membrane permeability and thus facilitate tissue healing and transdermal drug penetration. Therapeutic ultrasound may also facilitate calcium resorption, plantar wart resolution, and herpes zoster recovery. In order to achieve these treatment outcomes, the appropriate frequency, intensity, duty cycle, and duration of ultrasound must be selected and applied. Ultrasound should not be applied in situations where it may aggravate an existing pathology, such as a malignancy, or when it may cause tissue damage, such as a burn. When evaluating an ultrasound device for clinical application, one should consider the appropriateness of the available frequencies, pulsed duty cycles, sizes of sound heads, and BNRs to the types of problems expected to be treated with the device. The reader is referred to the Evolve website at http://evolve.elsevier.com/Cameron for study questions pertinent to this chapter.

References

1. Hill CR, Ter Haar G: Ultrasound and non-ionizing radiation protection, In Suess MJ, ed: WHO Regional Publication, European Series No. 10, Copenhagen, 1981, World Health Organization.
2. Goodman CE, Al-Karmi AM, Joyce JM et al: The biological effects of therapeutic ultrasound: frequency dependence. Proceedings of the 14th annual meeting of the Society for Physical Regulation in Biology and Medicine, Washington DC, 1994.
3. Kramer JF: Ultrasound: Evaluation of its mechanical and thermal effects, *Arch Phys Med Rehabil* 65:223-227, 1984.
4. Pye SD, Milford C: The performance of ultrasound physiotherapy machines in Lothian Region, Scotland, 1992, *Ultrasound Med Biol* 20(4):347-359, 1994.
5. Chapelon JY, Cathignol D, Cain C et al: New piezoelectric transducers for therapeutic ultrasound, *Ultrasound Med Biol* Jan;26(1):153-159, 2000.
6. Baker KG, Robertson VJ, Duck FA: A review of therapeutic ultrasound: biophysical effects, *Physical Therapy* 81(7):1351-1358, 2001.
7. Harvey EN: Biological aspects of ultrasonic waves: a general survey, *Biol Bull* 59:306-325, 1930.
8. Lehmann JF: *Ultrasound Therapy in Therapeutic Heat and Cold,* ed 4, Baltimore, 1990, Williams & Wilkins, 1990.
9. Lehmann JF, DeLateur BJ, Stonebridge JB et al: Therapeutic temperature distribution produced by ultrasound as modified by dosage and volume of tissue exposed, *Arch Phys Med Rehabil* 48:662-666, 1967.
10. Lehmann JF, DeLateur BJ, Warren G et al: Bone and soft tissue heating produced by ultrasound, *Arch Phys Med Rehabil* 48:397-401, 1967.
11. Nyborg WN, Ziskin MC: Biological effects of ultrasound, *Clin Diagn Ultrasound* 16:24, 1985.
12. Draper DO, Castel JC, Castel D: Rate of temperature increase in human muscle during 1 MHz and 3 MHz continuous ultrasound, *J Orthop Sport Phys Ther* 22(4):142-150, 1995.
13. Darlas Y, Solasson A, Clouard R et al: Ultrasonotherapie: Calcul de la thermogenese, *Annals Readaptation Med Phys* 32:181-192, 1989.
14. TerHaar G: Basic physics of therapeutic ultrasound, *Physiotherapy* 64(4):100-103, 1978.
15. Lehmann JF, Stonebridge JB, DeLateur BJ, et al: Temperatures in human thighs after hot pack treatment followed by ultrasound, *Arch Phys Med Rehabil* 59:472-475, 1978.
16. Draper DO, Schulties S, Sorvisto P et al: Temperature changes in deep muscle of humans during ice and ultrasound therapies: an in vivo study, *J Orthop Sport Phys Ther* 21(3):153-157, 1995.

17. Harle J, Salih V, Mayia F et al: Effects of ultrasound on the growth and function of bone and periodontal ligament cells in vitro, *Ultrasound in Medicine and Biology* 27(4):579-586, 2001.

18. Mortimer AJ, Dyson M: The effect of therapeutic ultrasound on calcium uptake in fibroblasts, *Ultrasound Med Biol* 14(6):499-506, 1988.

19. Dinno MA, Crum LA, Wu J: The effect of therapeutic ultrasound on electrophysiological parameters of frog skin, *Ultrasound Med Biol* 15(5):461-470, 1989.

20. Fyfe MC, Chahl LA: Mast cell degranulation: a possible mechanism of action of therapeutic ultrasound, *Ultrasound Med Biol* 8(Suppl 1):62, 1982.

21. Young SR, Dyson M: Macrophage responsiveness to therapeutic ultrasound, *Ultrasound Med Biol* 16(8): 809-816, 1990.

22. Harvey W, Dyson M, Pond JB et al: The stimulation of protein synthesis in human fibroblasts by therapeutic ultrasound, *Rheumatol Rehabil* 14:237, 1975.

23. Dinno MA, Al-Karmi AM, Stoltz DA et al: Effect of free radical scavengers on changes in ion conductance during exposure to therapeutic ultrasound, *Membr Biochem* 10(4):237-247, 1993.

24. Robertson VJ, Baker KG: A review of therapeutic ltrasound: effectiveness studies, *Phys Ther* Jul;81(7): 1339-1350, 2001.

25. van der Windt DAWM, van der Heijden GJMG, van der Berg SG et al: Ultrasound therapy for musculoskeletal disorders: a systematic review, *Pain* 81:257-271, 1999.

26. Warren CG, Lehmann JF, Koblanski JN: Elongation of rat tail tendon: effect of load and temperature, *Arch Phys Med* 52:465, 1971.

27. Lehmann JF, Masock AJ, Warren CG et al: Effects of therapeutic temperatures on tendon extensibility, *Arch Phys Med* 51:481, 1970.

28. Lehmann JF: Clinical evaluation of a new approach in the treatment of contracture associated with hip fracture after internal fixation, *Arch Phys Med Rehabil* 42:95, 1961.

29. Wessling KC, DeVane DA, Hylton CR: Effects of static stretch versus static stretch and ultrasound combined on triceps surae muscle extensibility in healthy women, *Phys Ther* 67(5):674-679, 1987.

30. Middlemast S, Chatterjee DS: Comparison of ultrasound and thermotherapy for soft tissue injuries, *Physiotherapy* 64(11):331-332, 1978.

31. Nwuge VCB: Ultrasound in treatment of back pain resulting from prolapsed disc, *Arch Phys Med Rehabil* 64:88-89, 1983.

32. Munting E: Ultrasonic therapy for painful shoulders, *Physiotherapy* 64(6):180-181, 1978.

33. Flemming K, Cullum N: Therapeutic ultrasound for venous leg ulcers, *Cochrane Database Syst Rev* (4):CD001180, 2000.

34. Flemming K, Cullum H: Therapeutic ultrasound for pressure sores, *Cochrane Database Syst Rev* (4): CD001275, 2000.

35. Dyson M, Suckling J: Stimulation of tissue repair by ultrasound: survey of the mechanisms involved, *Physiotherapy* 63:105-108, 1978.

36. McDiarmid T, Burns PN, Lewith GT et al: Ultrasound and the treatment of pressure sores, *Physiotherapy* 71(2):66-70, 1985.

37. Lundeberg T, Nordstrom F, Brodda-Jansen G et al: Pulsed ultrasound does not improve healing of venous ulcers, *Scand J Rehabil Med* 22:195-197, 1990.

38. Eriksson SV, Lundeberg T, Malm M: A placebo-controlled trial of ultrasound therapy in chronic leg ulceration, *Scand J Rehabil Med* 23:211-213, 1991.

39. TerRiet G, Kessels AGH, Knipschild P: A randomized clinical trial of ultrasound in the treatment of pressure ulcers, *Phys Ther* 76(12):1301-1312, 1996.

40. Young SR, Dyson M: The effect of therapeutic ultrasound on angiogenesis, *Ultrasound Med Biol* 16(3): 261-269, 1990.

41. Byl NN, McKenzie AL, West JM et al: Low dose ultrasound effects on wound healing: a controlled study with Yucatan pigs, *Arch Phys Med Rehabil* 73:656-664, 1992.

42. Byl NN, McKenzie AL, Wong T et al: Incisional wound healing: a controlled study of low dose and high dose ultrasound, *J Orthop Sport Phys Ther* 18(5):619-628, 1993.

43. Ferguson HN: Ultrasound in the treatment of surgical wounds, *Physiotherapy* 67(2):43, 1981.

44. Fieldhouse C: Ultrasound for relief of painful episiotomy scars, *Physiotherapy* 65(7):217, 1979.

45. Binder A, Hodge G, Greenwood AM et al: Is therapeutic ultrasound effective in treating soft tissue lesions? *Br Med J* 290:512-514, 1985.

46. Ebenbichler GR, Erdogmus CB, Resch KL et al: Ultrasound therapy for calcific tendinitis of the shoulder, *N Engl J Med* 340:1533-1538, 1999.

47. Lundeberg T, Abrahamsson P, Haker E: A comparative study of continuous ultrasound, placebo ultrasound and rest in epicondylalgia, *Scand J Rehab Med* 20:99-101, 1988.

48. Haker E, Lundeberg T: Pulsed ultrasound treatment in lateral epicondylitis, *Scand J Rehab Med* 23:115-118, 1991.

49. Downing DS, Weinstein A: Ultrasound therapy of subacromial bursitis: a double blind trial, *Phys Ther* 66(2): 194-199, 1986.

50. Enwemeka CS: The effects of therapeutic ultrasound on tendon healing, *Am J Phys Med Rehabil* 6:283-287, 1989.

51. Enwemeka CS, Rodriguez O, Mendosa S: The biomechanical effects of low intensity ultrasound on healing tendons, *Ultrasound Med Biol* 16(8):801-807, 1990.

52. Frieder SJ, Weisberg B, Fleming B et al: A pilot study: the therapeutic effect of ultrasound following partial rupture of Achilles tendons in male rats, *L Orthop Sport Phys Ther* 10:39-46, 1988.

53. Jackson BA, Schwane JA, Starcher BC: Effect of ultrasound therapy on the repair of Achilles tendon injuries in rats, *Med Sci Sport Exerc* 23(2):171-176, 1991.

54. Roberts M, Rutherford JH, Harris D: The effect of ultrasound on flexor tendon repairs in rabbits, *Hand* 14(1):17-20, 1982.

55. Turner SM, Powell ES, Ng CS: The effect of ultrasound on healing of repaired cockerel tendon: is collagen cross-linkage a factor? *J Hand Surg* [BR] 14(4):428-433, 1989.

56. Cline PD: Radiographic follow-up of ultrasound therapy in calcific bursitis, *Phys Ther* 43:16, 1963.

57. Gorkiewicz R: Ultrasound for subacromial bursitis: a case report, *Phys Ther* 64(1):46-47, 1984.

58. Griffin J, Karselis T: *Physical Agents for Physical Therapists,* Springfield, IL, 1982, Charles C Thomas.

59. Hecox B, Mehreteab TA, Weisberg J: *Physical Agents: A Comprehensive Text for Physical Therapists,* East Norwalk, CT, 1994, Appleton & Lange.

60. Fukada E, Yasuda I: On the piezoelectric effect of bone, *J Phys Soc Jap* 12:10, 1957.

61. Duarte LR: The stimulation of bone growth by ultrasound, *Archiv Orthop Trauma Surg* 101:153-159, 1983.

62. Pilla AA, Mont MA, Nasser PR et al: Non-invasive low-intensity ultrasound accelerates bone healing in the rabbit, *J Orthop Trauma* 4(3):246-253, 1990.

63. Kristiansen T, Pilla AA, Siffert RS et al: A multicenter study of Colles' fracture healing by noninvasive low intensity ultrasound. Presented at the 57th meeting of the American Association of Orthopedic Surgeons, New Orleans, February 1990.

64. Heckman JD, Ryaby JP, McCabe J et al: Acceleration of tibial fracture healing by non-invasive, low-intensity pulsed ultrasound, *J Bone Jt Surg* 76A(1):26-34, 1994.

65. Herrick JF: Temperatures produced in tissues by ultrasound: experimental study using various technics, *J Acoust Soc Am* 25:12-16, 1953.

66. Oztas O, Turan B, Bora I et al: Ultrasound therapy effect in carpal tunnel syndrome, *Arch Phys Med Rehabil* Dec;79(12):1540-1544, 1988.

67. Ebenbichler GR, Resch KL, Nicolakis P et al. Ultrasound treatment for treating the carpal tunnel syndrome: randomised "sham" controlled trial, *BMJ* 316:731-735, 1988.

68. McNeill SC, Potts RO, Francoer ML: Local enhanced topical drug delivery (LETD) of drugs: does it truly exist? *Pharm Res* 9:1422-1427, 1992.

69. Fellinger K, Schmid J: Klinik und Therapie des Chronischen Gelenkheumatismus. Vienna, 1954, Maudrich.

70. Griffin JE, Touchstone JC: Ultrasonic movement of cortisol into pig tissues, I: Movement into skeletal muscle, *Am J Phys Med* 42:77-85, 1963.

71. Griffin JE, Touchstone JC, Liu ACY: Ultrasonic movement of cortisol into pig tissues, II: Movement into paravertebral nerve, *Am J Phys Med* 44:20-25, 1965.

72. Griffin JE, Touchstone JC: Low intensity phonophoresis of cortisol in swine, *Phys Ther* 48:1336-1344, 1968.

73. Griffin JE, Touchstone JC: Effects of ultrasonic frequency on phonophoresis of cortisol into swine tissues, *Am J Phys Med,* 51:62-78, 1972.

74. Mitragotri S, Farrell J, Tang H et al: Determination of threshold energy dose for ultrasound-induced transdermal drug transport, *J Control Release* Jan 3;63(1-2):41-52, 2000.

75. Bommannan D, Okuyama H, Stauffer P et al: Sonophoresis, I: The use of high frequency ultrasound to enhance transdermal drug delivery, *Pharm Res* 9: 559-564, 1992.

76. Tang H, Mitragotri S, Blankschtein D et al: Theoretical description of transdermal transport of hydrophilic permeants: application to low-frequency sonophoresis, *J Pharm Sci* May;90(5):545-68, 2001.

77. Mitragotri S: Effect of therapeutic ultrasound on partition and diffusion coefficients in human stratum corneum, *J Control Release* Mar 12;71(1):23-29, 2001.

78. Franklin ME, Smith ST, Chenier TC et al: Effect of phonophoresis with dexamethasone on adrenal function, *J Orthop Sport Phys Ther* 22(3):103-107, 1995.

79. Byl NN: The use of ultrasound as an enhancer for transcutaneous drug delivery: phonophoresis, *Phys Ther* 75(6):539-553, 1995.

80. Kleinkort JA, Wood AF: Phonophoresis with 1% versus 10% hydrocortisone, *Phys Ther* 55:1320-1324, 1975.

81. Cameron MH, Monroe LG: Relative transmission of ultrasound by media customarily used for phonophoresis, *Phys Ther* 72:142-148, 1992.

82. Levy D, Kost J, Meshulam Y et al: Effect of ultrasound on transdermal drug delivery to rats and guinea pigs, *J Clin Invest* 83:2074-2078, 1989.

83. Brucks R, Nanavaty M, Jung D et al: The effect of ultrasound on the in vitro penetration of ibuprofen through human epidermis, *Pharm Res* 6(8):697-701, 1989.

84. Delacerda FG: Ultrasonic techniques for treatment of plantar warts in athletes, *J Orthop Sport Phys Ther* 1: 100-103, 1979.

85. Braatz JH, McAlistar BF, Broaddus MD: Ultrasound and plantar warts: a double blind study, *Milit Med* 139: 199-201, 1974.

86. Jones RJ: Treatment of acute herpes zoster using ultrasonic therapy, *Physiotherapy* 70:94-95, 1984.

87. Jones RJ, Silman GM: Trial of ultrasonic therapy for acute herpes zoster, *Practitioner* 231:1336-1340, 1987.

88. Sicard-Rosenbaum L, Lord D, Danoff JV et al: Effects of continuous therapeutic ultrasound on growth and metastasis of subcutaneous murine tumors, *Phys Ther* 75(1):3-11, 1995.

89. Marmor JB, Pounds D, Hahn GM: Treating spontaneous tumors in dogs and cats by ultrasound-induced hyperthermia, *Int J Radiat Oncol Biol Phys* 4:967-973, 1978.

90. Marmor JB, Hilerio FB, Hahn GM: Tumor eradication and cell survival after localized hyperthermia induced by ultrasound, *Cancer Res* 39:2166-2171, 1979.

91. Smachlo K, Fridd CW, Child SZ et al: Ultrasonic treatment of tumors, 1: Absence of metastases following treatment of a hamster fibrosarcoma, *Ultrasound Med Biol* 5:45-49, 1979.

92. Shista K: Neural tube defects and maternal hyperthermia in early pregnancy: epidemiology in a human embryo population, *Am J Med Genet* 12:281-288, 1982.

93. Kalter H, Warkany J: Congenital malformations: etiological factors and their role in prevention, *N Engl J Med* 308:424-431, 1983.

94. McLeod DR, Fowlow SB: Multiple malformations and exposure to therapeutic ultrasound during organogenesis, *Am J Med Genet* 34:317-319, 1989.

95. Carstensen EL, Gates AH: The effects of pulsed ultrasound on the fetus, *J Ultrasound Med* 3:145-147, 1984.

96. National Council of Radiation Protection and Measurements: Biological effects of ultrasound: Mechanisms and clinical implications. NCRP Report No. 74. Bethesda, MD, 1983, NCRP.

97. Normand H, Darlas Y, Solassol A et al: Etude experimentale de l'effet thermique des ultrasons sur le materiel prothetique, *Ann Readaptation Med Phys* 32:193-201, 1989.

98. Skoubo-Kristensen E, Sommer J: Ultrasound influence on internal fixation with rigid plate in dogs, *Arch Phys Med Rehabil* 63:371-373, 1982.

99. Deforest RE, Herrick JF, Janes JM: Effects of ultrasound on growing bone: an experimental study, *Arch Phys Med Rehab* 34:21, 1953.

100. Spadaro JA, Skarulis T, Albanese SA: Effect of pulsed ultrasound on bone growth in rats. Proceedings of the 14th Annual Meeting of the Society for Physical Regulation in Biology and Medicine, Washington DC, 1994.

101. Nyborg WL: Biological effects of ultrasound: development of safety guidelines. Part II: General review, *Ultrasound Med Biol* Mar;27(3):301-333, 2001.

102. Dyson M, Pond JB, Woodward B et al: The production of blood cell stasis and endothelial damage in blood vessels of chick embryos treated with ultrasound in a stationary wave field, *Ultrasound Med Biol* 63:133-138, 1974.

103. TerHaar GR, Dyson M, Smith SP: Ultrastructural changes in the mouse uterus brought about by ultrasonic irradiation at therapeutic intensities in standing wave fields, *Ultrasound Med Biol* 5:167-179, 1979.

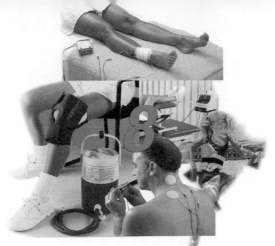

Electrical Currents

Sara Shapiro, MPH, PT

OBJECTIVES

Upon completion of this chapter, the reader will be able to

1. Define the basic settings for the use of electrical stimulation as they are applied in the management of neuromuscular and musculoskeletal dysfunctions and wound care.
2. Identify the physiological effects of electrical stimulation.
3. Be familiar with the multiple uses of electrical stimulation including muscle re-education and strengthening, gait training, spasticity reduction, wound care, and pain modulation.
4. Discuss the basic principles of electrode size and materials, and demonstrate appropriate placement techniques for each application.

5. Compare the basic similarities, differences, and functional applications of high volt, medium frequency and interferential, and DC for iontophoresis and then choose the appropriate device to obtain the desired treatment goals.
6. Be familiar with the guidelines, precautions, and contraindications in working with electrical stimulation devices.
7. When presented with a clinical case, analyze the clinical findings, propose goals of treatment, assess whether electrotherapy would be an appropriate treatment, and if so, formulate an effective treatment plan including the appropriate device and treatment parameters for achieving the goals of treatment.

INTRODUCTION AND HISTORY

An electrical current is a flow of charged particles. The charged particles may be either electrons or ions. Electrical currents have been applied to biological systems to change physiological processes dating back as far as 46 AD, when it was recorded that the electric discharge from torpedo fish was used to alleviate pain.[1,2]

In the late 18th and early 19th centuries there was a revival of interest in medical applications of electrical currents. In 1791, Galvani first recorded producing muscle contractions by touching metal to a frog's muscle. He called this effect animal electricity. A few years later, when Volta constructed the precursor to the battery, Galvani used the current put out by this device to produce muscle contractions. He named the current "Galvanic current." In an attempt to understand the mechanisms by which electrical currents cause muscle contractions, Duchenne mapped out the locations on the skin where electrical stimulation most effectively caused specific muscles to contract. He called these locations "motor points."[3] During the 1830s Faraday discovered that bidirectional electrical currents could be induced by a moving magnet. He called this current "Faradic current." Faradic current can be used to produce muscle contractions. In 1905, Lapicque developed the "law of excitation" relating the intensity and duration of a stimulus to whether it would produce a muscle contraction. Lapicque introduced the concept of the strength-duration curve, as described later in this chapter.

The use of electrical currents for controlling pain is derived from the gate control theory of pain perception developed by Melzack and Wall in the 1960s. For a more complete description of the historical development of electrical stimulation the reader is referred to Sidney Licht's *Electrodiagnosis and Electromyography*.[4]

Today, electrical stimulation has a wide range of clinical applications in rehabilitation. These include muscle strengthening,[5,6] pain control,[7,8] facilitating the healing of recalcitrant wounds,[9] and the resolution of edema and inflammatory reactions following injury or surgery.[10]

Many professionals, including physical therapists, occupational therapists, physicians, chiropractors, and others, have found electrical stimulation to be a valuable and effective component of their therapeutic armamentarium. In an ongoing effort to provide evidence-based treatment, researchers have evaluated the efficacy of electric stimulation for its common clinical applications. The proliferation of more sophisticated machines has also increased interest in the use of electric stimulation as an adjunct to rehabilitation treatment. These machines have multiple waveforms, allow a wide variety of parameter selection, and may include computer-generated images of body parts and electrode placement for specific diagnoses. The availability of small, patient-friendly units that can be used at home has also enhanced the effectiveness of electrical stimulation by allowing ongoing treatment between clinic visits.

Electrical stimulation can be applied to the body in a variety of ways. The electricity may be delivered by a stimulator implanted in the body, as occurs with a cardiac pacemaker, or an external stimulator can be used to deliver current to implanted or external surface transcutaneous electrodes. This chapter only describes the application of electrical stimulation by external stimulators that deliver current transcutaneously via surface electrodes applied to the skin.

TERMINOLOGY FOR ELECTRICAL CURRENTS

An issue that continues to complicate the use of electric stimulation is the varied use and misuse of terminology describing therapeutic electrical currents. In 1986 the Clinical Electrophysiology Section of the American Physical Therapy Association (APTA) published a terminology guide in an attempt to standardize the terminology used by clinicians, manufacturers, researchers, educators, and engineers to describe therapeutic electrical currents. A second edition of this guide was published in 2000.[11] This guide has helped to promote the consistent use of terminology. This chapter uses its terminology and definitions. Because not all manufacturers or clinicians use this terminology, any alternative commonly used terms are noted in parentheses.

General Terms

Electrical Current: The movement or flow of charged particles through a conductor in response to an applied electric field. Current is noted as I and is measured in Amperes (A).

Charge: One of the basic properties of matter, which either has no charge (is electrically neutral), or may be negatively (–) or positively (+) charged. Charge is noted as Q and is measured in Coulombs (C).

Polarity: The property of having two oppositely charged conductors, with the positive called the *anode*, and the negative called the *cathode*. In a conductor, free electrons flow from an area of excess electrons (negative pole) to an area deficient in electrons (positive pole).

Voltage: The electrical force capable of moving charged particles through a conductor between two regions or points. Voltage is also known as the *potential difference*. Voltage is noted as V and is measured in volts (V).

Resistance: The property of a conductor that resists or is in opposition to the flow of charged particles. Resistance is noted as R and is measured in Ohms (Ω).

Ohm's Law: $V = I \times R$ is the mathematical expression of how voltage (V), current (I), and resistance (R), relate.

Impedance: The total frequency-dependent opposition to current flow. Impedance is noted by Z and is measured in Ohms (Ω). For biological systems, impedance describes the ratio of voltage to current more accurately than resistance because it is a frequency-dependent measure that includes the effects of capacitance and resistance.

Electrical Stimulation Treatment Parameters—Waveforms

Direct Current (DC): A continuous unidirectional flow of charged particles is known as *direct current (DC)*. Direct current is used to for iontophoresis and for stimulating contraction of denervated muscle and also occasionally to facilitate wound healing (Fig. 8-1).

Alternating Current (AC): A continuous bidirectional flow of charged particles is known as *alternating current (AC)* (Fig. 8-2). Alternating current has equal ion flow in each direction, and as such no pulse charge remains in the tissues. Most commonly, AC is delivered as a sine wave. The wavelength is the duration of 1 cycle. A cycle is from the time that the current departs from the isoelectric line (zero current amplitude) in one direction and then crosses the isoelectric line in the opposite direction to when it returns to the isoelectric line.

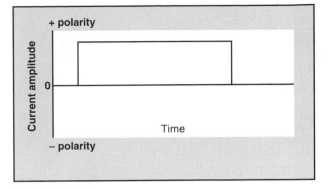

Figure 8-1. Direct current (DC).

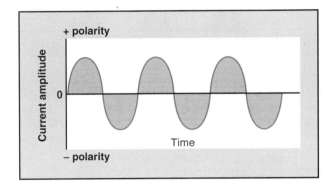

Figure 8-2. Alternating current (AC).

An inverse relationship between cycle duration and frequency is inherent to the AC waveform: when the frequency increases, the cycle duration decreases; and when the frequency decreases, the cycle duration increases (Fig. 8-3).

Pulsed Current or Pulsatile Current: Electrical current can be delivered discontinuously, in a series of pulses separated by periods when no current flows. This is known as *pulsed* or *pulsatile current*. The current pulses may be either uni- or bidirectional. A series of unidirectional pulses is known as a *monophasic pulsed current*. In this case, charged particles move only in one direction. A series of bidirectional pulses is known as a *biphasic pulsed current* (Fig. 8-4). With a biphasic pulsed current, charged particles move first in one direction and then in the opposite direction. A biphasic pulsed current may be symmetric or asymmetric, and if asymmetric, it may be balanced or unbalanced (Fig. 8-5). With a balanced pulse the charge of the phases are equal in amount and opposite in

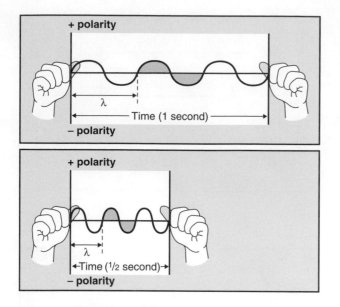

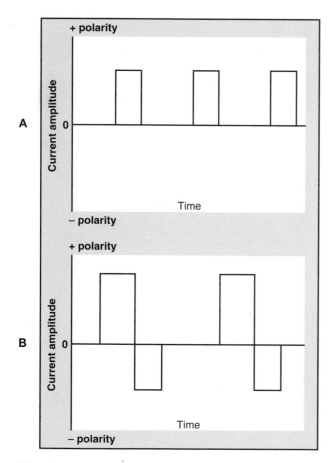

Figure 8-3. Illustration of the inverse relationship between frequency and cycle duration for an alternating current (λ=Wavelength)

Figure 8-4. **A,** Monophasic and **B,** biphasic pulsed currents.

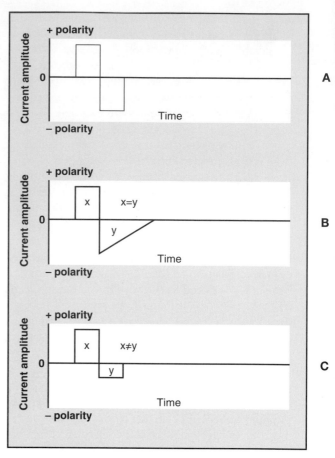

Figure 8-5. **A,** Symmetric, **B,** balanced asymmetric and **C,** unbalanced asymmetric biphasic pulsed currents.

polarity, resulting in a net charge of zero. With an unbalanced pulse the charge of the phases are not equal and the net charge is not zero.

Interferential Current: Interferential current is the waveform produced by the interference of two medium frequency (1,000 to 10,000 Hz) sinusoidal ACs of slightly different frequencies. These two waveforms are delivered through two sets of electrodes through separate channels in the same stimulator. The electrodes are configured on the skin so that the two AC currents intersect (Fig. 8-6). When the currents intersect they interfere, producing a higher amplitude when both currents are in the same phase and a lower amplitude when the two currents are in opposite phases. This produces envelopes of pulses known as *beats*. The beat frequency is equal to the difference between the frequencies of the two original ACs. The frequency of slower original AC is called the *carrier frequency*. For example, when a carrier frequency of 5000 Hz

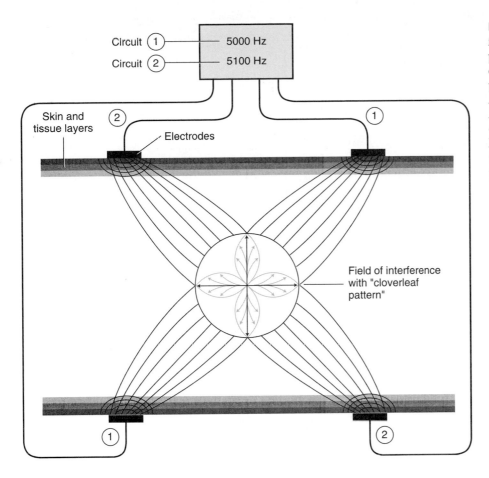

Figure 8-6. Intersecting medium frequency alternating currents producing an interferential current between two crossed pairs of electrodes. (From May H-U, Hansjürgens A: Nemectrodyn Model 7 Manual of Nemectron GmbH, Daimlerstr. 15, Karlsruche/ Germany, 1984. Used with permission.)

interferes with a current with a frequency of 5100 Hz a beat frequency of 100 Hz will be produced in the tissue (Fig. 8-7). Typically, electrical stimulation units that produce interferential stimulation allow the clinician to set the beat frequency and some also allow the clinician to select the carrier frequency.

It is proposed that interferential current is more comfortable than other waveforms because it allows a low amplitude current to be delivered through the skin, where most discomfort is produced, while delivering a much higher current amplitude to deeper tissues. Interferential current may also stimulate a larger area than other waveforms. Of note, there is no published research to verify these claims. Additionally, interferential current is a continuous AC and therefore has a higher average amplitude than pulsed waveforms.

Premodulated Current: Premodulated current is a waveform produced by one channel (two electrodes) that has the same form as the current produced by the interference of two medium-frequency sinusoidal ACs. Premodulated current has a continuous sinusoidal waveform with a medium frequency and a sequentially increasing and decreasing current amplitude. The advantages of interferential current, including a lower current amplitude being delivered to the skin and a larger area of stimulation, are not reproduced by premodulated current.

Russian Protocol: The Russian protocol is comprised of 2500 Hz carrier frequency AC sinusoidal wave modulated to produce 50 bursts per second (bps). Each burst (or envelope) is a polyphasic waveform delivered for 10 milliseconds followed by an interburst interval of 50 milliseconds (Fig. 8-8).

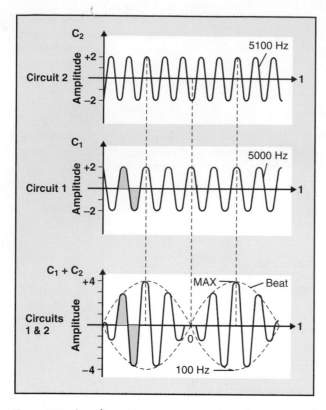

Figure 8-7. An alternating current with a frequency of 5000 Hz interfering with an alternating current with a frequency of 5100 Hz to produce an interferential current with a beat frequency of 100 Hz. (From May H-U, Hansjürgens A: Nemectrodyn Model 7 Manual of Nemectron GmbH, Daimlerstr.15, Karlsruche/ Germany, 1984. Used with permission.)

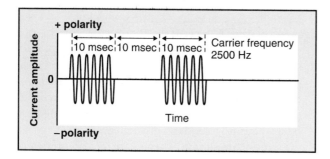
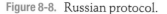

Figure 8-8. Russian protocol.

Time Dependent Parameters

Frequency: *Frequency* describes the number of cycles or pulses per second and is expressed as Hertz (Hz) for cycles or pulses per second (pps) for pulses (Fig. 8-9).

Pulse Duration/Phase Duration: Pulse duration is the time from the beginning of the first phase of a

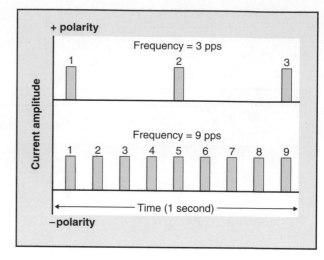

Figure 8-9. Monophasic pulsed current with frequencies of 3 pulses per second and 9 pulses per second.

pulse to the end of the last phase of a pulse. *Phase duration* refers to the duration of one phase of a pulse. Pulse and phase duration are generally expressed in microseconds (μs) or milliseconds (ms) (Fig. 8-10).

Interpulse Interval: The interpulse interval is the time between pulses (see Fig. 8-10).

Interphase Interval: The interphase interval is the time between phases of a pulse. This is sometimes referred to as intrapulse interval (Fig. 8-11).

Rise Time/Decay Time: Rise time is the time it takes for the current to increase from zero to its peak during any one phase. Decay time is the time it takes for the current to decrease from its peak level to zero during any one phase (Fig. 8-12). Note that this is different from ramp up and ramp down as described below.

On/Off Time: On time is the time during which a train of pulses occurs. Off time is the time between trains of pulses when no current flows. On and off times are usually only used when electrical stimulation is used to produce muscle contractions. During the on time the muscle contracts, and during the off time it relaxes. The off times are needed to reduce muscle fatigue during the stimulation session. The sequential on and off times also attempt to mimic the voluntary contract and relax phases of normal physiological exercise. The relationship of the on and off time is often expressed as a ratio. For example, if a muscle is stimulated for 10 seconds and then allowed to relax for 50 seconds,

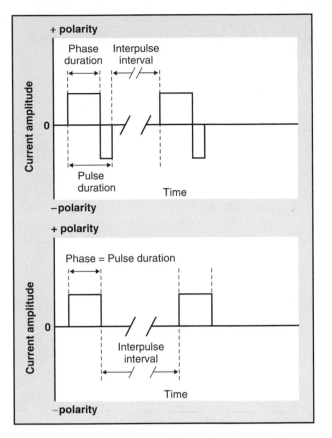

Figure 8-10. Pulse duration, phase duration, and interpulse interval for biphasic and monophasic pulsed currents.

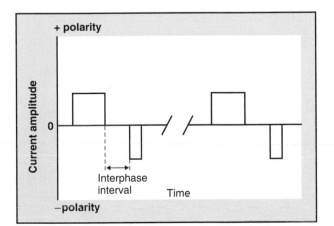

Figure 8-11. Interphase interval for a biphasic pulsed current.

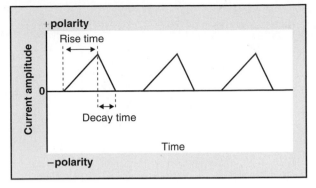

Figure 8-12. Rise and decay times.

this may be written as a 10:50 second on:off time or a 1:5 on:off ratio. The on:off ratio is a ratio of the on time to the off time (Fig. 8-13).

Duty Cycle: Duty cycle is the ratio of the on time to the total cycle time, where the total cycle time is the on time plus the off time. Because the term *duty cycle* is frequently misunderstood to mean on:off ratio, it is recommended that the clearer terminology of "on:off time" or "on:off ratio" be used.

Ramp Up Time/Ramp Down Time: The ramp up time is the time it takes for the current to increase from zero to its maximum amplitude for any one on time. This is in contrast to the rise time, which describes the time for the current amplitude to increase during one phase only. The ramp down time is the time it takes for the current to decrease from its maximum amplitude to zero during any one on time. This is in contrast to the decay time, which describes the time for the current amplitude to fall during one phase only (Fig. 8-14).

Ramping is used to produce a "soft start," allowing patients to become accustomed to the stimula-

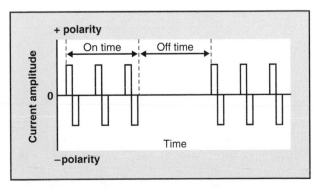

Figure 8-13. On and off times for a biphasic current.

Figure 8-14. Ramp up and ramp down times.

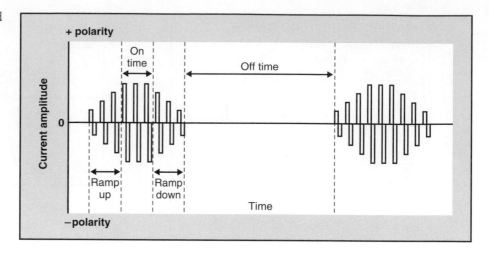

tion as it increases from a subsensory level to a sensory level and finally reaches motor threshold. Ramp up is generally included in the on time while the ramp down time is included in the off time.

Other Electrical Current Parameters

Amplitude: Amplitude is the magnitude of current or voltage. While the term intensity is frequently used interchangeably with amplitude, it is not the correct term to use in this context (Fig. 8-15).

Modulation: Modulation refers to any pattern of variation in one or more of the stimulation parameters. Modulation is used to limit neural adaptation to an electrical current. Modulation may be cyclic or random (Fig. 8-16).

Frequency Modulation: Frequency modulation refers to variation in the number of pulses or cycles per second delivered.

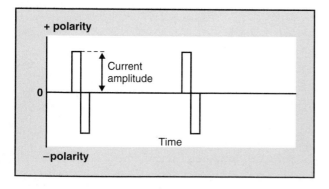

Figure 8-15. Current amplitude.

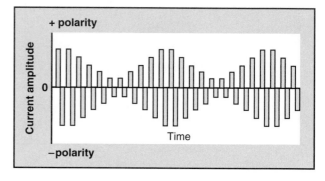

Figure 8-16. Current amplitude modulation.

Amplitude Modulation: Amplitude modulation refers to variation in peak current amplitude.

Phase Duration or Pulse Duration Modulation: Phase duration or pulse duration modulation refers to variation in the phase or pulse duration.

Note that modulation of interferential currents waveforms is similar to that of pulsed currents; however, the terminology used by most manufacturers is different. *Sweep* is generally used to describe frequency modulation and *scan* is used to describe current amplitude modulation. Current amplitude modulation makes the effective field of stimulation change, causing the patient to feel the focus of the stimulation moving. Manufacturers often claim that currents can be crossed at a precise location, allowing the clinician to *target* any area. However, due to differences in tissue conductivity, current will not generally flow through bone and thus cannot be precisely crossed at the center of a joint.

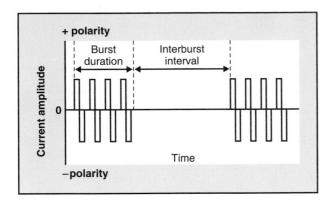

Figure 8-17. Burst mode.

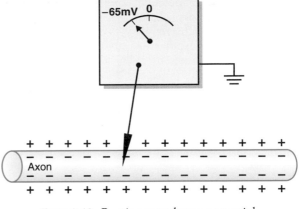

Figure 8-18. Resting membrane potential.

Burst Mode: Burst mode refers to a series of pulses delivered in a package or "envelope" as a single pulse. The burst is generally delivered with a present frequency and duration. *Burst duration* is the time from the beginning to the end of the burst. The time between bursts is called the *interburst interval* (Fig. 8-17).

EFFECTS OF ELECTRICAL CURRENTS

Nerve Depolarization

For most applications, electrical currents exert their physiological effects by depolarizing nerve membranes and thereby producing action potentials, the message unit of the nervous system. Electrical currents with sufficient amplitude, that last for a sufficient length of time, will cause enough of a change in nerve membrane potential to generate an action potential. Once that action potential is propagated along the axon, the human body responds to it in the same way as it does to action potentials that are initiated by physiological stimuli.

An *action potential* is the basic unit of nerve communication. When a nerve is at rest, without physiological or electrical stimulation, the inside is more negatively charged than the outside by –60 to –90 millivolts. This is known as the *resting membrane potential* (Fig. 8-18). When a stimulus of sufficient amplitude (strength) is applied over a sufficient length of time, the membrane rapidly depolarizes and then repolarizes. This rapid sequential depolarization and repolarization is known as an action potential (AP).

The resting membrane potential is maintained by most of the sodium ions being outside the cell and most of the potassium ions being inside the cell. When a sufficient stimulus is applied, sodium channels in the cell membrane open rapidly, while the potassium channels open slowly. Because of the high extracellular concentration of sodium, sodium ions rush into the cell though the open channels. This makes the inside of the cell become more positively charged, reversing the membrane potential. When the membrane potential reaches +30 mV, the permeability to sodium decreases and potassium channels rapidly open, increasing the permeability to potassium. Because there is a high intracellular concentration of potassium ions, potassium ions then flow out of the cell, returning the membrane polarization to its resting state of –60 to –90 mV. This sequential depolarization and repolarization of the cell membrane caused by the changing flow of ions across the cell membrane is the AP (Fig. 8-19).

While the nerve is depolarized, no additional APs can be generated. During this time the nerve cannot be further excited, however strong a stimulus is applied. This period is known as the *absolute refractory period*. After depolarization, prior to returning to the resting potential, there is a brief period of membrane hyperpolarization. During this period a greater stimulus than usual is required to produce another AP. This period of hyperpolarization is known as the *relative refractory period*.

Strength-duration curve

The amount of electrical current required to produce an AP in a specific type of nerve varies and can be

Figure 8-19. An action potential is the basic unit of nerve communication and is achieved by rapid sequential depolarization and repolarization in response to stimulation. Note that depolarization starts when the Na+ gate opens and Na+ flows into the cell causing a rapid change from the normal resting membrane potential to a more positively charged state. Sequential repolarization occurs as permeability to sodium decreases causing the K+ channels to open and K+ to flow out of the cell, returning the membrane polarization to its resting state.

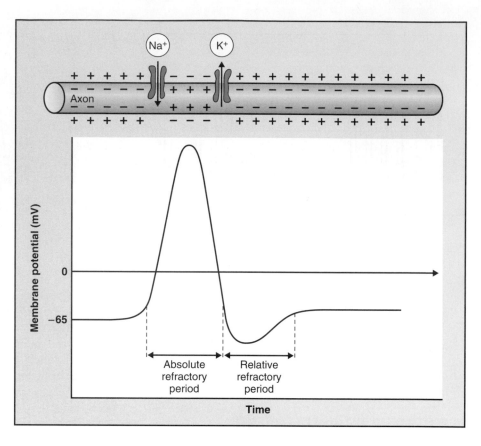

represented by the nerve's strength-duration curve (Fig. 8-20). The strength-duration curve for a nerve is a graphic representation of the minimum combination of current strength (amplitude) and pulse duration needed to depolarize that nerve. This interplay of amplitude and pulse duration is the basis for the specificity of the effect of electrical stimulation. In general, lower current amplitudes and shorter pulse durations can depolarize sensory nerves while higher amplitude or longer pulses are needed to depolarize motor nerves. Even higher amplitudes and longer pulses are needed to depolarize pain-transmitting C fibers. Thus, short pulses, generally of less than 80 μseconds (80 × 10^{-6} seconds), are used to produce sensory stimulation only, while longer pulses, of 150 to 350 μseconds, are used to produce muscle contractions. By keeping pulse durations below 1 ms (10^{-3} seconds), pain is minimized because C fibers are not depolarized. Pulses of greater than 10 msec. are required to produce muscle contraction in denervated muscle.

When the current amplitude and pulse duration fall below the curve for a particular nerve type, the stimulation is considered to be subthreshold and no response

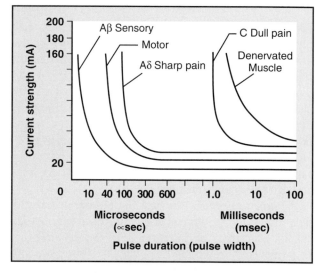

Figure 8-20. Strength-duration curve.

will occur. For any type of tissue, the minimum current amplitude, with a very long pulse duration, required to produce an action potential is called *rheobase*. The minimum duration it takes to stimulate that tissue at twice rheobase intensity is known as *chronaxie*. Rheobase is a measure of current amplitude, while chronaxie is a measure of time/duration (Fig. 8-21).

Increasing the current amplitude or pulse duration beyond that which is sufficient to stimulate an AP will not change the AP in any way. Neither a larger nor a faster AP occurs. All nerve APs are the same. They occur in an all-or-none fashion. The same AP occurs with any stimulus above threshold, and no AP will occur with any stimulus below threshold level.

In addition to sufficient current amplitude and pulse duration, the current amplitude must rise quickly for an AP to be triggered. If the current rises too slowly the nerve will accommodate to the stimulus. Accommodation is the process of a nerve gradually becoming less responsive to stimulation; a stimulus of sufficient amplitude and duration which usually produces a response no longer does so. Accommodation occurs with a slow rate of current rise because of the prolonged subthreshold stimulation.

Once an AP is generated, it triggers an AP in the adjacent area of the nerve membrane. This process is called *propagation* or *conduction* of the AP along the neuron. With normal physiological stimulation, AP propagation occurs in only one direction. With electrically stimulated APs, propagation occurs in both directions from the site of stimulation; however, only those APs transmitted in the usual physiological direction have an effect.

The speed at which an AP travels depends on the diameter of the nerve through which it travels, and whether or not the nerve is myelinated. The larger the nerve diameter the faster the AP will travel. For example, large-diameter myelinated A-alpha motor nerves conduct at between 60 and 120 meters/second, while smaller diameter myelinated A-gamma and A-delta nerves conduct at only 12 to 30 meters/second. Action potentials travel faster in myelinated nerves than in nonmyelinated nerves. Myelin is a fatty sheath that covers the length of certain axons. The sheath is not continuous, and the small gaps in it are called *nodes of Ranvier*. Action potentials propagate along myelinated nerve fibers by jumping from node to node—a process called *saltatory conduction* (Fig. 8-22). This movement or jumping of the AP between nodes increases the speed of conduction. For example, unmyelinated C-fibers that transmit slow pain and temperature conduct at only 0.5 to 2 meters/second, which is much slower than the 12 to 30 meters/second conduction speed of similar diameter myelinated A-gamma and A-delta nerves.[12]

Muscle Depolarization

In the late 1800s it was found that denervated muscles do not contract in response to the pulses of electricity that produce contractions in innervated muscles. Innervated muscles contract in response to electricity because the current causes depolarization of their motor nerves. Denervated muscles will contract in response to long pulses of electricity, lasting for 10 ms or longer. These longer duration pulses depolarize the muscle cell membrane directly. Because denervated muscle membrane does not accommodate, a slow rising stimulus can be used to produce a muscle contraction in it.[13]

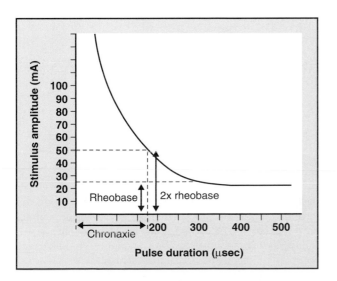

Figure 8-21. Chronaxie and rheobase.

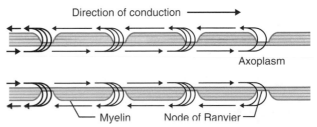

Figure 8-22. Saltatory conduction along a myelinated nerve. (From Burt AM: *Textbook of Neuroanatomy*, Philadelphia, 1997, WB Saunders.)

Ionic Effects of Electrical Currents

Most electrical currents used therapeutically have balanced biphasic waveforms. This type of waveform leaves no charge in the tissue and thus has no ionic effects. In contrast, DC pulsed monophasic currents and unbalanced biphasic waveforms, which are used occasionally for electrical stimulation, do leave a net charge in the tissue. This charge can produce ionic effects. The negative electrode (cathode) attracts positively charged ions and repels negatively charged ions while the positive electrode (anode) attracts negatively charged ions and repels positively charged ions (Fig. 8-23).

These ionic effects can be exploited therapeutically. For example, a DC can be used to repel ionized drug molecules and may thus provide a force to increase their transdermal penetration. This application of electrotherapy is known as *iontophoresis*. The ionic effects of electricity are also exploited for the treatment of inflammatory states and to facilitate tissue healing, as described in detail below.

CLINICAL APPLICATIONS OF ELECTRICAL CURRENTS

Muscle Contraction

Innervated muscle

When action potentials are propagated along motor nerves, the muscle fibers innervated by those nerves become depolarized, and contract. The muscle contraction produced by electrically stimulated APs is similar to that produced by physiologic generation of

APs; however, there are some important differences between these muscle contractions.

The primary difference between electrically stimulated muscle contractions and physiologically initiated muscle contractions is the order of recruitment of motor units. With electrical stimulation, nerve fibers with the largest axonal diameters, which innervate the larger, fast-twitch muscle fibers, are activated first and those with a smaller axonal diameter are recruited later.[14] In contrast, with physiological contractions, the smaller, slow-twitch muscle fibers are activated before larger fibers. The fast-twitch muscle fibers, which contract preferentially in response to electrical stimulation, fatigue rapidly while the slow-twitch muscle fibers, preferentially recruited physiologically, are more fatigue resistant. A clinical implication of this difference is that, since stimulated contractions are more fatiguing, longer rest times are needed between contractions (Fig. 8-24). In addition, because electrically stimulated contractions may affect different motor units than those affected by physiological contraction, it is recommended that patients perform both electrically stimulated and physiological contractions, if possible, to optimize their functional rehabilitation.

Another difference between electrically stimulated contractions and physiologically initiated contractions is the smoothness of the onset of the con-

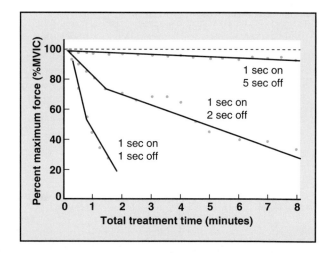

Figure 8-24. The effect of changing the on:off ratio on the force of contraction produced. Note that stronger contractions are produced when longer off times are used. (Adapted with permission from Benton LA, Baker LL, Bowman BR, et al: *Functional Electrical Stimulation: A Practical Clinical Guide.* Rancho Los Amigos, Rehabilitation Center, Rancho Los Amigos Hospital, 1981, Downey, CA.)

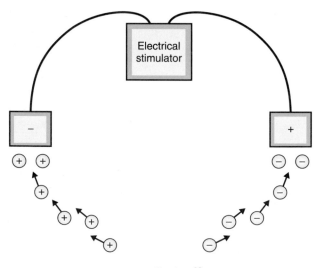

Figure 8-23. Ionic effects.

traction. Physiological contractions usually gradually increase in force in a smoothly graded manner. The force is regulated by physiological control of which motor units are recruited and the rate at which each motor unit is activated. The contraction is kept smooth by asynchronous recruitment of motor units. In contrast, electrically stimulated contractions generally have a rapid and often jerky onset because all motor units of a given size fire simultaneously when the stimulus reaches threshold.

Electrical stimulation is thought to strengthen muscles by two mechanisms: overload and specificity.[15] According to the overload principle, the greater the load placed on a muscle, and the higher force contraction it produces, the more strength that muscle will gain. This principle applies both to contractions produced by electrical stimulation and to those produced by physiological exercise.[16] In normal healthy human subjects it has been shown that combining electrical stimulation with a voluntary exercise regime does not cause greater strengthening than either intervention alone, if the same force of contraction is produced.[17] In addition, in healthy subjects, the gains in muscle strength are similar for electrically stimulated contractions and exercise when the same amount of force is produced.[18]

According to the specificity theory, since electrical stimulation causes larger, fast-twitch (type II) muscle fibers, which produce a greater level of force, to contract before smaller slow-twitch (type I) muscle fibers, electrical stimulation should be able to produce greater strength gains than exercise alone with the same force contractions. This theory is supported by the findings that, in weak patients with reduced muscle strength or after surgery, early use of electrical stimulation can result in a more rapid recovery and greater strength gains than exercise alone.[19,20,21] A recent study has also demonstrated that 4 weeks of electrical stimulation alone or in combination with voluntary exercise, applied after anterior cruciate ligament reconstruction, produced greater strength gains than exercise alone.[22] Although electrical stimulation appears to accelerate postoperative recovery of strength, research indicates that by 12 weeks after surgery strength is not significantly different for patients who exercise and those who receive electrical stimulation.[23]

Electrical stimulation can also assist in rehabilitation by recruiting a larger pool of motor units than physiological activity does. For example, electrical stimulation of the lower extremity in patients with hemiplegia has been shown to produce improved voluntary recruitment of motor units and improvements in gait following treatment.[24] The increased general excitability of the motor neuron pool produced by electrical stimulation may enhance descending control of muscle recruitment and augment sensory input. The sensory input may also provide a cue for the patient to initiate a movement or activate a muscle group.

Electrically stimulated muscle contraction can accelerate and improve patient rehabilitation by increasing muscle strength and endurance.[25] These can enhance the quality of motor recruitment and carry over to improved performance of functional activities. In order to produce strength gains in healthy muscle, the force of the stimulated contraction needs to be at least 50% of the maximum voluntary isometric contraction (MVIC), although the greatest strength gains will be achieved with the maximally tolerated force of contraction. To produce strength gains in injured patients, the stimulated contractions may have a force of as little as 10% of the MVIC, although stronger contractions will be more effective if they are tolerated. For the greatest gains in endurance, more prolonged periods of stimulation with lower force contractions are more effective.[12,26]

Electrically stimulated muscle contractions can also support or assist with joint positioning, functioning like an orthotic. For example, Baker and colleagues reported that an aggressive program of electrically stimulated contraction of the muscles surrounding the shoulder over a 6-week period reduced shoulder subluxation in patients with hemiplegia due to stroke more effectively than facilitation programs, slings, or sitting support.[27] A more recent smaller study in patients with hemiplegia due to stroke demonstrated that neuromuscular electrical stimulation (NMES) reduced shoulder subluxation slightly while the glenohumeral separation increased in the control group even though the affected arm was supported at all times.[28] Several studies have also reported an improvement in gait in children with cerebral palsy when NMES of the lower extremities has been included in their treatment regimen and an improvement in upper extremity function when NMES of the upper extremities has been included.[29-32]

Studies concerning the use of NMES in patients with spasticity have primarily focused on stimulating the antagonist muscles. However, stimulating the agonist and the antagonist sequentially, with brief rest periods after each contraction, may be more effective since this would more closely mimic normal motor activity. Individuals without central nervous system (CNS) dysfunction flex and extend the elbow by firing the biceps and triceps sequentially, with a brief latency period between them. Individuals with CNS dysfunction maintain some ongoing motor activity of both agonist and antagonist throughout the movement, and the latency period is absent.

Additionally, studies have shown that electrically stimulated muscle contraction can promote blood flow in healthy individuals and in patients with poor circulation.[33-36] This increase in circulation can accelerate tissue healing and has been demonstrated to help reduce the risk of deep venous thrombosis formation.[35,37-40] Some studies suggest that sensory level electrical stimulation may also augment peripheral blood flow, but this effect has been found to occur only in patients and not in healthy individuals.[33,34,41-43]

Another more recent use of electrically stimulated muscle contractions is for the treatment of urinary incontinence associated with pelvic floor dysfunction.[44,45] Electric stimulation for this purpose has been applied transcutaneously, percutaneously, and via intravaginal probes.[46,47] Most reports have focused on urinary incontinence in women, some review protocols for men. In 1996, the Agency for Health Care Policy and Research (AHCPR) Guidelines on urinary incontinence stated that pelvic floor electrical stimulation has been shown to decrease incontinence in women with stress urinary incontinence, and may be useful for urge and mixed incontinence.[48]

Denervated muscle

When a muscle becomes denervated by nerve injury or disease it no longer contracts physiologically, nor can a contraction be produced by the usual electrical stimulus used for NMES. However, if the electrical current has a longer pulse duration, of more than 10 ms, the denervated muscle will contract. Usually continuous DC is applied for a number of seconds to produce contractions in denervated muscle. The duration of stimulation is controlled directly by the clinician depressing a manually controlled switch on a DC stimulator. In order to produce a graded contraction in a denervated muscle, the current amplitude can be gradually ramped up to reach full amplitude over a number of seconds.

Denervation causes muscle to atrophy and fibrose. The entire muscle and the individual muscle fibers become smaller, and fibrous tissue forms between the muscle fibers. It has been suggested that electrical stimulation of denervated muscles may retard this atrophy and fibrosis; however, studies have shown that the final outcome of muscle denervation is not improved by this intervention.[49,50] In addition, there is evidence from studies in rats that electrically stimulated contractions of denervated muscles may retard motor nerve sprouting and muscle reinnervation.[51] Therefore we do not recommend stimulation of contractions in denervated muscles with DC. Direct current electrical stimulation has traditionally been used for treatment of Bell's palsy (facial paralysis due to damage to the seventh cranial nerve); however, evidence indicates that this treatment is no more effective than placebo.[52,53] Some studies have shown improved clinical recovery in patients with chronic facial palsy in response to long term sensory level electrical stimulation.[54,55]

Pain Modulation

A substantial body of research demonstrates that electrical stimulation can modulate pain.[56-59] Melzack and Wall first proposed that electrical stimulation may reduce the sensation of pain by interfering with its transmission at the spinal cord level.[7] This approach to pain control is known as the *gate control theory* of pain and is described in detail in Chapter 3 of this book.

Noxious stimuli are transmitted from the periphery along small myelinated A-delta nerves and small unmyelinated C nerve fibers. According to the gate control theory, activation of nonnociceptor A-beta nerve fibers can inhibit transmission of noxious stimuli from the spinal cord to the brain. Electrical stimulation, when applied with appropriate parameters, can selectively activate A-beta nerves. Because pain perception is determined by the relative activity of A-delta and C fibers compared with A-beta fibers, when greater A-beta activity is produced by electrical stimulation, pain perception is decreased.[60]

A-beta nerves can be activated by both short and long duration electrical current pulses.[61] However, short duration pulses, lasting for between 50 to 80 μseconds, and with a current amplitude that produces a comfortable level of sensation, selectively activate these nerves. Pulse frequencies of 100 to 150 pps are generally found to be most comfortable for this application. This application of electrical stimulation is known as *conventional* or *high rate TENS*. Because the primary pain-modulating effects of conventional transcutaneous electrical nerve stimulation (TENS) last only while the stimulation is being applied, this type of TENS should be applied at the time when the patient has pain and may be used 24 hours a day if necessary. Conventional TENS can also interrupt the pain-spasm-pain cycle, thereby resulting in some reduction of pain after the stimulation stops. The pain is reduced directly by the electrical stimulation, and this indirectly reduces muscle spasms, further reducing pain unless the muscle spasm recurs.

The stimulus used for conventional TENS is generally modulated to limit adaptation. Adaptation is a decrease in the frequency of action potentials, and a decrease in the subjective sensation of stimulation, while electrical stimulation is applied if there are no changes in the applied stimulus. Adaptation is a known property of sensory receptors caused by decreased excitability of the nerve membrane with repeated stimulation. Modulation of any of the stimulation parameters, including frequency, pulse duration, or current amplitude, is likely to equally effectively help prevent adaptation to the stimulus.

It has also been proposed that electrical stimulation may control pain by stimulating the production and release of endorphins and enkephalins. These substances, known as *endogenous opiates,* act in a manner similar to morphine and are known to modulate pain perception. They modulate pain by binding to opiate receptors in the brain and other areas and acting as neurotransmitters and neuromodulators.[62] They also activate descending inhibitory pathways that involve nonopioid (serotonin) systems. It has been shown that endorphin and enkephalin levels are increased following the application of electrical stimulation.[63] Stimulation with pulsed currents with frequencies of less than 10 pps have been found to most effectively increase endorphin and enkephalin levels,[64] and a recent study found that naloxone, a mu opioid receptor blocker, blocks the analgesia produced by low frequency TENS (4 pps) but not that produced by high frequency TENS (100 pps), whereas naltrindole, a delta opioid receptor blocker, blocks only the analgesia produced by high frequency TENS.[65]

It is thought that electrical stimulation can cause endogenous opiate production and release. This may be caused by repetitive muscle contraction or repetitive stimulation of nociceptive A-delta nerves. For this application a longer pulse duration and higher current amplitude than used for conventional TENS are required because motor nerves, and possibly A-delta nerves, must be depolarized. Lower frequencies of 2 to 10 pps are usually used for this application in order to minimize the risk of muscle soreness. This application of electrical stimulation is known as *low rate* or *acupuncture-like* TENS. Low rate TENS will usually control pain for 4 to 5 hours after a 20- to 30-minute treatment. It is effective for this amount of time because the half-life of the endogenous opiates released is approximately $4^1/_2$ hours. Low rate TENS should not be applied for more than 30 minutes at a time because prolonging the repetitive muscle contraction produced by the stimulus can result in delayed onset muscle soreness.

Another form of transcutaneous electrical stimulation also used for pain modulation is known as *burst mode* TENS. This mode of TENS is thought to work by the same mechanisms as low rate TENS but may be more effective or better tolerated. For burst mode TENS, the stimulation is delivered in bursts, or packages, composed of a number of pulses each (see Fig. 8-17).

Electrical stimulation may also control pain when the electrodes are placed on acupuncture points. This method of application is thought to stimulate energy flow along acupuncture meridians that connect acupuncture points in the body.[66,67]

Tissue Healing

A number of studies have shown that electric stimulation can promote tissue healing.[9,10] Gardner, Frantz, and Schmidt's recent metaanalysis of the effects of electrical stimulation on chronic wound healing found that in the majority of clinical trials, electrical stimulation was associated with faster healing.[68] They evaluated four different types of electrical currents for this application: low intensity direct current (LIDC), high voltage pulsed current (HVPC), AC, and TENS (i.e., sensory level pulsed biphasic current). For all types of electrical current, electrical stimulation was associated with faster wound healing. Although the usual control treatment in the clinical trials varied, the treatment of the control samples in at least 10 of the studies appeared to be standardized. Moist dressings were used on the majority of controls, and whirlpool was used in a few cases. At least a number of the control samples were treated with an electrical stimulation placebo. Fifteen studies were included in the final metaanalysis. The most common measure used to report change was percentage of healing per week. The net effect of electrical stimulation across all studies evaluated was 13% increased healing per week, which represents a 144% increase over the control rate of healing. When wounds were categorized by type it was found that electrical stimulation was most effective for accelerating the healing of pressure ulcers. The proposed mechanisms by which electrical stimulation promotes tissue healing include attraction of appropriate cell types to the area, activation of these cells by altering cell membrane function, modification of endogenous electrical potential of the tissue in concert with healing potentials, reduction of edema, enhancement of antimicrobial activity, and promotion of circulation.

Specific cells, including neutrophils, macrophages, lymphocytes and fibroblasts, can be attracted to an injured healing area by an electrical charge because the cells themselves carry a charge.[69,70] This process of attraction is known as *galvanotaxis*. Activated neutrophils, which are present when a wound is infected or inflamed, are attracted to the negative pole, while inactive neutrophils move toward the positive pole. Macrophages and epidermal cells are also attracted to the positive pole while lymphocytes, platelets, mast cells, keratinocytes, and fibroblasts are attracted to the negative pole. It is generally recommended that, in order to attract the most appropriate cell types, the negative electrode be used for treatment of infected or inflamed wounds and the positive electrode be used if there is necrosis without inflammation and when the wound is in the proliferative stage of healing.[71]

Not only can electrical stimulation attract cells to an injury site, it has also been shown to enhance fibroblast replication and increase the synthesis of DNA and collagen by fibroblasts.[72,73] Fibroblasts and the collagen they produce are essential for the proliferation phase of tissue healing. The proposed mechanism of enhanced cell function is the triggering of calcium channel opening in the fibroblast cell membrane by the electrical current pulse. The open channels allow calcium to flow into the cells, increasing intracellular calcium levels to induce exposure of additional insulin receptors on the cell surface. Insulin can bind to the exposed receptors, stimulating the fibroblasts to synthesize collagen and DNA.[74] This

sequence of events is voltage dependent, with a maximum calcium influx and protein and DNA synthesis occurring when a high volt pulsed current with a peak voltage in the range of 60 to 90 V is applied. Both higher and lower voltages have less effect. Electrical stimulation can also promote epidermal cell and lymphocyte migration, proliferation, and function.[75]

When skin and cell membranes are intact they have an electrical charge across them due to the action of the sodium/potassium pumps. When tissue is injured, thereby rupturing cell membranes, charged ions leak out of the cell, causing the wound and the adjacent area to become positively charged relative to the surrounding uninjured tissue.[76,77] This has been demonstrated in children with accidental finger amputations where the stump tips were positively charged relative to the uninjured forearm.[78] This electrical potential difference steadily declines over time, returning to normal only after the wound closes.

Electrical stimulation can also reduce the amount of edema formed with acute injury and inflammation.[79] This application of electrical stimulation has been studied extensively by Fish, Mendel and coworkers.[10,80-83] The application of electrical stimulation during the acute stage of tissue healing can retard edema formation but has not been shown to decrease the amount of edema already present. This effect has been demonstrated in animal studies with negative polarity high voltage pulsed current (HVPC) at below the threshold for motor contraction.[84] Positive polarity stimulation has been found not to affect edema formation.[83]

A number of theories have been suggested for how HVPC alters microvascular permeability to plasma proteins and reduces edema formation. One proposal suggests that the negative charge of cathodal stimulation repels the negatively charged serum proteins, essentially blocking their movement out of blood vessels. Another theory is that the current decreases blood flow by reducing microvessel diameter, although cathodal stimulation has not been shown to have an effect on microvessel diameter.[85] Still another suggested mechanism involves a reduction in pore size in the microvessel walls, thereby preventing large plasma protein leakage through pores. In the normal histamine response to acute trauma, these pores would be enlarged. Prior studies listed have found that both negative polarity and positive polarity HVPC decrease microvessel permeability, suggesting that some other mechanism is likely to underlie the reduced edema formation produced by negative polarity stimulation only.

Although it has been suggested that electrical stimulation may enhance tissue healing by having antimicrobial activity, studies suggest that this is unlikely. In order to inhibit bacterial growth, electrical currents must be applied either at much higher voltages or for much longer times than used in the clinical setting.[86-90]

It is also possible that electrical stimulation facilitates tissue healing by increasing circulation. However, studies have shown that a muscle contraction is generally required for electrical stimulation to increase circulation, while tissue healing has been shown to be enhanced by submotor levels of stimulation.[36,41,42,91]

Most studies use similar electrical stimulation parameters to promote wound healing. Negative polarity is generally used during the early inflammatory stage of healing, while positive polarity is generally used later to facilitate epithelial cell migration across the wound bed. Kloth recommends using negative polarity for the first 3 to 7 days of treatment and changing to positive polarity thereafter; however, some researchers recommend using negative polarity for all treatments.[41,42,92] Alternatively, it has been recommended that polarity be switched when wound healing reaches a plateau. Another recommendation is to use negative polarity initially and for 3 days after the wound bed becomes free of necrotic tissue and the drainage becomes serosanguinous, and thereafter to use positive polarity.[93,94]

The pulse duration recommended when using HVPC to promote wound healing is between 40 and 100 μseconds. This parameter is generally preset in the device by the manufacturer and cannot be changed by the clinician. The current amplitude should be sufficient to produce a comfortable sensation without a motor response. The pulse frequency should be between 100 and 125 pps. At this time, the majority of studies recommend treating for at least 5 days each week with each treatment lasting for 45 to 60 minutes.

Transdermal Drug Delivery

Transdermal drug delivery (Iontophoresis) is the use of a low voltage DC for moving charged ions across the dermal barrier. The use of iontophoresis was first reported in the early 1900s.[95,96] The primary route of ion transport across or through the skin is thought to be through the skin pores and hair follicles.[97,98] In the past, iontophoresis has been described as "driving the ions through the skin."[99] However, more recent studies suggest that iontophoresis may promote transdermal drug penetration primarily by increasing the permeability of the stratum corneum, the main barrier to transdermal drug uptake.[100-102]

The depth of drug delivery with iontophoresis is uncertain. Most studies have demonstrated penetration to a depth of 3 mm to 20 mm.[103] For example, in comparing iontophoretic delivery with passive delivery of salicylic acid and lidocaine to rats it was found that both drugs penetrated 3 to 4 mm below the skin when delivered by iontophoresis if the epidermis was intact or by passive delivery if the epidermis was removed.[104] Penetration was negligible with passive delivery when the epidermis was not removed. Passive delivery was the application of the drug to the skin without additional enhancement. The authors of this study concluded that iontophoresis allows salicylic acid and lidocaine to penetrate through the stratum corneum. Another study demonstrated that sodium ethanolamine and lidocaine could be detected up to 2 cm laterally away from the iontophoresis treatment electrode in the intact skin of rats.[105] Declining drug concentration with distance was thought to be due to clearance from the site of application by the skin's microcirculation, resulting in systemic uptake of the drug.

For an electrical current to be effective to facilitate transdermal drug penetration the current must be at least sufficient to overcome the combined resistance of the skin and the electrode being used.[106] The amount of electricity used for performing iontophoresis is described in milliamp minutes (mA.minutes). This is the product of the current amplitude, measured in millamps, and the time, measured in minutes. The number of mA.minutes to be used depends on the specific electrode being used and is determined by the manufacturer of the electrode. At this time most manufacturers recommend treating for 40 mA.minutes for each iontophoresis treatment. In the past the recommended dose has ranged from 28 to 80 milliamp minutes. Studies have shown effective drug delivery with a range of 40 to 80 mA. minute treatments.[107]

One can use a number of combinations to achieve the currently recommended 40 mA.minute dosage level. For example, a 1 milliamp current for 40 minutes, a 2 milliamp current for 20 minutes, or a 4 milliamp current for 10 minutes, all give a 40 mA.minute treatment (Table 8-1). In practice, one should set the current amplitude to patient comfort and then adjust the time to produce the desired product. Typical treatment current amplitudes reported are between 1.0 mA.minutes and 5.0 mA.minutes; however, currently available clinical devices only allow a maximum current amplitude of 4.0 mA.minutes.[108]

In order to promote continuous delivery of the ionized drug, a direct current must be used for iontophoresis. Unfortunately, this type of current can also produce undesirable chemical changes under the electrodes. Sodium hydroxide, which is caustic, can form under the negative electrode, causing discomfort, skin irritation, or chemical burns.[109] This is known as the *alkaline reaction*. Reducing the current density by making the negative electrode larger will help decrease the risk of adverse effects. Hydrochloric acid can form under the positive electrode. This is known as the *acidic reaction* and is generally less uncomfortable than the alkaline reaction.

Many different drugs can be delivered by iontophoresis as long as they can be ionized and are stable in solution, are not altered by the application of an electrical current, and are small or moderate in size. Different drugs have been used for the treatment of different pathologies (Table 8-2); however, at this time the manufacturers of iontophoresis elec-

TABLE 8-1 Current Amplitude and Treatment Duration for Iontophoresis Treatment

Current amplitude (mA)	Treatment time (minutes)	Dose in mA.minutes
1	40	40
2	20	40
3	13.3	40
4	10	40

trodes recommend using iontophoresis only for delivering dexamethasone or lidocaine.

Dexamethasone is a corticosteroid with antiinflammatory action that is recommended for treatment of inflammatory conditions such as tendonitis or bursitis. Dexamethasone is delivered by iontophoresis, using a 0.4% solution of dexamethasone sodium phosphate. The negative polarity electrode is used to promote the penetration of the negatively charged dexamethasone phosphate ion through the skin (Fig. 8-25).

Lidocaine is an anesthetic drug. In the past, dexamethasone and lidocaine were delivered together by iontophoresis, with a positive charge being used initially to promote lidocaine delivery and then a negative charge

TABLE 8-2 Ions Used Clinically for Iontophoresis, Including Ion Source, Polarity, Recommended Indications, and Concentration

Ion	Source	Polarity	Indications	Concentration (%)
Acetate	Acetic acid	−	Calcium deposits	2.5–5
Chloride	NaCl	−	Sclerolytic	2
Copper	$CuSO_4$	+	Fungal infection	2
Dexamethasone phosphate	$DexNa_2PO_3$	−	Inflammation	0.4
Hyaluronidase	Wydase	+	Edema reduction	
Iodine		−	Scar	5
Lidocaine	Lidocaine @ 1:50,000 with epinephrine	+	Local anesthetic	5
Magnesium	$MgSO_4$	+	Muscle relaxant, vasodilator	
Salicylate	NaSal	−	Inflammation, plantar warts	2
Tap water		±	Hyperhidrosis	
Zinc	ZnO_2	+	Dermal ulcers, wounds	

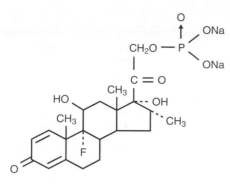

Figure 8-25. The molecular structure of dexamethasone sodium phosphate. Note that the negatively charged dexamethasone phosphate ion is moved across the dermal barrier by iontophoresis using the negatively charged electrode.

being used to promote dexamethasone delivery.[110] This combined procedure mimicked the combined application of lidocaine and dexamethasone by injection and provided chemical buffering. However, because ion-tophoresis should not be as painful as an injection, the lidocaine is not needed. Also, newer electrodes are buffered, adding to the safety of the treatment. It is therefore recommended that dexamethasone be delivered alone with the negative electrode only. The manufacturers of iontophoresis electrodes have recommended lidocaine iontophoresis for local anesthesia in children; however, this technique has not gained much popularity.

ELECTRICAL CURRENT IN CLINICAL PRACTICE

Contraindications, Precautions, and Application Techniques

The use and application of electrical stimulation is not without risks. There are widely accepted contraindications and precautions that have been established to ensure the best clinical practice and application of these tools. These contraindications and precautions are presented below:

CONTRAINDICATIONS
for Electrical Stimulation

- Demand cardiac pacemaker or arrhythmias
- Placement of electrodes over carotid sinus
- Areas of venous or arterial thrombosis or thrombophlebitis
- Pregnancy—over or around the abdomen or low back

The use of electric stimulation is contraindicated...

. . . in patients with a demand pacemaker or known arrhythmias

Electrical stimulation devices should not be used on patients with demand cardiac pacemakers as electrical stimulation may interfere with the functioning of this type of pacemaker and could alter the heart rate. Electrical stimulation may also aggravate an unstable arrhythmia that is not treated with a pacemaker.

ASK THE PATIENT:
- Do you have a cardiac pacemaker?
- Do you have a history of heart problems or have you been treated for heart problems?
- What type of heart problems?
- How recently has your doctor checked your heart? If the patient has a pacemaker, do not apply electrical stimulation.

If the patient is unsure of his/her cardiac status, or has recently had episodes of cardiac arrhythmias or pain, the therapist should consult with the referring physician to rule out the possibility of cardiac compromise during the use of electrical stimulation as a treatment modality.

. . . over the carotid sinus.

Care should be taken to avoid placement of electrodes on the anterior or lateral neck in the areas over the carotid sinuses as stimulation to these areas may induce a rapid fall in blood pressure that may cause the patient to faint.

. . . over areas of venous or arterial thrombosis or thrombophlebitis.

Stimulation should not be placed over areas of known venous or arterial thrombosis or thrombophlebitis because stimulation may increase circulation, increasing the risk of releasing emboli.

Continued

CONTRAINDICATIONS—cont'd

ASK THE PATIENT:
- Do you have a blood clot in this area?

ASSESS:
- Check the area for increased swelling, redness, and increased tenderness. If any of these are present, do not apply electrical stimulation until the possibility of a thrombus has been ruled out.

. . . over the pelvis, abdomen, trunk and low back area during pregnancy.

The effects of electrical stimulation on the developing fetus and on the pregnant uterus have not been determined. Therefore it is recommended that stimulation electrodes not be placed in any way that the current may reach the fetus. Electrodes should not be applied to the low back, abdomen, or hips (as might be the case for bursitis), where the path of the current might cross the uterus.

Occasionally, electric stimulation is used for pain control during labor and delivery as an alternative to general anesthesia or a spinal block.[111-113] Electrodes can be placed on the low back or on the anterior lower abdominal region, depending on where the pain is felt. The patient increases the current amplitude during a contraction and turns the amplitude down or off between contractions.

ASK THE PATIENT:
- Are you pregnant?
- Might you be pregnant?
- Are you trying to get pregnant?

The patient may not know if she is pregnant, particularly in the first few days or weeks after conception. Because damage may occur early during development, electrical stimulation should not be applied in any area where the current may reach the fetus of a patient who is or might be pregnant.

PRECAUTIONS
For Electrical Stimulation

- Cardiac disease
- In patients with impaired mentation or in areas with impaired sensation
- Malignant tumor
- Areas of skin irritation or open wounds
- Iontophoresis after other physical agents

Electrical stimulation should be applied with caution . . .

. . . to patients with a known history of cardiac disease, previous myocardial infarction, or other specifically known congenital or acquired cardiac abnormalities

ASK THE PATIENT:
- Do you have a known history of cardiac disease?
- Have you had a previous myocardial infarction?
- Have you ever had rheumatic fever as a child or an adult?
- Are you aware of having any cardiac problems at this time?

ASSESS:
- Check for surgical incisions in the thoracic area, both anteriorly and posteriorly.
- Check the patient's resting pulse and respiratory rate before initiating treatment and check for changes in these values during and/or after applying electrical stimulation.

. . . to patients with impaired mentation or in areas with impaired sensation

The patient's sensation and reporting of pain are usually used to limit the intensity of current applied to within safe limits. If the patient cannot report or feel pain, electrical stimulation must be applied with caution and close attention must be paid to any possible adverse effects. In addition, patients with impaired mentation may also be agitated and try to pull off the stimulation electrodes. Electrical stimulation may be used to treat chronic open wounds in areas with decreased sensation by first determining the appropriate current amplitude in an area with intact sensation.

ASSESS:
- Sensation in the area.
- Patient orientation and level of alertness.
- Patient agitation.

. . . to patients with known malignant tumors

Although there is no research concerning the effects of applying electrical stimulation to malignant tumors, since electrical currents can enhance tissue growth, in most cases it is recommended that electrical stimulation not be applied to patients with known or suspected malignant tumors. Electrical stimulation should not be applied to any area of the body of a patient with a malignancy because malignant tumors can metastasize to areas beyond where they are first found or known to be. Occasionally, electrical stimulation is used to control pain in patients with known malignancy. This is done when the improvement in quality of life afforded by this intervention is considered to be greater than the possible risks associated with the treatment.

ASK THE PATIENT:
- Have you ever had cancer? Do you have cancer now?
- Do you have fever, sweats, chills, or night pain?
- Do you have pain at rest?
- Have you had recent unexplained weight loss?

. . . over skin irritations or open wounds.

Electrodes should not be placed over abraded skin or known open wounds unless the electrical stimulation is being used to treat the wound. Open or damaged skin should be avoided because it has lower impedance and less sensation than intact skin and this may result in too much current being delivered to the area.

ASSESS:
- Inspect the patient's skin carefully prior to placing electrodes.
- Check for increased redness, swelling, warmth, rashes or broken and abraded areas.

. . . when iontophoresis is being considered after another physical agent.

It is recommended that iontophoresis not be applied after the application of any physical agent, such as heat, ice, or ultrasound, which may alter skin permeability. In addition, heat will cause vasodilation and increased blood flow that can accelerate dispersion of the drug from the treatment area.

ADVERSE EFFECTS OF ELECTRICAL STIMULATION:
- Electrical burns
- Skin reactions to the electrodes
- Pain

There are very few potential adverse effects from the clinical application of electrical currents. Careful evaluation of the patient and review of the patient's pertinent medical history and current medical status will minimize the likelihood of any adverse effects. In addition, patients should be monitored throughout the initial treatment with electrical stimulation for any adverse effects of the stimulation. If a patient is provided with an electrical stimulation unit for home use, the patient should be clearly instructed in its use and in early identification of potential adverse effects.

Electrical currents can cause burns. This effect is seen most commonly when a direct current is being applied. This is because direct current is always on, unlike pulsed current, resulting in high total charge delivery and high skin impedance. In addition, the chemical effects produced under direct current electrodes can be caustic. If there is not enough conduction medium on an electrode, as can occur with repeated use of self-adhesive electrodes or poorly applied nonadhesive electrodes, the risk of burns also increases due to the increased current density in the areas where there is adequate conduction.

Skin irritation or inflammation may occur in the area where electrical stimulation electrodes are applied because the patient is allergic to the contact surface of the electrode, such as the adhesive or foam rubber. If this occurs, a different type of electrode should be tried.

Some patients find electrical stimulation to be painful. In such patients, increasing the current amplitude slowly over a longer period of time may be better tolerated. In patients who find all forms of electrical stimulation painful, other treatment approaches should be used.

Additionally, the student and clinician should be aware of research-based application techniques that may be used across the spectrum of the modality.

This section provides guidelines for the sequence of procedures required for the safe and effective application of therapeutic electrical stimulation.

APPLICATION TECHNIQUE
Electrical Stimulation

1. Assess the patient and set treatment goals.
2. Determine if electrical stimulation is the most appropriate treatment modality.
3. Determine that electrical stimulation is not contraindicated for this patient or for the specific diagnosis you are treating. Check with the patient and review the patient's chart for contraindications or precautions regarding the application of electrical stimulation.
4. Select an electrical stimulation unit with the necessary waveform and adjustable parameters for the treatment (pain modulation, muscle contraction, tissue healing, etc.)
5. Explain treatment procedure to the patient, including an explanation of what he/she might expect to experience, and any instructions or directions regarding patient participation with the electrical stimulation.
6. Position the patient appropriately and comfortably for the treatment.
7. Inspect the skin where the treatment is to be applied for any signs of abrasions or skin irritation. Clean the skin and clip hair if necessary for good adhesion of the electrode to the skin, and thus good current flow. The hair should not be shaved as this can cause skin cuts or abrasions.
8. Check electrodes and lead wires for continuity or signs of excessive wear and replace any of those found faulty or of concern.
9. Apply the electrodes to the area being treated. Use conductive gel if electrodes are not pregelled. Use the appropriate size and number of electrodes to address the problem. For specific information on electrode selection and placement, please see the sections below on these topics.
10. Attach the lead wires to electrodes and to the stimulation unit.
11. Set optimal parameters for treatment including pulse frequency, pulse (phase) duration—if applicable to specific unit—, on/off time, ramp up/ramp down, and length of treatment time. For specific information on parameter selection for different treatment effects, please see Tables 8-3 to 8-5 and the section on parameter selection below.
12. Slowly advance the amplitude until the patient is just able to notice a sensation under the electrodes. If a muscle contraction is needed to achieve the treatment objectives, continue to increase the amplitude control until a visible contraction is apparent. If the patient complains of discomfort, decrease the current amplitude to a sensory level. It may take more than one treatment to familiarize a patient with the equipment and procedure and to make them comfortable with the necessary level of stimulation to produce the desired outcome. When electrical stimulation is applied to promote tissue healing, where a patient may be insensate, it is necessary to be more cautious and use an alternate area to establish sensory level prior to placing electrodes in or around a wound.
13. Observe the patient's reaction to the stimulation over the first few minutes of the treatment. If the treatment includes muscle strengthening, observe the amplitude and quality of the contraction. Question the patient regarding the expected outcome and adjust parameters based on the patient's response. The parameters may need to be adjusted or the electrodes may need to be moved slightly if the expected outcome is not achieved.
14. When the treatment is completed, remove the electrodes and inspect the patient's skin for any signs of adverse reaction to the treatment.
15. Document the treatment, including electrode placement, the parameters, waveform, and the patient's response to the treatment.

PATIENT POSTIONING

Patient positioning is dictated by the area to be treated, the goal(s) of the treatment, and the device used. Primary to these three issues are patient comfort and modesty. Upper extremity set-ups require short sleeves or a halter top for women, while men may or may not be comfortable with their shirts off. With neck, upper and lower back, and hip set-ups, primarily used in pain control, the art of appropriate draping is essential. The clinician should ask the patient if they feel protected or covered enough by their clothing or additional sheets or towels the clinician has in place. If in doubt, an additional covering may add to a patient's comfort. For lower extremity set-ups, shorts are generally adequate and allow the patient to perform voluntary exercise with the stimulation in place.

When applying electrical stimulation for muscle strengthening, the limb should be secured to prevent motion through the range, with the joint that the stimulated muscles cross in mid-range. This will allow the patient to perform a strong isometric contraction in mid-range rather than moving through the range and then applying maximum force at the end of the available ROM. The limb may be secured by placing a barrier to motion in either direction or by using cuff weights to overpower the strength of the muscle. In addition, most treatment tables have positioning straps that can be used to facilitate both appropriate and comfortable positioning for the patient, while maintaining the joint in a single position to facilitate an isometric contraction.

ELECTRODE TYPES

Many different types of electrodes are available for use with electrical stimulation devices. The electrodes serve as the interface between the patient and the stimulator. They are connected from the machine to the electrodes by cables or lead wires. While there are electrodes that can be implanted in the tissues, only surface electrodes are discussed here. There are a number of considerations when selecting electrodes for electrical stimulation including material, conductive gel if needed, size, shape, and the tissues to be treated.

The electrodes most commonly used today are disposable and flexible and have a self-adhesive gel coating that serves as the conduction medium (Fig. 8-26). The conduction medium decreases resistance between the electrode and the skin. These self-adhesive electrodes may be designed for single use or for multiple uses over a period a month or more. Although many electrodes on the market may appear to be made with similar material and conductive gel, their conductivity, impedance, and comfort may differ. How often an electrode can be used depends on the nature of the gel coating. Once this coating starts to dry out, the current density becomes less uniform, causing uneven current delivery. In areas where the electrode is still able to conduct, the current density will be high, and this can cause the skin under the electrode to burn. Therefore electrodes must be inspected regularly and dry or discolored ones should be discarded.

More long-lasting electrodes are made of carbon-impregnated silicone rubber, stainless steel or aluminum (see Fig. 8-26). The carbon rubber electrodes

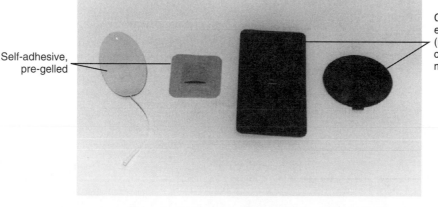

Self-adhesive, pre-gelled

Carbon-rubber electrodes (must add conductive medium)

Figure 8-26. Examples of different types of electrodes.

Continued

are used with a gel conduction medium, and the metal electrodes are used with a sponge soaked in normal tap water to promote conduction. Because these types of electrodes are not self-adhesive, they must be secured to the patient with tape, elastic straps, or bandages. Carbon rubber and other similar electrodes should be cleaned with warm, soapy water and not alcohol.

Selection of electrode size, shape, and type depends on the treatment goals, the area to be treated, and the amount of tissue or muscle bulk targeted. Because current density, which is the amount of current delivered per unit area, is inversely proportional to the size of the electrode, larger electrodes are more comfortable than smaller ones. However, large electrodes cannot target small areas.

ELECTRODE PLACEMENT

Electrode placement is critical to the outcome of treatment with electrical stimulation. Having determined the ideal electrode placement this should be documented, noting distance or approximation to bony landmarks or anatomical structures, so that follow-up sessions can replicate the placement. Diagrams are often helpful for this. In order to ensure even delivery of current, electrodes must lie smoothly against the skin with no wrinkles or gaps. Self-adhesive electrodes usually maintain good contact; however, with other types of electrodes, flexible bandaging is generally needed to maintain good electrode-to-skin contact. Electrodes should not be placed directly over bony prominences because the higher resistance of bone and the poor adhesion of electrodes to highly contoured surfaces increases the risk of discomfort and burns and is less likely to produce therapeutic benefits.

The distance or spacing between electrodes affects the depth and course of the current. The closer together electrodes are configured, the more superficially the current travels, and conversely, the greater the distance between them, the deeper the current travels (Fig. 8-27). When stimulating contraction of larger muscle groups such as the quadriceps, it is more comfortable and effective to place the electrodes over the proximal and distal ends of the muscle, so that the current travels parallel to the direction of the muscle fibers (Fig. 8-28). Electrodes should be at least two fingers' width, or one inch, apart when applied for pain control, and at least two inches apart when applied for motor contraction. Electrodes are placed further apart when stimulating a muscle contraction because the change in shape of the muscle during a contraction may move the electrodes close together.

When electrical stimulation is applied to produce a muscle contraction, one electrode should be placed over the motor point for the muscle. The motor point is the place where an electrical stimulus will produce the greatest contraction with the least amount of electricity and is the area of skin over the location where the motor nerve enters the muscle. Charts of motor points are available; however, because most motor points are over the middle of the muscle belly, it is generally easy and effective to place electrodes over the middle of the muscle belly. The second electrode should also be placed on the muscle to be stimulated, and, as noted above, with the two electrodes aligned parallel to the direction of the muscle fibers.

When electrical stimulation is used to control pain, a variety of electrode placements can be effective.[116] If two channels, and thus four electrodes are used, the electrodes can be placed to surround the area of pain.

Figure 8-27. The effect of electrode spacing. When the electrodes are closer together the current travels more superficially. When the electrodes are further apart the current goes deeper.

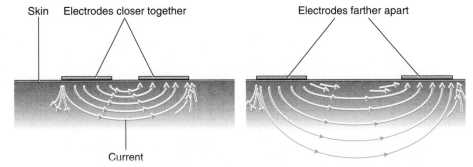

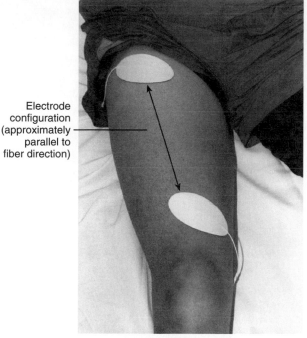

Electrode configuration (approximately parallel to fiber direction)

Figure 8-28. Electrodes placed over the proximal and distal ends of the quadriceps muscles for maximum efficacy.

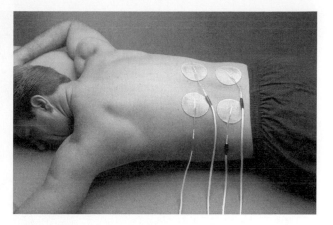

Figure 8-29. Electrodes placed over the low back for electrical stimulation treatment to control low back pain. (Courtesy Mettler Electronics, Anaheim, CA.)

The two channels can be placed so that they intersect, allowing the current to cross at the area of pain (Fig. 8-29) or they may be placed parallel, either horizontally or vertically. The two channels must intersect if an interferential current is desired. To change the flow of current, it is generally easier to switch the lead wires between electrodes rather than moving the electrodes themselves. Placement over trigger points or acupuncture points, which are generally areas of decreased skin resistance, has also been reported to be effective.[117] When the electrodes cannot be placed near or over the painful area, for example if the area is in a cast or local application of the electrodes is not tolerated, the electrodes can be placed proximal to the site of pain along the pathway of the sensory nerves supplying the area.[116]

When electrical stimulation is used for edema control, the therapist must determine whether the edema is due to acute inflammation or to lack of motion. For retarding the formation of edema due to acute inflammation, the negative polarity treatment electrode(s) should be placed directly over the area of edema, with the dispersive electrode more proximal if possible (Fig 8-30). To reduce edema caused by lack of motion, elec-

trically stimulated contractions of the muscles around the deep veins supplying the area can pump away the excess fluid. For this application the electrodes should be placed on the appropriate muscle in the same way as recommended for muscle contractions (Fig. 8-31).

For electrical stimulation to promote wound healing, the treatment electrodes may be placed in or around the wound (Fig. 8-32). One treatment electrode is used when stimulation is applied directly in the wound and two or more treatment electrodes may be used when the stimulation is applied to the area around the wound. If stimulation is applied directly to the wound, a single-use electrode constructed by the therapist should be used. This type of electrode is made of saline-soaked gauze placed directly in the wound. Aluminum foil or a single-patient, reusable electrode may be placed over the gauze. The electrode is attached to the lead wire with an alligator clip. If stimulation is applied to the intact tissue around the wound, the usual commercially available electrodes, as described above, may be used. One large dispersive electrode, of opposite polarity to the treatment electrode, should be placed close to the wound site to ensure delivery of current to the wound.

For iontophoresis the drug delivery electrode is placed over the area of pathology and the dispersive or return electrode is placed at least 6 inches away, at a site of convenience over a large muscle belly (Fig. 8-33). The drug delivery electrode should have the same polarity as the active ion of the drug to be delivered. Care should be taken to inspect the surrounding

Continued

APPLICATION TECHNIQUE—cont'd
Electrical Stimulation

Figure 8-30. Electrode placement to retard acute edema formation at the ankle.

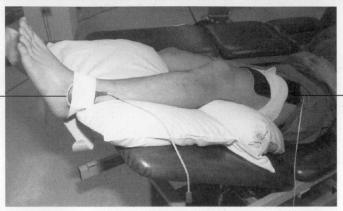

Negative treatment electrode

Positive polarity dispersive electrode

Figure 8-31. Electrode placement to reduce edema in the wrist and hand caused by lack of motion. (Courtesy Mettler Electronics, Anaheim, CA.)

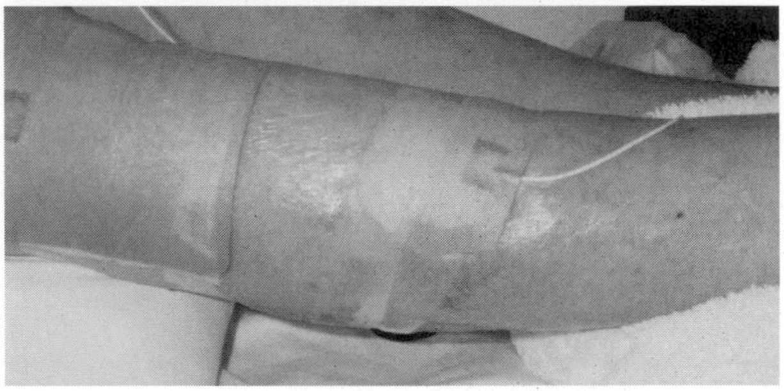

Figure 8-32. Electrode placement to promote tissue healing.

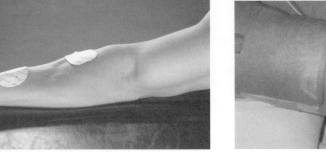

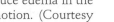

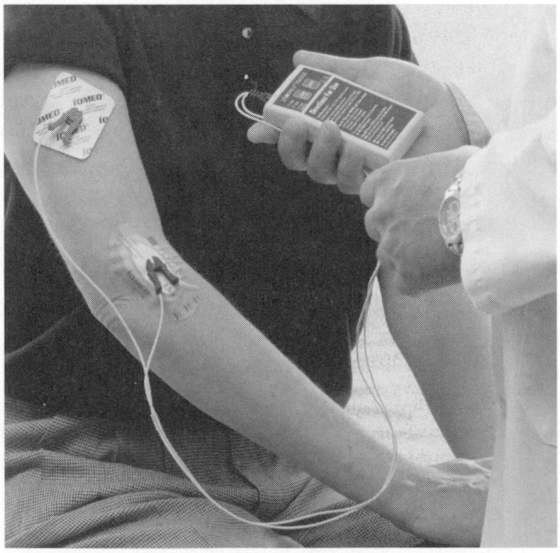

Figure 8-33. Electrode placement for iontophoresis. (Courtesy IOMED, Salt Lake City, Utah.)

skin area for abrasions. Current density must also be considered here. It is suggested in the literature that current density not exceed 0.5 mA/cm^2 when using the cathode as the delivery electrode and 1.0 mA/cm^2 if the anode is used.[41]

Parameter Selection

Although no one combination of electrical stimulation parameters will always be effective for a specific problem and treatment goal, with a thorough clinical assessment and an understanding of the effects of specific electrical currents parameters, the clinician can select parameters that are most likely to be effective (see Tables 8-3 to 8-5 for a summary of recommended treatment parameters). These parameters can then be rationally modified if the desired treatment goal is not achieved. The understanding of the contribution of each individual parameter and their interactions is essential for choosing the appropriate treatment regimen. A unit that allows manipulation of a variety of parameters is also necessary so that the clinician can select the most effective and comfortable stimulation parameters. Careful selection of treatment parameters will minimize discomfort while optimizing functional outcome with electrical stimulation.

Pulse duration

When using electrical stimulation to produce a muscle contraction in an innervated muscle, the pulse duration should be between 150 and 350 µs. Most units with an adjustable pulse duration allow a maximum duration of 300 µs, and many units intended to be used only for stimulation of muscle contractions have a fixed pulse duration of around 300 µs. If the pulse duration is adjustable, most patients find shorter pulse durations more comfortable when stimulating smaller muscles and longer pulsed durations more comfortable when stimulating larger muscles. In addition, for similar applications, smaller people and children also often find shorter pulse durations to be more comfortable and as effective as longer pulse durations. It is important to remember that as the pulse duration is shortened, a greater amplitude is required to achieve the same contraction as produced by a longer pulse duration. Selection of the ideal combination of pulse duration and current amplitude should be based both on patient comfort and achievement of the desired outcome of treatment.

Most clinical units with biphasic waveforms intended to be used for pain control, and most portable units intended for use for pain control (frequently called *TENS units*) allow the clinician to adjust the pulse duration of the symmetric or asymmetric biphasic waveform. When using a biphasic waveform for conventional TENS, the pulse duration should be between 50 and 80 µs in order to depolarize only the A-beta sensory nerves. When applying low rate acupuncture-like TENS, the pulse duration should be between 100 and 200 µs in order to depolarize the motor nerves and possibly the A-delta nerves. Interferential current is also frequently used for pain control. With interferential current the pulse duration is inversely proportional to the carrier frequency. If the carrier frequency is increased the pulse (cycle) duration will decrease, and if the carrier frequency is decreased the pulse duration will increase. Manufacturers may put a control for the carrier frequency but do not directly allow control of duration on units that deliver interferential current. When the carrier frequency is 2,500 Hz the cycle duration is 400 µs, when the carrier frequency is 4,000 Hz the cycle duration is 250 µs, and when the carrier frequency is 5,000 Hz the cycle duration is 200 µs. When using electrical stimulation to promote tissue healing or to inhibit the formation of edema during the acute inflammatory response, HVPC is the recommended waveform. Most units that can deliver HVPC do not allow the pulse duration to be altered. The pulse duration is fixed in the range of 40 to 100 µs and appears effective for these applications.

Frequency

Frequency determines the type of response or muscle contraction that electrical stimulation will produce. When a low frequency of less than approximately 30 pps is used to stimulate a motor nerve, each pulse will produce a separate muscle twitch contraction. As the frequency increases the twitches will occur more closely together, eventually summating to produce a smooth tetanic contraction. This requires approximately 35 to 50 pps. Increasing the frequency beyond the 35 to 50 pps range may produce greater muscle strengthening but will also result in more rapid fatigue during stimulation.[12,117,118]

Selection of frequency for pain control depends both on the selected mode (high rate or low rate TENS-like characteristics), as well as the waveform and parameter options available on the unit being used. With high rate TENS, the pulse frequency is selected in a range between 100 to 150 pps, while low rate requires the pulse frequency to be no greater than ten pps. Burst mode TENS units are generally preset

TABLE 8-3 Recommended Parameter Settings for Electrically Stimulated Muscle Contractions

Parameter settings/ treatment goal	Pulse frequency	Pulse duration	Amplitude	On/off times & ratio	Ramp time	Treatment time	Times/day
Muscle Strengthening	35-80 pps	150-200 µs for small muscles, 200-350 µs for large muscles.	To > 10% of MVIC* in injured, >50% MVIC in uninjured	6-10 sec on: 50-120 sec off, ratio of 1:5, initially. May reduce the off time with repeated treatments	At least 2 sec.	10-20 min to produce 10-20 repetitions	Every 2-3 hours when awake
Muscle Re-education (FES)	35-50 pps	150-200 µs for small muscles, 200-350 µs for large muscles.	Sufficient for functional activity	Depends on functional activity	At least 2 sec.	Depends on functional activity	N/A
Muscle Spasm Reduction	35-50 pps	150-200 µs for small muscles, 200-350 µs for large muscles.	To visible contraction	2-5 sec on: 2-5 sec off. Equal on:off times	At least 1 sec.	10-30 min	Every 2-3 hours until spasm relieved
Edema Reduction Using Muscle Pump	35-50 pps	150-200 µs for small muscles, 200-350 µs for large muscles.	To visible contraction	2-5 sec on: 2-5 sec off. Equal on: off times	At least 1 sec.	30 min	Twice a day

*MVIC = Maximum Voluntary Isometric Contraction

TABLE 8-4 Recommended Parameter Settings for Electrical Stimulation for Pain Control

Parameter settings	Pulse frequency (or beat frequency for interferrential)	Pulse duration	Amplitude	Modulation (of frequency, duration or amplitude)	Treatment time	Likely mechanism of action
Conventional (high rate)	100-150 pps	50-80 μs	To produce tingling	Use if available	May be worn 24 hours, as needed for pain control	Gating at the spinal cord
Acupuncture-like (low rate)	2-10 pps	100-200 μs	To visible contraction	None	20-30 minutes	Endorphin release
Burst mode	Generally preset in unit at 10 bursts	Generally preset and may have max of 100-300 μs	To visible contraction	Is generally not possible in burst mode	20-30 minutes	Endorphin release

TABLE 8-5 Recommended Parameter Settings for Electrical Stimulation for Tissue Healing, Edema Control and Iontophoresis

Parameter settings/ goal of treatment	Waveform	Pulse frequency	Pulse duration	Amplitude	Polarity	Treatment time
Tissue healing – inflammatory phase/infected	HVPC	60-125 pps	Usually preset for HVPC at 40-100 μs	To produce comfortable tingling	Negative	45–60 minutes
Tissue healing – proliferation phase/clean	HVPC	60-125 pps	Usually preset for HVPC at 40-100 μs	To produce comfortable tingling	Positive	45–60 minutes
Edema control – for edema due to inflammation	HVPC	120 pps	Usually preset for HVPC at 40-100 μs	To produce comfortable tingling	Negative	30 minutes
Edema control – for edema due to lack of motion	Biphasic (Can use interferential if on:off time available)	35-50 pps, 2-5 sec equal on:off times	150-350 μs	To visible contraction	N/A	30 minutes
Iontophoresis	DC	N/A	N/A	To patient tolerance, not greater than 4 mA	Same as drug ion. See Table 8-1	Depends on amplitude, to produce a total of 40 mA.minutes

by the manufacturer to provide 10 or fewer bursts each second, with the pulses within the burst being at 100 to 150 pps, thereby attempting to combine the effects of high rate and low rate TENS.

Pulse frequency for promoting tissue healing should be in a range of 60 to 125 pps. When electrical stimulation is used to control the formation of edema due to inflammation, the pulse frequency is set to 120 pps. However, when electrical stimulation is used to control more longstanding edema by muscle pumping, the parameters used are the same as those used for muscle reeducation with a frequency of 35 to 50 pps.

On:off time

Electrical stimulation is delivered continuously, throughout the treatment time, when applied for pain control, tissue healing, acute edema control and iontophoresis. When used to produce muscle contractions, an on:off time must be set in order to allow the muscles to both contract and relax during the treatment. The relaxation time is needed to limit fatigue.

When electrical stimulation is used for muscle strengthening, the recommended on time is in the range of 6 to 10 seconds and the recommended off time is in the range of 50 to 120 seconds, with an initial on:off ratio of 1:5. The long off time is required to minimize muscle fatigue. With subsequent treatments, as the patient gets stronger, the on:off ratio may be decreased to 1:4 or even 1:3. When the goal of electrical stimulation is to relieve a muscle spasm, the on:off ratio is set at 1:1, with both the on and off times being between 2 and 5 seconds, in order to produce muscle fatigue and relax the spasm. When the treatment is intended to pump out edema, the on:off ratio is also set at 1:1 with both the on and off times being between 2 and 5 seconds.

Ramp time

A ramp time may be needed when a muscle contraction is stimulated. The ramp time allows for a gradual increase and decrease of force rather than a sudden increase and decrease when switching from off time to on time. For most exercises and with longer on times, a ramp up and down of 1 to 4 seconds is recommended. However, some activities do not benefit and are actually impaired by a ramp time. For example, gait training or table activities, in which the muscles function for a very short time, may actually be completed before the stimulation reaches peak amplitude. In contrast, in a patient with spasticity, it may be necessary to have a long ramp time, of 4 to 8 seconds, in order to avoid stimulating a generalized increase in tone.

Current amplitude

When using electrical stimulation for muscle strengthening, the current amplitude is a critical parameter. An amplitude sufficient to produce a contraction of at least 50% of maximum voluntary isometric contraction (MVIC) strength is needed to increase strength in uninjured individuals. However, Snyder-Mackler and colleagues found that for patients recovering from anterior cruciate ligament reconstruction, those treated with a current amplitude that produced contractions of at least 10% of the MVIC of the uninjured limb had greater strength gains and faster functional recovery than controls who did not receive electrical stimulation.[119]

When electrical stimulation is used for muscle reeducation, the goal of treatment is functional outcome rather than maximum strength. Electrical stimulation can assist with functional recovery by providing sensory and proprioceptive feedback of normal motion as well as by enhancing muscle strength. For this purpose one may start with sensory level stimulation, which is the most comfortable, to allow the patient to become accustomed to the stimulation, and then increase the current amplitude to produce a contraction level within patient tolerance.

When electrical stimulation is used to reduce muscle spasms, the current amplitude need only be sufficient to produce a visible contraction.

In order to control pain with electrical stimulation, the treatment should be as comfortable as possible. For high rate TENS it is generally recommended that the amplitude be set to produce a gentle sensation only, likened to tingling or vibration. However, some authors recommend a strong or maximally tolerated level of sensory stimulation for this application. It is likely that different individuals respond best to different levels of sensory stimulation and that the ideal for a particular individual will need to be determined by the patient and the clinician. For low rate and burst TENS to be effective, the amplitude must be sufficient to produce a visible contraction.

When using electrical stimulation to promote tissue healing or to retard the formation of inflammatory edema, the current amplitude should be set to a comfortable sensory level. If the patient has decreased or altered sensation in the treatment area, the appropriate amplitude can be determined by first applying the electrode to another area with normal intact sensation.

Treatment time

The length of a particular treatment depends on patient tolerance and the goals of treatment. When using electrical stimulation for muscle strengthening, it is generally recommended that the treatment last long enough to allow for 10 to 20 contractions. This will usually take 10 to 20 minutes. This treatment session should be repeated multiple times throughout the day if the patient has an electrical stimulation device available for home use. When treating in the clinic, electrical stimulation is generally applied once for 10 to 20 minutes.

When electrical stimulation is used for muscle reeducation, the treatment time will vary base on the functional activity being addressed, but is generally no more than 20 minutes at a single session or less if a patients shows signs of inattentiveness or fatigue.

When using electrical stimulation for pain control using high rate TENS, a patient may wear a home unit at all times as needed to relieve pain. The low rate or burst mode TENS modes, if being used, should be applied for a maximum of 20 to 30 minutes every 2 hours. Low rate and burst mode TENS should not be used for longer periods because the muscle contractions they produce can cause delayed onset muscle soreness if the stimulation is applied for prolonged periods.

When electrical stimulation is used to promote tissue healing, whether in the infected or proliferation phase, it should be applied for 45 to 60 minutes per session, usually daily for at least 5 days per week. When used to control edema, whether inflammatory or due to lack of motion, electrical stimulation is generally applied for 30 minutes, but may be used more than once a day.

For iontophoresis the treatment time is affected by the current amplitude and should be adjusted to produce a total treatment dose of 40 mA.minutes. This is achieved by setting the amplitude to patient tolerance, although the amplitude should not exceed 4 mA, and then setting the treatment time to achieve the desired treatment dose (see Table 8-1). It is important to check the patient's skin during this treatment because the DC and the small electrodes used for iontophoresis produce a high current density, increasing the risk of burning the patient.

Documentation

Document the area of the body treated with electrical stimulation, the treatment duration, patient positioning, electrode placement, treatment parameters, and the response to treatment. Documentation is typically written in the SOAP note (Subjective, Objective, Assessment, Plan) format. The following examples only summarize the modality component of treatment and are not intended to represent a comprehensive plan of care.

EXAMPLES

When applying electrical stimulation (ES) to the right (R) knee for quadriceps muscle reeducation after right anterior cruciate ligament (ACL) reconstruction, document:

S: Pt. reports she is unable to independently perform the quad set exercise she was instructed to do last PT treatment.

O: ES to R quadriceps muscles × 20min. Electrodes placed over vastus medialis oblique muscle and proximal lateral anterior thigh. Biphasic waveform, pulse duration 300 msec, frequency 50 pps, on:off time 10sec:50sec, ramp up/ramp down 2sec/2sec, amplitude to produce maximum tolerated contraction. Pt instructed to attempt to contract quadriceps muscle with the ES.

A: Pt able to perform 2 visible quadriceps contractions independently following ES treatment.

P: D/C ES when pt can perform quad setting × 10 independently as part of home program.

When applying TENS for relief of acute pain in bilateral (B) upper trapezius and neck due to a motor vehicle accident (MVA), document:

S: Pt. c/o constant B trap area pain s/p MVA 10 days ago. He states he awakens 6–10 × each night secondary to neck pain. Pt. denies having pain, numbness, or tingling in his upper extremities.

O: TENS to B upper trap area × 30 min. 2 channels, 4 electrodes, 2 at level of cervical thoracic junction and 2 at level of proximal-medial scapulae, crossed channels. Biphasic waveform, pulse duration 70 msec, frequency 140 pps, with amplitude modulation. Pt set amplitude to his comfort. After 20 min of treatment pt notes a 50% decrease in his trap area discomfort. Pt instructed in appropriate application and use; he then correctly demonstrated set up and operation of unit. Given written instruction in use of TENS for independent home use. Pt to monitor the condition of his skin under the electrodes and D/C TENS if irritation or redness occurs. Pt to use TENS up to 24 hours/day for pain relief.

A: Decrease in pain intensity with TENS use. Pt demonstrated appropriate independent set up and use of TENS and understands precautions.

P: *Pt to use TENS independently at home up to 24 hrs/day for pain. Pt to call therapist at clinic if he has any questions or concerns re independent TENS use.*

When applying ES to a full thickness venous ulcer on the left lateral ankle, document:

S: *Pt alert and oriented × 3. She states she has been keeping her L lower extremity elevated as much as possible because the edema in her L ankle increases with dependent positioning.*

O: *Pt supine with 2 pillows under L leg for elevation. HVPC to L lower extremity × 1 hour. 2 treating electrodes placed peri-wound, 1dispersive electrode placed on proximal posterior calf. Frequency 100 pps, negative (−) polarity to treatment area, intensity to sensory level. Wound area decreased from 10 cm × 5 cm on first treatment 2/10/02 to 8 cm × 3 cm today month/day/year*

A: *Pt tolerated treatment well. Wound areas decreasing.*

P: *Continue HVPC to L lateral ankle area until wound closes. Change polarity if healing plateaus.*

▶ Clinical Case Studies ◀

The following case studies demonstrate the concepts of the clinical application of electrical stimulation discussed in this chapter. Based on the scenarios presented, an evaluation of the clinical findings and goals of treatment are proposed. These are followed by a discussion of the factors to be considered in the selection of electrical stimulation as the indicated treatment modality and in the selection of the ideal electrical stimulation parameters to promote progress toward the set goals.

Case 1

DS is a 28-year-old female who has been referred to physical therapy with a diagnosis of upper back and neck pain. DS complains of gradually increasing neck and upper trapezius pain over the past 6 weeks. She reports her pain is worse at the end of her work day as a supermarket checker. She notes that her pain has become more intense and frequent in the past month. DS states her pain increases with lifting, carrying, and any twisting motion of her neck. She has been evaluated by a physician, and her cervical spine x-rays were negative. She has no history of cardiac arrhythmias and does not have a pacemaker.

Significant objective findings include upper extremity active range of motion (ROM) within normal limits. Her upper extremity strength is 4+/5 bilaterally and is limited by neck pain. Her rhomboid and lower trapezius strength are 4–/5 bilaterally. Neck rotation and lateral flexion ROM are 75% of normal, with pain on overpressure bilaterally. Forward flexion is uncomfortable in the final 30% of the range. Extension is within normal limits. On palpation, there are significant nodules in bilateral upper trapezius and trigger points along the medial borders of both scapulae. DS denies numbness or tingling in her upper extremities.

EVALUATION OF CLINICAL FINDINGS
This patient presents with impairments of cervical and upper back pain, restricted cervical ROM, and decreased upper body strength. These impairments have resulted in difficulty with her normal functional activities, especially her work-related duties of lifting and carrying.

PREFERRED PRACTICE PATTERN
Impaired Posture, (4B)

PLAN OF CARE
Goals of treatment include controlling pain and regaining normal cervical ROM so the patient can perform her work duties and other functional activities. The goals of treatment would also include regaining normal upper body strength.

ASSESSMENT REGARDING THE APPROPRIATENESS OF ELECTRIC STIMULATION AS A COMPONENT OF THE OPTIMAL TREATMENT
TENS (transcutaneous electric nerve stimulation) is an indicated treatment for the reduction of pain. Other physical agents such as ultrasound or ice and heat might be used in conjunction with electrical stimulation. This patient has no contraindications to the use of electrical stimulation.

PROPOSED TREATMENT PLAN AND RATIONALE
It is proposed that electrical stimulation be used for the control of pain, with the patient being issued a unit to use at home following evaluation and instruction (Fig. 8-34). The following parameters are chosen:

Continued

❱ *Clinical Case Studies—cont'd* ❰

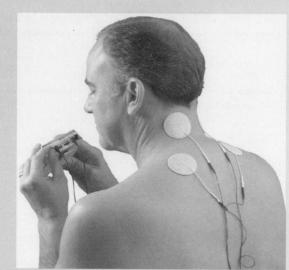

Figure 8-34. Treatment of upper back and neck pain with electrical stimulation. (Courtesy Rehabilicare, Inc., New Baighton, Minn.)

Electrode placement:	One pair of electrodes upper cervical, one pair lower cervical.
Waveform:	Pulsed biphasic (or interferential)
Pulse rate:	100-150 pps (or 100 bps-150 bps for interferential)
Pulse duration:	50-80 μseconds {suggest spell out as submitted}
Modulation:	Yes
Amplitude:	Sensory only – to patient comfort
Treatment duration:	The patient may wear the unit throughout the day for pain control.

The patient will initially feel a gentle humming or buzzing under the electrodes. Once comfortable, patient may switch the unit to modulation mode so there is little or no adaptation to the stimulus. Because the patient will have a home unit, she will be able to receive treatment throughout the day to minimize her pain at all times. DS will be reevaluated for revision of parameters as well as update of home exercise program weekly, with the frequency of visits decreasing as her problem is resolved. Use of the electrical stimulation is generally discontinued at the patient's request upon reaching tolerable resolution of pain.

If the patient is experiencing significant relief while wearing the TENS unit, she may use it at work. The lead wires can be placed under clothing, and the unit can be placed in a pocket or clipped onto a waistband. With present technology, amplitude controls are covered so that they cannot be accidentally moved, increasing or decreasing the current.

Case 2

VP is a 47-year-old male carpet layer who developed severe right medial knee pain 4 months ago. Arthroscopic surgery revealed a flap tear abrasion of the trochlear surface of the femur, which was then debrided. VP had his surgery 3 weeks ago and comes to your physical therapy clinic with an order from his surgeon to evaluate and treat. On palpation, there is mild warmth and tenderness of the patient's right knee. The surgical sites are healing well. His right patellar girth is 5 cm greater than his left. The right knee active ROM is from 10 to 50 degrees of flexion. VP is ambulating household distances without any assistive device but with his right knee in about 15 to 20 degrees of flexion during stance. He has 4/5 quadriceps strength on the right, within the available ROM.

EVALUATION OF CLINICAL FINDINGS

This patient presents with the impairments of pain, loss of motion, and increased girth of his right knee, resulting in the disabilities of limited ambulation and inability to work.

PREFERRED PRACTICE PATTERN

Impaired Joint Mobility, Motor Function, Muscle Performance, and Range of Motion Associated With Bony or Soft Tissue Surgery, (4I)

PLAN OF CARE

The goals of treatment at this time are to control pain and edema, and improve ROM, strength, and function.

ASSESSMENT REGARDING THE APPROPRIATENESS OF ELECTRICAL STIMULATION AS A COMPONENT OF THE OPTIMAL TREATMENT

Electric stimulation would be an appropriate treatment for this patient because it would facilitate the generation of a greater level of force than the patient would be able to generate of his own volition. This patient has no contraindications to the use of electrical stimulation. Electrically stimulated muscle contractions would help increase the patient's lower extremity strength and may assist in eliminating fluid from around his knee, both of which would contribute to functional improvements.

PROPOSED TREATMENT PLAN AND RATIONALE

It is proposed that electrical stimulation with either a biphasic square waveform or Russian protocol be used (Fig. 8-35). With a square wave the recommended parameters are:

Electrode placement:
> One channel is set up on the quadriceps with one electrode over the VMO and the second electrode at the proximal lateral anterior thigh. Placement may need to be varied slightly depending on quality of contraction and patient comfort. The second channel is placed on the hamstrings generally, also using large electrodes for comfort. The stimulation is applied alternately to the quadriceps and hamstrings, with a rest period in between. The channels should not run simultaneously as this would produce a cocontraction of the quads and hamstrings.

Pulse duration:
> 200-350 µs (based on patient comfort, with longer durations used for larger muscles).

Pulse frequency:
> 50 pps-80 pps to achieve a smooth tetanic contraction.

On/off time:
> 10 s on/50 s off to initiate treatment, moving to 10/30 as the patient progresses.

Ramp up/ramp down Time:
> 2-3 s ramp up/2 s ramp down for comfort.

Amplitude:
> 10%-50% of MVIC muscle contraction, as tolerated. The patient should be encouraged to actively contract with the stimulation if he is able.

Treatment time:
> Sufficient to produce 10 to 20 contractions. If available, the patient should use a portable stimulation device at home 3 to 4 times a day, in order to accelerate his recovery.

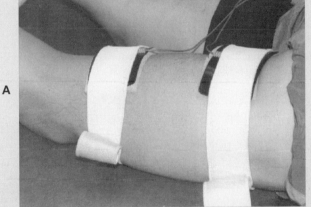

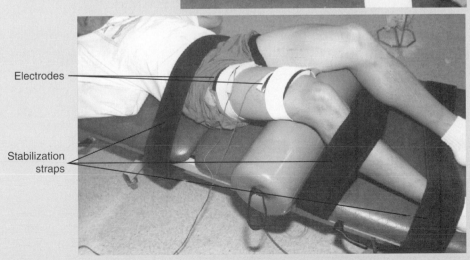

Figure 8-35. Electrical stimulation to increase hamstring **A**, and **B**, quadriceps strength.

Continued

▶ *Clinical Case Studies—cont'd* ◀

Case 3

MC is a 23-year-old student. He injured his left ankle during a soccer game at school. He was seen by the attending physician on the field and diagnosed with a Grade II lateral ankle sprain. MC's ankle was packed in ice and he was sent to the locker room for immediate physical therapy follow-up. Given the mechanism of injury, there is most likely an active inflammatory process occurring. The physician instructed MC to be nonweight bearing on crutches to rest the injured ankle. Visual inspection shows patient holding ankle in a single position with extreme hesitancy in allowing the therapist to move the joint. Gentle passive ROM reveals restrictions in all directions. There is minimal active ROM. The joint is tender to touch, with discoloration indicative of internal bleeding along the lateral surface and the inability to view the lateral malleolus due to swelling. The area is warm to the touch and slightly reddened. The student is otherwise healthy and denies a history of cancer, diabetes, or other significant health problems.

EVALUATION OF CLINICAL FINDINGS

The patient presents with impairments of pain, edema, and decreased ROM, resulting in limited ambulation.

PREFERRED PRACTICE PATTERN

Impaired Joint Mobility, Motor Function, Muscle Performance, and Range of Motion Associated With Connective Tissue Dysfunction, (4D)

PLAN OF CARE

The goals of treatment at this time are to control edema and pain, accelerate the resolution of the acute inflammatory phase of healing, and speed the recovery of ROM and function.

ASSESSMENT REGARDING THE APPROPRIATENESS OF ELECTRICAL STIMULATION AS THE OPTIMAL TREATMENT

Electrical stimulation using high voltage pulsed current would be an appropriate choice of treatment as it has been shown to retard the formation of edema during the inflammatory stage of injury. It is also known to help control pain. There is nothing in the patient's history to indicate a contraindication to using electrical stimulation.

PROPOSED TREATMENT PLAN AND RATIONALE

Electrical stimulation, using a high voltage pulsed current (HVPC) waveform, is chosen based on the literature indicating that it is effective at decreasing edema formation after injury (see Fig. 8-30). The following parameters are chosen:

Electrode placement:	One or two treating electrodes may be used over the swollen, discolored area. (Polarity is negative for treating electrodes.) The larger dispersive electrode is placed proximally over either the calf or the quadriceps. This may be based on comfort or other suspected areas of swelling. Ice may be added over the electrodes to further inhibit the formation of edema.
Pulse duration:	Generally fixed at 40-100 μs for HVPC.
Pulse frequency:	120 pps
Mode:	Continuous
Amplitude:	Sensory **ONLY**. Ask the patient to state when a tingling or vibratory sensation just begins to occur. Continue to increase the amplitude until it reaches the maximum tolerable level. If a contraction is seen, decrease the amplitude.
Treatment time:	30 minutes

Chapter Review

This chapter assists the clinician in understanding the basic principles of how electric stimulation works and how it can best be applied clinically for patient rehabilitation. The basis for most uses of electrical stimulation is its ability to excite nerves to produce an action potential (AP). Once an AP is generated by an electrical current, the body responds to it in the same way as it does to an AP that is physiologically generated. An electrically stimulated AP can produce a muscle contraction or it can produce a pleasant or noxious sensation. Electrically stimulated APs can be used for many purposes, including muscle strengthening, functional activities, and the control of pain and edema. Electrical currents can also have ionic effects. These may be used to facilitate tissue healing, control the formation of inflammatory edema, and promote transdermal drug penetration. By understanding the language and the effects of electric currents, the clinician can select the ideal treatment parameters to achieve the desired results. It is also important to have an understanding of the history of electric stimulation as well as the groundwork research that has examined its applications, benefits, and contraindications, and which support its continued inclusion in evidence-based patient care. The reader is referred to the Evolve website at http://evolve.elsevier.com/Cameron for study questions pertinent to this chapter.

References

1. McNeal DR: 2000 years of electrical stimulation. In: Hambrecht FT, Reswick JB, eds: *Functional Electrical Stimulation: Applications in Neural Prostheses*, New York, 1977, Marcel Dekker.
2. Cambridge NA: Electrical apparatus used in medicine before 1900, *Proc Roy Soc Med,* 70:635-641, 1977.
3. Duchenne G-B: *A Treatise on Localized Electrization and Its Applications to Pathology and Therapeutics,* London, 1871, Hardwicke.
4. Licht, S: History of electrodiagnosis. In Licht S, ed: *Electrodiagnosis and Electromyography,* ed 3, New Haven, CT, 1971, Elizabeth Licht.
5. Currier DP, Mann R: Muscular strength development by electrical stimulation in healthy individuals, *Phys Ther* 63:915-921, 1983.
6. Kralj A, Acimovic R, Stanic U: Enhancement of hemiplegic patient rehabilitation by means of functional electrical stimulation, *Prosthet Orthot Int* Aug;17(2):107-114, 1993.
7. Melzack R, Wall PD: Pain mechanisms: a new theory, *Science* 150:971-979, 1965.
8. Schuster G, Marsden B: Treatment of pain by transcutaneous electric nerve stimulation in general practice, *J Neurol Orthop Surg* 1:137-1141, 1980.
9. Kloth, LC, Feedar JA: Acceleration of wound healing with high voltage, monophasic, pulsed current, *Phys Ther* 68:503-508, 1988.
10. Mendel FC, Wylegala JA, Fish DR: Influence of high voltage pulsed current on edema formation following impact injury in rats, *Phys Ther* 72:668-673, 1992.
11. American Physical Therapy Association: Clinical Electrophysiology. In *Electrotherapeutic Terminology in Physical Therapy,* Alexandria, VA, 2000, APTA.
12. Baker LL, Wederich CL, McNeal DR et al. *Neuromuscular Electrical Stimulation,* ed 4, Downey, CA, 2000, LAREI.
13. Petrofsky JS, Petrofsky S: A wide-pulse-width electrical stimulator for use on denervated muscles, *J Clin Eng* 17:331-338, 1992.
14. Garnett R, Stephens JA: Changes in the recruitment threshold of motor units produced by cutaneous stimulation in man, *J Physiol* (London) 311:463-473, 1981.
15. Delitto A, Snyder-Mackler: Two theories of muscle strength augmentation using percutaneous electrical stimulation, *Phys Ther* 70:158-164, 1990.
16. DeLuca CJ, LeFever RS, McCue MP et al: Behavior of human motor units in different muscles during linearly varying contractions, *J Physiol* (London) 329:113-128, 1982.
17. Alon G, McCombe SA, Koutsantonis S et al: Comparison of the effects of electrical stimulation and exercise on abdominal musculature, *J Orthop Sports Phys Ther* 8:567-573, 1987.
18. Wolf SL, Gideon BA, Saar D et al: The effect of muscle stimulation during resistive training on performance parameters, *Am J Sports Med* 14:18-23, 1986.
19. Delitto A, Rose SJ, McKowen JM et al: Electric stimulation vs. voluntary exercise in strengthening thigh musculature after anterior cruciate ligament surgery, *Phys Ther* 68:660-663, 1988.
20. Eriksson E, Haggmark T: Comparison of isometric muscle training and electrical stimulation supplementing isometric muscle training in the recovery after major knee ligament surgery, *Am J Sports Med* 7:169-171, 1979.
21. Godfrey CM, Jayawardena H, Quance TA et al: Comparison of electrostimulation and isometric exercise in strengthening the quadriceps muscle, *Physiother Can* 31:265-267, 1979.
22. Snyder-Mackler L, Delitto A, Bailey S et al: Quadriceps femoris muscle strength and functional recovery after anterior cruciate ligament reconstruction: a prospective randomized clinical trial of electrical stimulation, *J Bone Joint Surg* 77(8):1166-1173, 1995.
23. Morrissey MC, Brewster CE, Shields CL et al: The effects of electrical stimulation on the quadriceps during postoperative knee immobilization, *Am J Sports Med* 13:40-45, 1985.
24. Mahdad M, Baker L: Effect of electrical stimulation on recruitment of motor units in patients with hemiparesis, *Phys Ther* 77:S17-S18, 1977.

25. Trimble MH, Enoka RM: Mechanisms underlying the training effects associated with neuromuscular electrical stimulation, *Phys Ther* 71:273-282, 1991.

26. Alon G, Dar A, Katz-Behiri D et al: Efficacy of a hybrid upper limb neuromuscular electrical stimulation system in lessening selected impairments and dysfunctions consequent to cerebral damage, *J Neuro Rehab* 12:73-80, 1988.

27. Baker L, Parker K: Neuromuscular electrical stimulation of the muscles surrounding the shoulder, *Phys Ther* 66:1930-1937, 1986.

28. Faghri PD, Rodgers MM, Glaser RM et al: The effects of functional electrical stimulation on shoulder subluxation, arm function recovery, and shoulder pain in hemiplegic stroke patients, *Arch Phys Med Rehabil* 75:73-79, 1994.

29. Carmick, J: Clinical use of neuromuscular electrical stimulation for children with cerebral palsy. Part I: Lower extremity, *Phys Ther* 73:505-613, 1993.

30. Comeaux P, Patterson N, Rubin M et al: Effect of neuromuscular electrical stimulation during gait in children with cerebral palsy, *Pediatr Phys Ther* 9:103-109, 1997.

31. Carmick, J: Clinical use of neuromuscular electric stimulation for children with cerebral palsy. Part 2:Upper extremity, *Phys Ther* 73:514-527, 1993.

32. Carmick, J: Guidelines for application of neuromuscular electric stimulation for children with cerebral palsy, *Pediatr Phys Ther* 9:128-136, 1997.

33. Walker DC, Currier DP, Threlkeld AJ: Effects of high voltage pulsed electrical stimulation on blood flow, *Phys Ther* 68:481-485, 1988.

34. Indergand HJ, Morgan BJ: Effects of high frequency transcutaneous electrical nerve stimulation on limb blood flow in healthy humans, *Phys Ther* 74:361-367, 1994.

35. Klecker N, Theiss W: Transcutaneous electric muscle stimulation: a "new" possibility for the prevention of thrombosis? *Vasa* 23(1):23-29, 1994.

36. Mohr T, Akers T, Wessman HC: Effect of high voltage stimulation on blood flow in the rat hind limb, *Phys Ther* 67:526-533, 1987.

37. Kaada B, Emru M: Promoted healing of leprous ulcers by transcutaneous nerve stimulation, *Acupunct Electrother Res* 13:165-170, 1988.

38. Finsen V, Persen L, Lovlin M et al: Transcutaneous electrical nerve stimulation after major amputation, *J Bone Joint Surg* (Br) 70-B:109-112, 1988.

39. Faghri PD, Van Meerdervort HF, Glaser RM et al: Electrical stimulation-induced contraction to reduce blood stasis during arthroplasty, *IEEE Trans Rehabil Eng* 5(1):62-9, 1997.

40. Merli GJ, Herbison GJ, Ditunno JF et al: Deep vein thrombosis: prophylaxis in acute spinal cord injured patients, *Arch Phys Med Rehabil* 69(9):661-664, 1988.

41. Lundeberg TC, Eriksson SV, Malm M: Electrical nerve stimulation improves healing in diabetic ulcers, *Ann Plast Surg* 29:328-331, 1992.

42. Lundeberg T, Kjartansson J, Samuelsson UE: Effect of electric nerve stimulation on healing of ischemic skin flaps, *Lancet* 24:712-714, 1988.

43. Bergslien O, Thereson M, Odemark H: The effects of three electrotherapeutic methods on blood velocities in human peripheral arteries, *Scand J Rehabil Med* 20: 29-33, 1988.

44. Siegel SW, Richardson DA, Miller KL et al: Pelvic floor electrical stimulation for the treatment of urge and mixed urinary incontinence in women, *Urology* 50(6):934-940, 1977.

45. Soomro NA, Khadra MH, Robson W et al: A crossover randomized trial of transcutaneous electrical nerve stimulation and oxybutynin in patients with detrusor instability, *J Urol* 166(1):146-149, 2001.

46. Govier FE, Litwiller S, Nitti V et al: Percutaneous neuromodulation for the refractory overactive bladder: results of a multicenter study, *J Urol* 165(4):1193-1198, 2001.

47. van Balken MR, Vandoninck V, Gisolf KW et al: Posterior tibial nerve stimulation as neuromodulative treatment of lower urinary tract dysfunction, *J Urol* 166(3):914-918, 2001.

48. Agency for Health Care Policy and Research : Guidelines on Urinary Incontinence, US Public Health Service Pub No, March 1992, US Department of Health and Human Services.

49. Girlanda P, Dattola R, Vita G et al: Effect of electrotherapy in denervated muscles in rabbits: an electrophysiological and morphological study, *Exp Neurol* 77:483-491, 1982.

50. Pachter BR, Eberstein A, Goodgold J: Electrical stimulation effect on denervated skeletal myofibers in rats: a light and electron microscopic study, *Arch Phys Med Rehabil* 63:427-430, 1982.

51. Schimrigk K, McLaughjlin J, Gruninger W: The effect of electrical stimulation on the experimentally denervated rat muscle, *Scand J Rehabil Med* 9:55-60, 1977.

52. Bisschop G, Aaron C, Bence G et al: Indications and limits of electrotherapy in Bell's palsy. In Portmann M, ed: *Facial Nerve,* New York, 1985, Masson.

53. Huizing EH, Mechelse K, Staal A: Treatment of Bell's Palsy. An analysis of the available studies, *Acta Otolaryngol* Jul-Aug;92(1-2):115-121, 1981.

54. Farragher D, Kidd G, Tallis R: Eutrophic electrical stimulation for Bell's palsy, *Clin Rehab* 1:265-271, 1987.

55. Targan RS, Alon G, Kay SL: Effect of long-term electrical stimulation on motor recovery and improvement of

clinical residuals in patients with unresolved facial nerve palsy, *Otolaryngol-Head Neck Surg* 122:246-252, 2000.

56. Chabal C, Fishbain A, Weaver M et al: Long term transcutaneous electrical nerve stimulation (TENS) use: impact on medication utilization and physical therapy costs, *Clin J Pain* 14(1):66-73, 1988.

57. Forster EL, Kramer JF, Lucy SD et al: Effect of TENS on pain, medications, and pulmonary function following coronary artery bypass graft surgery, *Chest* 106(5): 1343-1348, 1994.

58. Ali J, Yaffe GS, Serrette C: The effect of transcutaneous electric nerve stimulation on postoperative pain and pulmonary function, *Surgery* 89:507-512, 1981.

59. Dawood MY, Ramos J: Transcutaneous electrical nerve stimulation (TENS) for the treatment of primary dysmenorrhea: a randomized crossover comparison with placebo TENS and ibuprofen, *Obstet Gynecol* 75: 656-660, 1990.

60. Wall PD: The gate control theory of pain mechanisms: a re-examination and restatement, *Brain* 101:1-18, 1978.

61. Levin MF, Hui-Chan C: Conventional and acupuncture-like transcutaneous electrical nerve stimulation excite similar afferent fibers, *Arch Phys Med Rehabil* 74(1): 54-60, 1993.

62. Pert CB, Snyder SH.: Opiate receptor: demonstration in nervous tissue, *Science* 179:1011-1014, 1973.

63. Sjolund BH, Terenius L, Eriksson, M: Increased cerebrospinal fluid levels of endorphins after electroacupuncture, *Acta Physiol Scand* 100:382-384, 1977.

64. Mannheimer JS, Lampe GN, eds: *Clinical Transcutaneous Electrical Nerve Stimulation,* Philadelphia, 1984, FA Davis.

65. Kalra A, Urban MO, Sluka KA: Blockade of opioid receptors in rostral ventral medulla prevents antihyperalgesia produced by transcutaneous electrical nerve stimulation (TENS), *J Pharmacol Exp Ther* 298(1): 257-263, 2001.

66. Omura Y: Basic electrical parameters for safe and effective electro-therapeutics [electro-acupuncture, TES, TENMS (or TEMS), TENS and electro-magnetic field stimulation with or without drug field] for pain, neuromuscular skeletal problems, and circulatory disturbances, *Acupunct Electrother Res* 12(3-4):201-225, 1987.

67. Debreceni L: Chemical releases associated with acupuncture and electric stimulation: critical reviews, *Phys & Rehab Med* 5(3):247-275, 1993.

68. Gardner S, Frantz R, Schmidt F: Effect of electrical stimulation on chronic wound healing: a meta-analysis: *Wound Repair & Regen* 11:495-503, 1999.

69. Fukushima K, Senda N, Inui H et al: Studies on galvanotaxis of leukocytes. I. Galvanotaxis of human neutrophilic leukocytes and methods of its measurement, *Med J Osaka Univ* 4:195-208, 1953.

70. Erickson CA, Nuccitelli R: Embryonic fibroblast motility and orientation can be influenced by physiological electric fields, *J Cell Biol* 98:296-307, 1984.

71. Kloth LC: Electric stimulation in tissue repair. In Kloth L, Feedar J, eds: *Wound Healing Alternatives in Management,* ed 2, Philadelphia, 1995, FA Davis.

72. Cheng N, Van Hoof H, Bock E et al: The effects of electric currents on ATP generation, protein synthesis, and membrane transport in rat skin, *Clin Orthop* 171: 264-272, 1982.

73. Bourguignon GJ, Bourguignon LYW: Electric stimulation of protein and DNA synthesis in human fibroblasts, *FASEB J* 1:398-402, 1987.

74. Bourguignon GJ, Wenche JY, Bourguignon LYW: Electric stimulation of human fibroblasts causes an increase in Ca 2+ influx and the exposure of additional insulin receptors, *J Cell Physiol* 140:379-385, 1989.

75. Cooper MS, Schliwa M: Electrical and ionic controls of tissue cell locomotion in DC electric fields, *J Neurosci Res* 13:223-244, 1985.

76. Jaffe LF, Vanable JW Jr: Electric fields and wound healing, *Clin Dermatol* 2:34-44, 1984.

77. Borgens RB, Vanable JS, Jaffe LF: Bioelectricity and regeneration: large currents leave the stumps of regenerating newt limbs, *Proc Natl Acad Sci USA* 74: 4528-4532, 1977.

78. Illingworth CM, Barker AT: Measurement of electrical currents emerging during the regeneration of amputated finger tips in children, *Clin Phys Physiol Meas* 1:87, 1980.

79. Reed BV: Effect of high voltage pulsed electrical stimulation on microvascular permeability to plasma proteins: a possible mechanism in minimizing edema, *Phys Ther* 68:491-495, 1988.

80. Bettany JA, Fish DR, Mendel FC: The effect of high voltage pulsed direct current on edema formation following impact injury, *Phys Ther* 70:219-224, 1990.

81. Bettany JA, Fish DR, Mendel FC: The effect of high voltage pulsed direct current on edema formation following hyperflexion injury, *Arch Phys Med Rehabil* 71:677-681, 1990.

82. Bettany JA, Fish DR, Mendel FC: Influence of cathodal high voltage pulsed current on acute edema, *J Clin Electrophysiol* 2:724-733, 1990.

83. Fish DR, Mendel FC, Schultz AM et al: Effect of anodal high voltage pulsed current on edema formation in frog hind limbs, *Phys Ther* 71(10)724-730, 1991.

84. Taylor K, Mendel FC, Fish DR et al: Effect of high voltage pulsed current and alternating current on macromolecular leakage in hamster cheek pouch microcirculation, *Phys Ther* 77:1729-1740, 1997.

85. Karnes JL, Mendel FC, Fish DR et al: High voltage pulsed current: its influences on diameters of histamine-dilated arterioles in hamster cheek pouches, *Arch Phys Med Rehabil* 76:381-386, 1995.

86. Kincaid C, Lavoie K: Inhibition of bacterial growth in vitro following stimulation with high voltage, monophasic, pulsed current, *Phys Ther* 69:29-33, 1989.

87. Szuminsky NJ, Albers AC, Unger P et al: Effect of narrow, pulsed high voltages on bacterial viability, *Phys Ther* 74:660-667, 1994.

88. Barranco SD, Spadaro JA, Berger TJ et al: In vitro effect of weak direct current on *Staphylococcus aureus, Clin Orthop* 100:250-255, 1974.

89. Rowley BA, McKenna J, Chase GR: The influence of electrical current on an infecting microorganism in wounds, *Ann NY Acad Sci* 238:543-551, 1974.

90. Ong PC, Laatsch LJ, Kloth LC: Antibacterial effects of a silver electrode carrying microamperage direct current in vitro, *J Clin Electrophysiol* 6:14-18, 1994.

91. Sherry JE, Oehrlein KM, Hegge KS et al: Effect of burst-mode transcutaneous electrical nerve stimulation on peripheral vascular resistance, *Phys Ther* 81(6):1183-1191, 2001.

92. Griffin JW, Tooms RE, Mendius RE et al: Efficacy of high voltage pulsed current for healing of pressure ulcers in patients with spinal cord injury, *Phys Ther* 71:433-444, 1991.

93. Unger P, Eddy J, Raimastry S: A controlled study of the effect of high voltage pulsed current (HVPC) on wound healing, *Phys Ther* 71(suppl):S119, 1991.

94. Unger PC: A randomized clinical trial of the effect of HVPC on wound healing, *Phys Ther* 71(suppl): S118, 1991.

95. Leduc S: Introduction of medicinal substances into the depths of tissues by electrical current, *Ann Electrobiol* 3:545, 1900.

96. Leduc S: *Electric ions and their use in medicine,* London, 1908, Rebman.

97. Li SK, Ghanem AH, Teng CL et al: Characterization of the transport pathways induced during low to moderate voltage iontophoresis in human epidermal membrane, *J Pharm Sci* 87(1):40-48, 1998.

98. Singh J, Roberts MS: Transdermal delivery of drugs by iontophoresis: a review, *Drug Design Deliv* 4:1, 1989.

99. Starkey C: Electrical Agents. In *Therapeutic Modalities for Athletic Trainers,* ed 2, Philadelphia, 1999, FA Davis.

100. Chen T, Langer R, Weaver JC: Skin electroporation causes molecular transport across the stratum corneum through localized transport regions, *J Investig Dermatol Symp Proc* Aug;3(2):159-165, 1998.

101. Nimmo WS: Novel delivery systems: electrotransport, *J Pain Symptom Manage* 8:160, 1992.

102. Cullander C: What are the pathways of iontophoretic current flow through mammalian skin? *Adv Drug Del Dev* 9:119, 1992.

103. Glass JM, Stephen RL, Jacobsen SC: The quantity and distribution of radiolabeled dexamethasone delivered to tissue by iontophoresis, *Int J Dermatol* 19:519-525, 1980.

104. Singh J, Roberts MS: Iontophoretic transdermal delivery of salicylic acid and lidocaine to local subcutaneous structures, *J Pharm Sci* 82(2):127-131, 1993.

105. Lai PM, Anissimov YG, Roberts MS: Lateral iontophoretic solute transport in skin, *J Pharm Res* 16(1):46-54, 1999.

106. Bertolucci LE: Introduction of anti-inflammatory drugs by iontophoresis: a double blind study, *J Orthop Sport Phys Ther* 4:103-108, 1982.

107. Delacerda FG: A comparative study of three methods of treatment for shoulder girdle myofascial syndrome, *J Orthop Sport Phys Ther* 4:51-54, 1982.

108. Harris PR: Iontophoresis: Clinical research in musculoskeletal inflammatory conditions, *J Orthop Sports Phys Ther* 4:109-112, 1982.

109. Henley EJ: Transcutaneous drug delivery: iontophoresis and phonophoresis, *Crit Rev Phys Rehabil Med* 2:139-151, 1991.

110. Gangarosa LP, Mahan PE, Ciarlone AE: Pharmacologic management of temporo-mandibular joint disorders and chronic head and neck pain, *Cranio* 2:139-151, 1991.

111. Labrecque M, Nouwen A, Bergeron M et al: A randomized controlled trial of nonpharmacologic approaches for relief of low back pain during labor, *J Fam Pract* Apr;48(4):259-263, 1999.

112. Harrison RF, Woods T, Shore M et al: Pain relief in labour using transcutaneous electrical nerve stimulation (TENS): A TENS/TENS placebo-controlled study in two parity groups, *Br J Obstet Gynaecol.* Jul; 93(7):739-746, 1986.

113. Kaplan B, Rabinerson D, Lurie S et al: Transcutaneous electrical nerve stimulation (TENS) for adjuvant pain-relief during labor and delivery, *Int J Gynaecol Obstet.* Mar;60(3):251-255, 1988.

114. Mannheimer JS: Electrode placements for transcutaneous electrical nerve stimulation, *Phys Ther* 58: 1455-1462, 1978.

115. Melzack R, Stillwell DM, Fox EJ: Trigger points and acupuncture points for pain: correlations and implications, *Pain* 3:3-23, 1977.

116. Long DM: Stimulation of the peripheral nervous system for pain control, *Clin Neurosurg* 31:323-343, 1984.

117. Jones DA, Bigland-Ritchie B, Edwards RH: Excitation frequency and muscle fatigue: mechanical responses during voluntary and stimulated contractions, *Exp Neurol.* May;64(2):401-413, 1979.

118. Selkowitz DM: Improvement in isometric strength of the quadriceps femoris muscle after training with electrical stimulation, *Phys Ther* 65:186-196, 1985.

119. Snyder-Mackler L, Delitto A, Stralka SW et al: Use of electrical stimulation to enhance recovery of quadriceps femoris muscle force production in patients following anterior cruciate ligament reconstruction, *Phys Ther* 74:901-907, 1994.

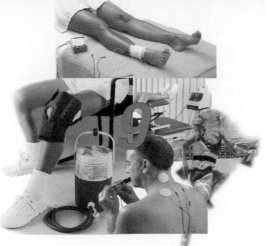

Hydrotherapy

OBJECTIVES

Upon completion of this chapter, the reader will be able to:

1. Discuss the physical properties of water, including heat transfer, buoyancy, resistance, and hydrostatic pressure.
2. Identify the physiological effects of cleansing with water and of water immersion.
3. Examine how the physical properties and physiological effects of hydrotherapy can be used for cleansing, musculoskeletal support and resistance, cardiovascular and respiratory training, and for psychological benefits.

4. Assess the indications, contraindications, and precautions for the use of hydrotherapy.
5. Choose and use the most appropriate hydrotherapy treatment technique to promote progress toward desired treatment goals.
6. Presented with a clinical case, evaluate the clinical findings, propose goals of treatment, assess whether hydrotherapy would be the best treatment, and, if so, formulate an effective treatment plan including the appropriate hydrotherapy treatment technique for achieving the goals of treatment.

Hydrotherapy, derived from the Greek words *hydro* and *therapeia,* meaning "water" and "healing," is the application of water, either internally or externally, for the treatment of physical or psychological dysfunction. This chapter concerns only the external application of water when used as a component of physical rehabilitation. Hydrotherapy can be applied externally, either by immersion of the whole body or of parts of the body in water, or without immersion by spraying or pouring water onto the body. The effects and applications of both immersion and nonimmersion hydrotherapy are discussed in this chapter.

Bathing in water has been considered healing since the beginning of recorded time and across many cultures, from Hippocrates in the 4th and 5th centuries B.C., who used hot and cold water to treat a variety of diseases, to the Romans at the beginning of the 1st century A.D., who constructed therapeutic baths across their empire, to the Japanese, who have used ritual baths from ancient times to the modern day.[1] The therapeutic use of water gained particular popularity in Europe in the late 19th century, with the development of health spas in areas of natural springs such as Baden-Baden and Bad Ragaz, and shortly thereafter in the United States in similar areas of natural hot springs. At this time, hydrotherapy was used for its effects on both the mind and the body: "It is readily shown that no remedy for lunacy exists which is at all comparable to the bath, owing to its purifying action on the blood."[2] The transition of hydrotherapy from a preventive and recreational role to a curative or rehabilitative role for diseases and their sequelae took place during the polio epidemic of the 1940s and 1950s, when Sister Kenny included activities in water as a component of her treatment of patients recovering from polio. She found that the unique properties of the water environment, including buoyancy, resistance, and support, allowed these weakened patients to perform a wide range of therapeutic activities with greater ease and safety than was possible on dry land.[3a]

Although hydrotherapy has been shown to have wide-ranging therapeutic effects and benefits, its use today continues to be limited in most clinical settings, largely due to the expenses associated with establishing and maintaining a safe hydrotherapy environment. Hydrotherapy is used today primarily as a component of the treatment of wounds or to provide an enhanced environment for therapeutic exercise. It is also used occasionally to control pain and/or edema. Rehabilitation professionals may also be involved in designing and instructing water exercise programs intended for health maintenance and/or disease prevention in the community rather than in the clinical setting.

PHYSICAL PROPERTIES OF WATER

Water has a number of unique physical properties that make it well-suited to a variety of rehabilitation applications. These properties include a relatively high specific heat and thermal conductivity, and the ability to provide buoyancy, resistance, and hydrostatic pressure to the body.

Specific Heat and Thermal Conductivity

Water can transfer heat by conduction and convection and can therefore be used as a superficial heating or cooling agent. It is particularly effective for this application because it has a high specific heat and thermal conductivity. The specific heat of water is approximately 4 times that of air, and its thermal conductivity is approximately 25 times that of air (Table 9-1). Thus water retains four times as much thermal energy as an equivalent mass of air at the same temperature, and it transfers this thermal energy 25 times more rapidly than air at the same temperature. More details regarding the effects of specific heat and thermal conductivity on heat transfer, and on the principles of heat transfer by conduction and convection, are provided in Chapter 6 in the section on modes of heat transfer.

TABLE 9-1	Comparison of Specific Heat and Thermal Conductivity of Water and Air	
	Specific heat (J/g/ ˚C)	**Thermal conductivity (Cal/sec)/(cm² × ˚C/cm)**
Water	4.19	0.0014
Air	1.01	0.000057
Water: air ratio	4.14	24.56

Clinically, during hydrotherapy, heat is generally transferred from warm water to a patient by placing the patient's limb in a whirlpool filled with warm water. Heat may also be transferred from the patient to cooler water by immersing a limb or part of a limb in a whirlpool filled with cold or ice water. The ability of water to transfer heat rapidly and efficiently is one of the advantages of performing exercises in a swimming pool that is colder than the patient's body temperature because, in such circumstances, immersion in the water helps to dissipate the heat generated by the patient through exertion and may also counteract the heat of a hotter climate.

Stationary water transfers heat by conduction; moving water also transfers heat by convection. As explained in detail in Chapter 6, the rate of heat transfer by convection increases as the rate of fluid flow relative to the body increases. Thus heating of a patient's limb in a whirlpool is accelerated with increasing agitation of the water, and cooling of a patient in a cold swimming pool is accelerated as the patient moves more quickly through the water in the pool.

Buoyancy

Buoyancy is a force experienced as an upward thrust on the body in the opposite direction to the force of gravity. According to Archimedes' principle, when a body is entirely or partially immersed in a fluid at rest, it experiences an upward thrust equal to the weight of the fluid it displaces. The amount of fluid it displaces depends on the density of the immersed body relative to the density of the fluid. If the density of the immersed body is less than the density of the fluid then it will displace a smaller volume of fluid and will float. Conversely, if the density of the immersed body is greater than the density of the fluid, it will displace a larger volume of fluid and will sink. Because the density of the human body is less than that of water, having a specific gravity of about 0.974 compared with that of water, it floats in water (Table 9-2). If the relative density of the body compared with the water is further decreased, either by the addition of salt to the water or by attaching air-filled objects such as a belt, vest, or arm bands to the patient, the body will float even higher in the water (Fig. 9-1). This effect is commonly experienced when a person swims in sea water or uses a life jacket.

The buoyancy of the body in water is used clinically to decrease stress and compression on weight-bearing joints, muscles, and connective tissue (Fig. 9-2). It may

TABLE 9-2	**Specific Gravity of Different Substances**
Substance	**Specific gravity**
Pure water	1
Salt water	1.024
Ice	0.917
Air	1.21×10^{-3}
Average human body	0.974
Subcutaneous fat	0.85

also be used to help raise weakened body parts against gravity or to assist the therapist in supporting the weight of the patient's body during therapeutic activities.

Resistance

The viscosity of water provides resistance to the motion of a body in water. This resistance occurs against the direction of the motion of the body and increases in proportion to the relative speed of the body's motion and the frontal area of the body part(s) in contact with the water[3] (Fig. 9-3). In the clinical setting, the relative speed of motion of the body can be increased by having the patient move faster in the water or by increasing the speed at which the water moves toward the patient. The frontal area of the body part in contact with the water can be increased by the use of paddles or fins and can be decreased by keeping the limbs more parallel to the direction of movement (Fig. 9-4). The velocity-dependent resistance provided by water makes it a safe and effective strengthening and conditioning medium for many patients. The fact that the resistance of the water falls to zero when motion stops provides safety, while the fact that the resistance can be readily increased by increasing the speed of motion or the frontal area in contact with the water provides effective training. The variable resistance, and thus pressure, provided by moving water can also be beneficial for debriding and cleansing wounds.

Hydrostatic Pressure

Hydrostatic pressure is the pressure exerted by a fluid on a body immersed in the fluid. According to Pascal's law, a fluid exerts equal pressure on all surfaces of

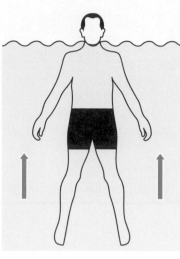
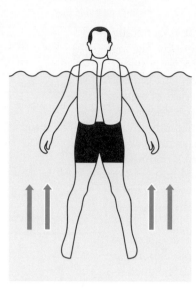
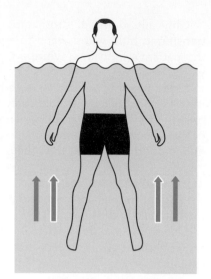

Person in water, floating head above water

Person with air-filled vest in water, floating head and shoulders above water

Person in water, with a high concentration of dissolved salt, floating head and shoulders above water

Figure 9-1. Buoyancy.

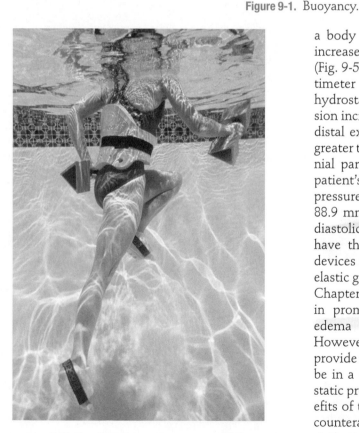

Figure 9-2. Patient exercising in water while wearing a foam vest to increase buoyancy. (Courtesy AQUAJOGGER®, Eugene, OR.)

a body at rest at a given depth, and this pressure increases in proportion to the depth of the fluid (Fig. 9-5). Water exerts 0.73 mm Hg pressure per centimeter of depth (22.4 mm Hg per foot).[4] Because hydrostatic pressure increases as the depth of immersion increases, the amount of pressure exerted on the distal extremities of an upright immersed patient is greater than that exerted on the more proximal or cranial parts of the body. Thus for example, when a patient's feet are immersed under 4 feet of water, the pressure exerted by the water will be approximately 88.9 mm Hg, which is slightly greater than normal diastolic blood pressure. This external pressure can have the same effects as the pressure exerted by devices intended to produce compression, such as elastic garments or bandages, as described in detail in Chapter 11. Therefore immersion in water can assist in promoting circulation or alleviating peripheral edema due to venous or lymphatic insufficiency. However, in contrast to most other devices used to provide external compression, since the limbs must be in a dependent position to maximize the hydrostatic pressure exerted by the water, some of the benefits of the compression produced by immersion are counteracted by the increase in circulatory hydrostatic pressure produced by placing a limb in this position. The increase in venous return that results from increasing external hydrostatic pressure on the limbs

Figure 9-3.
Resistance.

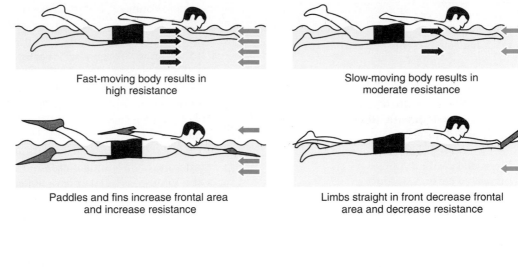

Fast-moving body results in
high resistance

Slow-moving body results in
moderate resistance

Paddles and fins increase frontal area
and increase resistance

Limbs straight in front decrease frontal
area and decrease resistance

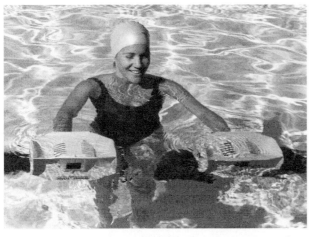

Figure 9-4. Patient exercising in water using hand-held devices to increase the frontal area and thus increase the resistance of the water.

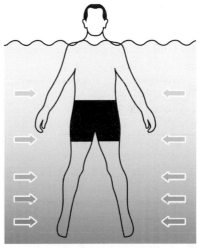

Figure 9-5. Hydrostatic pressure.

may also facilitate cardiovascular function, while the support provided by this external pressure may help to brace unstable joints or weak muscles.

It is important to note that since hydrostatic pressure increases with depth of immersion, the physiological and clinical benefits of the hydrostatic pressure of water will vary with patient positioning. The greatest effects will occur with vertical positioning, in which the feet are immersed deep in the water. The effects will be much less pronounced if the patient is swimming or performing other activities in more horizontal positions close to the water surface, where the limbs are kept at lower depths of immersion. There are also no hydrostatic pressure effects when nonimmersion hydrotherapy techniques are used.

PHYSIOLOGICAL EFFECTS OF HYDROTHERAPY

The physiological effects of water are the result of its physical properties, as described above. The physiological effects of superficial heating or cooling by warm or cold water are the same as the physiological effects of heating or cooling with other superficial heating or cooling agents and include hemodynamic,

Cleansing effects
  Pressure
  Dissolved surfactants and antimicrobials
Musculoskeletal effects
  Decreased weight bearing
  Strengthening
  Slowed bone density loss
  Less fat loss than with other forms of exercise
Cardiovascular effects
Increased venous circulation
  Increased cardiac volume
  Increased cardiac output
  **Decreased heart rate, systolic blood pressure,
     and VO$_2$ response to exercise**
Respiratory effects
  Decreased vital capacity
  Increased work of breathing
  Decreased exercise-induced asthma
Renal effects
  Diuresis
  Increased sodium and potassium excretion
Psychological effects
  Relaxing or invigorating, depending on temperature

neuromuscular, and metabolic changes and modification of soft tissue extensibility. For detailed descriptions of these effects, the reader is referred to the sections on the effects of heat and cold provided in Chapter 6. The physiological effects of water that are distinct from those of superficial thermal agents are described directly below. These effects include cleansing, as well as musculoskeletal, cardiovascular, respiratory, renal, and psychological changes.

Cleansing Effects

Water can be used as a cleanser because it can soften materials and exert pressure. Water is most commonly used for cleansing intact skin; however, in rehabilitation, its cleansing properties are most often used as a component of the treatment of open wounds where there are exposed areas of subcutaneous tissue and the skin is no longer intact. In this circumstance, the hydrating effects and friction of water are used to soften and remove debris that is lodged in a wound or adhered to the tissue. Water is well-suited to this application because the force it exerts is proportional to its rate of flow, and can thus be readily controlled. In addition, water can quickly and easily get into and out of the contoured areas of open wounds. Water is used clinically both as a debriding agent, to remove endogenous debris such as wound exudate or necrotic tissue, and as a cleanser, to remove exogenous waste, such as gravel or adhered dressing materials, and to reduce bacterial burden. The presence of necrotic tissue and contamination by microorganisms delay wound healing.[5,6]

Products can be added to water to increase its cleansing power. Such additives are generally antimicrobials or surfactants. Antimicrobials reduce the microbe count in the water and thus on the surface of the wound, while surfactants, such as soap or detergent products, reduce surface tension and thereby reduce the adhesion of debris to the tissue. A number of clinical benefits and risks are associated with putting additives in the water used for treating open wounds. These are discussed in detail later in this chapter in the section on the clinical use of hydrotherapy for wound care.

Musculoskeletal Effects

The buoyancy of water unloads the weight-bearing anatomical structures and can thus allow patients with load-sensitive joints to perform exercises with less trauma and pain. This effect can help patients with arthritis, ligamentous instability, cartilage breakdown, or other degenerative or traumatic conditions of the articular or periarticular structures of the weight-bearing joints to progress more rapidly with rehabilitation activities. For example, since at 75% immersion weight bearing on the lower extremities is reduced by 75%, patients may be able to perform weight-bearing exercises or walk unassisted with a normal gait pattern in a pool, although they can perform such activities on dry land only with the support of crutches.[7]

Buoyancy can also be particularly helpful for obese patients for whom land-based exercise places extreme stresses on the weight-bearing joints. Because such individuals are more buoyant in water than average, having more subcutaneous fat (see Table 9-2), they have greatly reduced joint loading with water-based activities. Therefore, water-based exercises may be used to restore fitness in obese patients who have difficulty with other forms of exercise, although paradoxically, exercise in water has been shown to produce less weight and fat loss than exercise of similar intensity and duration on dry land.[8-10] Therefore, water-based exercise is recommended for improving the fitness and function of obese patients but is not generally recommended for weight loss.

The velocity-dependent resistance provided by water can also be used to provide a force against which muscles can work in order to gain or maintain strength. For example, water-based exercises have been shown to result in increased upper and lower extremity strength in patients with neuromuscular diseases, such as multiple sclerosis, and to maintain strength in healthy individuals.[11,12] If the direction of water flow is adjusted to be in the same direction as the patient's motion, the resistance of the water can also be used to aid the patient's motion.

The hydrostatic pressure exerted by water has also been shown to increase resting muscle blood flow by 100% to 225% during immersion of the body up to the neck.[13] This is proposed to be the result of reduced peripheral vasoconstriction or increased venous return produced by the external compression provided by the water. This increase in muscular blood flow may improve muscular performance by increasing oxygen availability and accelerating the removal of waste products and may thus promote more effective muscular training.

Cardiovascular Effects

The cardiovascular benefits of hydrotherapy are primarily due to the effects of hydrostatic pressure. The hydrostatic pressure exerted on the distal extremities with upright immersion in water displaces venous blood proximally from the extremities and thus enhances venous return by shifting blood from the periphery to the trunk vessels and thence to the thorax and the heart. It has been shown that central venous pressure rises with immersion to the chest and continues to increase until the body is fully immersed.[14,15] With immersion to the neck, central blood volume increases by about 60%, and cardiac volume increases by nearly 30%.[15,16] This increase in cardiac volume results in an increase in right atrial pressure of 14 to 18 mm Hg, to which the heart responds, according to Starling's law, with an increase in the force of cardiac contraction and an increase in stroke volume.[14] This results in approximately 30% increased cardiac output over baseline in response to upright immersion up to the neck[14] (Fig. 9-6).

The increase in cardiac work associated with this increased cardiac output is in contrast to the decrease in heart rate that occurs in response to immersion in water, and counters the reduced heart rate and reduced systolic blood pressure that occur when exercise at the same metabolic rate or perceived level of exertion is performed in water rather than on dry land.[15,17-19] $\dot{V}O_2$ (rate of oxygen consumption) is also lower when exercise is performed in water than when exercise at the same level of perceived exertion is performed on dry land, and $\dot{V}O_{2\,max}$ (maximum rate of oxygen consumption) has been found to be slightly lower with maximal running in water than with maximal running on dry land.[20-22] Because of these reduced physiological responses, exercise in water

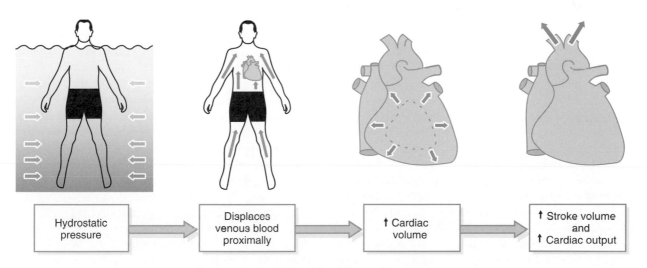

| Hydrostatic pressure | → | Displaces venous blood proximally | → | ↑ Cardiac volume | → | ↑ Stroke volume and ↑ Cardiac output |

Figure 9-6. Cardiovascular effects of immersion.

has often been considered to be less effective for cardiac conditioning than similar exercise on dry land. However, it is important to realize that these reduced physiological responses are accompanied by an increase in stroke volume and cardiac output, which may increase myocardial efficiency. Thus there is a physiological basis for using exercise in water for cardiac conditioning and rehabilitation. Also, a number of studies have shown that cardiovascular training effects, including an increased $\dot{V}O_{2\,max}$ and a decreased resting heart rate, do occur in healthy individuals in response to water-based exercise programs.[22,23]

Because the heart rate response to exercise is blunted in water, clinically the target heart rate may not provide an appropriate guideline for water exercise intensity prescription. Therefore when a patient exercises in water, it is recommended that the level of perceived exertion, rather than the heart rate response, be used as a guide for exercise intensity. The reader should also note that the blunting of heart rate and systolic blood pressure in response to exercises that occur with water immersion may be obscured if warm water is used, because increasing the body's temperature may elevate the heart rate and reduce the systolic blood pressure.[15,24]

The velocity-dependent resistance to motion provided by water also increases the metabolic rate and energy expenditure, as measured by $\dot{V}O_2$, by approximately a factor of 3 when an activity is performed at the same speed in water as on dry land.[25] Thus exercise performed in water at one-half to one-third of the speed with which similar exercise is performed on dry land has the same effect on the metabolic rate.[26] This altered response can allow individuals with musculoskeletal conditions that limit their speed of movement to perform exercise in water to maintain or improve their cardiovascular fitness.

Respiratory Effects

Immersion of the whole body in water increases the work of breathing because the shift of venous blood from the peripheral to the central circulation increases the circulation in the chest cavity, and the hydrostatic pressure on the chest wall increases the resistance to lung expansion[14] (Fig. 9-7). Immersion in water up to the neck has been shown to decrease expiratory reserve volume by about 50% and to decrease vital capacity by 6% to 12%; these effects, combined,

increase the total work of breathing by about 60%.[27-29] Thus the workload challenge to the respiratory system that occurs when exercise is performed in water can be used to improve the efficiency and strength of the respiratory system. However, since this additional respiratory challenge may be detrimental to patients with respiratory or cardiovascular impairments that prevent or limit adaptation to this additional workload, such patients should always be carefully monitored during water-based exercise.[26]

Water-based exercise is also often recommended for patients with exercise-induced asthma because several studies have shown that water-based exercise is less likely to cause asthma in these individuals than exercise on dry land.[30,31] Various properties of water, including the absence of pollen over the water, hydrostatic pressure on the chest, hypoventilation, hypercapnia, peripheral vasoconstriction, and the high humidity of the inspired air in the pool environment, have been proposed as mechanisms for this effect.[32] Although most of these factors have not been studied experimentally, it appears that the high humidity of the air inspired during water exercise, which prevents drying and/or cooling of the respiratory mucosa, is the most important factor in reducing exercise-induced asthma.

Renal Effects

Immersion of an individual up to the neck in water has been shown to increase urine production and urine, sodium, and potassium excretion[18,33,34] (Fig. 9-8). It is proposed that these effects are the result of increased renal blood flow and decreased antidiuretic hormone (ADH) and aldosterone production.[33,35] Water immersion is thought to cause these circulatory and hormonal changes in response to the redistribution of blood volume and the relative central hypervolemia that result from the hydrostatic pressure that water exerts on the periphery. These renal effects can be taken advantage of in the treatment of patients with hypervolemia, hypertension, and/or peripheral edema.

Psychological Effects

As is well known to those who bathe or exercise in water, water immersion can be invigorating and/or relaxing. The variations in these psychological effects

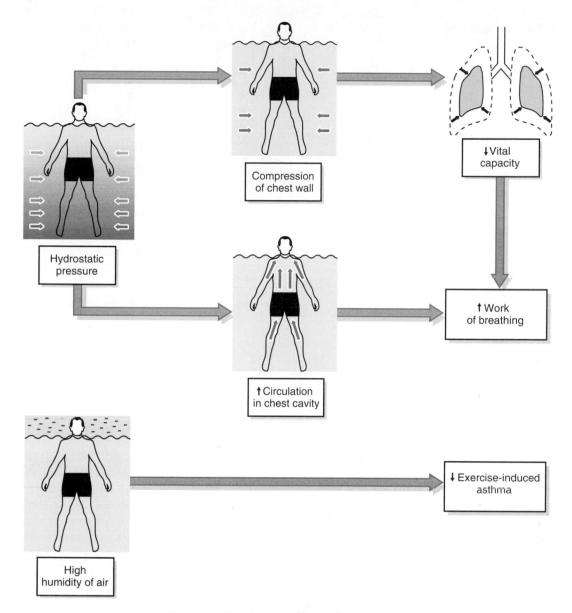

Figure 9-7. Respiratory effects of immersion.

appear to depend primarily on the temperature of the water. While soaking in warm water is generally relaxing, cold water immersion is found by most persons to be invigorating and energizing. Thus the neutral stimulation and support of warm water can be used clinically to provide a comforting and calming environment for overstimulated or agitated patients, while the invigorating effects of cold water can be used to facilitate more active exercise participation by those who are generally less active or responsive.[36] Although there is no published research that has directly evaluated the effects of water-based exercise on mood, it has been proposed that the clinically observed psychological effects mentioned above may be mediated by a central process within the reticular activating system.[4]

Figure 9-8. Renal effects of immersion.

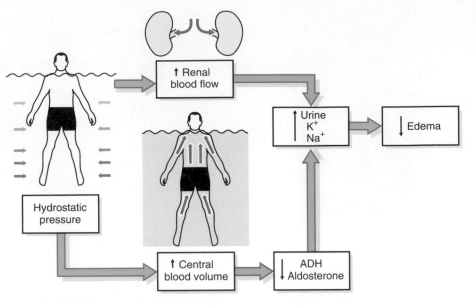

USES OF HYDROTHERAPY

> **Superficial heating or cooling**
> **Wound care**
> **Water exercise**
> **Pain control**
> **Edema control**

Superficial Heating or Cooling

Warm or cold water can be used clinically to heat or cool superficial tissues. Warm water and cold water transfer heat primarily by conduction, while warm and cold whirlpools transfer heat both by conduction and by convection.[37] The effects and clinical applications of heating or cooling superficial tissues with water are the same as those produced when other superficial heating or cooling agents are used and are described in detail in Chapter 6. Water has a number of advantages over most other superficial thermal agents. It provides perfect contact with the skin, even in very contoured areas, does not need to be fastened to the body, and allows movement during heating or cooling. Its primary disadvantage is that, when it is applied to the extremities only, the distal extremity must be in a dependent position, which may aggravate edema. However, the edema-producing effect of the dependent position is somewhat counteracted during immersion in water by the compression provided by the hydrostatic pressure of the water.

Wound Care

Hydrotherapy has been shown to accelerate the healing of wounds of various etiologies including diabetes mellitus, pressure, vascular insufficiency, or burns.[38-41] Hydrotherapy may also be used in the care of wounds due to trauma, surgery, abscesses, dehisced incisions, necrotizing fasciitis, or cellulitis. Hydrotherapy is used for wound care because its cleansing properties facilitate the rehydration, softening, and debridement of necrotic tissue and the removal of exogenous wound debris, while the hydrostatic pressure of water immersion and the heat of warm water improve circulation[42] (Fig. 9-9). The use of hydrotherapy is also consistent with the current understanding that it is important to maintain a moist rather than a dry wound environment in order to optimize wound healing.[44]

The use of hydrotherapy for wound care is not new. As early as 1734, a German physician, Dr. Johann Hahn, recommended prolonged immersion in water for the treatment of leg sores[44]. Traditionally, a whirlpool has been used for the application of hydrotherapy for wounds; however, recently nonimmersion techniques of hydrotherapy have become more popular for applying this type of treatment. This change in practice is due in part to concern regarding the potentially damaging effects of placing excessive pressures on the regenerating tissue in wounds by water agitated by a whirlpool turbine and is also due, in part, to concern regarding the potential for wound

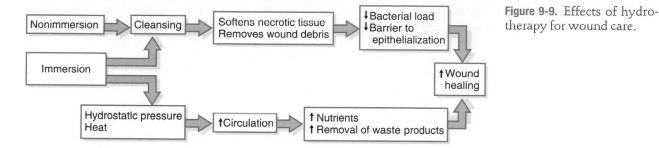

Figure 9-9. Effects of hydrotherapy for wound care.

infection if a wound is allowed to soak in contaminated tank water for a prolonged period of time.

It has been shown that excessive fluid pressure can cause wound trauma and drive bacteria into a wound, and that therefore, because the pressure of the water being directed at a wound in a whirlpool cannot be accurately controlled, there is a risk of applying too much or too little pressure with this type of device.[45] Although the pressure of the water being applied to a wound in a whirlpool can be modified to some extent by moving the turbine output toward or away from the wound or by changing the degree of aeration, the absolute amount of pressure being exerted is not known and cannot be controlled. Therefore it is generally recommended that whirlpool treatments be used only for cleansing wounds that contain extensive thick exudate, slough or necrotic tissue, gross purulence, or dry eschar when other, nonimmersion hydrotherapy devices may be ineffective or when nonimmersion hydrotherapy devices are not available, and it is recommended that all forms of hydrotherapy treatment be discontinued when a wound is clean.[18]

Concerns regarding the potential for wound infection with immersion hydrotherapy are the result of reports of outbreaks of wound infection, most commonly due to *Pseudomonas aeruginosa* but also occasionally due to *Staphylococcus aureus, Acinetobacter baumannii* or *Candida albicans,* after whirlpool treatments.[46-50] Reports of contamination of hydrotherapy equipment with these microorganisms have been a cause for concern; however, a recent report found that only about 10% of whirlpools tested were contaminated.[47,49,51] Whirlpool tank water may become contaminated by microorganisms from the patient being treated at that time, or by microorganisms that become lodged in the crevices of the tank from prior treatments or between treatments. In order to reduce the risk of wound infection with hydrotherapy, a number of authors recommend the addition of antimicrobial additives to the water when treating

wounds; however, this practice is controversial at this time.[46,49-54] This controversy is based on the conflict between the potential benefits of improved infection control when antimicrobials are used and the potential for adverse effects, since it has been found that many antimicrobial products are cytotoxic to normal tissue unless used at very dilute concentrations[55-61] (Table 9-3). These conflicting findings on the benefits of using antimicrobial additives in hydrotherapy water lend support to the practice of either using an antimicrobial at the lowest effective

TABLE 9-3 Toxicity Index for Wound and Skin Cleansers

Test agent	Toxicity index*
Biolex	1:100
Saf Klenz	1:100
Ultra Klenz	1:100
Clinical Care	1:1,000
Uniwash	1:1,000
Ivory Soap (0.5%)	1:1,000
Constant Clens	1:10,000
Dermal wound cleanser	1:10,000
Puri Clens	1:10,000
Hibiclens	1:10,000
Betadine surgical scrub	1:10,000
Technicare scrub	1:100,000
Bard Skin Cleanser	1:100,000
Hollister	1:100,000

From Foresman PA, Payne DS, Becker D et al: A relative toxicity index for wound cleaners, *Wounds* 5(5): 226-231, 1993.
*The dilution required to maintain white blood cell viability and phagocytic efficiency.

concentration or using only clean water without additives when using a whirlpool to treat open wounds. The policy for the use of antimicrobials in whirlpools in most facilities is set by the infection control department of the facility, in accordance with regulatory guidelines, and should always be followed. Whether or not additives are used during whirlpool treatment of open wounds, the tank and turbine should always be thoroughly cleaned and disinfected between uses. Recommendations for whirlpool cleaning procedures are provided in this chapter in the section on safety issues regarding hydrotherapy. In order to avoid the infection risks associated with whirlpool use, many facilities use nonimmersion hydrotherapy techniques for wound care because, with these techniques, the wound does not soak in potentially contaminated water inside a potentially contaminated tank.

A variety of devices can be used to apply hydrotherapy without immersion to wounds. In order to be safe and effective for this application, such devices must deliver fluid at a pressure of between 4 and 15 psi (pounds per square inch) because, below this level, bacteria and debris are not effectively removed, while at higher pressures, wound trauma may occur or bacteria may be driven into the tissue.[43,62,63] A number of devices have been shown to deliver fluid within this pressure range (Table 9-4). These include a saline squeeze bottle with an irrigation cap or a 35-mL syringe with a 19-gauge needle. Electric pulsatile irrigation devices can also be set to deliver pressure within this range.

Generally, nonimmersion hydrotherapy is recommended for the treatment of wounds containing necrotic, nonviable tissue or debris. This type of treatment has been shown to facilitate the removal of

TABLE 9-4 Irrigation Pressure Delivered by Various Devices

Device	Irrigation pressure (psi)
Spray bottle—Ultra Klenz* (Carrington Laboratories Inc., Dallas, TX)	1.2
Bulb Syringe* (Davol Inc., Cranston, RI)	2.0
Piston Irrigation Syringe, 60 mL, with catheter tip[†] (Premium Plastics Inc., Chicago)	4.2
Saline Squeeze Bottle, 250 mL, with irrigation cap[†] (Baxter Healthcare Corp., Deerfield, IL)	4.5
Water Pik at lowest setting[†] (Teledyne Water Pik, Fort Collins, CO)	6.0
Irrijet DS Syringe with tip[†] (Ackrad Laboratories, Inc., Cranford, NJ)	7.6
35-mL syringe with 19 gauge needle or angiocatheter[†]	8.0
Water Pik at middle setting[‡] (Teledyne Water Pik, Fort Collins, CO)	42
Water Pik at highest setting[‡] (Teledyne Water Pik, Fort Collins, CO)	50
Pressurized Cannister Dey Wash[‡] (Dey Laboratories, Inc., Napa, CA)	50

From U.S. Department of Health and Human Services: *Treatment of Pressure Ulcers: Clinical Practice Guidelines*. Rockville, MD, 1994, U.S. Department of Health and Human Services.
*Too little pressure for effective wound cleansing <4 psi.
[†]Appropriate pressure for safe and effective wound cleansing at 4 to 15 psi.
[‡]Too much pressure for safe wound cleansing >15 psi.

necrotic tissue, promote healing, and increase patient comfort in both hospital and homebound patients. [64] It is recommended that nonimmersion hydrotherapy be continued until all necrotic, nonviable material has been removed and a full granulation bed is present.[65] A combination of immersion hydrotherapy, using a whirlpool to soften debris followed by nonimmersion hydrotherapy with a spray to remove this debris and bacteria, has also been shown to be particularly effective for the removal of bacteria from wounds.[66]

When applying hydrotherapy to wounds, whether using immersion or nonimmersion techniques, it is important to balance the potential benefits to the wound with the potential for damaging regenerating granulation tissue in the wound bed by mechanical disruption, or for damaging the intact skin surrounding the wound by maceration as a result of excessive moisture. Therefore all forms of hydrotherapy should be discontinued when the wound base is fully covered with granulation tissue, and the intact skin surrounding a wound should always be thoroughly, though gently, dried immediately after completion of any hydrotherapy treatment.

Special concerns regarding the use of hydrotherapy in the treatment of burns

Hydrotherapy is considered to be an important component of the treatment of acute burn injuries in most burn centers in the United States.[48,67-69] The purposes and uses of hydrotherapy in burn care are generally the same as those for other types of wounds, except for a few noteworthy differences. As with other types of wounds, hydrotherapy is used as a component of early treatment in order to cleanse, soften, and loosen necrotic tissue before debridement, and to reduce bacterial colonization. However, in contrast to most other types of wounds, where such debridement is relatively painless, the debridement of burn wounds is frequently extremely painful because the wounds are less deep and many of the sensory nerves are still intact. Therefore high-dose analgesics are generally used during this procedure, necessitating closer monitoring of the patient during the treatment. Also, because burn wounds are often extensive, covering a large area of the body, the larger Hubbard tank whirlpools have traditionally been used for this application, and, with the increasing concern for and awareness of the risks of nosocomial infections with the use of immersion hydrotherapy, special nonimmersion techniques for the treatment of burns have been developed.[48,68] These generally involve showering the patient while the patient is lying on a sur-

face, such as a mesh net stretcher or trauma table, that allows the water to pour off into a suitable drain.[70] This type of treatment setup has the additional advantages of being less painful for the patient and allowing more rapid treatment and greater ease in patient handling. If immersion techniques are used for the hydrotherapy treatment of burns, it has been recommended that salt be added to the water in order to reduce sodium loss from the patient to the water and to reduce the risk of hyponatremia associated with the soaking of some patients with extensive burns in water.[71,72]

Hydrotherapy is used not only in the early treatment of burn wounds, when necrotic tissue is present, but also in the later stages of recovery after reepithelialization has occurred. In this circumstance, the risk of wound infection is eliminated and the water is used to provide a comfortable environment for exercise and for active and passive range of motion (ROM), helping to prevent contractures and to facilitate increased ROM in scarred areas.

Water Exercise

Types of water exercise

Various types of exercise, including swimming, running with or without a vest or belt, walking, cycle ergometry, and other forms of upright exercise can be performed in water (Fig. 9-10). In general, patients are free to move about the pool while exercising, although they may be tethered to the side, as for example during in-place water running. The tether may be used to facilitate monitoring of the exercise by the therapist or to increase resistance and allow a wider range of activities, particularly in a small pool. The principles, mechanisms of action, and rationales for performing exercise in water are discussed below; however, specific water exercise programs are not covered since they are described in detail in other texts devoted to aquatic therapy.[72]

General uses of water exercises

Exercise in water can be used to increase circulation, muscle strength, joint viscoelasticity, flexibility, and ROM; to improve ambulation, coordination, cardiovascular and respiratory conditioning and psychological well-being; and to decrease pain, muscle spasm, and stiffness. The specific contributions of the unique physical properties of water, including its ability to retain and conduct heat, and its buoyancy, resistance, and hydrostatic pressure in producing these effects, are discussed in detail directly following.

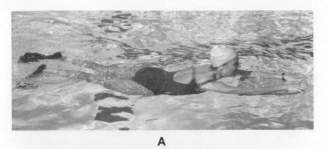

A

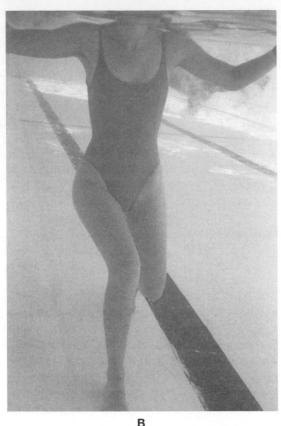

B

Figure 9-10. Water exercise in a swimming pool. **A,** Swimming, and **B,** jogging.

The ability of water to retain and conduct heat is used clinically when a patient, or a part of a patient, exercises while immersed in warm water. The combination of heat transfer and exercise is particularly effective in certain cases because increasing the temperature of soft tissue can augment the vasodilation, increased circulation, decreased joint stiffness, increased joint ROM, and enhanced functional abilities that result from exercise.[74,75] The relaxing effects of immersion in warm water may also improve the psychological well-being of the patient during and after water-based exercise.

Because the buoyancy of water decreases the gravitational forces placed on weight-bearing structures, patients with weakened limbs or load-sensitive joints can often perform strengthening, conditioning, and coordination exercises in water that they would not be able to perform on dry land. This can contribute to improved functional mobility and strength. The resistance provided by water during movement can also serve as a force against which muscles can work in order to develop strength or, when applied in the direction of patient movement, can be used to assist weakened muscles in the production of movement.[76]

Because the hydrostatic pressure provided by immersion in water can facilitate venous return from the extremities, circulation may be enhanced during exercise in water compared to similar exercise performed on dry land. As described previously, the circulatory changes produced by the hydrostatic pressure of water on the extremities during water-based exercise can also facilitate cardiovascular and respiratory conditioning, and help to reverse and control the formation of peripheral edema.

Specific uses of water exercise

Orthopedic problems
  Decreased weight bearing on joints
  Velocity-dependent resistance
  Closed or open chain exercises
  Slowed bone density loss
Neurological problems
  Proprioceptive input
  Increased safety
  Improved balance
Cardiac fitness
  **Cardiac conditioning in patients with poor
    tolerance for land-based exercise**
Exercise in water during pregnancy
  Decreased weight bearing
  Less elevation of heart rate with exercise
  Decreased risk of maternal hyperthermia
Exercise-induced asthma
  **Less exercise-induced asthma than with other
    forms of exercise**

Orthopedic problems

The water environment can be used to provide graded weight bearing and patient-controlled resistance to help individuals with spinal and/or peripheral musculoskeletal dysfunction perform exercises they would have difficulty performing on dry land.[77,78] This can allow for earlier exercise participation following injury, surgery, or immobilization and greater exercise participation by patients with load-sensitive conditions such as osteoarthritis or spinal disc displacement.[79] Such exercise participation may also result in earlier recovery of and greater final functional mobility in these individuals.

Weight bearing can be graded by varying the depth of water immersion or by the use of flotation devices, such as belts, arm bands, or hand-held floats, with deeper immersion or more flotation devices providing more unloading. Flotation devices also allow greater muscular relaxation in the water by eliminating or reducing the amount of work required by the patient to stay afloat. Therefore the use of such devices is particularly appropriate for the patient who can benefit from both decreased joint loading and decreased muscular activity. For example, patients with load-sensitive spinal conditions such as disc bulges or herniations or nerve root compression may benefit from relaxed vertical floating in water, supported by a flotation belt, to allow unloading of the spinal intraarticular structures and relaxation of the paraspinal muscles (Fig. 9-11).

Varying the resistance provided by water during exercise, by altering the speed or direction of the motion of the water or the speed of movement of the patient, can alter the clinical effects of the exercise. The faster the water moves toward the patient, against the patient's direction of movement, or the faster the patient moves in the water, the greater the resistance against the patient's movement and thus the greater the strengthening or endurance-building

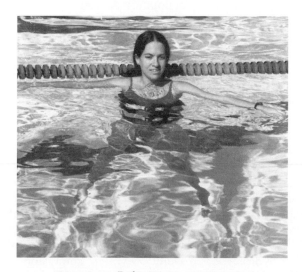

Figure 9-11. Relaxing in a water vest.

effect of the activity. Exercise intensity can thus be graded by modifying the speed of water motion in a pool that allows control of water motion or by altering the speed at which the patient is moving while exercising. If the flow of the water can be directed to be in, rather than against, the direction of the patient's motion, the resistance of the water can also be used to assist with motion when muscles are weak in order to allow strengthening through a greater ROM.

The types of exercises performed in water must be carefully designed and selected to address different conditions and to avoid exacerbating existing problems or causing new ones. The patient can perform either closed-chain or open-chain exercises in water. Closed-chain exercises can be performed using the bottom of the pool to fix the distal extremity when the patient is in shallow water (Fig. 9-12) or using the side of the pool to fix the distal extremity when the patient is in deeper water. Open-chain exercises can also be performed in either deep or shallow water, depending on the area of the body involved and the type of exercise to be performed (Fig. 9-13). It is important to select the appropriate exercise for a particular problem and to be aware of the changes in biomechanics if an exercise usually performed on dry land is transferred to a water environment. For example, running on dry land is primarily a closed-chain activity, whereas when running is performed in deep water using a flotation vest, it is entirely an open-chain activity. This change may reduce pain from tibiofemoral joint compression by decreasing the weight bearing on this joint, but it may increase patellofemoral joint pain by producing increased compression at this joint during open-chain knee extension.

When designing rehabilitation programs that involve swimming, it is particularly important to guard against adverse effects of compensatory motions because such motions can cause problems in other areas.[77] For example, if the patient has limited shoulder ROM and increases lumbar or cervical motion to bring the shoulder out of the water during freestyle swimming, the result may be problems in these spinal areas. In a similar manner, a patient with hypomobility of the thoracic spine may overuse the shoulder during freestyle or breast stroke swimming and increase subacromial compression of the rotator cuff, causing tendon breakdown.

Because exercise in water results in reduced weight bearing on the bones, it has generally been assumed that exercise in this environment does not assist in maintaining bone density in postmenopausal women.

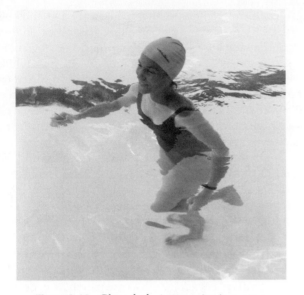

Figure 9-12. Closed-chain exercise in water.

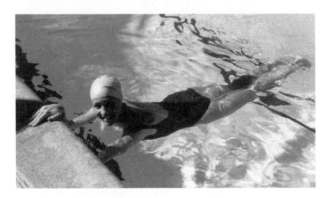

Figure 9-13. Open-chain exercise in water.

However, because a recent cross-sectional and longitudinal study has shown that water in exercise can slow bone mineral density loss in the lumbar spine in this population, water-based exercise is recommended for slowing bone mineral density loss.[80]

Neurological problems

Water-based exercise has been recommended to address the impairments, disabilities, and handicaps resulting from neurological dysfunction because it provides proprioceptive input, weight relief, and a safe environment for movement.[81] The proprioceptive input may be particularly beneficial for patients with central sensory deficits, such as those that can

occur after a stroke or traumatic brain injury, while the weight relief can increase ease of movement and reduce the risk of falling to facilitate greater movement exploration, functional activity training, and strengthening in patients with weakness or impaired motor control.[82] It has been proposed that the greater movement exploration and the increased production of movement errors that occur in water-based exercise are responsible for the balance enhancement that has been shown to result from water-based exercise programs.[83] Reduced loading due to buoyancy, and the increased abdominal support from the hydrostatic pressure of water, may also provide assistance for breathing in patients with a weak diaphragm, as can occur after a spinal cord injury or with amyotrophic lateral sclerosis (ALS), although this must be balanced against the increased breathing workload produced by the shift of fluids to the central circulation. The decreased patient weight caused by the buoyancy of the patient's body in water, and the support provided by the buoyancy and hydrostatic pressure of water, may also contribute to patient progress by allowing for easier patient handling by the therapist.

Exercise in water using a variety of specific approaches, such as neurodevelopmental training (NDT) or the Bad Ragaz method, has been recommended for improving function in patients with neurological problems.[84,85] These methods use verbal instructions and tactile cues to guide the patient to practice normal movement progression and sequencing. The challenge of the activities can then be modified by varying the depth of the water or by using the support of one or more flotation devices. These methods are particularly recommended for improving stability and motor control.

Cardiac fitness

Because water-based exercise programs have been shown to maintain and increase aerobic conditioning, exercise in water can be used to provide general conditioning for deconditioned patients or for those who wish to increase their cardiovascular fitness.[22,86] This form of exercise can be particularly beneficial for cardiac conditioning in patients with conditions such as osteoarthritis, postoperative recovery, or joint instability that are aggravated by joint loading and thus limit land-based exercise.

The increased cardiac output resulting from the hydrostatic pressure of water immersion, as described previously, has led some to investigate the effects of exercise in water for cardiac rehabilitation. Two recent studies of patients with a history of myocardial infarction or ischemic heart disease have demonstrated improvement in heart function of about 30% in patients performing exercise in water for a month.[87,88] Exercise in water has also been shown to reduce the resting heart rate and increase VO_{2max}, maximum heart rate, and work capacity in healthy older adults and to improve respiratory function in patients with chronic obstructive pulmonary disease.[10,16]

A novel form of water exercise consisting of immersion in water in combination with expiring into water has been found to increase cardiac ejection fraction and to decrease left ventricular end-diastolic and systolic dimensions at rest in patients with emphysema. This exercise also resulted in an increase in the ratio of forced expired volume in one second to forced vital capacity (FEV_1:FVC) and a decrease in $PaCO_2$. These results suggest that this type of water exercise may improve both the breathing and cardiac function of patients with emphysema.[90]

Exercise in water during pregnancy

A number of studies on the effects of exercise in water during pregnancy indicate that this form of exercise may be particularly appropriate for pregnant women.[17,18,89] Exercise in water provides the benefits of unloading the weight-bearing joints, controlling peripheral edema, and causing less elevation of heart rate, blood pressure, and body temperature than similar exercise performed on dry land. The American College of Obstetricians and Gynecologists recommends that women keep their heart rate below 140 beats per minute throughout pregnancy. Thus, given the lower heart rate response to exercise in water, women may be able to perform exercise in water at a higher level of perceived exertion, and at a higher metabolic rate, than they could on dry land while staying within safe heart rate limits.[17,91] Exercise in water is also thought to pose less risk to the fetus than land-based exercise because it has been shown that the incidence of postexercise fetal tachycardia is lower with this type of exercise than with land-based exercise.[18,89]

Immersion in water, and thus upright exercise, or even immersion in an upright position in water, places hydrostatic pressure on the immersed areas and can therefore be used to help reduce peripheral edema in pregnant patients. This effect is the result of improved venous and lymphatic flow and renal-influenced diuresis caused by the hydrostatic pressure of water on the lower extremities. Because hydrostatic pressure increases at increasing depths of water, control of peripheral edema is most marked when the patient exercises in an upright position to produce the greatest pressure on the distal lower extremities.

Exercise-induced asthma

Water-based exercise, including swimming, is particularly suited to patients with exercise-induced asthma because the water environment has been found to reduce the incidence of asthma in these individuals compared with land-based exercise.[30,31] Also, a number of studies have shown decreased symptoms of asthma and increased fitness in individuals with asthma, particularly children, in response to swimming exercise.[92,93]

Pain Control

Hydrotherapy is often recommended as a treatment for the control of pain. Although there is little data regarding this application of hydrotherapy, hydrotherapy is thought to control pain by providing a high level of sensory stimulation to the peripheral mechanoreceptors to gate the transmission of pain sensations at the spinal cord. Such a mechanism is consistent with the reports by many clinicians that forms of hydrotherapy that provide the greatest sensory stimulation, such as contrast baths, or water at a high temperature with a high level of agitation, are particularly effective in reducing pain. Cold water may also contribute to the reduction of pain by reducing acute inflammation. Pain control may also result from the decreased weight bearing and increased ease of movement produced by water immersion.

Edema Control

Water immersion has been shown to reduce peripheral edema. It is proposed that this effect is due to the hydrostatic pressure of water and the resulting changes in circulation and renal function. Therefore water immersion has been recommended for the treatment of peripheral edema with a variety of etiologies including venous or lymphatic insufficiency, renal dysfunction, and postoperative inflammation.[4,94] In addition to the effects of hydrostatic pressure on postoperative edema, the cooling effects of cold water may also contribute to edema reduction by causing vasoconstriction and reducing vascular permeability. Therefore cold water immersion of a limb, or part of a limb, is frequently used as a component of the treatment of edema due to recent trauma when other signs of acute inflammation are present. Immersion in warm or hot water is not recommended in such circumstances because heating the area and placing it in a dependent position can increase tissue temperature and intravascular pressure, resulting in increased inflammation and peripheral arterial flow, and thus increased rather than decreased edema.[95] In such cases it has been found that the higher the temperature of the water, the greater the amount of edema.[95]

Contrast baths are frequently recommended and clinically used to control edema, with the rationale that the alternating vasodilation and vasoconstriction produced by the alternating immersion in hot and cold water may help to train or condition the smooth muscles of the blood vessels. However, because there are no research data on the efficacy or mechanisms of this effect, it is recommended that clinicians carefully assess the effect of such treatment on the individual patient when considering using this form of hydrotherapy treatment.

CONTRAINDICATIONS AND PRECAUTIONS FOR HYDROTHERAPY

Although hydrotherapy is a relatively safe treatment modality, its use is contraindicated in some circumstances and it should be applied with caution in others.[96] When applying hot or cold water to a patient, all the contraindications and precautions that apply to the use of other superficial heating or cooling agents, described in detail in Chapter 6, apply to this mode of superficial heating or cooling. In addition, a number of contraindications and precautions apply specifically to the application of hydrotherapy, either by local immersion in a whirlpool or contrast bath, or by whole body immersion in a pool or Hubbard tank, or by nonimmersion methods. These are listed in the boxes and discussed in detail in the text that follows.

CONTRAINDICATIONS
for Local Immersion Forms of Hydrotherapy

- Maceration around a wound
- Bleeding

The use of local forms of hydrotherapy is contraindicated . . .

. . . when there is maceration around a wound

Immersion hydrotherapy is contraindicated when there is maceration of intact skin around a wound because it is likely to increase the maceration and thus increase the size of the wound.

ASSESS:
- Inspect the skin around the wound for signs of maceration, including pallor or other early indications of breakdown.

When there is maceration around a wound, and when the cleansing benefits of hydrotherapy are desired, nonimmersion techniques should be used to avoid excessive or prolonged soaking of the macerated tissues.

. . . when there is bleeding

Immersion hydrotherapy should not be applied if there is bleeding in or near an area being considered for treatment because immersion hydrotherapy may increase bleeding by increasing venous circulation as a result of the hydrostatic pressure and may increase arterial circulation as a result of vasodilation if warm or hot water is used.

ASSESS:
- Check for bleeding in or near the area being considered for treatment.

If bleeding is mild and has been determined not to be dangerous to the patient, nonimmersion hydrotherapy may be used.

PRECAUTIONS
for Local Immersion Forms of Hydrotherapy

- Impaired thermal sensation in the area to be immersed

- Infection in the area to be immersed
- Confusion or impaired cognition
- Recent skin grafts

Use local immersion forms of hydrotherapy with caution . . .

. . . when there is impaired thermal sensation in the area to be immersed

Areas with impaired thermal sensation are at increased risk for thermal burns. Therefore in order to minimize this risk, the temperature of the water to be used for hydrotherapy should always be checked with a thermometer before the patient enters the water. It is also recommended that the clinician check the water temperature directly by placing a hand, wearing a clean rubber glove, in the water before the patient enters. Thermostatically controlled mixing valves should also be used to control the temperature of the incoming water.

ASK THE PATIENT:
- Can you feel heat and cold in this area?

ASSESS:
- Thermal sensation can be tested by applying test tubes filled with cold or warm water to the area and asking the patient to report the sensation of the stimulus.

If the patient has impaired thermal sensation, only water at a temperature close to body temperature should be used for applying hydrotherapy.

. . . when there is infection in the area to be immersed

Hydrotherapy is frequently applied to wounds when an infection is present in the area to be immersed. In such circumstances, use the additional infection control measures described in the section of this chapter concerning the use of hydrotherapy for the treatment of wounds and in the section of this chapter concerning safety issues regarding the application of hydrotherapy.

ASSESS:
- Check the area to be treated for signs of infection. Signs of infection include induration, fever, erythema, and edema. Since all open wounds are colonized with bacteria, when treating open wounds with immersion hydrotherapy, one should take the same precautions as when an infection is known to be present.[97]

. . . with patients experiencing confusion or impaired cognition

Hydrotherapy is frequently applied when patients are confused or have impaired cognition. For example, many patients have open wounds, to some degree as a result of their impaired mental status, and many patients with burns are given high-dose analgesics to control pain during the debridement performed during or directly after hydrotherapy, which also results in impairment of mental status.

ASSESS:
- Assess the patient's level of cognition and alertness. Check if the patient can effectively communicate discomfort.

When a patient is confused or is unable to effectively report discomfort or other problems for any other reason, one should provide direct supervision throughout hydrotherapy treatment and only use water at a temperature close to body temperature.

. . . in areas with recent skin grafts

Extra care should be taken when treating recent skin grafts with hydrotherapy because a graft may not tolerate the mechanical agitation of a whirlpool or may not have a sufficient vascular response to compensate for extreme heat or cold. Therefore, the whirlpool agitator should always be directed away from the area of a graft, and water with neutral warmth (33° to 35.5° C; 92° to 96° F) or mild warmth (35.5° to 37° C; 96° to 98° F) should be used when treating recent skin grafts.

Full Body Immersion Hydrotherapy

All the contraindications and precautions for partial body immersion hydrotherapy apply to full body immersion hydrotherapy.[98] In addition, a number of contraindications and precautions, due to the risks associated with deep water and the fact that most full body immersion occurs in a pool where the water is not changed between uses, apply uniquely to full body immersion hydrotherapy.

CONTRAINDICATIONS
for Full Body Immersion Hydrotherapy

- Cardiac instability
- Infectious conditions that may be spread by water
- Bowel incontinence
- Severe epilepsy
- Suicidal patients

The use of full body immersion hydrotherapy is contraindicated . . .

. . . for patients with cardiac instability

Full body immersion is contraindicated in cases of cardiac instability, such as uncontrolled hypertension or heart failure, because in such circumstances the heart may not be able to adapt sufficiently in response to the changes in circulation produced by the hydrotherapy to maintain cardiac homeostasis.

ASSESS:
- Check with the patient's physician and review the patient's chart to determine if any cardiac instability is present. Heart rate and blood pressure should also be monitored during and after immersion in all patients with a history of cardiac problems.

. . . for patients with infectious conditions that may be spread by water

Patients with infectious conditions that may be spread by water should not use any type of hydrotherapy where the water is not changed between uses. Thus such patients should not use a pool but may use a Hubbard tank, where the water is changed between treatments, for full body immersion. Infectious conditions that may be spread by water include urinary tract infections, tinea pedis, plantar warts, and infections present in open wounds.

ASK THE PATIENT:
- Do you have a urinary tract infection, athlete's foot, plantar warts, or any open wounds? This question may be asked most readily in a written checkoff sheet given to all patients before any pool activities.

. . . for patients with bowel incontinence

Patients with bowel incontinence may not be immersed in water that will be used by other patients. In patients with bowel incontinence and open wounds, care should also be taken to avoid contaminating the water used for hydrotherapy, and thus the wound, with bacteria from the patient's own feces.

ASSESS:
- Check the patient's chart for any notation regarding bowel incontinence.
  Nonimmersion forms of hydrotherapy are recommended for the treatment of open wounds in patients with bowel incontinence.

. . . for patients with severe epilepsy

Full body immersion hydrotherapy should not be applied to patients with severe epilepsy because such patients have an increased risk of drowning.

. . . for suicidal patients

Full body immersion hydrotherapy should also not be applied to suicidal patients because they have an increased risk of drowning.

PRECAUTIONS
for Full Body Immersion Hydrotherapy

- Confusion or disorientation
- After ingestion of alcohol by the patient
- Limited strength, endurance, balance, or ROM
- Medications
- Urinary incontinence
- Fear of water
- Respiratory problems

Use full body immersion hydrotherapy with caution . . .

. . . with patients experiencing confusion or disorientation

Full body immersion is occasionally used for the treatment of confused or disoriented patients who have multiple or large open wounds or wounds that are difficult to access by other means. In such cases, extra care should be taken to monitor the water temperature and to be sure that the patient is well and safely secured, with the head above the water.

. . . after ingestion of alcohol by the patient

Full body water immersion should be avoided after the ingestion of alcohol because the impairment of judgment and cognitive functions that occurs with intoxication and the hypotensive effects of alcohol ingestion can increase the risk of drowning.

ASK THE PATIENT:

- If you suspect that a patient has recently been drinking alcohol—for example, if you smell alcohol on the patient's breath, ask, "Have you drunk alcohol in the last few hours?"

. . . with patients with limited strength, endurance, balance, or range of motion

Although hydrotherapy is frequently used for treating limitations of strength, endurance, balance, or ROM, extreme limitations in any of these areas can be a safety hazard for full body immersion hydrotherapy. Therefore, for full body immersion hydrotherapy treatment, a patient must have the ability to maintain the head above water or, if unable to do so, must be well and safely secured so as to keep the head

above water. Direct, hands-on assistance, with the therapist in the water, can also be provided for patients who have difficulty keeping their heads above water.

ASSESS:

- Check strength, balance, and ROM before the patient enters the water. If any of these are significantly limited, secure the patient so that the head cannot enter the water or accompany the patient into the water, at least for the first treatment, to assess the patient's safety in the water.

. . . with patients taking medications

Some medications, particularly those used to treat cardiovascular disease, alter the cardiovascular response to exercise. It is therefore recommended that a physician be consulted to establish safe limits of cardiovascular response for each patient before initiating an aquatic exercise program with any patient taking medications.

. . . with patients who have urinary incontinence

A patient with urinary incontinence may be catheterized to allow full body immersion hydrotherapy; however, this is generally not recommended because immersion may increase the risk of urinary tract infection in a catheterized patient.

. . . with patients who have a fear of water

Patients with a fear of water will generally refuse to participate in immersion hydrotherapy. For such patients, alternative treatments such as immersing only the area requiring treatment, using nonimmersion hydrotherapy, or using an intervention, such as dry land exercise, which does not involve the use of water, should be considered.

CONTRAINDICATIONS—cont'd

. . . with patients who have respiratory problems

Although water-based exercise can provide respiratory and general conditioning for patients with exercise-induced asthma or other breathing problems, since water immersion increases the work of breathing, one should carefully monitor patients with respiratory problems for signs of respiratory distress throughout the water immersion treatment.

PRECAUTIONS
for Full Body Immersion in Hot or Very Warm Water[71]

- Pregnancy

- Multiple sclerosis
- Poor thermal regulation

Use full body immersion in hot or very warm water with caution . . .

. . . with pregnant patients

Because maternal hyperthermia has been found to be teratogenic and is associated with a variety of central nervous system abnormalities in the child, in order to minimize the possibility of maternal hyperthermia, full body immersion in a hot pool should be avoided during pregnancy, particularly during the first trimester, when the effects of heat are most hazardous to the fetus.[99] Full body immersion in normal-temperature pool water is recommended during pregnancy because, as explained above, this can be an ideal environment for exercise by the pregnant woman.

ASK THE PATIENT:
- Are you pregnant?
- Do you think you might be pregnant?

. . . with patients who have multiple sclerosis

Patients with multiple sclerosis should not be placed in a hot or warm pool because temperatures above 31° C (88° F) may cause increased fatigue and weakness in these patients.

. . . with patients who have poor thermal regulation

Thermal regulation in response to body heating is generally accomplished by a combination of conduction, convection, radiation, and evaporation. If a small area of the body is immersed in hot water, the patient with impaired thermal regulation may still be able to dissipate heat by conduction to areas in direct contact with the heated area and by direct radiation of heat from the skin; however, the dissipation of heat by convection by blood circulating through the area from other areas that have not been heated and the production of sweat may be impaired. Because all of these mechanisms are impaired when large areas of the body are heated, as occurs with full body immersion in hot or warm water, a patient with poor thermal regulation may be at risk for thermal shock if large areas of the body are immersed in hot water.

ASSESS:
- Check for any history of thermal shock or any other signs of poor thermal regulation. Because thermal regulation is frequently impaired in the elderly and in infants, warm or hot water hydrotherapy should be limited to small areas in these individuals.

PRECAUTIONS
for Nonimmersion Hydrotherapy

- Maceration
- May be ineffective

Use nonimmersion hydrotherapy with caution . . .

. . . when there is maceration around a wound

Caution should be taken to minimize the wetting of intact skin surrounding a wound due to the risk of causing or aggravating maceration. The intact skin should also be gently and thoroughly dried after any type of hydrotherapy in order to minimize the risk of macerating this tissue.

. . . because it may be ineffective

Because nonimmersion hydrotherapy does not provide buoyancy or hydrostatic pressure, it is effective for only a limited number of problems that can be addressed by immersion hydrotherapy. Thus it can be used for cleansing but should not be used when the cardiovascular, respiratory, musculoskeletal, or renal effects of immersion are desired. Nonimmersion hydrotherapy also produces little heat transfer because the water is in contact with the tissue for too brief a period. Therefore when considering the use of nonimmersion hydrotherapy, one must weigh these disadvantages against the advantages of reduced infection risk, increased ease of application, and reduced treatment times.

ADVERSE EFFECTS OF HYDROTHERAPY

Drowning
Burns
Fainting
Bleeding
Hyponatremia
Infection
Aggravation of edema

Drowning

The most severe potential adverse effect of hydrotherapy is death by drowning, and it is imperative that adequate precautions be taken to minimize this risk. The American Red Cross has identified the three most common causes of drowning to be failure to recognize hazardous conditions and practices, inability to get out of dangerous situations, and lack of knowledge of the safest ways to aid a drowning person.[100] Specific recommendations for safety precautions to be taken to minimize the risk of drowning are provided below in the section on safety issues regarding hydrotherapy.

Burns, Fainting, and Bleeding

Treatment by immersion in a warm or hot whirlpool has the risks associated with other forms of superficial thermotherapy, including burning, fainting, and bleeding. To minimize the possibility of any of these adverse effects, the temperature of the water used for hydrotherapy should be kept within the appropriate range and should always be checked with a thermometer before the water touches the patient. Additionally, the therapist may check the water temperature by placing a gloved hand into the water. Because certain populations, including the elderly, the very young, and those with impaired sensation or other neurological deficits, are at an increased risk of suffering burns, the use of hot water should be avoided when treating these patients.[101]

The risk of fainting due to hypotension is greatest when large areas of the patient's body are immersed in warm or hot water. This risk may be further increased in patients taking antihypertensive medications. Therefore in order to minimize the possibility of fainting, only the parts of the body requiring treatment in warm water should be immersed, and all patients taking antihypertensive medications should be closely monitored. Also, all patients should be well-supported during warm water immersion in order to prevent falling should the patient faint.

Hyponatremia

Immersion hydrotherapy has been associated with hyponatremia in patients with extensive burn wounds.[71] Hyponatremia occurs because these patients can lose salt from the open wound areas into the whirlpool water when the salinity of the water is lower than that of the tissue fluids. Therefore to minimize the possibility of this adverse consequence of hydrotherapy, salt should be added to the whirlpool water when treating patients with extensive burns or other extensive wounds.[72]

Infection

A number of reports have documented the association of hydrotherapy with infections in patients.[46-48]

Such a risk can be minimized by using nonimmersion hydrotherapy techniques or, when using immersion techniques, strictly adhering to appropriate cleaning protocols and using antimicrobials in the water.

Aggravation of Edema

Immersion in hot or warm water has been shown to increase edema[102] in the hands of patients with upper extremity disorders, and this effect becomes more pronounced as the temperature of the water increases.[95] Therefore in order to avoid aggravation of edema, only cool water should be used and dependency of the extremity in the water should be minimized when signs of acute inflammation are present.

APPLICATION TECHNIQUES

This section provides guidelines for the sequence of procedures required for the safe and effective application of hydrotherapy.

APPLICATION TECHNIQUE
Hydrotherapy

1. Evaluate the patient and set the goals of treatment.
2. Determine if hydrotherapy is the most appropriate treatment.

    Hydrotherapy may be an appropriate treatment when progress toward the goals of treatment can be achieved by the use of superficial heat or cold, wound cleansing and debridement, or exercise in a water environment, or where the goals of treatment include controlling pain or edema. Hydrotherapy is a particularly appropriate means of applying superficial heat or cold when the area to be treated is a distal extremity with varied contouring and when dependency of the limb will not aggravate the patient's symptoms. Hydrotherapy is the ideal intervention for wound cleansing and debridement when there is a moderate amount of debris or necrotic tissue in a wound. When a wound is clean, hydrotherapy is not indicated; when there is a large amount of necrotic tissue, more aggressive treatment, as can be provided by surgical debridement, may be required. Exercise in water is indicated for patients with load-sensitive conditions or where the benefits of resistance or hydrostatic pressure of water, as described

above, can promote progress toward the goals of treatment.

3. Determine that hydrotherapy is not contraindicated for this patient or this condition.

    The treatment area should be inspected for the presence of any open wounds, rash, or other signs of infection, and sensation in the area should be assessed. The patient's chart should also be checked for any record of previous adverse responses to hydrotherapy, and the patient should be asked the appropriate questions regarding contraindications. It is also recommended that heart rate and blood pressure be measured and recorded if a large area of the body is going to be immersed.

4. Select the appropriate form of hydrotherapy according to the condition to be treated and the desired treatment effects.

    Select from the following list:

    Whirlpool
    Hubbard tank
    Contrast bath   (See applications for each
    Nonimmersion   hydrotherapy agent on
       irrigation device   the following pages.)
    Pool

The form of hydrotherapy selected should be one that produces the desired treatment effects, is appropriate for the size of the area to be treated, allows for adequate safety and control of infection, and is cost effective. The advantages and disadvantages of the different forms of hydrotherapy, based on treatment goals, are provided below, together with the directions for their application. Detailed information on safety and infection control is provided in the section on safety issues toward the end of this chapter.

Because most clinical settings have only a limited selection of forms of hydrotherapy, it is recommended that the available form be used if it is effective and safe. For example, if no nonimmersion devices are available for treating a small open wound on a patient's ankle, a whirlpool may be used as long as appropriate infection control measures are taken; however, treatment of this condition should not be provided in an exercise pool or Jacuzzi, where the same water will be used by other patients. In contrast, if hydrotherapy is being considered for cardiovascular conditioning but only nonimmersion hydrotherapy devices are available, hydrotherapy should not be performed because it will be ineffective. In this case, a land-based exercise program should be considered.

5. Explain to the patient the procedure, the reason for applying hydrotherapy, and the sensations the patient can expect to feel.

During the application of hydrotherapy the patient may feel a sensation of warmth or cold, depending on the temperature of the water used. The patient will also feel gentle pressure if the water is being agitated. The patient should not feel excessively hot or cold, or excessive pressure, nor should the patient feel faint during the application of hydrotherapy. In general, hydrotherapy is not a painful procedure unless it is being used for the treatment of burns or other sensate wounds in conjunction with debridement. The pain associated with this procedure can usually be controlled to some extent by the administration of high-dose analgesics before the hydrotherapy treatment.

6. Apply the appropriate form of hydrotherapy.
7. When hydrotherapy is completed, assess the outcome(s) of the treatment. Remeasure and assess progress relative to the initial patient evaluation and the goals of treatment.
8. Document the treatment.

Whirlpool

A whirlpool is composed of a tank that can hold water and a turbine that provides agitation and aeration in order to produce movement of the water in the tank. The tank is usually made of stainless steel, although fiberglass and plastic tanks are also available. Whirlpools are available in a number of different shapes and sizes in order to allow for treatment of different body parts (Figs. 9-14 and 9-15). Extremity tanks are suitable for immersion of a distal extremity, such as a hand or a foot, whereas low-boy and high-boy tanks are intended for immersion of larger parts of the extremities and may be used for immersion up to the waist.

A whirlpool turbine is composed of a motor bracketed securely to the side of the whirlpool and pipes for air and water circulation suspended in the water (Fig. 9-16). The height and direction of the turbine can be adjusted to project the water pressure toward or

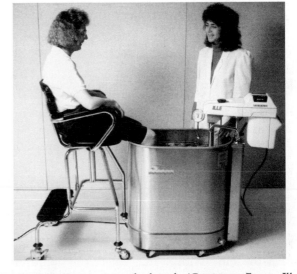

Figure 9-14. Extremity whirlpool. (Courtesy Ferno Ille, Wilmington, OH.)

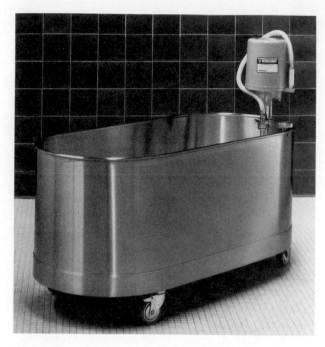

Figure 9-15. Low-boy whirlpool. (Courtesy Whitehall Manufacturing, City of Industry, CA.)

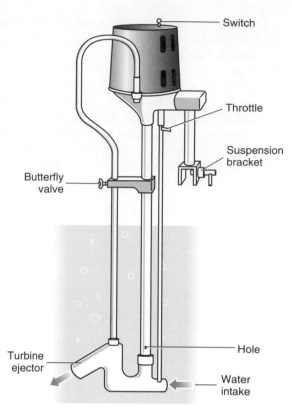

Figure 9-16. Whirlpool turbine.

away from the involved area. The turbine may be directed toward the involved area in order to achieve maximum stimulation, as may be desired to control pain or to remove tightly adhered wound debris. The turbine should be directed away from the involved area if the area is hypersensitive or if granulation tissue is present because the high direct pressure of water from the turbine can adversely affect such conditions. Most turbines also allow the clinician to open or close the aeration valve in order to further modify the pressure of the water flow.

Whirlpools are generally used for the treatment of open wounds, or for exercise or pain control, in limited areas of the body, such as the leg and foot or arm and hand.

APPLICATION TECHNIQUE
Whirlpool

Equipment Required
- Hot and cold water mixing valves
- Thermometer for checking the temperature of the water in the tank
- A turbine to agitate and aerate the water
- Seat or stretcher for the patient to sit either in or out of the water, depending on the area being treated and the configuration of the whirlpool
- Gravity drain
- Heated, well-ventilated space
- Towels and blankets

PROCEDURE

1. Fill the tank with water. Select the appropriate temperature range according to the condition and treatment objectives (Table 9-5).

A cold whirlpool, at 0° to 26° C (32° to 79° F), should be used for the treatment of acute inflammatory conditions of the distal extremities. Low temperatures can be achieved by adding ice to the whirlpool water; however, very low temperatures should not be used on large areas due to the increased risk of tissue damage.

A tepid whirlpool, at 26° to 33 °C (79° to 92 °F), should be used if the water is being used solely as a medium for exercise, because warmer temperatures are likely to produce fatigue and colder temperatures can inhibit muscle contraction. A tepid whirlpool may also be used when an inflammatory condition is present if lower temperatures are not tolerated.

A neutral warmth whirlpool, at 33° to 35.5 °C (92° to 96 °F), should be used for the treatment of open wounds and in patients with circulatory, sensory, or cardiac disorders. Neutral warmth may

shown to increase the temperature of subcutaneous tissue to within the range required to produce these effects.[103] The higher end of this temperature range is recommended for the treatment of chronic conditions, such as osteoarthritis or rheumatoid arthritis in the nonacute phases, when small areas are being treated, while the lower end of this range is recommended when large areas of the body are to be immersed.

The whirlpool temperature should not exceed 43 °C (110 °F) at any time because higher temperatures may cause burns.

The tank should be filled with water immediately before it is used in order to prevent the water

TABLE 9-5	Clinical Applications and Sensations of Whirlpool Treatment at Different Temperature Ranges	
Temperature range (°C/°F)	**Sensation**	**Clinical applications**
0 to 26/32 to 79	Cold	Acute inflammation
26 to 33/79 to 92	Tepid	Medium for exercise Acute inflammation if colder temperature not tolerated
33 to 35.5/92 to 96	Neutral warmth	Open wounds Medically compromised patients with circulatory, sensory, or cardiac disorders Decrease tone
35.5 to 37/96 to 98	Mild warmth	Increase mobility in burn patients
37 to 40/99 to 104	Hot	Control pain
40 to 43/104 to 110	Very hot	Increase soft tissue extensibility Chronic conditions Limited body area only
>43/>110		Should not be used

also be used to control tone in patients with neurologically based hypertonicity.

Mild warmth, at 35.5° to 37 °C (96° to 98 °F), may be used for the treatment of burns once epithelialization has begun. Such treatment promotes mobility and relaxation and minimizes energy loss by cooling or shivering.[72]

A hot whirlpool, at 37° to 40 °C (99° to 104 °F), or a very hot whirlpool, at 40° to 43 °C (104° to 110 °F), is recommended for the control of pain and/or to increase soft tissue extensibility because this temperature range of whirlpool water has been

temperature from changing excessively between filling and patient immersion. If an antimicrobial is being used, it should be added to the water as the whirlpool is being filled.

2. Allow the patient to undress the area to be treated, and provide a gown or halter and pants as necessary for modesty. Do not allow any clothing to enter the water because it may be sucked into the turbine.

When treating an open wound, the clinician must wear gloves, a waterproof gown, goggles, and a mask as universal precautions to protect the patient and the clinician from cross-infection by

Continued

APPLICATION TECHNIQUE—cont'd
Whirlpool

microorganisms that may be carried in the water or in airborne water droplets.

3. Remove wound dressings if any are present and if they are easy to remove without causing pain or damaging the tissue. Because adhered dressings may be easier to remove after brief soaking in the water, this may be done as long as the dressings are removed before the agitator turbine is turned on to avoid clogging the turbine. Inspect the skin and test it for thermal sensitivity. Vital signs should be checked and recorded before immersing any area of a patient with a current or recent cardiovascular abnormality in a whirlpool.

4. Position the patient comfortably, with the affected area immersed in the water. Try to avoid pressure of the limb on the edge of the whirlpool in order to avoid impairing circulation or nerve function or causing discomfort. Dry padding, such as a folded towel, may be placed on the rim of the tank to distribute pressure (Fig. 9-17). Do not allow the patient's fingers or toes to be near the turbine ejector.

5. Adjust the direction and aeration of the turbine. The entire turbine can be moved from side to side and up and down to adjust its direction. The butterfly valve at the top of the shaft of the turbine adjusts the aeration of the water (see Fig. 9-16). The hole at the lower end of the pipe through which air is forced should always be immersed at least 2 inches below the surface of the water in order to avoid overheating of the turbine.

6. Turn on the turbine.

7. Stay with the patient throughout the hydrotherapy treatment and monitor the patient's vital signs before, during, and after treatment as necessary. It is generally recommended that patients not be left alone during warm or hot hydrotherapy treatments due to the risk of fainting or other heat-related distress. Treatment should be discontinued if there are any abnormal or unsafe changes in vital signs.

8. The patient may exercise the affected part during the treatment. Movement is recommended when treatment is for joint stiffness or impaired ROM or when edema without acute inflammation is present.

9. Whirlpools are generally applied for 10 to 30 minutes, although shorter periods may be sufficient for softening wound eschar, while longer periods will increase the amount of heat transferred to the patient.

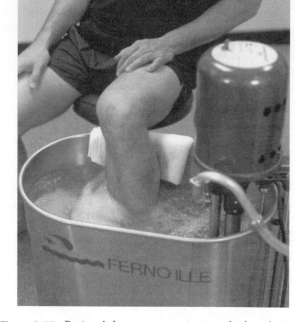

Figure 9-17. Patient's lower extremity in whirlpool. Note towel padding on edge of tank to disperse pressure.

10. When the treatment is completed, remove the limb from the water, dry the intact skin thoroughly, and inspect the treated area. Keep the body covered or wrapped after treatment to avoid chilling the patient.

11. If the whirlpool is being used for the treatment of an open wound, a clean, pressurized rinse is recommended after the whirlpool in order to remove bacteria more effectively.

12. Reapply wound dressings if open wounds are present.

13. Drain, rinse, and clean the whirlpool according to the directions given in the section on safety issues regarding hydrotherapy.

ADVANTAGES
- Can be used for heat transfer, for cleansing and debriding open wounds, or for exercise.
- Patient can be positioned securely and comfortably.
- Weaker muscles can move more freely than on dry land.

- Allows movement while heat is being applied, unlike other conductive thermal agents such as hot packs.

DISADVANTAGES
- Size of tank limits the amount of exercise and the size of the area that can be treated.
- Large quantity of water used.
- Risk of infection.
- Costs associated with cleaning.
- Costs associated with heating water.
- Time expended assisting the patient to dress and undress.

Hubbard Tank

A Hubbard tank, named after the engineer who invented it, is a large whirlpool intended for full body immersion. These tanks vary somewhat in size but are generally about 8 feet long by 6 feet wide and 4 feet deep, and they hold approximately 425 gallons of water (Fig. 9-18). The tank is equipped with turbines, a stretcher, and a hoist to raise and lower the stretcher. This large tank is particularly suitable for debridement of burns covering large areas of the body and for the treatment of other painful conditions that affect large areas of the body. Hubbard tanks can also be used for ROM exercises for multiple areas or for ambulation if a walking trough is added; however, these procedures are more often performed in a pool, except in cases where pool use is specifically contraindicated due to the risk of infection.

The popularity of the Hubbard tank has waned in recent years because of the considerable expense associated with providing such a large volume of warm water and because of the time involved in cleaning this large pool. Hubbard tanks must be cleaned between each use in the same manner as whirlpools of other sizes, as described in the section on safety issues regarding hydrotherapy.

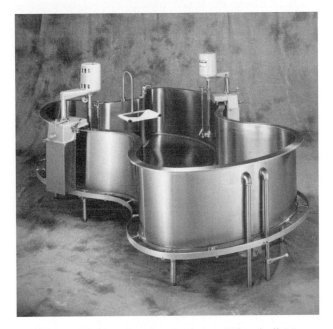

Figure 9-18. Hubbard tank. (Courtesy Whitehall Manufacturing, City of Industry, CA.)

APPLICATION TECHNIQUE
Hubbard Tank

Equipment Required
- Hot and cold water mixing valves
- Thermometer for checking the temperature of the water in the tank
- A turbine to agitate and aerate the water
- Seat or stretcher for the patient to sit either in or out of the water, depending on the area being treated and the configuration of the whirlpool
- Gravity drain
- Heated, well-ventilated space
- Towels and blankets

Continued

APPLICATION TECHNIQUE—cont'd
Hubbard Tank

PROCEDURE

Treatment in a Hubbard tank is applied in a similar manner to treatment in a whirlpool of any other size, as described above, except that the water temperature is generally kept in the slightly lower range of 36° to 39° C (97° to 100° F) because patients cannot dissipate the increase in tissue temperature as effectively when heat is applied to such a large area. Specific instructions for placing patients in a Hubbard tank and removing them from the tank are as follows:

1. Place the patient on the stretcher next to the tank, with the patient's weight evenly distributed.
2. Attach the hoist to the rings on the four corners of the stretcher.
3. Remove dressings if present and easy to remove without causing pain or damaging the tissue. If the dressings are adhered, they can be removed after brief soaking in the water before the turbines are turned on.
4. Raise the hoist to lift the patient. Gently swing the patient on the stretcher over the water and then slowly lower the patient to just above the water level.
5. Attach the head end of the stretcher to the support bracket.
6. Slowly lower the hoist until the foot end of the stretcher touches the bottom of the tank.
7. Remove the hoist.
8. Adjust the force and direction of the agitators.
9. Stay with the patient throughout the treatment to monitor the physiological responses to the treatment and to be sure that the patient does not slide down the stretcher into the water (Fig. 9-19).
10. Patients generally stay in a Hubbard tank for about 20 minutes or until the procedure, such as debridement, is completed.
11. When the treatment is completed, reattach the hoist to the stretcher and remove the patient from the water.
12. Dry the patient quickly and thoroughly.

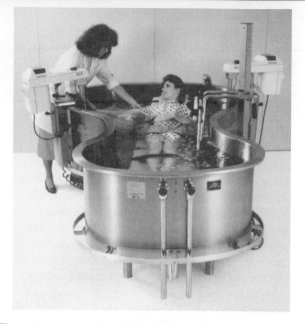

Figure 9-19. Patient in the Hubbard tank. (Courtesy Ferno Ille, Wilmington, OH.)

13. Wrap or cover the patient immediately to avoid chilling, leaving exposed any open wound areas requiring dressing.

ADVANTAGES

- Can treat large areas or multiple areas of the body.
- Can be used for heat transfer, for cleansing and debriding open wounds, or for water exercise.

DISADVANTAGES

- Costly to provide treatment.
- Costly equipment and space requirements.
- Uses large amount of warm water.
- Time-consuming to fill, empty, and clean tank and to place patient in the tank.
- Requires extra caution with regard to possible systemic effects of overheating with a large body area exposed.

Contrast Bath

Contrast baths are applied by alternately immersing an area, generally a distal extremity, first in warm or hot water and then in cool or cold water. Although there are no published research data on the effects of contrast baths, since this form of hydrotherapy is thought to train the vascular system by inducing alternating vasodilation and vasoconstriction, it is frequently used clinically when a goal of treatment is to decrease edema. The varying sensory stimulus is also thought to promote pain relief and desensitization. Thus treatment with a contrast bath may be considered when patients present with chronic edema; subacute trauma; inflammatory conditions such as sprains, strains, or tendonitis; or hyperalgesia or hypersensitivity due to reflex sympathetic dystrophy or other conditions.

APPLICATION TECHNIQUE
Contrast Bath

Equipment Required
- Two water containers
- Thermometer
- Towels

PROCEDURE
1. Fill two adjacent containers with water. The containers may be whirlpools, buckets, or tubs. Fill one container with warm or hot water, at 38° to 44 °C (80° to 104 °F), and the other with cold or cool water, at 10° to 18 °C (55° to 67 °F). When using contrast baths for the control of pain or edema, it is recommended that the temperature difference between the warm and cold water be large; when using contrast baths for desensitization, it is recommended that the temperature difference between the two baths initially be small and then gradually increased for later treatments as the patient's sensitivity decreases.
2. First, immerse the area to be treated in the warm water for 3 to 4 minutes; then immerse the area in the cold water for 1 minute (Fig. 9-20).
3. Repeat this sequence five or six times to provide a total treatment time of 25 to 30 minutes and end with immersion in the warm water.
4. When the treatment is completed, dry the area quickly and thoroughly.

ADVANTAGES
- May promote a more vigorous circulatory effect than heat or cold alone.

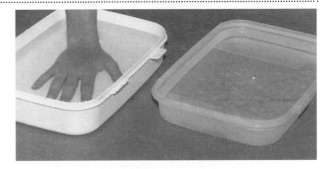

Figure 9-20. Contrast bath.

- Provides good contact with contoured distal extremities compared with other thermal agents.
- May help to provide pain control without aggravating edema.
- Allows movement in water for increased circulatory effects.

DISADVANTAGES
- Limb is in a dependent position, which may aggravate edema.
- Some patients do not tolerate cold immersion.
- Lack of research evidence to support the effect of contrast baths on circulation.

Nonimmersion Irrigation Devices

A variety of devices, including hand-held showers, syringes, and purpose-designed pulsatile irrigation units, can apply hydrotherapy without immersion of the area to be treated.[48,70,104] These devices apply water by spraying it on the treatment area. Nonimmersion irrigation devices are particularly well-suited for the application of hydrotherapy to open wounds because they involve less risk of infection than whirlpools and because some, although not all, of these devices can spray fluid onto an open wound within the appropriate, safe, and effective pressure limits of 4 to 15 psi (see Table 9-4). However, because without immersion water does not produce buoyancy or hydrostatic pressure, and therefore does not reduce weight bearing or edema or increase circulation, the use of nonimmersion hydrotherapy is limited to situations where these are not required to achieve the goals of treatment.

Because electric pulsatile irrigation devices both deliver fluid at a controlled pressure and provide suction to remove contaminated fluid, they are ideally suited to the treatment of open wounds.[104] These devices pump an intermittent stream of fluid from an irrigation bag or bottle. The fluid is delivered via tubing to a handpiece that directs the flow of fluid onto the wound.

The used and contaminated irrigation fluid is then removed from the treatment area by suction. The handpiece has a trigger to control the flow of fluid and can be fitted with a variety of tips to vary the fluid dispersion. With most of these devices, the tubing, handpiece, and tips are all intended to be discarded after each treatment in order to minimize the risk of cross-infection. Electric pulsatile irrigation devices are available in both portable and clinical models. This type of treatment is known as *pulsed lavage*.

APPLICATION TECHNIQUE
Nonimmersion Irrigation Device

Equipment Required
- Nonimmersion irrigation device
- Irrigation fluid—usually bags of sterile saline
- Towels

PROCEDURE

When applying nonimmersion irrigation, the following guidelines should be used. The clinician should always wear gloves, a waterproof gown, and eye, nose, and mouth protection during treatment because this type of treatment can spray contaminated fluid toward the clinician. In order to maximize comfort and optimize healing, clean, warm fluid should always be used for irrigation. Clean, warm water can be used for shower treatments, while sterile normal saline is recommended when irrigation is provided with other devices. It is recommended that treatment be applied once a day for 5 to 15 minutes or long enough to hydrate hard eschar or loosen debris. The appropriate frequency and duration of treatment will depend primarily on the size of the wound and the amount of necrotic tissue, exudate, or other debris present. In addition, when using an electric pulsatile irrigation device, the following treatment guidelines should be followed. Further specific directions for the use of different brands and models of these devices are provided by the manufacturers.

1. Although patients may be treated at the bedside with this type of device, in order to reduce the risk of transmitting infection, all irrigation treatments should be performed in an enclosed area separated from other patients. Pulsatile irrigation is also generally performed using sterile technique.

2. Sterile normal saline in 1000-ml bags is generally used as the irrigation fluid; in cases of wound infection, antimicrobials may be added to this fluid. It is recommended that the saline be warmed before it is used by placing it in a basin of hot tap water. Hang the bag(s) of fluid on the device.

3. Attach the tubing, suction canister, handpiece, and irrigation tip to the device.
4. Turn on the pump.
5. Select the treatment pressure. Most devices can spray fluid at pressures of between 0 and 60 psi and have a half-switch to limit the maximum pressure to 30 psi. Pressures of 4 to 8 psi are generally sufficient for cleansing or debriding most wounds; however, the pressure can be adjusted according to the nature of the wound, the tip used, and the sensitivity of the patient. It is recommended that the lowest pressure that effectively loosens and removes debris be used and that the pressure be decreased if the patient complains of pain, if bleeding occurs, or if the tip is near a major or exposed vessel. The pressure may need to be increased in the presence of tough eschar or when there is a large amount of necrotic tissue.
6. Apply the treatment until adequate hydration and/or debridement is achieved (Fig. 9-21).
7. This form of treatment may be followed by sharp debridement if necessary to remove adhered necrotic tissue.
8. Reapply the appropriate wound dressing.
9. Pulsatile irrigation treatments are generally applied once a day but may be applied more frequently to wounds that have greater than 50% necrotic, nonviable tissue with purulent drainage or a foul odor and, less frequently, if the wound does not have purulent drainage or odor. Treatment with this type of device should result in a decrease in necrotic tissue and/or an increase in granulation within 1 week of initiating treatment. If this does not occur, the treatment approach should be reevaluated.

ADVANTAGES
- Control of fluid pressure to stay within a safe and effective range for application to open wounds.
- Reduced infection risk because the fluid and wound debris are removed from the wound by gravity and suction.
- Jet of fluid can be directed to stay within the wound bed.

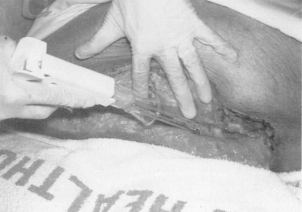

Figure 9-21. Using a nonimmersion hydrotherapy device to cleanse and debride a wound. (Courtesy Zimmer, Warsaw, IN.)

- Less time-consuming to apply than a whirlpool.
- Saves the expense of filling, draining, and cleaning a whirlpool.
- Does not require the patient to be transferred to the whirlpool area.
- Uses less fluid than a whirlpool.
- Normal saline rather than water applied to the open wound reduces the risk of hyponatremia.
- Can be used where whirlpool treatment is not recommended, such as with an unresponsive or incontinent patient.
- Faster granulation of the wound bed reported in one study comparing pulsatile irrigation with whirlpool treatment of wounds.[105]

DISADVANTAGES
- Treatment with pulsatile irrigation device incurs the additional expense of using new tubing, handpiece, and tip for each application. These components cost about $50 per treatment.
- Does not provide the therapeutic benefits associated with the buoyancy and hydrostatic pressure of immersion hydrotherapy.

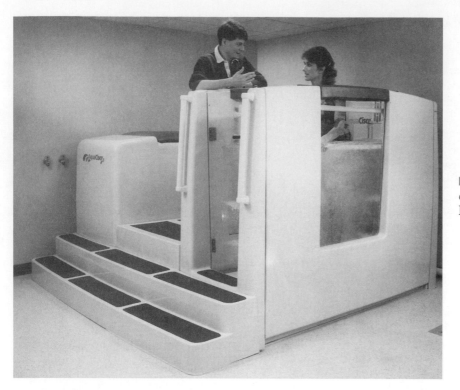

Figure 9-22. Purpose-designed exercise pool with treadmill. (Courtesy Ferno Ille, Wilmington, OH.)

Exercise Pool

To optimize the cardiovascular, respiratory, renal, or psychological benefits of hydrotherapy, the use of an exercise pool, which allows full body immersion and exercise, is recommended unless immersion in water that will be used by other individuals is contraindicated. An exercise pool is also generally the optimal means for applying hydrotherapy to achieve the musculoskeletal benefits associated with water immersion, although a whirlpool may be used when only the extremities require immersion.

Both swimming pools and purpose-designed hydrotherapy pools can be used for the application of hydrotherapy. Most swimming pools are at least 100 feet long and 25 feet wide and have a maximum depth of 8 feet, with a sloping bottom to produce a gradual descent. Most purpose-designed hydrotherapy pools are smaller and position the patient in the middle or at the edge of the pool to allow performance of specific types of exercises. Some hydrotherapy pools are equipped with an underwater treadmill,[107] an adjustable rate-of-water flow, and/or adjustable depths with movable floors in order to provide graded exercise activity[107] (Fig. 9-22). An exercise pool may be available for use in the clinical setting or the patient may be able to use a public or private swimming pool. Either type of pool may be used for individual or group treatment, depending on its size, with a therapist present, and/or for independent home exercise programs.

Pool temperature

The temperature of the water in an exercise pool should be kept at 26° to 36 °C (79° to 97 °F). The amount of movement expected to be performed by the patient should be used to determine the optimal temperature within this range. The warmer end of the range, 34° to 36 °C (93° to 97 °F), should be used when low-intensity activities, such as light exercise by elderly deconditioned patients or by patients with arthritis, will be performed. This is because warmer temperatures are more comfortable and help patients who move less to conserve body heat while in the water. The cooler end of the range, 26° to 28° C (79° to 82 °F), is recommended for recreational pools or where more intense exercise will be performed because the cooler temperature dissipates heat produced by the patients and therefore allows them to perform more exercise, or more vigorous exercise, with less fatigue. The water temperature should not be allowed to be below 18.5 °C (65 °F) because such low temperatures can impair the muscles' ability to contract.

APPLICATION TECHNIQUE
Pool

Equipment Required

- Appropriate space for the pool—adequate size, support, ventilation, and heating
- Space to store auxiliary equipment, including chemicals and mechanical systems
- Space for patients to shower and change clothes
- Water supply

- Nonslip area around pool
- Safety equipment
- Infection control equipment, including pump and filter, chemicals, and testing kit
- Towels
- Thermometer

PROCEDURE

1. The patient and the therapist should wear a bathing suit for pool exercise. The therapist may wear other light clothing over the bathing suit if not planning to enter the water except in the case of an emergency.
2. The therapist should assist the patient to enter the pool if necessary. Provide ramps, stairs, a ladder, or a lift to help patients get into and out of the pool.
3. The patient may perform activities to improve strength, cardiovascular fitness, endurance, or functional activities, as determined by the evaluation and plan of care. Activities may include upright exercise, walking in the pool, swimming, or other forms of exercise. The patient may use flotation devices, a tether, or other objects to alter the resistance or buoyancy effects of the water. Water-based exercise programs can be progressed by increasing the number of repetitions of an activity, increasing the speed of the activity, changing the length of the lever arm, decreasing the degree of stabilization provided, or using larger floats to increase resistance. More detailed descriptions of water exercise programs are beyond the scope of this text and can be found in books devoted to aquatic therapy.
4. The therapists should stay with the patient throughout the treatment and monitor vital signs during exercise if the patient has risk factors or any history indicating that this may be necessary. For example, heart rate and blood pressure should be monitored in patients recovering from myocardial infarction, and heart rate should be monitored in pregnant patients.
5. After completion of the water activities, the therapist should help the patient to get out of the pool if necessary. The patient should dry the body and wrap up immediately to avoid chilling.

ADVANTAGES

- Patient can move freely, with less risk of falling.
- Decreases weight bearing on joints. With immersion in water 60 inches deep, weight bearing on the lower extremities is reduced by 88to95%.
- Buoyancy may assist weak muscles to allow increased performance of active exercise.

DISADVANTAGES

- Risk of falling when the patient gets into and out of the water because water around the pool can make the floor slippery.
- Risk of infection from other individuals who have been in the water.
- Difficulty stabilizing or isolating body parts during exercise.
- Risk of drowning.
- Fear among some patients of water immersion.

Documentation

Documentation of hydrotherapy should include the type of hydrotherapy used, the patient's position and/or activities, the water temperature, the duration of the treatment, and the outcome of or response to the treatment. The fluid pressure and any water additives used should also be noted if applicable. Documentation is typically written in the SOAP note format. The following examples only summarize the modality component of treatment and are not intended to represent a comprehensive plan of care.

Examples

When applying a warm whirlpool to the right ankle to promote increased motion, document:

S: Pt c/o R ankle stiffness and difficulty with walking.

O: Warm WP, 36 °C, R ankle, 15 min. Pt performed AROM during immersion.

A: PROM DF increased from −10° to −5°, increased duration of heel strike during gait.

P: Continue WP as above followed by gait training and ther ex

When applying pulsatile irrigation to a sacral pressure ulcer, document:

S: Pt oriented to name but not date or place.

O: Pulsatile irrigation, 1000 cc warm saline, pressure 25% of max to sacral pressure ulcer. Pt left side lying on gurney.

A: Area of wound necrosis decreased from 50% to 20% since last week.

P: Decrease treatment frequency of pulsatile irrigation from 2× per day to 1× per day.

When using pool exercise to increase the fitness of a patient with exercise-induced asthma and obesity, document:

S: Pt reports ambulation continues to be limited by asthma.

O: Pool ex, pool at 30 °C, forward and backward walking across pool, 20 minutes at slow pace with 1 minute rest at each end of the pool.

A: Tol. ex without onset of asthma. Functional ambulation tolerance increased from 30 minutes to 1 hour.

P: Continue pool ex program as above, increasing time from 20 to 25 minutes next session.

SAFETY ISSUES REGARDING HYDROTHERAPY, INCLUDING INFECTION CONTROL AND POOL SAFETY

In order to optimize safety and infection control during hydrotherapy, it is recommended that the following general guidelines be adhered to. A facility hydrotherapy safety and infection control program that addresses the specific needs of the facility should be developed in conjunction with an infection control specialist or in conjunction with the facility infection control committee. This program should take into account the specific safety hazards associated with this type of treatment and the types of microorganisms most commonly encountered at that time and place. The program must also be in compliance with the guidelines, rules, and regulations of the local public health department. Infection control experts should also be consulted if a problem with infection control, such as frequent patient infections after the use of hydrotherapy, arises.

Safety Precautions and Infection Control for Whirlpools

These recommendations apply for whirlpools of all sizes and shapes, including Hubbard tanks.

Safety

1. The tank should be properly grounded, and the turbine must have a hospital-grade plug. The motor must be securely fastened to the outside of the tank. Whirlpools should also be inspected regularly for any breaks in wiring or insulation because of the high risk of severe electrical injury should any breach of electrical safety occur with this type of equipment.[109]
2. Do not run the turbine without water in the whirlpool because this can damage the turbine motor.
3. The treatment room should be comfortably warm and well-ventilated but not drafty. Ventilation is required in order to control the humidity of the room and to remove aerosolized additives or infectious agents from the air. A room temperature of 25° to 30° C (77° to 86° F) with a relative humidity of 50% is recommended.[110]

Infection control

Hydrotherapy tanks, having numerous crevices and being in frequent contact with warm contaminated water under pressure, provide an ideal breeding ground for infectious organisms and are therefore particularly likely purveyors of infection. The primary goal of infection control is to reduce the number of microorganisms in the environment and thus to reduce the potential for infection.[110] For optimal infection control there must be appropriate cleaning protocols and culturing of all relevant equipment, and protective garments should be worn by the individuals providing hydrotherapy care. Many facilities also add antimicrobials to the water being used for treatment in an attempt to reduce contamination with microorganisms. All of these precautions are intended to reduce the risk of patient or clinician contamination from water-borne bacteria, aerosolized mist, fomites, or blood-borne pathogens.

1. Generally, it is recommended that only clean water, without any antimicrobial, be used in a whirlpool when treating any type of open wound. As discussed previously, the use of antimicrobials in the water when treating open wounds is controversial because although these chemicals offer improved control of infection and cross-contamination, most have been found to be cytotoxic to healing tissue cells even when applied at low concentrations. When infection control is a priority, antimicrobials should be used only at the lowest concentration stated by the manufacturer to be effective for antimicrobial action. Soaps, detergents, or povidone-iodine should not be used for this application because their efficacy is reduced in the presence of blood or tissue debris.[112] Sodium hypochlorite, in the form of household bleach, can provide some control of infection during hydrotherapy; however, its application is limited because it corrodes stainless steel tanks and releases chlorine vapors, which are irritating to many individuals. The chloramine form of chlorine has been recommended for use as an antimicrobial in whirlpool water because it does not corrode stainless steel or release noxious vapors and is not inactivated in the presence of blood or tissue debris.

2. The whirlpool tank and turbines should be properly drained and cleaned after each use. Although there are slightly varying cleaning procedures at different facilities, all protocols are designed to optimize patient and clinician safety and minimize the risk of infection. In general the cleaning procedure is as follows:

    a. The person cleaning the whirlpool should wear rubber gloves and goggles throughout the cleaning procedure.

    b. Drain the tank. Various drainage configurations or sumps are available to minimize the amount of water left at the bottom of the tank.

    c. Rinse the tank with clean water directly from a hose.

    d. Scrub the inside of the tank with a brush and detergent and then rinse the tank again.

    e. Disinfect the tank. A detergent must be used before the application of the disinfectant because most disinfectants are inactivated in the presence of blood or tissue debris.[112] At present there is no conclusive evidence to support the recommendation of one disinfectant over another; however, one should note that certain disinfectants are more effective against particular microorganisms and that some bromine-based disinfectants can cause allergic dermatitis.[113] It is also generally recommended that disinfecting agents be changed occasionally to reduce the risk of promoting the development of resistant strains. If the whirlpool was used only to treat areas with intact skin, then low-level disinfection of the whirlpool, using 70% to 90% ethyl or isopropyl alcohol, 100 parts per million (ppm) sodium hypochlorite (the active ingredient of household bleach), a phenolic germicidal detergent solution, or a quaternary ammonium germicidal solution, is sufficient. However, if areas where the skin was not intact have been treated, intermediate-level disinfection, using 70% to 90% ethyl or isopropyl alcohol, a phenolic germicidal detergent solution, or an iodophor germicidal detergent solution, has been recommended.[111] Chlorine-based products should not be used to clean stainless steel tanks because, with repeated use, these products corrode the tank surface. To apply the disinfectant, fill the tank with hot water, add the appropriate amount of disinfecting agent, and expose all the inside surfaces of the tank to the solution for 10 minutes.

    f. Clean and disinfect the turbine by running it for 5 minutes in a bucket with a detergent and then for 10 minutes in a bucket with disinfectant solution.

    g. Drain the tank.

    h. Rinse the tank with clean water.

    i. Dry the tank thoroughly with clean towels.

    j. Wipe all tank stretchers, hoist cables, and seats with disinfectant after each use.

3. Culture samples should be obtained periodically from the tank, the turbine, the tank drains, and the water supply in accordance with facility and governmental guidelines.[47]

Safety Precautions and Infection Control for Exercise Pools

Safety

Personnel training

Individuals who are responsible for maintaining and cleaning an exercise pool must be trained in the use and hazards of the disinfecting and pesticide chemicals used. They should also be provided with the necessary protective clothing for handling these substances.

Staff working with individuals in the pool should have lifesaving and rescue training and knowledge of personal water safety techniques. At a minimum they should be certified to perform cardiopulmonary resuscitation (CPR) and to provide advanced first aid. Ideally, a certified lifeguard should be present whenever anyone is in the pool. Staff should also be trained in emergency evacuation procedures and should know the emergency action plan.

Safety in and around the pool

In order for the area around an exercise pool to be safe, and to minimize the risk of a patient slipping and falling, the area surrounding the pool should have nonslip surfaces. Pool regulations, the water depth, and emergency procedures and phone numbers should all be clearly posted in the pool area. Means of entering the pool should be appropriate for patients' ambulatory ability and may include stairs, ramps, ladders, or lifts for nonambulatory or impaired patients. For safety in the pool, the depth of the water should be clearly marked at intervals around the pool edge, and there should be hand grip bars all the way around the edge of the pool.

The pool should be evacuated during power outages and floods, and outdoor pools should not be used during electrical storms. Emergency equipment should be kept near the pool at all times, and all such equipment should be inspected regularly. Emergency equipment should include a shepherd's crook, a life ring, a rescue tube, resuscitation equipment, a spine board, a blanket, and scissors. A first-aid kit should also be available.

Keep all chemicals for use in the pool in their original containers, off the floor, and in a locked cabinet. Material Safety Data Sheets for all chemicals must be maintained and filed to be in compliance with Occupational Safety and Health Administration (OSHA) and Environmental Protection Agency (EPA) regulations. Avoid electrical shocks by keeping electrical equipment, such as hair dryers, electrotherapy devices, and heaters, out of the wet environment of the pool and poolside.

Infection control

Because water is not drained from an exercise pool between uses, the pool water must be filtered and treated with chemical additives at all times in order to prevent infection transmission. Coliform bacteria, *Giardia lamblia, Pseudomonas aeruginosa*, and various types of staphylococcal bacteria, which can cause intestinal, skin, or ear infections in exposed individuals, are commonly found in water, and the risk of excessive bacterial growth is elevated if the water is warm. Airborne endotoxins around a pool may also cause respiratory problems in susceptible individuals.

Adequate infection control of a pool can be achieved with continuous filtering and chemical disinfection of the pool water with chlorine or bromine. The pH and chlorine or bromine levels of the pool water should be tested at the beginning of each day and at least at two additional times during the day. The total alkalinity and calcium hardness of the water should also be checked twice a month. Chemical testing kits designed for this application indicate the safe levels for these tests. In order to minimize the risk of high bacterial levels in a pool, it is also essential that, as detailed in the section on contraindications above, patients with conditions that may be a source of infection not be allowed to use an exercise pool that would be reused by themselves or by others.

▶ *Clinical Case Studies* ◀

The following case studies summarize the concepts of hydrotherapy discussed in this chapter. Based on the scenarios presented, an evaluation of the clinical findings and goals of treatment are proposed. These are followed by a discussion of the factors to be considered in the selection of hydrotherapy as a treatment modality, and guidelines for the selection of the appropriate hydrotherapy device and application technique.

Case 1

FR is a 45-year-old female who has been diagnosed with osteoarthritis of both knees. She complains of bilateral knee pain that is worse on the right than on the left, and that worsens with standing or walking for more than 5 minutes. She uses a cane in her left hand to control her knee pain and to assist with balance during community and most household ambulation. She is able to walk approximately one-half block on a flat, level surface with her cane. She does not tolerate anti-inflammatory medications due to gastric complaints. The pain in her right knee started about 5 years ago, without any known aggravating activity, and has gradually worsened since that time. The pain in her left knee started about 2 years ago, also without any known aggravating activity. She has had no prior treatment for her knee pain. The objective exam is significant for obesity, postural and gait deviations of bilateral genu valgum, bilateral foot pronation, and weakness and shortness of the quadriceps and hamstring muscles. Knee passive ROM is –5° extension to 95° flexion on the right and 0° extension to 120° flexion on the left. FR uses a step to gait for ascending and descending stairs.

EVALUATION OF THE CLINICAL FINDINGS

This patient has impairments of knee pain, abnormal lower extremity alignment, reduced lower extremity strength, reduced knee ROM, and excessive body weight resulting in the functional limitations of reduced standing and decreased ambulation tolerance.

PREFERRED PRACTICE PATTERN

Impaired Joint Mobility, Motor Function, Muscle Performance, and Range of Motion Associated with Connective Tissue Dysfunction, (4D)

PLAN OF CARE

The goals of treatment include decreasing knee pain and increasing lower extremity strength and knee ROM to increase this patient's standing tolerance to 20 minutes and increase her walking tolerance to two blocks. The anticipated goals of treatment may also include discontinuing the use of a cane, increasing cardiovascular fitness, and losing weight.

ASSESSMENT REGARDING THE APPROPRIATENESS OF HYDROTHERAPY AS THE OPTIMAL TREATMENT

Although many forms of exercise could be used to increase this patient's lower extremity strength and knee ROM, given her body weight and the reported degeneration of her knee joints, in order to avoid aggravation of her symptoms, treatment with exercises with limited weight bearing on her lower extremities is proposed. This could be achieved by the use of a water environment, although other non–weight-bearing exercises, such as straight leg raises, or reduced weight-bearing exercises, such as stationary cycling, could be used. Water-based exercises are recommended because they have a number of advantages over non–weight-bearing, land-based exercises. These advantages include allowing the patient to perform normal functional activities, such as walking without an assistive device, in order to train the muscles and develop the balance skills required for normal function, providing some pain control during the exercise, allowing fine grading of joint loading by varying the depth of the water, and allowing fine grading of resistance by varying the speed of patient movement. Should the patient have lower extremity edema, as is common in inactive obese individuals, the hydrostatic pressure provided by immersion may also provide the additional benefit of edema reduction. From the subjective and objective evaluation reported above, it does not appear that hydrotherapy would be contraindicated for this patient; however, before initiating hydrotherapy, one should ascertain that the patient is not afraid of being in water and that she does not have any infections that may be spread by water or any other medical conditions that would contraindicate the use of this form of treatment.

PROPOSED TREATMENT PLAN AND RATIONALE

Pool exercise is the only form of hydrotherapy that would address all of the proposed goals of treatment for this patient. Although soaking in a warm whirlpool may be comfortable and may temporarily decrease this patient's pain, and although lower extremity active exercise in an extremity whirlpool may promote ROM to some degree, neither of these forms of hydrotherapy treatment is likely to provide sufficient resistance to motion to increase the patient's lower extremity strength and thus her functional standing and ambulation tolerance. For this patient's treatment the pool water should be kept slightly warmer than generally used for recreation, at 34° to 36 °C (93° to 95° F), in order to allow her to exercise comfortably at the slow pace to which she will probably be limited. A pool exercise program may include forward and backward walking, either holding or not holding on to the hand rail, as necessary for balance, partial squats, kicking, and a variety of other closed- and open-chain lower extremity activities. This water-based exercise program is likely to be most effective if provided in conjunction with land-based exercises, active and passive stretching, joint mobilization, and a home exercise program.

Case 2

ST is an 85-year-old female with stage IV pressure ulcers in the areas of both femoral greater trochanters and a

Continued

) *Clinical Case Studies—cont'd* (

stage II pressure ulcer over her sacrum. The ulcer in the area of her right greater trochanter is approximately 8 cm long and 8 cm wide and has no undermining. The ulcer in the area of her left greater trochanter is approximately 9 cm long and 10 cm wide and has approximately 1 cm of undermining along the proximal border. Both of these wounds have yellow necrotic tissue and a heavy, thick exudate; no granulation tissue is visible. The ulcer over the sacrum is approximately 5 cm by 10 cm and has no necrotic tissue. No tunnels or sinus tracts are apparent in any of these wounds. The patient is bedridden, oriented to name and place, and noncombative. She has a history of two strokes, one 3 years ago and the other 8 years ago, resulting first in right and then in left hemiplegia, with hypertonicity that is moderately severe and has not changed significantly in the last 2 years. She also has hypertension that is controlled by medication and generally keeps her blood pressure at or below 145/100.

EVALUATION OF THE CLINICAL FINDINGS

This patient presents with impairments of soft tissue integrity and abnormal muscle tone and has reduced functional mobility. She is also at risk for the development of further pressure ulcers and infection.

PREFERRED PRACTICE PATTERN

Impaired Integumentary Integrity Associated With Skin Involvement Extending Into Fascia, Muscle, or Bone and Scar Formation, (7E)

PLAN OF CARE

The goals of treatment at this time include softening and removing the necrotic tissue that is present in the two wounds in the trochanteric areas and removing debris from these wounds in order to facilitate wound closure, and to reduce the risk of infection and further tissue breakdown. Improving circulation in the areas of the wounds may also facilitate wound closure.

ASSESSMENT REGARDING THE APPROPRIATENESS OF HYDROTHERAPY AS THE OPTIMAL TREATMENT

Hydrotherapy is indicated for this patient because this treatment can soften and debride necrotic tissue, cleanse wound debris, and, if provided by immersion with warm water, facilitate improved circulation. Removal of necrotic tissue from a wound bed and improving the local circulation can accelerate wound healing and closure. In order to optimize the treatment outcome, other forms of treatment, such as pressure relief, electrical stimulation, exercise, appropriate wound dressings, and

possibly other forms of debridement should also be applied in conjunction with the hydrotherapy. The evaluation of this patient does not indicate that hydrotherapy would be contraindicated; however, the infection risk and safety concerns limit the types of hydrotherapy that would be appropriate. Also, hydrotherapy is indicated only for the trochanteric wounds, where necrotic tissue is present, not for the sacral wound, where no necrotic tissue is apparent. Neither whirlpool immersion nor nonimmersion irrigation would be contraindicated, although care should be taken to ascertain that the patient can feel and report heat in the areas to be treated before warm or hot water is used. Since it is most likely that this patient has impaired sensation and circulation in the areas of the pressure ulcers, the water temperature should be no higher than 35.5° C (96° F).

PROPOSED TREATMENT PLAN

Either immersion or nonimmersion techniques could be used to apply hydrotherapy to this patient. Immersion techniques have the advantages of allowing all the wounds to receive hydrotherapy at the same time and providing potential circulatory benefits due to heat transfer if warm water is used and due to hydrostatic pressure if the extremities are sufficiently immersed; however, because immersion techniques increase the risk of maceration of the intact tissue around the wounds, have a high infection risk, do not allow control of the water pressure at the wound bed, cannot restrict the hydrotherapy treatment to the trochanteric wounds, and require monitoring of vital signs during treatment, a nonimmersion technique would be more appropriate. A nonimmersion form of hydrotherapy would also be easier, quicker, and less costly to apply, although it would not have the circulatory benefits associated with immersion. Although nonimmersion hydrotherapy can be provided by the use of either a mechanical or an electrical device, the use of an electric pulsatile irrigation device is recommended for the treatment of this patient because this will allow close control of fluid pressure and removal of contaminated fluid from the wound bed during treatment. Antimicrobials may be added to the fluid for either form of hydrotherapy. It is recommended that treatment with pulsatile irrigation be provided once each day until the wound bed is fully granulated. Hydrotherapy of these wounds should be discontinued if bleeding occurs, if the amount of necrotic tissue does not decrease, or if the amount of granulation does not increase within 1 week. Should sharp debridement of necrotic tissue be indicated, it is recommended that this be performed after the hydrotherapy, when the necrotic tissue is likely to be softer and easier to remove.

Case 3

FS is a 65-year-old female who sustained a closed Colles' fracture of her right arm 6 weeks ago. The fracture was initially treated with a closed reduction and cast fixation. This cast was removed 3 days ago, when radiographic reports indicated callus formation and good alignment of the fracture site. FS has been referred to therapy with an order to evaluate and treat. She has not received any prior rehabilitation treatment for this injury. FS complains of severe pain, stiffness, and swelling of her right wrist and hand. She is wearing a wrist splint and is not using her right hand for any functional activities at this time because she is afraid that any activity may cause further damage. FS is retired and lives alone. She is unable to drive at this time because of the dysfunctions of her right hand and wrist. The objective exam is significant for decreased active and passive ROM of the right wrist. Active wrist flexion is 30° on the right and 80° on the left. Wrist extension is 25° on the right and 70° on the left. Wrist ulnar deviation is 10° on the right and 30° on the left, and wrist radial deviation is 25° on the right and 0° on the left. There is also moderate nonpitting edema of the right hand, and the skin of the right hand and wrist appears shiny. FS's functional grip on the right is limited by both muscle weakness and restricted joint ROM. The patient is wearing a splint and is holding her hand across her abdomen. She reports severe pain when her hand is touched, even lightly. All other objective measures, including shoulder, elbow, and neck ROM, upper extremity sensation, and left upper extremity strength, are within normal limits for this patient's age and gender.

EVALUATION OF THE CLINICAL FINDINGS

This patient presents with impairments of pain, hypersensitivity, restricted ROM, abnormal skin appearance, and increased volume of her right hand and wrist. These impairments, in conjunction with her fear, have resulted in total disuse of this distal extremity for all functional activities and an inability to drive. Although this patient's signs and symptoms are consistent with disuse after a fracture and immobilization, they also indicate that she has stage I reflex sympathetic dystrophy.

PREFERRED PRACTICE PATTERN

Impaired Joint Mobility, Muscle Performance, and Range of Motion Associated With Fracture, (4G)

PLAN OF CARE

The anticipated long-term goals of treatment are to achieve normal sensation, function, ROM, strength, and volume of the right hand and wrist. In order to achieve these goals, the proposed short-term goals for the first 2 weeks of treatment are to decrease this patient's pain, hypersensitivity, and fear sufficiently to allow her to initiate use of her right hand to assist with functional activities and to increase her right wrist ROM by 20% to 50% in all planes.

ASSESSMENT REGARDING THE APPROPRIATENESS OF HYDROTHERAPY AS THE OPTIMAL TREATMENT

Immersion hydrotherapy, using either a low level of water agitation in a neutral warmth whirlpool or a contrast bath with warm and cool water of similar temperatures, may reduce the hypersensitivity and hypalgesia of this patient's hand while providing a suitable environment for active exercise to increase the ROM and functional use of her hand. The hydrostatic pressure provided by water immersion and the alternating vasoconstriction and vasodilation produced by a contrast bath may also contribute to reducing the edema in this extremity. The use of a warm or hot water whirlpool would not be recommended because the resulting increase in tissue temperature, in conjunction with the dependent position of the extremity, is likely to aggravate the edema already present in this patient's hand. Although the evaluation of this patient does not indicate any contraindication for the use of hydrotherapy, since hot water may be used for the contrast bath during the later stages of desensitization, her ability to sense temperature should be assessed before initiating treatment with a contrast bath.

PROPOSED TREATMENT PLAN

Since immersion in water is required to provide the heat transfer, resistance, and hydrostatic pressure that will produce the therapeutic benefits of hydrotherapy for this patient, only immersion hydrotherapy techniques would be appropriate for her treatment. As noted above, a contrast bath is likely to be most effective because it may assist with desensitization and edema reduction while providing a comfortable environment for active exercise. It is recommended that contrast bath treatments be provided both in the clinic and by the patient as part of her home program. It is recommended that the water temperature of the two baths initially be similar and, as the patient progresses, that the temperature difference gradually be increased.

Chapter Review

Hydrotherapy is the application of water for therapeutic purposes. The unique physical properties of water, including its high specific heat and thermal conductivity, buoyancy, resistance, and hydrostatic pressure, all contribute to its therapeutic efficacy. Water can be used as a cleanser, and immersion in water also produces a wide range of cardiovascular, respiratory, musculoskeletal, renal, and psychological benefits. These beneficial effects of hydrotherapy include reducing the bacterial load and the presence of debris during wound care, and controlling pain, modifying muscular demands, and reducing edema during water-based exercise. Hydrotherapy can be applied by immersion in water in a whirlpool, Hubbard tank, contrast bath, or exercise pool or by nonimmersion methods using a shower or a specialized irrigation device. Immersion methods provide all the above-mentioned benefits of hydrotherapy; however, because immersion can be associated with increased risks of infection or drowning and can be time-consuming to apply, nonimmersion hydrotherapy techniques that provide only cleansing effects have been developed for the treatment of open wounds when only these effects are required. In order to optimize the outcome of hydrotherapy treatments, the treatment plan and equipment selection should take into account both the risks and benefits associated with the various means of applying hydrotherapy, and all appropriate precautions should be taken to provide a safe environment for such treatment. The reader is referred to the Evolve website at http://evolve.elsevier.com/Cameron for study questions pertinent to this chapter.

References

1. Bettmann OL: City life: beware of contagion. In: Bettmann OL, Hench PC, eds: *A Pictorial History of Medicine.* Springfield, IL, 1956, Charles C Thomas.
2. Shepard CH: Insanity and the Turkish bath, *JAMA* 34:604-606, 1900.
3. Roberts P: Hydrotherapy: its history, theory and practice, *Occup Health Saf* 33(5):235-244, 1982.
3a. Kenney E, Ostenso M: *And they shall walk.* New York, 1943, Dodd Mead and Co.
4. Becker BE: The biological aspects of hydrotherapy, *J Back Musculoskel Rehabil* 4(4):255-264, 1994.
5. Robson MC, Heggers JP: Bacterial quantification of open wounds, *Mil Med* 134:19-24, 1969.
6. Winter GD: Formation of scab and the rate of epithelialization in superficial wounds of the domestic pig, *Nature* 193:293-294, 1962.
7. Wade J: Sports splash, *Rehab Mgmt* 10(4):64-70, 1997.
8. Gwinup G: Weight loss without dietary restriction: efficacy of different forms of aerobic exercise, *Am J Sport Med* 15:275-279, 1987.
9. Kieres J, Plowman S: Effect of swimming and land exercises on body composition of college students, *J Sport Med Phys Fitness* 31:192-193, 1991.
10. Ruoti RG, Troup JT, Berger RA: The effects of nonswimming water exercises on older adults, *J Orthop Sports Phys Ther* 19(3):140-145, 1994.
11. Gehlsen GM, Grigsby S, Winant D: The effects of an aquatic fitness program on the muscular strength and endurance of patients with multiple sclerosis, *Phys Ther* 64(5):653-657, 1984.
12. Henker L, Provast-Craig M, Sestili P et al: Water running and the maintenance of maximum oxygen consumption and leg strength in runners, *Med Sci Sport Exerc* 24:3-5, 1991.
13. Balldin UI, Lundgren CEG, Lundvall J et al: Changes in the elimination of 133 Xenon from the anterior tibial muscle in man induced by immersion in water and by shifts in body position, *Aerospace Med* 42(5):489-493, 1971.
14. Arborelius M, Balldin UI, Lilja B et al: Hemodynamic changes in man during immersion with the head above water, *Aerospace Med* 43(3):593-599, 1972.
15. Risch WD, Koubenec HJ, Beckmann U et al: The effect of graded immersion on heart volume, central venous pressure, pulmonary blood distribution and heart rate in man, *Pfleugers Arch* 374:115-118, 1978.
16. Haffor AA, Mohler JG, Harrison AAC: Effects of water immersion on cardiac output of lean and fat male subjects at rest and during exercise, *Aviation, Space Environ Med* 62:123-127, 1991.
17. McMurray RG, Katz VL, Berry MJ et al: Cardiovascular responses of pregnant women during aerobic exercise in water: a longitudinal study, *Int J Sports Med* 9(6):443-447, 1988.
18. Katz VL, McMurray R, Goodwin WE et al: Nonweight-bearing exercise during pregnancy on land and during immersion; a comparative study, *Am J Perinatol* 7(3):281-284, 1990.
19. Svendenhag J, Serger J: Running on land and in water: comparative exercise physiology, *Med Sci Sports Exerc* 24:1155-1160, 1992.
20. Butts NK, Tucker M, Smith R: Maximal responses to treadmill and deep water running in high school female cross country runners, *Res Q Exer Sports* 62:236-239, 1991.
21. Butts NK, Tucker M, Greening C: Physiologic responses to maximal treadmill and deep water running in men and women, *Am J Sports Med* 19:612-614, 1991.

1843

22. Michaud T, Brennan D, Wilder R et al: Aquarun training and changes in treadmill running maximal oxygen consumption, *Med Sci Sports Exerc* 24:5-7, 1991.
23. Hamer TW, Morton AR: Water-running: training effects and specificity of aerobic, anaerobic and muscular parameters following an eight week interval training programme, *Aust J Sci Med Sport* 22(1):13-22, 1990.
24. Abramson D, Brunnet C, Bell Y et al: Changes in blood flow, oxygen uptake, and tissue temperatures produced by a topical application of wet heat, *Arch Phys Med Rehabil* 42:305-318, 1961.
25. Gleim GW, Nicholas JA: Metabolic costs and heart rate responses to treadmill walking in water at different depths and temperatures, *Am J Sports Med* 17(2):248-252, 1989.
26. Evans BW, Cureton KJ, Purvis JW: Metabolic and circulatory responses to walking and jogging in water, *Res Q* 49(4):442-449, 1978.
27. Hong SK, Cerretelli P, Cruz JC et al: Mechanics of respiration during submersion in water, *J Appl Physiol* 27(4):535-536, 1969.
28. Perk J, Perk L, Boden C: Adaptation of COPD patients to physical training on land and in water, *Eur Respir J* 9(2):248-252, 1996.
29. Agostoni E, Gurtner G, Torri G et al: Respiratory mechanics during submersion and negative pressure breathing, *J Appl Physiol* 21(1):251-258, 1966.
30. Bar-Yishay E, Gur I, Inbar O et al: Differences between swimming and running as stimuli for exercise-induced asthma, *Eur J Appl Physiol* 48:387-397, 1982.
31. Fitch KD, Morton AR: Specificity of exercise in exercise-induced asthma, *Br Med J* 4:577-581, 1971.
32. Bar-Or O, Inbar I: Swimming and asthma benefits and deleterious effects, *Sports Med* 14:397-405, 1992.
33. Epstein M: Cardiovascular and renal effects of head out water immersion in man, *Circ Res* 39(5):620-628, 1976.
34. Katz VL, McMurray R, Berry MJ et al: Renal responses to immersion and exercise in pregnancy, *Am J Perinatol* 7(2):118-121, 1990.
35. Epstein M, Pins DS, Silvers W et al: Failure of water immersion to influence parathyroid hormone secretion and renal phosphate handling in normal man, *J Lab Clin Med* 87(2):218-226, 1976.
36. Braslow JT: Punishment or therapy: patients, doctors, and somatic remedies in the early twentieth century: *Psych Clin North Am* 17(3):493-513, 1994.
37. Holmes G: Hydrotherapy as a means of rehabilitation, *Br J Phys Med* 5:93-95, 1942.
38. Feedar JA, Kloth LC: Conservative management of chronic wounds. In Kloth LC, McCulloch JM, Feedar JA, eds: *Wound Healing: Alternatives in Management,* Philadelphia, 1990, FA Davis.
39. Neiderhuber S, Stribley R, Koepke G: Reduction in skin bacterial load with the use of therapeutic whirlpool, *Phys Ther* 55(5):482-486, 1975.
40. Walter PH: Burn wound management, *AACN Clin Issues Crit Care Nurs* 4(2):378-387, 1993.
41. Burke DT, Ho CH, Saucier MA et al: Effects of hydrotherapy on pressure ulcer healing, *Am J Phys Med Rehabil* 77(5):394-398, 1998.
42. McCulloch J: Physical modalities in wound management: ultrasound, vasopneumatic devices and hydrotherapy, *Ostomy Wound Mgmt* 41(5):30-32, 35-37, 1995.
43. Winter GD: Formation of a scab and the rate of epithelialization of superficial wounds in the skin of the young domestic pig, *Nature* 193:293-294, 1962.
44. Hahn JS: Lecture on the power and effect of fresh water on the human body. 1734, Germany.
45. Wheeler CB, Rodeheaver GT, Thacker JG et al: Side effects of high-pressure irrigation, *Surg Gynecol Obstet* 143(5):775-778, 1976.
46. McGuckin M, Thorpe R, Abrutyn E: Hydrotherapy: an outbreak of *Pseudomonas aeruginosa* wound infections related to Hubbard tank treatments, *Arch Phys Med Rehabil* 62:283-285, 1981.
47. Tredget EE, Shankowsky HA, Joffe AAM et al: Epidemiology of infections with *Pseudomonas aeruginosa* in burn patients: the role of hydrotherapy, *Clin Infect Dis* 15(6):641-649, 1992.
48. Shankowsky HA, Callioux LS, Tredget EE: North American survey of hydrotherapy in modern burn care, *J Burn Care Rehabil* 15(2):143-146, 1994.
49. Richard P, LeFoch R, Chamoux C, et al: *Pseudomonas aeruginosa* outbreak in a burn unit: role of antimicrobials in the emergence of multiply resistant strains, *J Infect Dis* 170(2):377-383, 1994.
50. Wisplinghoff H, Perbix W, Seifert H: Risk factors for nosocomial bloodstream infections due to *Acinetobacter baumannii*: a case-control study of adult burn patients, *Clin Infect Dis* 28(1):59-66, 1999.
51. Stanwood W, Pinzur MS: Risk of contamination of the wound in a hydrotherapeutic tank, *Foot Ankle Int* 19(3):173-176, 1998.
52. Myers RS: *Saunders Manual of Physical Therapy Practice,* Philadelphia, 1995, WB Saunders.
53. Walsh MT: Hydrotherapy: the use of water as a therapeutic agent. In Michlovitz SL, ed: *Thermal Agents in Rehabilitation,* ed 3, Philadelphia, 1996, FA Davis.
54. Steve L, Goodhart P, Alexander J: Hydrotherapy burn treatment: use of chloramine-T against resistant microorganisms, *Arch Phys Med Rehabil* 60(7):301-303, 1979.
55. Custer J, Edlich RF, Prusak M et al: Studies in the management of the contaminated wound: V. An assessment of the effectiveness of pHisoHex and Betadine surgical scrub solutions, *Am J Surg* 121:572-575, 1971.

56. Johnson AR, White AC, McAnalley B: Comparison of common topical agents for wound treatment: cytotoxicity for human fibroblasts in culture, *Wounds* 1(3): 186-192, 1989.

57. Rodeheaver GT, Kurtz L, Kircher BJ et al: Pluronic F-68: a promising new wound cleanser, *Ann Emerg Med* 9(11):572-576, 1980.

58. Rydberg B, Zederfeldt B: Influence of cationic detergents on tensile strength of healing skin wounds in the rat, *Acta Chir Scand* 134(5):317-320, 1968.

59. Burkey JL, Weinberg C, Branden RA: Differential methodologies for the evaluation of skin and wound cleansers, *Wounds* 5(6):284-291, 1993.

60. Foresman PA, Payne DS, Becker D et al: A relative toxicity index for wound cleansers, *Wounds* 5(5):226-231, 1993.

61. Henderson JD, Leming JT, Melon-Niksa DB: Chloramine-T solutions: effect on wound healing in guinea pigs, *Arch Phys Med Rehabil* 70(8):628-631, 1989.

62. Bhaskar SN, Cutright DE, Gross A: Effect of water lavage on infected wounds in the rat, *J Periodontol* 40(11):671-672, 1969.

63. Brown LL, Shelton HT, Bornside GH et al: Evaluation of wound irrigation by pulsatile jet and conventional methods, *Ann Surg* 187(2):170-173, 1978.

64. Morgan D, Hoelscher J: Pulsed lavage: promoting comfort and healing in home care, *Ostomy Wound Manage* 46(4):44-49, 2000.

65. University Medical Center Physical Therapy Department: *Wound Care Protocol Using the Pulsavac Wound Debridement System,* Lubbock, TX, 1994, University Medical Center.

66. Bohannon RW: Whirlpool versus whirlpool rinse for removal of bacteria from a venous stasis ulcer, *Phys Ther* 62(3):304-308, 1982.

67. Bingham HG, Hudson D, Popp J: A retrospective review of the burn intensive care unit admissions for a year, *J Burn Care Rehabil* 16(1):56-58, 1995.

68. Thomson PD, Bowden ML, McDonald K et al: A survey of burn hydrotherapy in the United States, *J Burn Care Rehabil* 11(2):151-155, 1990.

69. Staley M, Richard R: Management of the acute burn wound: an overview, *Adv Wound Care* 10(2):39-44, 1997.

70. Neville C, Dimick AR: The trauma table as an alternative to the Hubbard tank in burn care, *J Burn Care Rehabil* 8(6):574-575, 1987.

71. Said RA, Hussein MM: Severe hyponatremia in burn patients secondary to hydrotherapy, *Burns Incl Thermal Inj* 13(4):327-329, 1987.

72. Headley BJ, Robson MC, Krizek TJ: Methods of reducing environmental stress for the acute burn patient, *Phys Ther* 55(1):5-9, 1975.

73. Bates A, Hanson N: *Aquatic Therapy: A Comprehensive Approach to Use of Aquatic Exercise in Treatment of Orthopaedic Injuries,* Westbank, British Columbia, Canada, 1992, Swystun & Swystun.

74. Hoyrup G, Kjorvel L: Comparison of whirlpool and wax treatments for hand therapy, *Physiother Can* 38: 79-82, 1986.

75. Templeton MS, Booth DL, O'Kelly WD: Effects of aquatic therapy on joint flexibility and functional ability in subjects with rheumatic disease, *J Orthop Sport Phys Ther* 23(6):376-381, 1996.

76. Genuario SE, Vegso JJ: The use of a swimming pool in rehabilitation and reconditioning of athletic injuries, *Contemp Orthop* 4:381-387, 1990.

77. Cole AJ, Eagleston RE, Moschetti M et al: Spine rehabilitation aquatic rehabilitation strategies, *J Back Musculoskel Rehabil* 4(4):273-286, 1994.

78. Triggs M: Orthopedic aquatic therapy, *Clin Mgmt* 11:30-31, 1991.

79. Konlian C: Aquatic therapy: making a wave in the treatment of low back injuries, *Orthop Nurs* 18(1):11-18, 1999.

80. Tsukahara N, Toda A, Goto J et al: Cross-sectional and longitudinal studies on the effect of water exercise in controlling bone loss in Japanese postmenopausal women. *J Nutr Sci Vitaminol Tokyo* 40(1):37-47, 1994.

81. Hurley R, Turner C: Neurology and aquatic therapy, *Clin Mgmt* 11:26-29, 1991.

82. Johnson CR: Aquatic therapy for an ALS patient, *Am J Occup Ther* 42(2):115-120, 1988.

83. Simmons V, Hansen PD: Effectiveness of water exercise on postural mobility in the well elderly: an experimental study on balance enhancement, *J Gerontol A Biol Sci Med Sci* 51(5):M233-M238, 1996.

84. Harris SR: Neurodevelopmental treatment approach for teaching swimming to cerebral palsied children, *Phys Ther* 58(8):979-983, 1978.

85. Boyle AM: The Bad Ragaz ring method, *Physiotherapy* 67:265-268, 1981.

86. Eyestone ED, Fellingham G, George J et al: Effect of water running and cycling on the maximum oxygen consumption and 2 mile run performance, *Am J Sports Med* 21:41-44, 1993.

87. McMurray RG, Fieselman CC, Avery KE et al: Exercise hemodynamics in water and on land in patients with coronary artery disease, *Cardiopulm Rehabil* 8:69-75, 1986.

88. Tei C, Tanaka N: Thermal vasodilation as a treatment of congestive heart failure: a novel approach, *J Cardiol* 21(1):29-30, 1996.

89. Watson WJ, Katz VL, Hackney AC et al: Fetal response to maximal swimming and cycling exercise during pregnancy, *Obstet Gynecol* 77(3):382-386, 1991.

90. Kurabayashi H, Machida I, Kubota K: Improvement in ejection fraction by hydrotherapy as rehabilitation in patients with chronic pulmonary emphysema, *Physiother Res Int* 3(4):284-291, 1998.

91. American College of Obstetricians and Gynecologists: *Exercise during Pregnancy and Postnatal Period ACOG Home Exercise Programs,* Washington, DC, 1985, ACOG.

92. Huang SW, Veiga R, Sila U et al: The effect of swimming in asthmatic children participants in a swimming program in the city of Baltimore, *J Asthma* 26:117-121, 1989.

93. Svenonius E, Kautto R, Arborelius M Jr: Improvement after training of children with exercise-induced asthma, *Acta Paediatr Scand* 72:23-30, 1983.

94. Tovin BJ, Wolf SL, Greenfield BH et al: Comparison of the effects of exercise in water and on land on the rehabilitation of patients with intraarticular anterior cruciate ligament reconstructions, *Phys Ther* 74(8): 710-719, 1994.

95. Magnes J, Garret T, Erickson D: Swelling of the upper extremity during whirlpool baths, *Arch Phys Med Rehabil* 51:297-299, 1970.

96. Gleck J: Precautions for hydrotherapeutic devices, *Clin Mgmt* 3:44, 1983.

97. U.S. Department of Health and Human Services: *Treatment of Pressure Ulcers: Clinical Practice Guidelines,* Rockville, MD, 1994, U.S. Department of Health and Human Services.

98. Moschetti M: Aquatics risk management strategies for the therapy pool, *J Back Musculoskel Rehabil* 4(4): 265-272, 1994.

99. McMurray RG, Katz VL: Thermoregulation in pregnancy: implications for exercise, *Sports Med* 10(3): 146-158, 1990.

100. American National Red Cross: *Lifesaving Rescue and Water Safety,* Washington, DC, 1989, Water Safety Program.

101. Hwang JCF, Himel HN, Edlich RF: Bilateral amputations following hydrotherapy tank burns in a paraplegic patient, *Burns* 21(1):70-71, 1995.

102. Byl N, Cameron M, Kloth L et al: Treatment and prevention goals and objectives. In Myers RS, ed: *Saunders Manual of Physical Therapy Practice,* Philadelphia, 1995, WB Saunders.

103. Borell PM, Parker R, Henley EJ et al: Comparison of in vivo temperatures produced by hydrotherapy paraffin wax treatment and Fluidotherapy, *Phys Ther* 60: 1273-1276, 1980.

104. Loehne HB: Enhanced wound care using the pulsavac system: case studies, *Acute Care Perspect* 3(2), 1995.

105. Luedtke-Hoffman KA, Schafer DS: Pulsed lavage in wound cleansing, *Phys Ther* 80(3):292-300, 2000.

106. Haynes LJ, Brown MH, Handley BC et al: Comparison of pulsavac and sterile whirlpool regarding the promotion of tissue granulation, *Phys Ther* 74(5S):S4 (PO-012-M), 1994.

107. Hall J, MacDonald IA, Maddison PJ et al: Cardiorespiratory responses to underwater treadmill walking in healthy females, *Eur J Apply Physiol* 77(3):278-284, 1998.

108. Edlich RF, Abidin MR, Becker DG et al: Design of hydrotherapy exercise pools, *J Burn Care Rehabil* 9(5):505-509, 1998.

109. Arledge RL: Prevention of electrical shock hazards in physical therapy, *Phys Ther* 58(10):1215-1217, 1978.

110. Atkinson G, Harrison A: Implications of the Health and Safety At Work Act in relation to hydrotherapy departments, *Physiotherapy* 67:263-265, 1981.

111. American Physical Therapy Association: *Hydrotherapy/Therapeutic Pool Infection Control Guidelines,* Alexandria, VA, 1994, APTA.

112. Bloomfield SF, Miller EA: A comparison of hypochlorite and phenolic disinfectants for disinfection of clean and soiled surfaces and blood spillages, *J Hosp Infect* 13:231-239, 1989.

113. Loughney E, Harrison J: Irritant contact dermatitis due to 1-bromo-3-chloro-5,5-dimethylhydantoin in a *hydrotherapy* pool. Risk assessments: the need for continuous evidence-based assessments, *Occup Med* (Lond) 48(7):461-463, 1998.

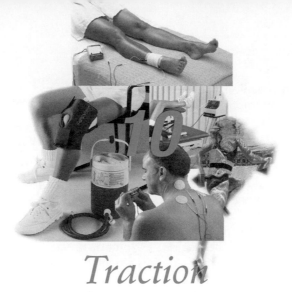

Traction

OBJECTIVES

Upon completion of this chapter, the reader will be able to:

1. Discuss the physical properties of traction.
2. Identify the physiological effects of traction.
3. Examine how the physical properties and physiological effects of traction can promote particular treatment goals.
4. Assess the indications, contraindications, and precautions for the use of traction with respect to different patient management situations.
5. Design appropriate methods for selecting traction devices and treatment parameters to produce desired physical and physiological effects.

6. Choose and use the most appropriate traction device and treatment parameters to obtain the desired treatment goals.
7. Evaluate different traction devices with respect to their potential application for treating different patient problems.
8. Presented with a clinical case, evaluate the clinical findings, propose goals of treatment, assess whether traction would be the best treatment, and, if so, formulate an effective treatment plan including the appropriate device and treatment parameters for achieving the goals of treatment.

Traction is the application of a mechanical force to the body in a way that separates, or attempts to separate, the joint surfaces and elongate the surrounding soft tissues. Traction can be applied manually by the clinician or mechanically by a machine. Traction can also be applied by the patient using body weight and the force of gravity to exert a force. Traction can be applied to the spinal or peripheral joints. This chapter focuses on the application of mechanical traction to the cervical and lumbar spine and briefly discusses the application of traction to the spine by other means. Information on the application of traction to the peripheral joints is not provided in this book since such traction is generally provided manually by the therapist and is therefore considered to be manual therapy rather than a physical agent. For further information on the application of traction to the peripheral joints, the reader should consult a manual therapy text.

Spinal traction gained popularity in the 1950s and 1960s in response to James Cyriax's recommendations regarding the efficacy of this technique for the treatment of back and leg pain caused by disc protrusions.[1] A range of studies suggest that spinal traction is more effective for reducing back pain and returning patients to activity that infrared radiation, corset and bed rest, hot packs and rest, hot packs, massage and mobilization, and bed rest.[2-5] A number of studies, however, have failed to demonstrate that traction is more effective than other treatments such as isometric exercises or that high force traction is any more effective than low force traction.[6,7] Although at this time controversy remains regarding the effectiveness of traction, this chapter presents what is known about the efficacy of traction and makes recommendations for treatment approaches that are most likely to be effective.

It has been stated that spinal traction can distract joint surfaces, reduce protrusions of nuclear discal material, stretch soft tissue, relax muscles, and mobilize joints.[1,8] Low-force traction, of 10 to 20 lb, applied for a long duration, ranging from hours to a few days, can also be used to temporarily immobilize a patient. All of these effects may reduce the pain associated with spinal dysfunction. The stimulation of sensory mechanoreceptors that occurs with the application of traction may also gate the transmission of pain along afferent neural pain pathways.

EFFECTS OF SPINAL TRACTION

> **Joint distraction**
> **Reduction of disc protrusion**
> **Soft tissue stretching**
> **Muscle relaxation**
> **Joint mobilization**
> **Patient immobilization**

Joint Distraction

Joint distraction is defined as "the separation of two articular surfaces perpendicular to the plane of the articulation."[9] Distraction of the spinal apophyseal joints may prove beneficial for the patient who has signs and symptoms related to loading of these joints or compression of the spinal nerve roots as they pass through the intervertebral foramina. Joint distraction reduces compression on the joint surfaces and widens the intervertebral foramina, potentially reducing pressure on articular surfaces, intraarticular structures, or the spinal nerve roots.[10] Thus joint distraction may reduce pain originating from joint injury or inflammation or from nerve root compression.

It has been proposed that the application of a traction force to the spine can cause distraction of the spinal apophyseal joints.[1] For distraction to occur, the force applied must be great enough to cause sufficient elongation of the soft tissues surrounding the joint to allow the joint surfaces to separate. Smaller amounts of force will increase the tension on, or elongate the soft tissues of, the spine without separating the joint surfaces. For example, a force equal to 25% of the patient's body weight has been shown to be sufficient to increase the length of the lumbar spine; however, a force equal to 50% of the patient's body weight has been found to be necessary to distract the lumbar zygapophyseal joints.[11,12] The amount of force required to distract the spinal joints also varies with the location and health of the joints. In general, the larger lumbar joints, which have more and tougher surrounding soft tissues, require more force to achieve joint distraction than do the smaller cervical joints. As mentioned above, distraction of the lumbar apophyseal joints has been demonstrated with a force equal to 50% of total body weight; in contrast, a force equal to approximately 7% of total body weight has been reported to be sufficient to distract the cervical vertebrae.[13] It has also been shown that the same magnitude of force produces greater vertebral separation in healthy spines than in spines with signs of disc degeneration.[14]

Reduction of Disc Protrusion

According to Cyriax, "traction is the treatment of choice for small nuclear protrusions."[1] The proposed mechanisms for disc realignment include clicking back of a disc fragment, suction due to decreased intradiscal pressure pulling displaced parts of the disc back toward the center, or tensing of the posterior longitudinal ligament at the posterior aspect of the disc, thereby pushing any posteriorly displaced discal material anteriorly toward its original position[1,15] (Fig. 10-1).

A number of studies have shown that spinal traction can reduce spinal discal protrusions, and a number of authors have proposed that the relief of back pain and related symptoms that occurs with the application of traction is the result of a reduction in protrusions of nuclear discal material.[16,17] Studies using a variety of diagnostic imaging techniques, including discography, epidurography, and computed tomography (CT), have demonstrated that lumbar traction, using a force of 27 to 55 kg (60 to 120 lb), can reduce a disc prolapse, cause retraction of herniated discal material, and result in clinical improvement in those patients in whom the discal defects are reduced.[15,18–20] It has been reported that symptoms generally fail to improve when traction is applied to patients with large discal herniations that fill the spinal canal or to those with calcification of the disc protrusion.[15]

Although studies support the belief that high-force traction can reduce nuclear discal protrusions, some reports indicate that lower forces may not produce this effect.[17] Andersson et al reported that intradiscal

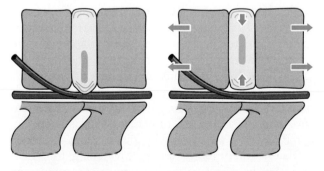

Figure 10-1. Suction due to traction causing realignment of nuclear discal material.

pressure was not reduced when self-traction was applied by the patient pulling on an overhead bar while lying down, wearing a pelvic harness attached to a spring force scale, or when manual traction was applied by one therapist pulling on the subject's pelvis while another pulled under the arms.[21] Also, Lundgren and Eldevik found that auto-traction, in which the traction force is limited by the patient's ability to pull with the arms, caused no change in the appearance of herniated lumbar discs on CT scan.[22]

Although the evidence for the effects of traction on discal protrusions is not entirely conclusive, it appears that with sufficient traction force, of at least 27 kg (60 lb) to the lumbar spine, some disc protrusions are reduced by spinal traction, and that traction can reduce symptoms in patients with local back or neck pain, or radicular spinal symptoms caused by a disc protrusion, if the protrusion is reduced. These symptomatic improvements may be the result of reducing the discal protrusion or may be due to concurrent changes in other associated structures, such as increased size of the neural foramina, changes in the tension on soft tissues or nerves, or modification of the tone of the low back muscles.

Soft Tissue Stretching

Traction has been reported to elongate the spine and increase the distance between the vertebral bodies and the facet joint surfaces.[23-25] It is proposed that these effects are due to increased length of the soft tissues in the area, including the muscles, tendons, ligaments, and discs. Soft tissue stretching using a moderate-load, prolonged force, such as that provided by spinal traction, has also been shown to increase the length of tendons and to increase joint mobility.[26-28] Increasing the length of the soft tissues of the spine may provide clinical benefits by contributing to spinal joint distraction or reduction of disc protrusion, as described above, or by increasing spinal range of motion (ROM) and decreasing the pressure on the facet joint surfaces, discs, and intervertebral nerve roots even when complete joint surface separation is not achieved.

Muscle Relaxation

Spinal traction has been reported to facilitate relaxation of the paraspinal muscles.[16,29] It has been proposed that this effect may be the result of pain reduction due to reduced pressure on pain-sensitive structures or gating of pain transmission by stimulation of mechanoreceptors by the oscillatory movements produced by intermittent traction.[30] As explained in detail in Chapter 3, reduction of pain by any means can facilitate muscle relaxation and a reduction of muscle spasms by interrupting the pain-spasm-pain cycle. It has also been proposed that static traction may cause muscle relaxation as a result of the depression in monosynaptic response caused by stretching the muscles for several seconds, and that intermittent traction may cause small changes in muscle tension to produce muscle relaxation by stimulating the Golgi tendon organs (GTOs) to inhibit alpha motor neuron firing.[31]

Joint Mobilization

Traction has been recommended as a means to mobilize joints in order to increase joint mobility or decrease joint-related pain.[32,33] Joint mobility is thought to be increased by high-force traction due to stretching of the surrounding soft tissue structures. When lower levels of force are applied, the repetitive oscillatory motion of intermittent spinal traction may also move the joints sufficiently to stimulate the mechanoreceptors and thus decrease joint-related pain by gating the afferent transmission of pain stimuli. In this manner, the effects of spinal traction may be similar to those produced by manual joint mobilization techniques, except that with most traction techniques a number of joints are mobilized at one time, whereas with manual techniques the mobilizing force can be more localized.

Patient Immobilization

Very low-load, prolonged static traction, using 4.5 to 9 kg (10 to 20 lb) applied for long periods of hours to days, can be used to temporarily immobilize a symptomatic spinal area and thereby relieve symptoms that would be aggravated by spinal motion.[12] The benefits of such treatment are thought to be the result of the enforced limited mobility and bed rest produced by the belts and harnesses used to apply the traction, rather than being a direct effect of the traction force.[34] Although the application of traction in the hospital for this purpose was popular only a decade or two ago, it has fallen out of favor at this time due to the growing awareness that most patients with back pain do not benefit from prolonged bed rest and inactivity.[35] The significant cost of providing this treatment has also limited its application. When this form of traction is used today, it is generally applied at home and seldom under the direction or supervision of a physical therapist.

CLINICAL INDICATIONS FOR THE USE OF SPINAL TRACTION

> **Disc bulge or herniation**
> **Nerve root impingement**
> **Joint hypomobility**
> **Subacute joint inflammation**
> **Paraspinal muscle spasm**

The clinical indications for the use of spinal traction include back or neck pain, with or without radiating symptoms when due to a disc bulge or herniation, nerve root impingement, joint hypomobility, subacute joint inflammation, or paraspinal muscle spasm. Although substantial evidence demonstrates the mechanical effects of spinal traction, limitations in the data from clinical studies concerning its use for the treatment of back and neck pain have caused its use for these problems to be somewhat controversial.[36]

Because treatment with traction has frequently been associated with a reduction or elimination of spinal pain, with or without radiating symptoms, and because spinal traction has been shown to reduce mechanical dysfunctions associated with such symptoms, the use of spinal traction is recommended for consideration as a treatment option for such problems. The indications and recommendations for the selection of traction as a treatment modality, provided following, and the guidelines for selection of treatment parameters, are based on the available data and an understanding of the spinal pathologies that can cause signs and symptoms in patients. If a patient's signs and symptoms are known to be due to a disc bulge or herniation, nerve root impingement, subacute joint inflammation, or paraspinal muscle spasm, and if these are aggravated by joint loading and eased by distraction or reduction of joint loading, then traction may be effective in reducing or controlling the symptoms. Traction is less likely to be effective when there is a large disc herniation that protrudes into the spinal canal or when herniated or protruding discal material has become calcified.

Disc Bulge or Herniation

In a number of clinical studies, spinal traction has been shown to relieve symptoms associated with a disc bulge or herniated nucleus pulposus.[2,15,37] The primary proposed mechanism of this beneficial effect is reduction of the disc bulge or protrusion and thus reduction of compression on the spinal nerve roots. Traction is most likely to improve the patient's outcome if it is applied soon after a discal injury when there is protrusion of soft nuclear discal material. This is because traction can reduce not only the protrusion that has occurred but can also reduce the risk of further protrusion.[17]

In contrast, a number of studies have failed to demonstrate a significant clinical benefit in response to the application of traction to patients with discal injuries.[4,6,38] This lack of positive effect may be related to the severity of the disc protrusions in the subjects studied, the use of insufficient traction force, or the use of sample sizes that were too small to detect a treatment effect. Despite these equivocal findings, spinal traction remains a common intervention for treating patients with discal protrusions and back or neck pain with or without radicular symptoms.

Because it is likely that any correction of a discal protrusion produced by spinal traction may be quickly lost if the patient returns to his or her prior activities, it is recommended that all patients be instructed in other techniques for reducing stresses on the spine after treatment with traction in order to avoid a rapid recurrence of symptoms. Such techniques may include correction of posture and body mechanics, lumbar stabilization by exercise or a corset, self-traction, and a cautious, gradual return to prior activities. Other exercises and mobilization techniques may also assist in maintaining the symptom relief and correction of discal positioning achieved with spinal traction.

Nerve Root Impingement

Traction has been reported to help alleviate signs and symptoms associated with spinal nerve root impingement, particularly if it is applied shortly after the onset of such symptoms.[2] Traction is generally recommended as the treatment of choice for patients with neurological deficits from spinal nerve root impingement.[39] Such impingement may be caused by bulging or herniation of discal material, as described above, or by ligament encroachment, narrowing of the intervertebral foramen, osteophyte encroachment, spinal nerve root swelling, or spondylolisthesis (Fig. 10-2). In the latter cases, if sufficient traction force is applied, the size of the neural foramen may temporarily be increased, reducing pressure on the spinal nerve root.[12,14,40] For example, when cervical lateral flexion and rotation to the same side, which both narrow the intervertebral foramen, are markedly limited by arm pain on the same side, indicating impingement of cervical nerve roots, the application of traction may effectively reduce the arm pain by increasing the size of the neural foramen and decreasing pressure on the involved nerve(s).

Some studies have reported good results when using traction for the treatment of pain and other related neurological symptoms associated with nerve root impingement, while others have failed to

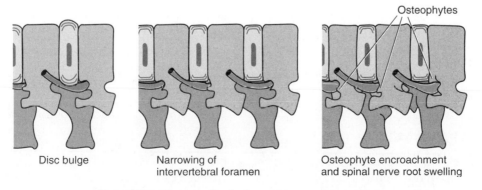

Disc bulge

Narrowing of intervertebral foramen

Osteophytes

Osteophyte encroachment and spinal nerve root swelling

Figure 10-2. Causes of spinal nerve root compression.

demonstrate greater benefits with traction than with sham traction.[38,41-43] Although the available data do not readily indicate which patients will benefit from spinal traction, clinically, in general, those patients who report aggravation of symptoms with increased spinal loading and easing of symptoms with decreased spinal loading are more likely to respond well to treatment with traction. It has also been recommended that traction be considered for patients with symptoms of radiating pain or paresthesia that do not improve with trunk movements.[44]

Joint Hypomobility

Because longitudinal spinal traction can glide and distract the spinal facet joints and stretch the soft tissues surrounding these joints, spinal traction may prove beneficial in the treatment of symptoms caused by joint hypomobility. However, spinal traction is not generally the optimal treatment if only individual segments are hypomobile because it applies a mobilizing force to multiple rather than single spinal levels. Such nonspecific mobilization could prove deleterious to the patient with hypomobility of one segment and hypermobility of adjoining segments. In such patients, the mobilizing force applied by traction would most probably cause the greatest increase in motion in the most extensible areas, the hypermobile segments, resulting in joint laxity, while having no effect on the mobility of the less mobile segments causing the patient's symptoms. Adjusting the degree of spinal flexion during the application of traction localizes the mobilizing effect of the force to some degree and thus may help to alleviate this problem.[45] For example, positioning the lumbar spine in more flexion localizes the force to the upper lumbar and lower thoracic spine, while positioning it in neutral or extension localizes the force to the lower lumbar area. Similarly, for the cervical spine, the flexed position focuses the forces on the lower cervical area, while the neutral or slightly extended position focuses the forces on the upper cervical area.[45] More detailed recommendations for patient positioning are provided in the section below regarding application techniques.

Subacute Joint Inflammation

Traction has been recommended for reducing the pain and limitations of function associated with subacute joint inflammation.[33] The force of traction can be used to reduce the pressure on inflamed joint surfaces, while the small movements of intermittent traction may control pain by gating transmission at the spinal cord level. These movements may also help to maintain normal fluid exchange in the joints to relieve edema in or around the joints caused by chronic inflammation.[46] Spinal traction can be used safely in the subacute or chronic stages of joint inflammation; however, intermittent traction should be avoided immediately after an injury, during the acute inflammatory phase, when the repetitive motion may cause further injury or amplify the inflammatory response.

Paraspinal Muscle Spasm

The maintained stretch of static traction or the repetitive motion of low-load, intermittent traction may help to reduce paraspinal muscle spasm.[16,29] As noted previously, this effect may be secondary to a reduction in pain and the consequent interruption of the pain-spasm-pain cycle or may be caused by inhibition of alpha motor neuron firing due to depression of the monosynaptic response or stimulation of the GTOs.[30] Higher load spinal traction may also alleviate protective paraspinal muscle spasms by reducing the underlying cause of pain, such as a disc protrusion or herniation, or a nerve root impingement, thus interrupting the pain-spasm-pain cycle.

CONTRAINDICATIONS AND PRECAUTIONS FOR SPINAL TRACTION

The application of spinal traction is contraindicated in some circumstances, and it should be applied with extra caution in other circumstances;[47] however, in all cases, in order to minimize the probability of adverse consequences, when traction is first applied, it should be applied in a less aggressive manner, using a small amount of force, and the patient's response to treatment should be closely monitored. Also, if the patient's condition worsens in response to traction, with symptoms becoming more severe, peripheralizing, increasing in distribution, or progressing to other domains (e.g., from pain to numbness or weakness), the treatment approach should be reevaluated and changed. If the patient's signs or symptoms do not improve within two or three treatments, the treatment approach should also be reevaluated and changed or the patient should be referred to a physician for further evaluation.

CONTRAINDICATIONS
for the Use of Traction

- Where motion is contraindicated
- With an acute injury or inflammation
- Joint hypermobility or instability
- Peripheralization of symptoms with traction
- Uncontrolled hypertension (for inversion traction)

The use of spinal traction is contraindicated . . .

. . . where motion is contraindicated

Traction should not be used if motion is contraindicated in the area to be affected; for example, with an unstable fracture, in cases of cord compression, or shortly after spinal surgery.

ASK THE PATIENT:

- Have you been instructed not to move your neck or back? If so, by whom?
- If wearing a brace or corset: Have you been instructed not to remove your brace at any time?
- How recent was your injury or surgery?

   Do not use any form of traction if motion in the area is contraindicated. Consider direct treatment with other physical agents, such as heat or cold, or treat other involved areas where motion is allowed.

. . . with an acute injury or inflammation

Acute inflammation may occur immediately after trauma or surgery, or as the result of an inflammatory disease such as rheumatoid arthritis or osteoarthritis. Since intermittent or static traction may aggravate acute inflammation or interfere with the healing of an acute injury, traction should not be applied under these conditions.

ASK THE PATIENT:

- When did your injury occur?
- When did your pain start?

   If the injury or onset of pain was within the last 72 hours, the injury is likely to still be in the acute inflammatory phase, and traction should not be used. As inflammation resolves, static traction may be used initially, with progression to intermittent traction as the area tolerates more motion.

ASSESS:

- Palpate and inspect the area to detect signs of inflammation, including heat, redness, and swelling.
- If signs of acute inflammation are present, it is recommended that the application of traction be delayed until they resolve.

. . . to a hypermobile or unstable joint

High-force traction should not be used in areas of joint hypermobility or instability because it may further increase the mobility of the area. Therefore the mobility of joints in the area to which one is considering applying traction should be assessed before the traction is applied. Joint hypermobility may be the result of a recent fracture, joint dislocation, or surgery, or it can be due to an old injury, high relaxin levels during pregnancy and lactation, poor posture, or congenital ligament laxity. Joint hypermobility and instability, particularly of the C1-C2 articulations, is also common in patients with rheumatoid arthritis, Down's syndrome, and Marfan's syndrome due to degeneration of the transverse atlantar ligament. Therefore cervical traction should not be applied to patients with these diagnoses until the integrity of the transverse atlantar ligament and the stability of the C1-C2 articulations have been ascertained.

ASK THE PATIENT:

- Have you dislocated a joint in this area?
- Do you have rheumatoid arthritis or Marfan's syndrome?
- Are you pregnant?

ASSESS:

- Assess joint mobility in the area that will be affected by the traction.

   All levels of the cervical or lumbar spine, depending on which is being treated, should be assessed, not just the symptomatic ones, since traction can affect the mobility of multiple levels.

Continued

CONTRAINDICATIONS—cont'd

- Check the patient's chart for any diagnosis of rheumatoid arthritis, Marfan's syndrome, or Down's syndrome and request radiographic studies to rule out C1-C2 instability before applying traction.
- Do not apply traction in areas where joint hypermobility is detected on manual or radiographic examination or to areas that have been previously dislocated.

    When some segments are hypomobile and adjacent segments are hypermobile, it is recommended that the hypomobile segments be treated with manual techniques rather than mechanical traction since manual techniques can mobilize individual spinal segments more specifically.

The use of spinal traction is contraindicated . . .

. . . with peripheralization of symptoms

Traction should be discontinued or modified immediately if it causes peripheralization of symptoms because, in general, progression of spinal symptoms from a central area to a more peripheral area is indicative of worsening nerve function and increasing compression. Continuing treatment when symptom peripheralization occurs could result in aggravation of the initial injury and prolonged worsening of signs and symptoms.

TELL THE PATIENT:

- Let me know immediately if you get more pain or other symptoms further down your arms or legs. Stop the traction if this occurs.

ASSESS:

- Recheck sensation, motor function, and reflexes in the appropriate extremity(ies) if the patient complains of peripheralization of symptoms.
- Discontinue or modify traction if signs or symptoms peripheralize.

    Traction may be modified by decreasing the load or changing the patient's position. Modified traction may be continued if peripheralization of symptoms no longer occurs. Mild aggravation of central symptoms alone in a patient with prior central and peripheral symptoms should not be a cause for discontinuation of treatment.

PRECAUTIONS
for the Use of Traction

In cases where traction should be applied with caution, check with the referring physician before initiating traction, start with a low level of force, progress slowly, and monitor the patient's response to the treatment closely at all times.

Precautions include:

- Structural diseases or conditions affecting the spine (e.g., tumor, infection, rheumatoid arthritis, osteoporosis, or prolonged systemic steroid use)
- When pressure of the belts may be hazardous (e.g., with pregnancy, hiatal hernia, vascular compromise, osteoporosis)
- Displacement of annular fragment
- Medial disc protrusion
- Severe pain fully relieved by traction
- Claustrophobia
- Patients who cannot tolerate the prone or supine position
- Disorientation
- Temporomandibular joint (TMJ) problems
- Dentures

Use traction with caution for . . .

. . . patients with a structural disease or condition affecting the bones of the spine

Traction should be applied with caution when the structural integrity of the spine may be compromised. Such structural compromise most commonly occurs due to a tumor, infection, rheumatoid arthritis, osteoporosis, or prolonged systemic steroid use. In these circumstances, the spine may not be strong enough to sustain the forces of the traction, and therefore injury may result from the application of strong traction forces. Radiographic reports and other studies that may indicate the nature and severity of the structural compromise should be checked before deciding to apply traction to patients with these conditions.

ASK THE PATIENT:
- Do you have any disease affecting your bones or joints?
- Do you have cancer, an infection in your bones, rheumatoid arthritis, or osteoporosis?
- Do you take steroid medications? If so, how long have you taken them?

Low-force traction only should be applied to patients with structural compromise of the spine. Therefore, in many cases, manual traction, which allows more direct monitoring of patient response, may be more appropriate in these patients.

. . . patients for whom the pressure of the belts may be hazardous

The pelvic belts used for the application of mechanical lumbar traction may apply excessive abdominal pressure to pregnant patients or to those with hiatal hernia and may place excessive pressure on the inguinal region on those with femoral artery compromise. Compression in the area of the femoral arteries in the inguinal region can be avoided by ensuring that the pelvic belt is positioned with its lower edge superior to the femoral triangle and by tightly securing the belt and keeping it in direct contact with the skin to prevent it from slipping down during treatment. There is also concern that the pelvic or thoracic belts may apply excessive pressure to the pelvis or ribs of patients with osteoporosis. Because the thoracic belts used for fixation of the patient during the application of lumbar traction may constrict respiration, it is also recommended that lumbar traction be applied with caution to patients with cardiac or pulmonary disorders.[48]

Cervical traction should be applied with caution to patients with cerebrovascular compromise, as indicated by a positive vertebral artery test, because poor placement of the halter may further compromise circulation to the brain. The halter should also be positioned away from the carotid arteries in patients with compromise of these arteries. This is most easily achieved by using a halter that distracts via the occiput rather than one that applies force to both the occiput and the mandible.

ASK THE PATIENT:
- Are you pregnant?
- Do you have a hiatal hernia?
- Have you had any trouble with blocked arteries?
- Do you get pain in your calves when walking a short distance? This is a sign of intermittent claudication, indicating possible arterial insufficiency to the lower extremities.
- Do you have osteoporosis?
- Do you have problems with your breathing?
- Have you had a stroke?
- Do you get dizzy when you put your head back?

If compression by the belts used for mechanical traction is hazardous to the patient, one should consider using other forms of traction, such as self-traction or manual traction, that do not require the use of these belts. Fastening the belts less tightly is generally not recommended because this will allow them to slip during treatment, rendering the treatment ineffective or increasing pressure in the inguinal region. If the patient's responses indicate possible compromise of the cervical or lower extremity vessels, it is essential that the halter or belts used for traction be positioned in such a manner that they do not compress these vessels.

. . . patients with a displacement of a fragment of annulus

Once a fragment of annulus has become displaced and is no longer connected to the body of the disc, traction is not likely to change the position of the disc fragment, and therefore treatment with traction is also not likely to improve the patient's symptoms.

ASK THE PATIENT:
- Has a magnetic resonance imaging (MRI) or computed tomography (CT) scan of your spine been performed? Please bring me the report(s) from that (those) test(s).

Continued

PRECAUTIONS—cont'd

Traction should not be used to treat symptoms resulting from a displaced disc fragment that is no longer attached to the body of the disc.

... patients with a medial disc protrusion

It has been proposed that traction may aggravate symptoms caused by a medial disc protrusion because, in such circumstances, the medial movement of the nerve root caused by a traction force may increase the impingement of the disc on the nerve root[49] (Fig. 10-3).

ASK THE PATIENT:

• Has an MRI or CT scan of your spine been performed? Please bring me the report(s) from that (those) test(s).

... patients for whom severe pain resolves fully with traction

If severe pain resolves fully with traction, this may indicate that the traction has increased rather than decreased compression on a nerve root, causing a complete nerve block.

ASK THE PATIENT:

• After a few minutes of traction: Have your symptoms changed?
• If the patient had severe pain and reports that the pain has decreased: Has the pain completely gone away or is it just less severe?

ASSESS:

• Test sensation, reflexes, and strength before treatment. Also, if the patient reports complete resolution of severe pain during treatment, check these again and assess for any changes.

Should severe pain be fully relieved by traction, it is recommended that the clinician immediately recheck other indicators of nerve conduction, including sensation, reflexes, and strength, to rule out increasing nerve compression. If these are worse, traction should be stopped immediately. If these are not worse, the force of traction may be reduced by 50%, or the direction of the traction force modified, and traction may be continued. If traction is maintained at a level that causes a nerve block, the patient may sustain a severe nerve injury as the result of the treatment.

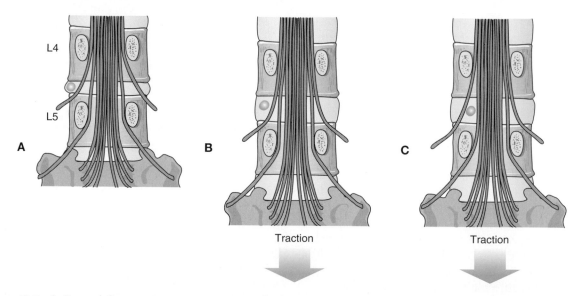

Figure 10-3. **A,** Lateral disc protrusion compressing the L4 nerve root. **B,** L4 nerve root compression by lateral disc protrusion relieved by traction due to elongation of the lumbar spine and a consequent medial movement of the nerve root. **C,** L4 nerve root compression by medial disc protrusion aggravated by traction due to medial movement of the nerve root.

. . . patients experiencing claustrophobia or other psychological aversion to traction

A number of patients are psychologically averse to the use of traction because this procedure generally involves considerable restriction of movement and loss of control. In particular, patients with claustrophobia may not tolerate the restriction of movement required for the application of mechanical lumbar traction. In such cases, other forms of traction that do not require immobilization with belts, such as manual or positional traction, may be better tolerated.

. . . patients who cannot tolerate the prone or supine position

A number of patients cannot tolerate the prone or supine position for the period of time necessary for the application of traction. Such limitations may be the result of their spinal condition or other medical problems such as reflux esophagitis. In such cases, the use of supports such as a lumbar roll may allow the patient to tolerate the position; cervical traction may be applied in the sitting position; or, for lumbar traction, some of the self-traction techniques may be effective.

ASK THE PATIENT:
- Does lying on your back with your knees bent for 15 to 20 minutes cause any problems for you?
- Does lying on your stomach for 15 to 20 minutes cause any problems for you?

. . . disoriented patients

It is recommended that mechanical traction not be applied to disoriented patients since they may move in the halter or belts, becoming entangled or altering the amount of force they receive. It is recommended that only manual traction techniques be used to treat disoriented patients.

Use cervical traction with caution for . . .

. . . patients with temporomandibular joint (TMJ) problems

In patients with TMJ problems, or a history of such problems, it is recommended that a halter that only applies pressure through the occiput be used rather than one that applies pressure through both the mandible and the occiput, because the latter may place pressure on the TMJs and thus aggravate preexisting joint pathology. Many clinicians use an occipital halter with all patients in order to avoid the possibility of causing TMJ problems in patients who did not have such problems previously.

ASK THE PATIENT:
- Do you have problems with your jaw?

. . . patients who wear dentures

The patient who wears dentures should be instructed to keep the dentures in place during treatment with cervical traction because their removal can alter the alignment of the TMJs and may cause problems if pressure is applied to these joints through the mandible. To protect dentures and the teeth, as well as the TMJs, an occipital halter should be used.

ASK THE PATIENT:
- Do you wear dentures?
- Do you have them in now?

Patient Recommendations and Instructions

Instruct the patient to try to avoid sneezing or coughing while on full traction because these activities increase intraabdominal pressure and can thus increase intradiscal pressure. It is also recommended that the patient empty the bladder and not have a heavy meal before lumbar traction since the constriction of the pelvic belts may cause discomfort on a full bladder or stomach.

ADVERSE EFFECTS OF SPINAL TRACTION

Although no systematic research has been performed on the adverse effects of spinal traction, some case reports suggest that prior symptoms may be increased by the application of lumbar traction exceeding 50% of the patient's total body weight or by the application of cervical traction exceeding 50% of the weight of the patient's head.[33,50] These reports stand in contrast to the finding that the force of traction must be at least 50% of the patient's body weight in order to achieve separation of the lumbar vertebrae.[12] Because a rebound increase in pain after the initial application of high-force traction can occur, it is generally recommended that traction force be kept low for the initial treatment and then be gradually increased until maximum benefit is obtained. Specific recommendations for the amount of traction force to be used for different regions of the spine and different spinal conditions are given below in the section on application techniques.

It has been reported that some patients experience lumbar radicular discomfort after receiving treatment with intermittent cervical traction for cervical radicular symptoms.[51] Thirty-three percent of the patients who were reported to experience this adverse effect had transitional lumbar vertebrae on roentgenograms, and 83% had evidence of spinal osteoarthritis. Their onset of lumbar radiculopathy after cervical traction suggests that axial tension induced in the spinal cord's dural covering was transmitted from the cervical spine to the lumbar nerve roots, and that limitations in nerve root excursion caused by structural abnormalities and degenerative changes in these patients probably resulted in excessive tension being placed on the nerve roots, provoking lumbar radicular symptoms.

Other adverse effects of spinal traction have been described in detail above in the sections describing contraindications and precautions.

APPLICATION TECHNIQUES

Traction can be applied in a variety of ways. Treatment with traction at this time includes the use of electric and weighted mechanical devices, self-traction, positional traction, and manual traction. In the past, traction was also applied using inversion techniques and purpose-built auto-traction tables.

Inversion traction, which is applied by placing the patient in a device that requires a head-down position, uses the weight of the patient's upper body to apply traction to the lumbar spine. This form of traction was fairly popular in the past 10 to 20 years; however, most inversion traction devices have recently been removed from the U.S. market by their manufacturers due to concerns regarding potential adverse effects in patients with hypertension. Significant increases in systolic and diastolic blood pressure and ophthalmic artery pressure have been documented in subjects without cardiovascular disease or a history of hypertension in response to the application of inversion traction; therefore, it is thought that the application of this type of traction could increase the risk of a cardiovascular accident or myocardial infarction in the patient with uncontrolled hypertension.[52-54] Because of these possible risks, the use of inversion traction is not recommended, and therefore instructions for its application are not provided in this book.

Auto-traction, a form of self-traction that requires the use of a purpose-built table with sections that can be moved apart by the patient during treatment, was also popular for a number of years; however, this type of table is no longer being manufactured, and therefore directions for its application are also not provided in this book.

When selecting the type of spinal traction, patient position, traction force, and duration and frequency of treatment to be used, the effects of these different parameters of treatment, the nature of the patient's problem, and the patient's response to prior treatments should be considered. Guidelines for the standard application technique for each of the above types of traction, and the advantages and disadvantages of each, are provided following. However, if the clinician understands the principles underlying the application of this type of treatment, many of these techniques can be modified or adapted by the clinician to suit individual clinical situations, such as when a patient does not tolerate the standard position(s) used for treatment or when preferred equipment is not available.

For all forms of traction, the clinician should first determine if the presenting symptoms and problems are likely to respond to treatment with traction. The clinician should also determine that traction is not contraindicated for this patient or condition. Traction can be applied to the lumbar or cervical spine; however, some forms of traction are appropriate for only one area or the other, while others can be applied to either with appropriate modifications.

Mechanical Traction

Mechanical traction can be applied to the lumbar or cervical spine. A variety of belts and halters, and a number of different patient treatment positions, can be used to apply traction to different areas of the spine and to focus the effect on different segments or structures. Electric mechanical traction units can apply static or intermittent traction of varying force. With static traction, the same amount of force is applied throughout the treatment session. With intermittent traction, the traction force alternates between two set points every few seconds throughout the treatment session. The force is held at a maximum for a number of seconds, the hold period, and is then reduced, usually by about 50%, for the following relaxation period.

Weighted mechanical traction units apply static traction only, with the amount of force being determined by the amount of weight used.

In order to apply mechanical traction safely and effectively, the following procedure should be followed.

APPLICATION TECHNIQUE
Mechanical Traction

Equipment Required
For Electrical Mechanical Traction
- Traction unit
- Thoracic and pelvic belts, cervical halters
- Spreader bar
- Extension rope

- Split traction table (optional)

For Weighted Mechanical Traction
- Traction device (ropes, pulley, weights)
- Thoracic and pelvic belts, cervical halters
- Spreader bar
- Weight bag for water, weights, or sand

PROCEDURE

Electrical Mechanical Traction Units

Most clinics have one or more electric mechanical traction units available. These units use a motor to apply traction forces to the lumbar or cervical spine, statically or intermittently, and can be used to apply forces of up to 70 kg (150 lb). These units have the advantage of being able to apply static or intermittent traction to the lumbar or cervical spine, and they allow fine, accurate control of the forces being applied. These units also allow considerable variation in patient position. The most significant limitations of electric mechanical traction devices are their cost and size (Fig. 10-4).

Over-the-Door Cervical Traction Devices

Over-the-door cervical traction units can be used for the application of static cervical traction only. The limited treatment flexibility of these devices makes them appropriate primarily for home use. In this setting, they have the additional advantages of being inexpensive, easy to set up, and compact. The patient should be educated regarding their position, and the amount and duration of force to use prior to using such a device at home.

Other Home Traction Devices

A number of other spinal traction devices are also available for home application of static or intermittent lumbar or cervical traction (Fig. 10-5, *A* and *B*). These devices offer more treatment options but are

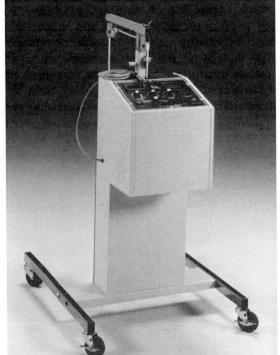

Figure 10-4. Mechanical traction unit. (Courtesy Chattanooga Group, Inc., Hixson, TN.)

Continued

APPLICATION TECHNIQUE—cont'd
Mechanical Traction

generally considerably more expensive than over-the-door devices, are more complex to use, and generally take up more space in the home.

Mechanical Lumbar Traction Procedure

1. Select the appropriate mechanical traction device.

   Various devices are available for applying mechanical traction to the lumbar spine in the clinic or home setting. The choice depends on the amount of force to be applied, whether static or intermittent traction is desired, and the setting in which the treatment will be applied.

2. Determine optimal patient position.

   When positioning the patient, try to achieve a comfortable position that allows muscle relaxation while maximizing the separation between the involved structures. The relative degree of flexion or extension of the spine during traction determines which surfaces are most effectively separated.[33] The flexed position results in greater separation of the posterior structures, including the facet joints and intervertebral foramina, whereas the neutral or extended position results in greater separation of

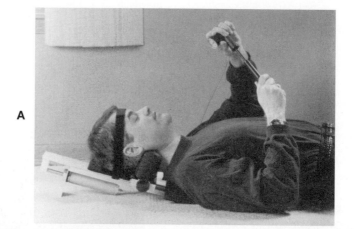

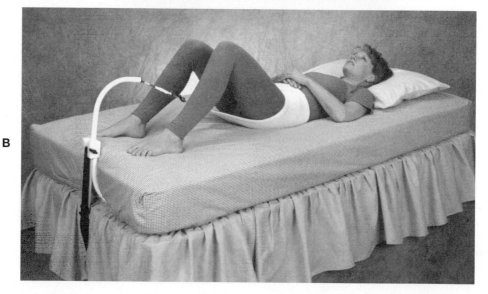

Figure 10-5. Examples of home traction devices. (**A,** Courtesy Chattanooga Group, Inc., Hixson, TN; **B,** Courtesy Elastatrac, San Jose, CA.)

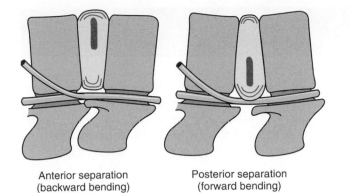

Anterior separation   Posterior separation
(backward bending)   (forward bending)

Figure 10-6. Effects of anterior and posterior separation on the spinal disc.

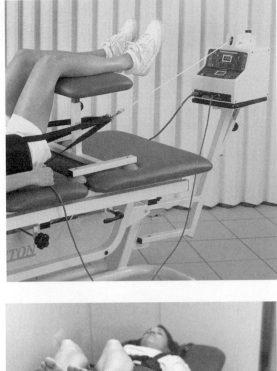

A

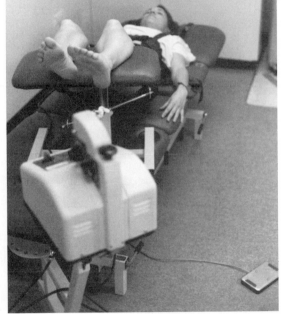

B

the anterior structures, including the disc spaces (Fig. 10-6). In most cases, a symmetrical central force is used, in which the direction of force is in line with the central sagittal axis of the patient (Fig. 10-7, *A*); however, if the patient presents with unilateral symptoms, a unilateral traction force that applies more force to one side of the spine than to the other may prove to be more effective.[55] A unilateral force can be applied by offsetting the axis of the traction in the direction that most reduces the patient's symptoms. For example, if the patient presents with right low back and lower extremity pain that is aggravated by right side bending and is relieved by left side bending, the traction should be offset so as to apply a left side bending force (Fig.10-7,*B*).

For the application of traction to the lumbar spine, the patient may be positioned prone or supine (Figs. 10-8 and 10-9). Supine positioning is more commonly used; however, prone positioning may be advantageous if the patient does not tolerate flexion or being supine, or if the symptoms are reduced by extension or by being in the prone position. Greater lumbar paraspinal muscle relaxation and less EMG activity have also been reported during traction in the prone rather than the supine position.[56] Clinically, symptoms of discal origin are also usually most reduced in the prone position, when the lumbar spine is in neutral or extension and the disc space is most separated (see Fig. 10-6), while symptoms due to facet joint dysfunction are most reduced when the patient is positioned supine with the hips flexed, when the lumbar spine is flexed and the facet joints are most separated.[33] Prone neutral positioning of the lumbar spine also localizes the force of the

Figure 10-7. Lumbar traction. **A,** Central axis lumbar traction. **B,** Unilateral lumbar traction. (**A,** Courtesy Chattanooga Group, Inc., Hixson, TN.)

traction to the lower lumbar segments, whereas supine flexed positioning localizes the traction force to the upper lumbar and lower thoracic segments.

The patient should lie on a split traction table, with the area of the spine to be distracted positioned over

Continued

APPLICATION TECHNIQUE—cont'd
Mechanical Traction

the split, and, if supine, with the lower extremities supported on a suitable stool that does not interfere with the motion of the traction rope. A split traction table separates into two sections, with one section sliding away from the other when the sections are unlocked and traction is applied (Fig. 10-10). This type of table reduces the amount of traction force lost to friction between the patient and the table because the lower half of the patient's body moves with the lower section of the table. Thus less trac-

tion force is needed when a split table is used than when a nonsplit table is used in order to provide the same amount of distractive force to the lumbar spine.[57] Initially the patient should be positioned with the sections of the table locked together so that the table does not move as the patient moves into the treatment position. The sections should then be slowly unlocked, after the traction force has been applied, in order to control the speed at which the initial traction force is applied.

3. Apply the appropriate belts or halter.

   Heavy-duty non-slip thoracic and pelvic belts should be used to secure the patient during the application of mechanical lumbar traction (Fig. 10-11). These belts must be placed with the non-slip surface directly in contact with the patient's skin, and not over the clothing, and both belts must be securely tightened in order to prevent slipping when the traction force is applied. The belts can either be placed on the table at the appropriate level, and then adjusted when the patient lies down on them, or they can be secured around the patient first and then secured to the table after the patient lies down. The thoracic belt is used to stabilize the upper body above the level at which traction force is desired in order to prevent the patient from being

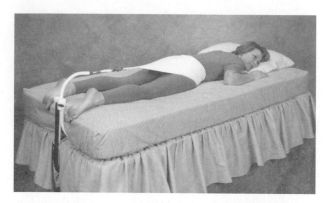

Figure 10-8. Prone lumbar traction with spine in neutral or slight extension. (Courtesy Elastatrac, San Jose, CA.)

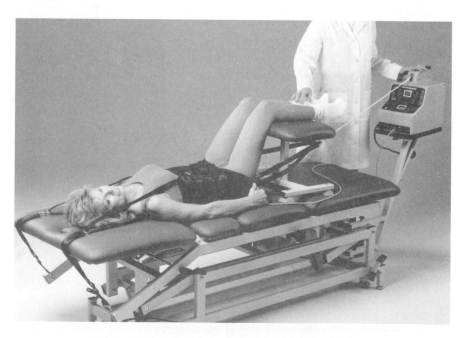

Figure 10-9. Supine lumbar traction with spine in flexion. (Courtesy Chattanooga Group, Inc., Hixson, TN.)

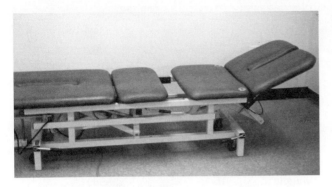

Figure 10-10. Split traction table.

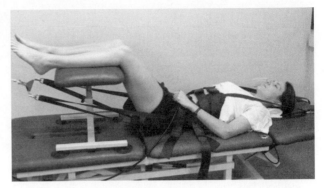

Figure 10-12. Positioning of belts for lumbar traction.

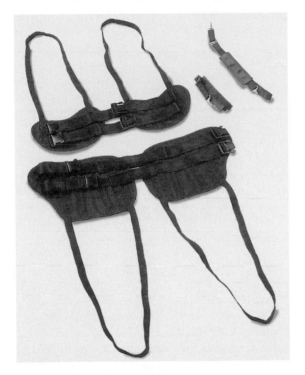

Figure 10-11. Traction belts. (Courtesy Chattanooga Group, Inc., Hixson, TN.)

pulled down the table by the force on the pelvic belt and in order to isolate the traction force to the appropriate spinal segments. The thoracic belt should be placed so that its lower edge aligns with the superior limit at which the traction force is desired, and with its upper edge aligned approximately with the xiphoid immediately below the greatest diameter of the thorax. The pelvic belt should be placed so that its superior edge aligns with the inferior limit at which traction force is

desired, generally just superior to the iliac crests (or superior to the superior edge of the sacrum if the patient is prone) (Fig. 10-12).

When the patient is supine with the lumbar spine in slight flexion, as indicated to maximize distraction of the posterior spinal structures, the pelvic belt should be placed with the fastening anteriorly and the rope posteriorly so that the pull is primarily from the posterior aspect of the pelvis (see Fig. 10-9). When the patient is prone, with the lumbar spine in neutral or slight extension, as indicated to maximize distraction of the anterior spinal structures, the pelvic belt may be placed with the fastening posteriorly and the rope anteriorly so that the pull is primarily from the anterior aspect of the pelvis.[58]

4. Connect the belts or halter to the traction device.

Fasten the thoracic belt to the table above the patient's head and connect the pelvic belt to the traction unit using a rope and a spreader bar.

5. Set the appropriate traction parameters (Table 10-1).

Select static or intermittent traction and then, for static traction, set the maximum traction force and the total traction duration, or, for intermittent traction, set the maximum and minimum traction force, hold and relax times, and the total traction duration.

Static or Intermittent Traction

Mechanical traction may be administered statically, with the same force throughout the treatment, or intermittently, with the force varying every few seconds throughout the treatment. Some authors recommend that only static traction be applied in order to avoid a stretch reflex of the muscles;[10] however, others report that static and intermittent traction are equally effective but that higher forces can be used with intermittent traction.[59] No differences in lumbar sacrospinalis

Continued

APPLICATION TECHNIQUE—cont'd
Mechanical Traction

TABLE 10-1 Recommended Parameters for the Application of Spinal Traction

Area of the spine and goals of treatment	Force	Hold/relax times (seconds)	Total traction time (minutes)
Lumbar			
Initial/acute phase	13-20 kg	Static	5-10
Joint distraction	22.5 kg; 50% of body weight	15/15	20-30
Decrease muscle spasm	25% of body weight	5/5	20-30
Disc problems or stretch soft tissue	25% of body weight	60/20	20-30
Cervical			
Initial/acute phase	3-4 kg	Static	5-10
Joint distraction	9-13 kg; 7% of body weight	15/15	20-30
Decrease muscle spasm	5-7 kg	5/5	20-30
Disc problems or stretch soft tissue	5-7 kg	60/20	20-30

EMG activity or vertebral separation have been found when static and intermittent traction of the same force have been compared.[60,61] It is generally recommended that static traction be used if the area being treated is inflamed, if the patient's symptoms are easily aggravated by motion, or if the patient's symptoms are related to a disc protrusion.[10] Intermittent traction with long hold times may also be effective for treatment of symptoms related to disc protrusion, while shorter hold and relax times are recommended for symptoms related to joint dysfunctions.

Hold/Relax Times

If intermittent traction is selected, the maximum traction force is applied during the hold time and a lower traction force is applied during the relax time. The recommended ratio and duration of the hold and relax times depend on the patient's condition and tolerance. In general, if intermittent traction is used for treatment of a disc problem, longer hold times, of approximately 60 seconds, and shorter relax times, of approximately 20 seconds, are recommended, whereas if traction is being used to treat a spinal joint problem, shorter hold and relax times of approximately 15 seconds each are recommended.[11] Symptom severity should also be used as a guide for determining hold and relax times. When the patient's symptoms are severe, both long hold and long relax times are recommended in order to limit the amount of

movement. As the symptoms become less severe, the relax time can gradually be decreased, and when the discomfort has decreased to a local ache rather than a pain, the hold time can also be reduced so that when the symptoms are mild, the traction produces an oscillatory motion with very short hold and relax times of approximately 3 to 5 seconds each.

Force

Different authors vary in their recommendations with regard to the amount of force to be used for traction; however, most agree that the optimal amount of force depends on the patient's clinical presentation, the goals of treatment, and the patient's position during treatment.[10,17,18] For all applications, the force should be kept low during the initial traction session in order to reduce the risk of reactive muscle guarding and spasms and to determine if traction is likely to aggravate the patient's symptoms. The traction force can be increased gradually in subsequent sessions as the patient becomes used to the procedure. It is recommended that, for all applications, the traction force to the lumbar spine start at between 13 and 20 kg (25 to 50 lb).

When the goal is to decrease compression on a spinal nerve root or facet joint, sufficient force to separate the facet joints in the area being treated must be used. In the lumbar spine, it has been shown that this requires a force of between 22.5 kg (50 lb) and approximately 60% of the patient's body weight.[11,60,62]

When the goal is to decrease muscle spasm, stretch soft tissue, or exert a centripetal force on the disc by spinal elongation without joint surface separation, lower forces of 25% of total body weight for the lumbar spine are generally effective. When this is the goal, the application of a hot pack in conjunction with the traction may result in greater spinal elongation and thus more effective relief of symptoms.

Higher traction forces are needed when patient positioning, or the harness or table, requires the traction force to overcome gravity or friction between the patient and the table. For example, when lumbar traction is applied without a split table and the traction has to overcome the friction between the patient's body and the surface of the table, higher traction forces may be necessary, whereas when gravity and friction are reduced, as occurs with lumbar traction when a split table is used, lower traction forces may be sufficient.

The force of traction can be adjusted during or between treatments. The force should be decreased during the treatment if there is any peripheralization of signs or symptoms or, as mentioned above in the section on precautions, if there is complete relief of severe pain. If the patient's symptoms are moderately decreased by traction, the force can be increased, by 2 to 5 kg (5 to 15 lb) for lumbar traction, at each subsequent treatment session until maximal relief of symptoms is achieved. Traction force to the lumbar spine should generally not exceed 50% of the patient's body weight.

When intermittent traction is used, the relaxed force should be approximately 50% of the maximum force or less; however, total release of the force during the relaxed phase of intermittent traction is not recommended since this can result in a rebound aggravation of the patient's symptoms.

Total Treatment Duration

There are no published studies comparing the effects of different treatment durations; however, most authors recommend that the duration of a patient's first treatment with traction be brief; that is, about 5 minutes if the initial symptoms are severe and 10 minutes if the initial symptoms are moderate, in order to assess the patient's response.[11,63] If severe symptoms are significantly relieved by brief low-force traction, the duration of treatment should be kept short; otherwise, symptom exacerbation after the treatment is likely. If the patient's symptoms are partially relieved after 10 minutes of traction, it is recommended that the duration of the initial treatment not be extended; however, if symptoms are unchanged after 10 minutes, the hold force may be increased slightly or the angle of pull modified, and treatment may be continued for a further 10 minutes. Recommendations for the duration of subsequent treatments vary from as short as 8 to 10 minutes for treatment of a disc protrusion[11] to as long as 20 to 40 minutes for this and other indications.[38] Treatment for longer than 40 minutes is generally thought to provide no additional benefit.

Treatment Frequency

Some authors state that spinal traction must be administered daily to be effective; however, there are no published studies evaluating the outcome of different treatment frequencies.[11,38]

6. Start the traction.

When applying traction to the lumbar spine, if a split table is being used, first allow the traction to pull for one hold cycle to take up the slack in the belt and rope and then, during the following relaxation of the traction, release the sections of the table slowly. If static traction is being used, the sections of the table may be released after the traction force is applied. The therapist should manually control the rate of separation of the sections in order to prevent sudden motion of the patient and the lower section of the table. If a split table is not available, the traction device will take up the slack in the belt and rope during the first hold cycle. When using a split table, once the sections are released, the force of the traction pulls the patient and the lower section of the table simultaneously, and so does not have to overcome friction between the patient and the surface of the table. For this to occur, it is essential that the lower section of the table actually move back and forth during the hold and relax cycles, rather than being stationary at its position of maximal excursion, where it will act as a static surface. The clinician should observe the traction being applied, and the movement of the table for a few cycles, and then make any necessary adjustments to ensure that the traction is producing the desired effect.

7. Assess the patient's response.

It is recommended that the clinician assess the patient's initial response to the application of traction within the first 5 minutes of treatment so that any adjustments can be made at that time if needed.

8. Give the patient a means to call you and to stop the traction.

Continued

APPLICATION TECHNIQUE—cont'd
Mechanical Traction

Most electric mechanical traction units are equipped with a patient safety cutoff switch that turns off the unit and rings a bell when activated. Instruct the patient to use this switch if he or she experiences any increase in, or peripheralization of, pain or other symptoms.

9. Release traction and assess the patient's response.

When the traction time is completed, lock the split sections of the table, release the tension on the traction ropes, and allow the patient to rest briefly before getting up and recompressing the joints. Then reexamine the patient's signs and symptoms.

ADVANTAGES

- Force and time well-controlled, readily graded, and replicable.
- Once applied, does not require the clinician to be with the patient throughout the treatment.
- Electrical mechanical traction units allow the application of static or intermittent traction.
- Static weighted devices such as over-the-door cervical traction are inexpensive and convenient for independent use by the patient at home.

DISADVANTAGES

- Expensive electric mechanical devices.
- Time-consuming to set up.
- Lack of patient control or participation.
- Restriction by belts or halter poorly tolerated by some patients.
- Mobilizes broad regions of the spine rather than individual spinal segments, potentially inducing hypermobility in normal or hypermobile joints.

MECHANICAL CERVICAL TRACTION PROCEDURE[64]

1. Select the appropriate mechanical traction device.

Various devices are available for applying mechanical traction to the cervical spine in the clinic or home setting. The choice depends on the region of the body to be treated, the amount of force to be applied, whether static or intermittent traction is desired, and the setting in which the treatment will be applied.

2. Determine optimal patient position.

When positioning the patient, try to achieve a comfortable position that allows muscle relaxation while maximizing the separation between the involved structures. The relative degree of flexion or extension of the spine during traction determines which surfaces are most effectively separated.[33] The flexed position results in greater separation of the posterior structures, including the facet joints and intervertebral foramina, whereas the neutral or extended position results in greater separation of the anterior structures, including the disc spaces (see Fig. 10-6). In most cases, a symmetrical central force is used, in which the direction of force is in line with the central sagittal axis of the patient; however, if the patient presents with unilateral symptoms, a unilateral traction force that applies more force to one side of the spine than to the other may prove to be more effective.[55] A unilateral force can be applied by offsetting the axis of the traction in the direction that most reduces the patient's symptoms. For example, if the patient presents with right neck or arm pain that is aggravated by right side bending and is relieved by left side bending, the traction should be offset so as to apply a left side bending force.

For the application of traction to the cervical spine, the patient may be in the supine or the sitting position (Figs. 10-13 and 10-14). Certain cervical traction devices can only be used in one of these positions, while others can be used in either position. For example, over-the-door cervical traction units must be applied with the patient sitting, whereas the Saunders occipital cervical traction halter can only be used with the patient supine. In the supine position, the cervical spine is supported and non–weight-bearing, resulting in increased patient comfort and muscle relaxation and greater separation between the cervical segments than when the same amount of traction force is applied with the patient in the sitting position.[13] When the patient is supine, cervical flexion, rotation, and side bending can be adjusted for patient comfort and to focus the traction force on the involved area (Fig. 10-15). When cervical traction is applied in the sitting position, cervical flexion and extension can be controlled to a limited degree by placing the patient facing toward (more flexion) or away from (neutral or more extension) the traction force; however, cervical side bending and rotation are difficult to

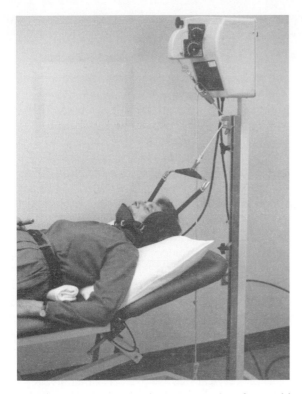

Figure 10-13. Supine cervical traction with soft mandibular halter with approximately 20- to 30-degree angle of pull to maximize separation of the intervertebral foramina and disc spaces.

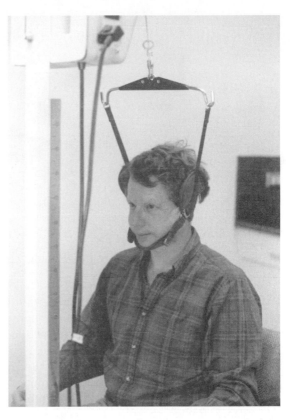

Figure 10-14. Sitting cervical traction, set up with the cervical spine in neutral.

adjust in the sitting position. Placing the cervical spine in a neutral or slightly extended position focuses the traction forces on the upper cervical spine, while placing the cervical spine in a flexed position focuses the traction forces on the lower cervical spine.[45,65] Maximum posterior elongation of the cervical spine is achieved when the neck and angle of pull are at approximately 25 to 35 degrees of flexion, as shown in Figure 10-13.[45,66]

3. Apply the appropriate belts or halter.

A number of different cervical halters have been developed to maximize patient comfort and avoid excessive pressure on the TMJs during the application of cervical traction (Fig. 10-16). There are soft fabric halters that apply pressure through both the mandibles and the occiput and soft fabric halters that apply pressure only through the occiput. The Saunders frictionless traction halter, which is solid and padded, is also designed to apply pressure only through the occiput. The adjustability of the halter, the patient position, and the status of the TMJs

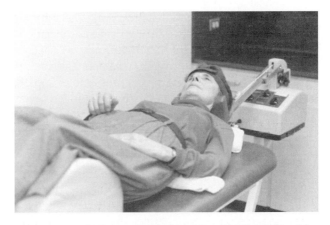

Figure 10-15. Supine cervical traction with right side-bending and rotation.

should all be considered in selecting the most appropriate cervical halter for a particular patient. The halter should be adjustable to accommodate variations in the shape and size of patients' heads

Continued

APPLICATION TECHNIQUE—cont'd
Mechanical Traction

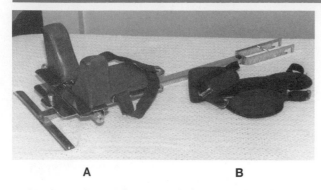

A   B

Figure 10-16. Cervical traction halters. **A,** Saunders halter. **B,** Mandibular halter.

and necks and to allow for different angles of traction pull. A halter that applies force through the mandibles and the occiput should allow adjustment of the distance between the occiput and spreader bar, the chin and spreader bar, and the mandibles and occiput. The tension on the straps should be adjusted so that the pull is comfortably and evenly applied to both the occiput and the mandibles. A halter that only applies pressure through the occiput should allow size adjustment and should be adjusted to fit snugly enough to stay on during the application of traction. The soft halters can be used in the sitting or supine position, whereas the Saunders halter can only be used in the supine position; however, the soft halters that apply pressure through the occiput tend to slip off the patient's head when traction is applied, even when appropriately adjusted for size, whereas the Saunders halter, which also avoids pressure on the TMJs, generally remains securely in place when traction is applied. The Saunders halter is also designed with a low-friction sliding component for the patient's head so that the traction force does not have to overcome friction between the patient's head and the table. Therefore, slightly less force should be applied when using this type of halter than when using a soft fabric halter.

4. Connect the belts or halter to the traction device.

    For cervical traction, all types of soft fabric halters are connected to the traction device by a rope and spreader bar, and the Saunders halter is connected directly to the traction device by a rope.

5. Set the appropriate traction parameters (see Table 10-1).

    Select static or intermittent traction and then, for static traction, set the maximum traction force and the total traction duration, or, for intermittent traction, set the maximum and minimum traction force, hold and relax times, and the total traction duration.

Static or Intermittent Traction

Mechanical traction may be administered statically, with the same force throughout the treatment, or intermittently, with the force varying every few seconds throughout the treatment. Some authors recommend that only static traction be applied in order to avoid a stretch reflex of the muscles;[10] however, others report that static and intermittent traction are equally effective but that higher forces can be used with intermittent traction;[59] and others have found intermittent traction to be most effective for reducing pain and increasing cervical ROM.[67] It is generally recommended that static traction be used if the area being treated is inflamed, if the patient's symptoms are easily aggravated by motion, or if the patient's symptoms are related to a disc protrusion.[10] Intermittent traction with long hold times may also be effective for treatment of symptoms related to disc protrusion, while shorter hold and relax times are recommended for symptoms related to joint dysfunctions.

Hold/Relax Times

If intermittent traction is selected, the maximum traction force is applied during the hold time and a lower traction force is applied during the relax time. The recommended ratio and duration of the hold and relax times depend on the patient's condition and tolerance. In general, if intermittent traction is used for treatment of a disc problem, longer hold times, of approximately 60 seconds, and shorter relax times, of approximately 20 seconds, are recommended, whereas if traction is being used to treat a spinal joint problem, shorter hold and relax times of approximately 15 seconds each are recommended.[11] Symptom severity should also be used as a guide for determining hold and relax times. When the patient's symptoms are severe, both long hold and long relax times are recommended in order to limit the amount of movement. As the symptoms become less severe, the relax time can gradually be decreased, and when the discomfort has decreased to a local ache rather than a pain, the hold time can also be reduced so that when the symptoms are mild, the traction produces an oscillatory motion with very short hold and relax times of approximately 3 to 5 seconds each.

Force

Different authors vary in their recommendations with regard to the amount of force to be used for traction; however, most agree that the optimal amount of force depends on the patient's clinical presentation, the goals of treatment, and the patient's position during treatment.[10,17] For all applications, the force should be kept low during the initial traction session in order to reduce the risk of reactive muscle guarding and spasms and to determine if traction is likely to aggravate the patient's symptoms. The traction force can be increased gradually in subsequent sessions as the patient becomes used to the procedure. It is recommended that, for all applications, the traction force to the cervical spine start at between 3 and 4 kg (8 to 10 lb).

When the goal is to decrease compression on a spinal nerve root or facet joint, sufficient force to separate the facet joints in the area being treated must be used. In the cervical spine, 9 to 13 kg (20 to 30 lb), or approximately 7% of the patient's body weight, is generally sufficient.[11,60,62]

When the goal is to decrease muscle spasm, stretch soft tissue, or exert a centripetal force on the disc by spinal elongation without joint surface separation, 5 to 7 kg (12 to 15 lb) for the cervical spine are generally effective. When this is the goal, the application of a hot pack in conjunction with the traction may result in greater spinal elongation and thus more effective relief of symptoms.

Higher traction forces are needed when patient positioning, or the harness or table, requires the traction force to overcome gravity or friction between the patient and the table. For example, when cervical traction is applied with the patient in the sitting position and the traction has to overcome the force of gravity on the patient's head, higher traction forces may be necessary, whereas when gravity and friction are reduced, as occurs with supine cervical traction, particularly if the Saunders frictionless halter is used, lower traction forces may be sufficient.

The force of traction can be adjusted during or between treatments. The force should be decreased during the treatment if there is any peripheralization

of signs or symptoms or, as mentioned above in the section on precautions, if there is complete relief of severe pain. If the patient's symptoms are moderately decreased by traction, the force can be increased, by 1.5 to 2 kg (3 to 5 lb) for cervical traction, at each subsequent treatment session until maximal relief of symptoms is achieved. Traction force to the cervical spine should generally not exceed 50% of the weight of the patient's head or 13.5 kg (30 lb).

When intermittent traction is used, the relaxed force should be approximately 50% of the maximum force or less; however, total release of the force during the relaxed phase of intermittent traction is not recommended since this can result in a rebound aggravation of the patient's symptoms.

Total Treatment Duration

There are no published studies comparing the effects of different treatment durations; however, most authors recommend that the duration of a patient's first treatment with traction be brief, about 5 minutes if the initial symptoms are severe and 10 minutes if the initial symptoms are moderate, in order to assess the patient's response.[11,63] If severe symptoms are significantly relieved by brief low-force traction, the duration of treatment should be kept short; otherwise, symptom exacerbation after the treatment is likely. If the patient's symptoms are partially relieved after 10 minutes of traction, it is recommended that the duration of the initial treatment not be extended; however, if symptoms are unchanged after 10 minutes, the hold force may be increased slightly or the angle of pull modified, and treatment may be continued for a further 10 minutes. Recommendations for the duration of subsequent treatments vary from as short as 8 to 10 minutes for treatment of a disc protrusion[11] to as long as 20 to 40 minutes for this and other indications.[38] Treatment for longer than 40 minutes is generally thought to provide no additional benefit.

Treatment Frequency

Some authors state that spinal traction must be administered daily to be effective; however, there are no published studies evaluating the outcome of different treatment frequencies.[11,36]

6. Start the traction.

The patient should be observed for the first few cycles of cervical traction to ensure that the halter

Continued

APPLICATION TECHNIQUE—cont'd
Mechanical Traction

is staying in place and exerting force through the appropriate areas and to ensure that the patient is comfortable and not experiencing any adverse effects from the treatment.

7. Assess the patient's response.

    It is recommended that the clinician assess the patient's initial response to the application of traction within the first 5 minutes of treatment so that any adjustments can be made at that time if needed.

8. Give the patient a means to call you and to stop the traction.

    Most electric mechanical traction units are equipped with a patient safety cutoff switch that turns off the unit and rings a bell when activated.

    Instruct the patient to use this switch if he or she experiences any increase in, or peripheralization of, pain or other symptoms.

9. Release traction and assess the patient's response.

    When the traction time is completed, lock the split sections of the table, release the tension on the traction ropes, and allow the patient to rest briefly before getting up and recompressing the joints. Then reexamine the patient's signs and symptoms.

ADVANTAGES

Force and time well controlled, readily graded, and replicable.

- Once applied, does not require the clinician to be with the patient throughout the treatment.
- Electrical mechanical traction units allow the application of static or intermittent traction.
- Static weighted devices such as over-the-door cervical traction are inexpensive and convenient for independent use by the patient at home.

DISADVANTAGES

- Expensive electric mechanical devices.
- Time-consuming to set up.
- Lack of patient control or participation.
- Restriction by belts or halter poorly tolerated by some patients.
- Mobilizes broad regions of the spine rather than individual spinal segments, potentially inducing hypermobility in normal or hypermobile joints.

Self-Traction

Self-traction is a form of traction that uses gravity and the weight of the patient's body, or force exerted by the patient, to exert a distractive force on the spine. Self-traction can be used for the lumbar but not the cervical spine. Self-traction of the lumbar spine is appropriate for home use by the patient whose symptoms are relieved by low loads of mechanical traction or that are associated with mild to moderate compression of spinal structures. Because the amount and duration of force that can be applied by self-traction is limited by the upper body strength of the patient and the weight of the lower body, self-traction is not generally effective when high forces are required to relieve symptoms with mechanical traction or when distraction of the spinal joints is necessary. Self-traction can be applied in a number of different ways, a few of which are described following. All methods of applying self-traction attempt to fix the patient's upper body and use

APPLICATION TECHNIQUE
Examples of Self-Traction

SITTING SELF-TRACTION

The patient should:

1. Sit in a sturdy chair with arms.
2. Hold on to the arms of the chair and push down with the arms, lifting the trunk to reduce the weight on the spine (Fig. 10-17). The patient may grade the force of the traction by varying the force of the downward pressure on the arms of the chair and thus the degree of unweighting of the spine; however, the patient should keep the feet on the floor at all times in order to control lumbopelvic position.

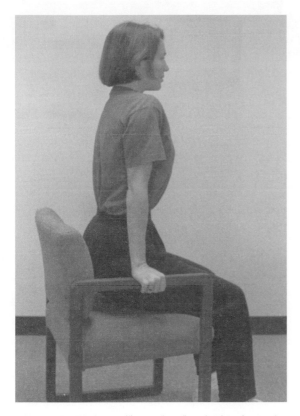

Figure 10-17. Sitting self-traction for the lumbar spine.

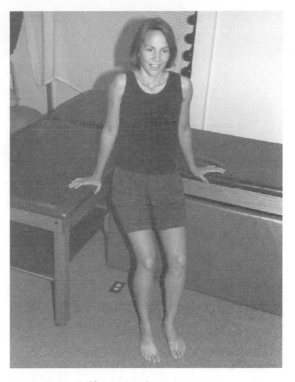

Figure 10-18. Self-traction between corner counters.

SELF-TRACTION BETWEEN CORNER COUNTERS

The patient should:

1. Stand in a corner with solid counter surfaces behind the patient.
2. Place the forearms on the counter and push down with the arms in order to decrease the weight on the spine by unweighting the feet (Fig. 10-18). The patient should leave the feet on the ground in order to control lumbopelvic position.

SELF-TRACTION WITH OVERHEAD BAR

The patient should:

1. Stand in a partial squat under a horizontal bar.
2. Hold on to the bar and pull to reduce the weight on the spine (Fig. 10-19). The patient should leave the feet on the ground in order to control lumbopelvic position.

ADVANTAGES

- Minimal or no equipment needed.
- Easy for patient to perform.

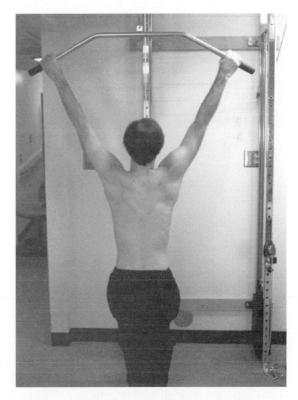

Figure 10-19. Self-traction with overhead bar.

Continued

APPLICATION TECHNIQUE—cont'd
Examples of Self-Traction

- Easy for patient to control.
- Can be performed in many environments and thus many times during the day.

DISADVANTAGES
- Low maximum force; therefore may not be effective.

- Requires strong, injury-free upper extremities.
- Cannot be used for the cervical spine.
- No research data to support the efficacy of this form of traction.
- Patient must have adequate postural awareness and control to position the body appropriately for maximum benefit.

---

either the body weight or the force of the arms to pull on the lumbar spine. Positions and ways to apply self-traction other than those described below can be developed by the clinician or the patient who is familiar with the principles of self-traction.

Positional Traction

Positional traction involves prolonged placement of the patient in a position that places tension on one side of the lumbar spine only (Fig. 10-20). This type of traction gently stretches the lumbar spine by applying a prolonged low-load longitudinal force to one side of the spine. Although the low force associated with this form of traction is unlikely to cause joint distraction, it may effectively decrease

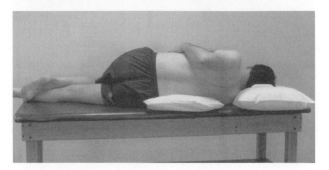

Figure 10-20. Positional traction to stretch and distract the left lumbar area.

muscle spasm, stretch soft tissue, or exert a centripetal force on the disc by spinal elongation without joint surface separation. Positional traction may be

APPLICATION TECHNIQUE
Positional Lumbar Traction

Equipment Required
- Pillow(s)

PROCEDURE

The patient should:
1. Lie on the side, with the involved side up and a pillow under the waist at approximately the level of the dysfunction. The pillow acts to side-bend the lumbar spine away from the involved side, opening the joints and disc spaces on the involved side.
2. Rotate toward the involved side by moving the lower shoulder forward and the upper shoulder back.
3. Rotate further toward the involved side by straightening the inferior lower extremity, bending the superior lower extremity, and hooking the superior foot behind the inferior leg. Rotation toward the involved side further stretches and opens the involved area.

4. Adjust flexion/extension to the position of greatest comfort and symptom relief.
5. Maintain the position for 10 to 20 minutes.

ADVANTAGES
- Requires no equipment or assistance.
- Inexpensive.
- Can be applied by the patient at home.
- Low force; thus not likely to aggravate an irritable condition.
- Position readily adjustable.

DISADVANTAGES
- Low force; therefore not likely to be effective where joint distraction is required.

- Requires agility and skill by the patient to perform correctly.
- No research data to support the efficacy of this form of traction.

used to treat unilateral symptoms originating from the lumbar spine and can be a valuable component of a patient's home program during the early stages of recovery when symptoms are severe and irritable.

Manual Traction

Manual traction is the application of force by the therapist in the direction of distracting the joints. It can be used for the cervical and lumbar spine as well as for the peripheral joints. There are many techniques for applying manual traction; however, since manual traction is generally classified as manual therapy rather than as a physical agent, only a few basic techniques for applying manual traction to the spine are described in this book. For more detailed descriptions of these and other techniques for applying manual traction to the spine or to the peripheral joints, please consult a manual therapy text.[10,68]

APPLICATION TECHNIQUE
Manual Traction

MANUAL LUMBAR TRACTION

1. Position the patient in the position of least pain. This is usually supine, with the hips and knees flexed.
2. Position yourself. Kneel at the patient's feet, facing the patient.
3. Place your hands in the appropriate position, behind the patient's proximal legs, over the muscle belly of the triceps surae (Fig. 10-21).
4. Apply traction force to the patient's spine by leaning your body back and away from the patient, keeping your spine in a neutral position.

   Adjust the force of the traction according to the desired outcome and the patient's report. Manual traction may be static, of constant force, or intermittent, of varying force.

MANUAL CERVICAL TRACTION
PATIENT SUPINE

1. Position the patient supine.
2. Position yourself. Stand at the head of the patient, facing the patient.
3. Place your hands in the appropriate position. Supinate your forearms so your hands are faced up; place the lateral border of your second finger in contact with the patient's occiput and your thumbs behind the patient's ears.
4. Apply traction. Apply force through the occiput by leaning back, keeping your spine in a neutral position (Fig. 10-22).

PATIENT SITTING

1. Position the patient in the sitting position.
2. Stand behind the patient.
3. Place your hands in the appropriate position. With your arms in a neutral position, place your thumbs under the patient's occiput and the rest of your hands along the side of the patient's face.
4. Apply traction. Apply traction through the patient's occiput by lifting up (Fig. 10-23).

   Adjust the force of the traction according to the desired outcome and the patient's report. Manual traction to the cervical spine may be static, of constant force, or intermittent, of varying force.

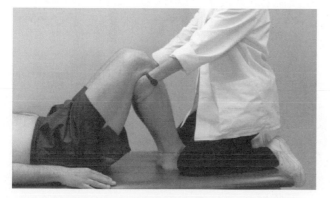

Figure 10-21. Manual lumbar traction.

Continued

APPLICATION TECHNIQUE—cont'd
Manual Traction

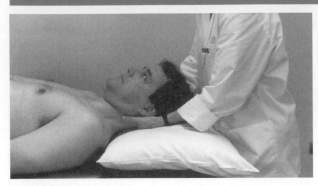

Figure 10-22. Manual cervical traction—supine.

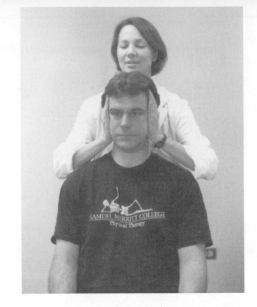

Figure 10-23. Manual cervical traction—sitting.

ADVANTAGES
- No equipment required.
- Short setup time.
- Force can be finely graded.
- Clinician is present throughout treatment to monitor and assess the patient's response.
- Can be applied briefly, prior to setting up mechanical traction, to help determine if longer application of traction will be beneficial.
- Can be used with patients who do not tolerate being placed in halters or belts.

DISADVANTAGES
- Limited maximum traction force, probably not sufficient to distract the lumbar facet joints.
- Amount of traction force cannot be easily replicated or specifically recorded.
- Cannot be applied for a prolonged period of time.
- Requires a skilled clinician to apply.

Documentation

When applying traction, document the type of traction, the area of the body the traction is applied to, the patient's position, the type of halter if one is used, the maximum force and the total treatment time, and the response to treatment. When using intermittent traction, the force during the relax time and the hold and relax times should also be recorded. Documentation is typically written in the SOAP note format. The following examples only summarize the modality component of treatment and are not intended to represent a comprehensive plan of care.

EXAMPLES

When applying intermittent mechanical cervical traction, document:

S: Pt c/o R UE pain from shoulder to wrist
O: Int mech cerv txn, pt supine, soft occipital halter. 10 kg/5 kg, 60 sec/20 sec, 15 min.
A: R UE pain from shoulder to wrist prior to treatment, from shoulder to elbow after treatment. Cervical AROM increased, forward bend from 40% to 60%, R side bend from 20% to 50%.
P: Increase force to 12 kg/7 kg next treatment

When instructing a patient in the application of self-traction, document:

S: Pt c/o low back and L LE pain that increases with sitting.
O: Pt instructed in self-traction in chair with arms. Pt unweighted approx 50% of body weight, 30 sec hold/relax × 3.
A: Low back and L LE pain decreased 50% for 2 to 3 hours after self-traction, pt able to continue working in sitting position for 4 hours.

P: Pt advised to perform self-traction as above every 2 hours at work.

When applying lumbar positional traction, document:

S: Pt c/o low back pain that awakens her 3-5× per night

O: Lumbar positional traction, R side lying with pillow at waist, R side bend, L rot H 20 minutes.

A: Pain decreased 30% after trial of positional traction.

P: Pt to perform traction as above at home 2-3× per day, including right before sleeping.

▶ *Clinical Case Studies* ◀

The following case studies summarize the concepts of spinal traction discussed in this chapter. Based on the scenario presented, an evaluation of the clinical findings and goals of treatment are proposed. These are followed by a discussion of the factors to be considered in the selection of spinal traction as the indicated treatment modality and in selection of the ideal patient position, traction technique, and traction parameters to promote progress toward the goals.

Case 1

TR is a 45-year-old male who has been referred to physical therapy with a diagnosis of a right L5, S1 radiculopathy. He complains of constant mild to moderately severe right low back pain that radiates to his right buttock and lateral thigh after sitting for more than 20 minutes and that is relieved to some degree by walking or lying down. He reports no numbness, tingling, or weakness of the lower extremities. The pain started about 6 weeks ago, the morning after TR spent a day stacking firewood, at which time he woke up with severe low back pain and right lower extremity pain down to his lateral calf; he also had difficulty standing up straight. He had similar problems in the past; however, they always resolved fully after a couple of days of bed rest and a few aspirins. TR first saw his doctor regarding his present problem 5 weeks ago, and at that time was prescribed a nonsteroidal anti-inflammatory drug and a muscle relaxant and was told to take it easy. His symptoms improved to their current level over the following 2 weeks but have not changed since that time. He has also been unable to return to his job as a telephone installer since the onset of symptoms 6 weeks ago. An MRI scan last week showed a mild posterolateral disc bulge at L5-S1 on the right. The patient has had no prior physical therapy for his back problem. The objective exam is significant for a 50% restriction of lumbar AROM in forward bending and right side bending, both of which cause increased right low back and lower extremity pain. Left side bending decreases the patient's pain. Passive straight leg raising is 35° on the right, limited by right lower extremity pain, and 60° on the left, limited by

hamstring tightness. Palpation reveals stiffness and tenderness to right unilateral posterior-anterior pressure at L5-S1 and no notable areas of hypermobility. All other tests including lower extremity sensation, strength, and reflexes are within normal limits.

EVALUATION OF THE CLINICAL FINDINGS

This patient presents with the impairments of restricted lumbar forward-bending and right side-bending motion, pain, restricted lumbar nerve root mobility on the right, as indicated by the restricted passive straight leg raising test, and bulging of the L5-S1 disc. These impairments have resulted in a limitation in sitting tolerance and an inability to return to work.

PREFERRED PRACTICE PATTERN

Impaired Joint Mobility, Motor Function, Muscle Performance, Range of Motion, and Reflex Integrity Associated With Spinal Disorders, (4F)

PLAN OF CARE

The goals of treatment at this time are to reduce pain and increase sitting tolerance sufficiently for the patient to be able to return to limited duty work. The anticipated long-term goals of treatment are to alleviate pain fully; to return lumbar ROM, passive straight leg raising, and sitting tolerance to within normal limits; and to have the patient return to his full work duties.

ASSESSMENT REGARDING THE APPROPRIATENESS OF SPINAL TRACTION AS THE OPTIMAL TREATMENT

The distribution of this patient's pain and its response to changes in loading indicate that his symptoms are probably related to the mild posterolateral disc bulge at L5-S1 on the right noted on his MRI scan. Traction is an indicated treatment for reducing symptoms associated with a disc bulge or lumbar nerve root compression and therefore should be considered as a treatment option for this patient. Studies have shown that lumbar traction can reduce disc protrusions and effectively relieve related symptoms. Traction is most likely to be effective for this patient if it is applied in conjunction with other

Continued

◗ *Clinical Case Studies—cont'd* ◖

treatment techniques including strengthening, stabilization and stretching exercises, joint mobilization, and body mechanics training. Treatment in the clinic should also be integrated with a complete home program. The use of spinal traction is not contraindicated in this patient since there is no displaced fragment of annulus or areas of hypermobility, and there are no indications of a hiatal hernia or a cardiac or pulmonary condition that may be aggravated by use of the belts for mechanical traction.

PROPOSED TREATMENT PLAN AND RATIONALE
It is proposed that electric mechanical traction be used to treat this patient since this type of traction device allows the greatest control of lumbar traction force and the application of sufficient force to distract the lumbar vertebrae. Prone positioning is recommended, if tolerated, to place the spine in a neutral or slightly extended position, and thus to provide greater separation of the disc spaces anteriorly and to localize the force to the lower lumbar segments.

A traction force of 25% of the patient's body weight may be sufficient to progress this patient toward the set goals of treatment, since this amount of traction force can produce a centripetal force on the lumbar disc and reduce a disc displacement. However, traction force of as much as 50% of the patient's body weight may be needed if joint distraction is required to alleviate this patient's symptoms. It is recommended that the initial treatment be with a low force, of approximately 25% of the patient's body weight, or 13 to 20 kg (25 to 50 lb), in order to allow assessment of the patient's response to the treatment and minimize the risk of protective muscle spasms. The traction force may then be increased for subsequent treatments, if necessary, until a level is reached at which the patient responds with approximately a 50% reduction in symptom severity after treatment. The application of a hot pack in conjunction with the traction may further improve the patient's response to the treatment by increasing superficial tissue extensibility and decreasing pain.[27,28]

Because intermittent traction with a long hold time, of approximately 60 seconds, and a short relax time, of approximately 20 seconds, is likely to have most effect on the discs, these times are recommended. Static traction may also be effective. The initial treatment should be limited to 10 minutes if the patient reports some reduction of symptoms in this time. If this is insufficient to reduce the patient's symptoms, the treatment time may be extended to up to 20 to 40 minutes for subsequent treatments.

If the application of mechanical traction in the manner described above relieves this patient's symptoms, and particularly if lower forces and lower durations of treatment are effective, the use of self-traction or positional traction at home, with the patient lying on the left side, with the left side bent and right rotation, may also help this patient progress toward the goals of treatment.

Case 2
AW is a 75-year-old female who has been referred to physical therapy with a diagnosis of osteoarthritis with moderately severe facet joint degeneration at C4 through C6 observed on x-ray. She complains of bilateral neck pain that is worse on the right than on the left. She also reports that her neck is very stiff first thing in the morning, loosening up throughout the day but becoming stiff and very sore late in the afternoon and for the rest of the evening. She has no complaints of upper extremity pain or stiffness; however, the neck stiffness makes her feel unsafe while driving, and when the pain is severe, she is unable to participate in her sewing class at the local senior center. She has had similar but gradually worsening symptoms intermittently for the past 20 years, and her symptoms are always more severe during the winter. In the past, AW has been referred to physical therapy for treatment of these symptoms, and her treatment has included traction, heat, massage, and a few exercises. Within four to six visits this combination of interventions has helped relieve her symptoms for about a year until the following winter.

At this time, the objective exam reveals a kyphotic thoracic posture with a forward head position. Cervical AROM is restricted by approximately 50% in all planes, and there is moderate hypertonicity of the cervical paraspinal muscles and stiffness of all the cervical facet joints on passive intervertebral motion testing, with the lower cervical joints being stiffer than the upper cervical joints. Shoulder flexion and abduction AROM are limited to 140° bilaterally, and all other objective tests, including upper extremity sensation, strength, and reflexes, are within normal limits for this patient's age.

EVALUATION OF THE CLINICAL FINDINGS
This patient presents with the impairments of an abnormal kyphotic thoracic posture, loss of neck movement in all planes, and pain. These have caused functional difficulties with driving and reduced participation in social activities.

PREFERRED PRACTICE PATTERN
Impaired Posture, (4B)

PLAN OF CARE

The goals of treatment at this time are to reduce AW's neck pain by at least 50%, so that she can return to full participation in her sewing class, and to increase her active and passive cervical ROM and soft tissue mobility sufficiently to allow her to drive safely. Goals of treatment should also include improving AW's posture and educating her in a home program to prevent, or at least limit, recurrences of her present symptoms.

ASSESSMENT REGARDING THE APPROPRIATENESS OF SPINAL TRACTION AS THE OPTIMAL TREATMENT

The application of spinal traction to the cervical spine is indicated for the treatment of joint hypomobility, particularly when multiple spinal segments are involved, and for the relief of symptoms caused by subacute joint inflammation. Spinal traction may also help alleviate this patient's spinal pain by gating its transmission at the spinal cord or by reducing joint compression and inflammation. The movement of intermittent traction may help to reduce symptoms resulting from inflammation by facilitating normal fluid exchange in the joints to relieve edema caused by chronic inflammation. This change, combined with stretching of the periarticular soft tissue structures, may increase spinal joint and soft tissue mobility and cervical active ROM. The application of a deep or superficial heating agent to this patient's neck, prior to or during the application of traction, may optimize the benefits of the treatment by increasing soft tissue extensibility to facilitate greater increases in soft tissue length. As in prior years, the application of traction and other passive modalities alone is likely to result in only temporary control of this patient's symptoms; however, more long-lasting benefits may be achieved by additionally addressing her posture and thoracic mobility and by modifying her home activities.

At the age of 75, this patient should be cleared for impairment of vertebral or carotid artery circulation and for osteoporosis prior to the application of cervical traction. One should also ascertain if she wears dentures; if so, she should be instructed to wear them during the treatment. It is also important not to assume that because this patient has tolerated traction well in the past, she will necessarily tolerate it equally well at this time, particularly if she has experienced any medical events, such as a cerebrovascular accident, since she was last treated with traction.

PROPOSED TREATMENT PLAN AND RATIONALE

Once this patient is cleared for the application of traction, a trial of manual traction is recommended to allow assessment of her response to traction and to help determine the ideal position prior to considering the use of other forms of traction. If manual traction affords her some relief of symptoms, then electric mechanical traction would be recommended for treatment in the clinic to provide optimal efficiency and consistency of treatment. An occipital halter should be used in order to avoid compression on the temporomandibular joints (TMJs), and the patient should be positioned supine, with her cervical spine in about 24° of flexion, in order to achieve maximum separation of the lower cervical joints and elongation of the posterior spinal structures.

As with all traction treatments, the force of traction should initially be low, at approximately 4 kg (10 lb), for the first session. The amount of force may then be increased by 1.5 to 2 kg (3 to 5 lb) at each subsequent session until optimal symptom control is achieved. A low amount of force, of 5 to 7 kg (12 to 15 lb), which can elongate the cervical spine without distracting the joints, will probably be sufficient to alleviate this patient's symptoms, and the use of more force will probably not provide greater benefit. The traction force should not exceed 13 kg (30 lb) at any time. Intermittent traction, with short hold and relax times of approximately 15 seconds each, are recommended since this ratio is generally effective at reducing symptoms associated with the joints. The total duration of the traction treatment should be between 10 and 40 minutes, depending on the patient's response.

Because this patient is presenting with recurrent symptoms that are probably due to progressive and chronic osteoarthritis, it is also recommended that she obtain and be instructed in the use of a simple mechanical traction device, such as an over-the-door cervical traction unit, for use at home. She may then use this device to treat aggravations of similar symptoms that she may experience in the future.

Case 3

MS is a 30-year-old female high school teacher. She was diagnosed with rheumatoid arthritis at the age of 22 and has been referred to physical therapy for treatment of neck pain. She complains of constant and severe pain in her neck that is aggravated by all neck movement, and she reports intermittent dizziness that is brought on by moving from sitting to standing or by looking up. The neck pain started about 3 or 4 years ago and has gradually become more severe, while the dizziness started only a few weeks ago. MS reports that at this time the pain keeps her awake at night and the dizziness interferes with her ability to write on the chalkboard when she is at work. MS has no numbness or tingling of her extremities and reports that no x-ray films have been taken of her neck in the last 3 years. Her objective exam reveals postural abnormalities, including standing with approximately 20° of hip and knee flexion bilaterally,

Continued

Clinical Case Studies—cont'd

bilateral genu valgum, a moderately increased lumbar lordosis, a flat thoracic spine, and a forward head position. The flat thoracic spine and forward head position are maintained in sitting. Cervical ROM testing was deferred at the initial evaluation due to the severity of the patient's reports of pain with motion. Her upper extremity strength was 4+/5 throughout within the available ROM, and her upper extremity sensation and reflexes were within normal limits.

EVALUATION OF CLINICAL FINDINGS

This patient presents with impairments of stiffness and loss of motion of her neck, neck pain, dizziness, and abnormal posture. These have resulted in an inability to sleep throughout the night and have limited her ability to perform her normal job-related activity of writing on the chalkboard.

PREFERRED PRACTICE PATTERN

Impaired Joint Mobility, Motor Function, Muscle Performance, and Range of Motion Associated With Connective Tissue Dysfunction, (4D)

PLAN OF CARE

Although goals of treatment could include resolving any of the above impairments or functional limitations, this patient's reports of dizziness associated with neck pain and the diagnosis of rheumatoid arthritis should alert the clinician to the possibility that this patient may have an unstable C1-C2 articulation due to ligamentous instability or osteoporosis as a result of prolonged systemic steroid use. Because instability at C1-C2 poses a significant risk to the patient, and because the presence of osteoporosis requires special caution with the application of traction, the initial goal, prior to applying traction or any other treatment, should be to ascertain the ligamentous stability and bony integrity of her upper cervical spine. Because these both require radiographic studies that must generally be ordered by a physician, the patient should be referred back to her physician for further evaluation.

Should all radiographic reports indicate that her upper cervical spine is stable and that she does not have osteoporosis, she may return to physical therapy for treatment of her complaints. The proposed goals of treatment would then be to relieve her pain and dizziness and to increase her cervical ROM sufficiently to allow full participation in job-related activities. Because this patient has a systemic disease that affects the joints and that appears to have caused permanent changes in other joints, including her hips and knees, it would not be expected that complete relief of symptoms or return of ROM would be achieved.

ASSESSMENT REGARDING THE APPROPRIATENESS OF SPINAL TRACTION AS THE OPTIMAL TREATMENT

If all tests indicate that spinal traction is not contraindicated, then such treatment may improve this patient's cervical mobility, increasing her cervical ROM, and decrease her neck pain. These effects may be achieved by distraction or mobilization of the cervical joints or by relaxation of the cervical paraspinal muscles. It is also possible that cervical traction may help alleviate this patient's dizziness since she associates this symptom with neck motion; however, her dizziness may be due to an inner ear or vestibular dysfunction, which would also be affected by head position, in which case this symptom would probably not respond to treatment with traction. Although traction may reduce this patient's symptoms sufficiently to allow her to write on a chalk board, it is recommended that job site adaptations, such as the use of an overhead projector, also be instituted to reduce the stresses on her cervical spine.

PROPOSED TREATMENT PLAN AND RATIONALE

It is proposed that in order to provide constant monitoring of this patient's severe symptoms, and to allow adjustment of the traction force and direction during the treatment, manual traction be used initially to treat this patient. Should the patient report moderate relief of her pain with the application of manual traction, then once optimal cervical positioning for traction has been determined, static mechanical traction may be substituted if it is thought that a longer duration of treatment would be more beneficial. Static cervical traction may be provided by an electrical or weighted device, but in either case it is recommended that the patient be treated supine rather than sitting, to achieve maximum muscle relaxation, and it is recommended that low forces be used initially due to the severity of the patient's symptoms.

As treatment progresses, the force of traction may be increased up to a maximum of 13 kg (30 lb) to achieve joint distraction if necessary, and intermittent traction may be used if this proves to be more comfortable as the patient tolerates more motion. Treatment with spinal traction should be provided in conjunction with postural education and recommendations for home or work site modifications in order to minimize the risk of symptom re-aggravation or progression.

Chapter Review

The application of a distracting mechanical force to the body is known as *traction*. Traction applies tension to the tissues, and when applied to the spine it can result in joint surface distraction, soft tissue stretching, muscle relaxation, joint mobilization, or patient immobilization. The effects and clinical benefits of spinal traction depend on the amount of force used, the direction of the force, and the status of the area to which the traction is applied. Spinal traction can be used for the treatment of a disc bulge or herniation, nerve root impingement, joint hypomobility, subacute joint inflammation, or paraspinal muscle spasm. Selection of a spinal traction technique depends on the nature of the problem being treated, specific contraindications, and whether the treatment is to be applied in the clinic or at home. The reader is referred to the Evolve website at http://evolve.elsevier.com/ Cameron for study questions pertinent to this chapter.

References

1. Cyriax J: *Textbook of Orthopedic Medicine, Volume I: Diagnosis of Soft Tissue Lesions,* London, 1982, Bailliere Tindall.
2. Mathews JA, Mills SB, Jenkins YM et al: Back pain and sciatica: controlled trials of manipulation, traction, sclerosant and epidural injections, *Br J Rheumatol* 26: 416-423, 1987.
3. Larsson U, Choler U, Lindstrom A et al: Auto-traction for treatment of lumbago-sciatica, *Acta Orthoped Scand* 51:791-798, 1980.
4. Lidstrom A, Zachrisson M: Physical therapy on low back pain and sciatica, *Scan J Rehabil Med* 2:37-42, 1970.
5. Moret NC, van der Stap M, Hagmeijer R et al: Design and feasibility of a randomized clinical trial of vertical traction in patients with a lumbar radicular syndrome, *Manual Therapy* 3:203-211, 1998.
6. Weber H, Ljunggren E, Walker L: Traction therapy in patients with herniated lumbar intervertebral discs, *J Oslo City Hosp* 34:61-70, 1984.
7. Beurskens AJ, de Vet HC, Koke AJ et al: Efficacy of traction for nonspecific low back pain: 12-week and 60-month results of a randomized clinical trial, *Spine* 22:2756-2762, 1977.
8. Goldish GD: Lumbar traction. In Tolison CD, Kriegel ML, eds: *Interdisciplinary Rehabilitation of Low Back Pain,* Baltimore, 1989, Williams & Wilkins.
9. Paris SV, Loubert PV: *Foundations of Clinical Orthopedics,* St Augustine FL, 1990, Institute Press.
10. Maitland GD: *Vertebral Manipulation,* ed 5, London, 1986, Butterworth.
11. Judovich B, Nobel GR: Traction therapy: a study of resistance forces, *Am J Surg* 93:108-114, 1957.
12. Judovich B: Lumbar traction therapy, *JAMA* 159:549, 1955.
13. Deets D, Hands KL, Hopp SS: Cervical traction: a comparison of sitting and supine positions, *Phys Ther* 57:255-261, 1977.
14. Twomey LT: Sustained lumbar traction: an experimental study of long spine segments, *Spine* 10:146-149, 1985.
15. Onel D, Tuzlaci M, Sari H et al: Computed tomographic investigation of the effect of traction on lumbar disc herniations, *Spine* 14:82-90, 1989.
16. Grieve GP: *Mobilization of the Spine,* ed 4, New York, 1984, Churchill Livingstone.
17. Cyriax J: *Textbook of Orthopaedic Medicine,* vol II, ed 11, Eastbourne, UK, 1984, Balliere Tindall.
18. Krause M, Refshauge KM, Dessen M et al: Lumbar spine traction: evaluation of effects and recommended application for treatment, *Man Ther* 5(2):72-81, 2000.
19. Mathews J: Dynamic discography: a study of lumbar traction, *Ann Phys Med* 9:275-279, 1968.
20. Gupta R, Ramarao S: Epidurography in reduction of lumbar disc prolapse by traction, *Arch Phys Med Rehabil* 59:322-327, 1978.
21. Andersson GBJ, Schultz AB, Nachemson AL: Intervertebral disc pressures during traction, *Scand J Rehabil Med* 9: 88-91, 1983.
22. Lundgren AE, Eldevik OP: Auto-traction in lumbar disc herniation with CT examination before and after treatment, showing no change in appearance of the herniated tissue, *J Oslo City Hosp* 36:87-91, 1986.
23. Basmajian JV: *Manipulation, Traction and Massage,* ed 3, Baltimore, 1985, Williams & Wilkins.
24. Coalchis SC, Strohm BR: Cervical traction relationship of time to varied tractive force with constant angle of pull, *Arch Phys Med Rehabil* 46:815-819, 1965.
25. Worden RE, Humphrey TL: Effect of spinal traction on the length of the body, *Arch Phys Med Rehabil* 45: 318-320, 1964.
26. LaBan MM: Collagen tissue: Implications of its response to stress in vitro, *Arch Phys Med Rehabil* 43: 461-466, 1962.
27. Lehmann J, Masock A, Warren C et al: Effect of therapeutic temperatures on tendon extensibility, *Arch Phys Med Rehabil* 51:481-487, 1970.
28. Lentall G, Hetherington T, Eagan J et al: The use of thermal agents to influence the effectiveness of a low-load prolonged stretch, *J Orthop Sport Phys Ther* 16(5): 200-207, 1992.
29. Mathews JA: The effects of spinal traction, *Physiotherapy* 58:64-66, 1972.
30. Wall PD: The mechanisms of pain associated with cervical vertebral disease. In Hirsch C, Zollerman Y, eds: Cervical Pain: Proceedings of the International

Symposium in Wenner-Gren Center, Oxford, 1972, Pergamon.

31. Seliger V, Dolejs L, Karas V: A dynamometric comparison of maximum eccentric, concentric and isometric contractions using EMG and energy expenditure measurements, *Eur J Apply Physiol* 45:235-244, 1980.

32. Swezey RL: The modern thrust of manipulation and traction therapy, *Semin Arthritis Rheum* 12:322-331, 1983.

33. Saunders HD: Use of spinal traction in the treatment of neck and back conditions, *Clin Orthop* 179:31-38, 1983.

34. Cheatle MD, Esterhai JL: Pelvic traction as treatment for acute back pain, *Spine* 16:1379-1381, 1991.

35. Pal B, Mangion P, Hossain MA et al: A controlled trial of continuous lumbar traction in the treatment of back pain and sciatica, *Br J Rheumatol* 25:181-183, 1986.

36. Van der Heijden GJMG, Beurskens AJHM, Assendelft WJJ et al: The efficacy of traction for back and neck pain: a systematic, blinded review of randomized clinical trial methods, *Phys Ther* 75(2):93-104, 1995.

37. Hood LB, Chrisman D: Intermittent pelvic traction in the treatment of the ruptured intervertebral disc, *Phys Ther* 48:21-30, 1968.

38. Weber H: Traction therapy in sciatica due to disc prolapse, *J Oslo City Hosp* 23:167-176, 1973.

39. Grieve G: *Common Vertebral Joint Problems,* Edinburgh, 1981, Churchill Livingstone.

40. Saunders HD, Saunders R: *Evaluation, Treatment and Prevention of Musculoskeletal Disorders,* Bloomington, MN, 1993, Educational Opportunities.

41. Mathews JA, Hickling J: Lumbar traction: a double-blind controlled study of sciatica, *Rheum Rehabil* 14:222-225, 1975.

42. Buerskens AJ, de Vet HC, Koke AJ et al: Efficacy of traction for non-specific low back pain: a randomized clinical trial, *Lancet* 346(8990):1596-1600, 1995.

43. Buerskens AJ, van der Heijden GJ, de Vet HC et al: The efficacy of traction for lumbar back pain: design of a randomized clinical trial, *J Manip Physiol Ther* 18(3):141-147, 1995.

44. Pellecchia GL: Lumbar traction: A review of the literature, *J Orthop Sports Phys Ther* 20(5):262-267, 1994.

45. Coalchis SC, Strohm BR: A study of tractive forces and angle of pull on vertebral interspaces in the cervical spine, *Arch Phys Med Rehabil* 46:820-824, 1965.

46. McDonough A: Effect of immobilization and exercise on articular cartilage: a review of the literature, *J Orthop Sport Phys Ther* 3:2-9, 1981.

47. Yates DAH: Indications and contraindications for spinal traction, *Physiotherapy* 54:55-57, 1972.

48. Quain MB, Tecklin JS: Lumbar traction: its effect on respiration, *Phys Ther* 65:1343-1346, 1985.

49. Frymoyer JW, Moskowitz RW: Spinal degeneration: pathogenesis and medical management. In Frymoyer JW, ed: *The Adult Spine: Principles and Practice,* New York, 1991, Raven Press.

50. Eie N, Kristiansen K: Complications and hazards of traction in the treatment of ruptured lumbar intervertebral disks, *J Oslo City Hosp* 12:5-12, 1962.

51. LaBan MM, Macy JA, Meerschaert JR: Intermittent cervical traction: a progenitor of lumbar radicular pain, *Arch Phys Med Rehabil* 73:295-296, 1992.

52. Haskvitz EM, Hanten WP: Blood pressure response to inversion traction, *Phys Ther* 66:1361-1364, 1986.

53. Giankopoulos G, Waylonis GW, Grant PA et al: Inversion devices: their role in producing lumbar distraction, *Arch Phys Med Rehabil* 66(2):100-102, 1985.

54. Zito M: Effect of two gravity inversion methods on heart rate, systolic brachial pressure, and ophthalmic artery pressure, *Phys Ther* 68:20-25, 1988.

55. Saunders HD: Unilateral lumbar traction, *Phys Ther* 61:221-225, 1981.

56. Weatherell VF: Comparison of electromyographic activity in normal lumbar sacrospinalis musculature during static pelvic traction in two different positions, *J Orthop Sport Phys Ther* 8:382-390, 1987.

57. Goldish GD: A study of mechanical efficiency of split table traction, *Spine* 15:218-219, 1989.

58. Saunders HD: Lumbar traction, *J Orthop Sport Phys Ther* 1:36-41, 1979.

59. Rogoff JB: Motorized intermittent traction. In Basmajian JV, ed: *Manipulation, Traction, and Massage,* Baltimore, 1985, Williams & Wilkins.

60. Coalchis SC, Strohm BR: Effects of intermittent traction on separation of lumbar vertebrae, *Arch Phys Med Rehabil* 50:251-253, 1969.

61. Hood CJ, Hart DL, Smith HG et al: Comparison of electromyographic activity in normal lumbar sacrospinalis musculature during continuous and intermittent pelvic traction, *J Orthop Sports Phys Ther* 2:137-141, 1981.

62. Meszaros TF, Olson R, Kulig K et al: Effect of 10%, 30%, and 60% body weight traction on the straight leg raise test of symptomatic patients with low back pain, *J Orthop Sports Phys Ther* Oct;30(10):595-601, 2000.

63. Hickling J: Spinal traction technique, *Physiotherapy* 58:58-63, 1972.

64. Harris PR: Cervical traction:review of literature and treatment guidelines, *Phys Ther* Aug;57(8):910-914, 1977.

65. Daugherty RJ, Erhard RE: Segmentalized cervical traction. In Kent BE, ed: *International Federation of Orthopaedic Manipulative Therapists Proceedings,* Vail, CO., 1977.

66. Hseuh TC, Ju MS, Chou YL: Evaluation of the effects of pulling angle and force on intermittent cervical traction with the Saunder's Halter, *J Formos Med Assoc* Dec;90(12):1234-9, 1991.

67. Zylbergold RS, Piper MC: Cervical spine disorders: a comparison of three types of traction, *Spine* Dec, 10(10):867-71, 1985.

68. Maitland GD: *Peripheral Manipulation,* ed 3, London, 1991, Butterworth.

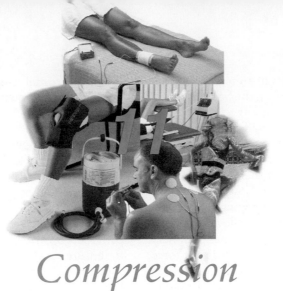

Compression

OBJECTIVES

Upon completion of this chapter, the reader will be able to:

1. Discuss the physical properties of compression.
2. Identify the physiological effects of compression.
3. Examine how the physical properties and physiological effects of compression can promote particular treatment goals.
4. Assess the indications, contraindications, and precautions for the use of compression with respect to different patient management situations.
5. Design appropriate methods for selecting compression devices and treatment parameters to produce desired physical and physiological effects.

6. Choose and use the most appropriate compression device and treatment parameters to obtain the desired treatment goals.
7. Evaluate different compression devices with respect to their potential application for treating different patient problems.
8. Presented with a clinical case, evaluate the clinical findings, propose goals of treatment, assess whether compression would be the best treatment, and, if so, formulate an effective treatment plan including the appropriate device and treatment parameters for achieving the goals of treatment.

Compression is the application of a mechanical force that increases external pressure on the body or a body part. Compression is generally used to improve fluid balance and circulation or to modify scar tissue formation. Compression improves fluid balance by increasing the hydrostatic pressure in the interstitial space so that it becomes greater than that in the vessels. This can limit or reverse outflow of fluid from blood vessels and lymphatics. Keeping fluid in the vessels, or returning it to the vessels, allows it to circulate rather than to accumulate in the periphery. Compression can be static, exerting a constant force, or intermittent, with the force varying over time. With intermittent compression the pressure may be applied to the entire limb all at one time, or it may be applied sequentially, starting distally and progressing proximally.

The primary clinical application of compression is for the control of peripheral edema due to vascular or lymphatic dysfunction; however, this physical agent can also be applied to help prevent the formation of deep venous thromboses, for residual limb shaping after amputation, or to facilitate the healing of venous ulcers.[1-3]

EFFECTS OF EXTERNAL COMPRESSION

Improved venous and lymphatic circulation
Limits the shape and size of tissue
Increased tissue temperature

Improved Venous and Lymphatic Circulation

The controlled application of external compression has a variety of effects on the body. The nature and extent of these effects vary with the pressure applied and with the nature of the device used.[4] Both static and intermittent compression devices can increase circulation since both can increase the hydrostatic pressure in the interstitial space outside the blood and lymphatic vessels. An increase in extravascular pressure can limit the outflow of fluid from the vessels into the interstitial space, where it tends to pool, keeping it in the circulatory system, where it can circulate. Intermittent compression may improve circulation more effectively than static compression because the varying amount of pressure is thought to milk fluids from the distal

to the proximal vessels.[5,6] Milking is thought to be achieved because, when the venous and lymphatic vessels are compressed, the fluid in them is pushed proximally, and then, when compression is reduced, the vessels can open and refill with new fluid from the interstitial space, ready to be pushed proximally at the next compression cycle. Sequential compression is thought to provide even more effective milking than single-chamber, intermittent compression because it can cause a wave of vessel constriction moving in a proximal direction to ensure that fluid is pushed along the vessels toward the heart rather than in a distal direction.[5-7] Improving circulation can benefit patients with edema, may help prevent the formation of deep venous thromboses in high-risk patients, and may facilitate the healing of ulcers caused by venous stasis.

Limits the Shape and Size of Tissue

Static compression garments or bandaging can provide a form to limit the shape and size of new tissue formation. This type of compression device acts as a second skin, which, having an elastic compression element or being less extensible than skin, limits the shape and size of the tissue. This effect of compression is exploited when compression bandaging or garments are used over residual limbs after amputation, when compression garments are applied over burn-damaged skin, and when compression bandaging or garments are applied to edematous limbs.

Increased Tissue Temperature

Most compression devices, except those with built-in cooling mechanisms, increase superficial tissue temperature because the device insulates the area to which it is applied. A heavy compression stocking or an air-filled sleeve will act as an insulator, preventing loss of body heat, thereby increasing local superficial tissue temperature. Although the increase in temperature produced by compression garments is not a direct effect of the compressive forces, it has been proposed that the increased activity of temperature-sensitive enzymes such as collagenase, which breaks down collagen, produced by these garments, may be the mechanism by which they control scar formation.[8]

CLINICAL INDICATIONS FOR THE USE OF EXTERNAL COMPRESSION

Edema
   Edema due to venous insufficiency
   Lymphedema
Deep venous thrombosis
Venous stasis ulcers
Residual limb shaping after amputation
Control of hypertrophic scarring

Edema

Causes of edema

Edema is the presence of abnormal amounts of fluid in the extracellular tissue spaces of the body. Normal fluid equilibrium in the tissues is maintained by the balance between the hydrostatic and osmotic pressure inside and outside the blood vessels. The hydrostatic pressure is determined by blood pressure and the effects of gravity, while the osmotic pressure is determined by the concentration of proteins inside and outside the vessels. The higher hydrostatic pressure inside the vessels acts to push fluid out of the vessels, whereas the higher protein concentration, and thus osmotic pressure, inside the vessels acts to keep fluid inside the vessels (Fig. 11-1). Under normal circumstances, the hydrostatic pressure pushing fluid out of the veins is slightly higher than the osmotic pressure keeping fluid in, resulting in a slight loss of fluid into the interstitial space. The fluid that is pushed out of the veins into the interstitial space is then taken up by the lymphatic capillaries, to be returned to the venous circulation at the subclavian veins. This fluid, known as *lymphatic fluid* or *lymph*, is rich in protein, water, and macrophages.

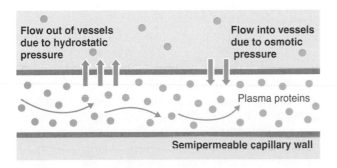

Figure 11-1. Effects of hydrostatic and osmotic pressure on tissue fluid balance.

A healthy diet, vascular system, and level of muscular contraction act together to ensure that the appropriate amount of fluid exits the veins and flows back toward the heart. Dysfunction in any of these mechanisms can result in increased extravasation of fluid from the vessels into the interstitial extravascular space or reduced flow of venous blood or lymph back toward the heart, and thus the formation of edema.

The most common reasons patients develop edema are venous insufficiency or dysfunction of the lymphatic system. These are discussed in detail in the following sections. Edema may also occur after exercise, trauma, surgery, or burns, or in conjunction with infection due to the increased vascular capillary permeability that occurs with the acute inflammation associated with these events. Increased vascular capillary permeability increases the fluid flow out of the capillaries, causing an accumulation of fluid at the site of trauma or infection. The formation of edema due to acute inflammation is described in detail in Chapter 2. Congestive heart failure, liver failure, acute renal disease, diabetic glomerulonephritis, malnutrition, and radiation injury may also contribute to peripheral edema formation because these abnormal states can alter circulation or osmotic pressure balance.

Edema due to venous insufficiency

The peripheral veins' function is to carry whole deoxygenated blood from the periphery back to the heart. In a healthy vascular system the resting hydrostatic venous pressure at the entrance to the right atrium of the heart averages 4.6 mm Hg, and this pressure increases by 0.77 mm Hg for each centimeter below the right atrium to reach an average of 90 mm Hg at the ankle.[9] When the calf muscles contract, they exert a pressure of about 200 mm Hg on the outside of the veins, which pushes the blood through the veins. Then, following the contraction, the pressure falls to about 10 mm Hg to 30 mm Hg, allowing the veins to refill. A healthy amount of skeletal muscle activity, such as occurs with walking or running, or even with just rhythmic isometric muscle contraction, provides a milking action to propel the blood in the veins from the periphery back toward the heart. Muscle contraction is the primary factor propelling both lymphatic and venous flow, and valves within the vessels prevent backflow of the fluid, ensuring that it moves proximally toward the heart rather than being pushed distally toward the distal extremities (Fig. 11-2).

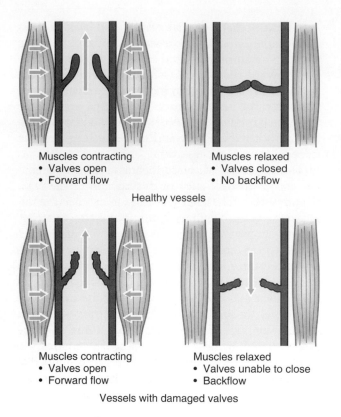

Muscles contracting
• Valves open
• Forward flow

Muscles relaxed
• Valves closed
• No backflow

Healthy vessels

Muscles contracting
• Valves open
• Forward flow

Muscles relaxed
• Valves unable to close
• Backflow

Vessels with damaged valves

Figure 11-2. Valves in venous and lymphatic vessels preventing backflow.

Lack of physical activity, dysfunction of the venous valves due to degeneration, or mechanical obstruction of the veins by a tumor or inflammation can result in venous insufficiency and accumulation of fluid in the periphery. The most common cause of venous insufficiency is inflammation of the veins, known as *phlebitis*, which causes thickening of the vessel walls and damage to the valves. Thickening and loss of elasticity of the vessel walls elevates the hydrostatic pressure in the venous system, and damage to the valves allows blood to flow in both proximal and distal directions, rather than just proximally through the veins, when the muscles contract (see Fig. 11-2). The retrograde flow reduces circulation of deoxygenated blood out of the veins and thus increases pressure in the venous system if fluid inflow from the arterial system is unchanged. The elevated venous pressure increases the amount of fluid that enters the extravascular space and thus causes edema. If the limbs are then placed in a dependent position, the edema will worsen because of increased hydrostatic pressure due to gravity.

Lymphedema

As explained above, the hydrostatic pressure that pushes fluid out of the veins normally exceeds the osmotic pressure keeping fluid inside them. This results in a net flow of fluids and proteins into the interstitial space, producing lymph. To prevent the lymph from accumulating in the interstitial space, the lymphatic system, acting as an accessory channel, returns it to the blood circulation. The lymphatic system consists of a large network of vessels and nodes through which the lymphatic fluid flows. Lymphatic vessels are found in almost every area where there are blood vessels, and lymph flows along these vessels, passing through numerous lymph nodes, to empty into the subclavian veins (Fig. 11-3). The lymph nodes are concentrated in the axillary, throat, groin, and paraaortic areas and act to filter the fluid, removing bacteria and other foreign particles. The lymphatic vessels of the right arm terminate in the right lymphatic duct and empty into the right subclavian vein, whereas the lymphatic vessels from all other areas terminate in the thoracic duct and empty into the left subclavian vein. Once the lymphatic fluid reenters the circulatory system it is processed through the kidneys, along with other fluids, waste product, and electrolytes, and is eliminated.

Fluid flows into the lymphatic system because the concentration of proteins inside the lymphatics is generally higher than in the interstitial space. As with the veins, flow along the lymphatic vessels in a proximal direction depends on muscle activity, such as walking or running, which compresses the vessels and valves within the vessels and prevents backflow. Decreased levels of plasma proteins, particularly albumin, mechanical obstruction of the lymphatics, abnormal distribution of lymphatic vessels or lymph nodes, or reduced activity can result in reduced lymphatic flow and the formation of lymphedema. Decreased levels of plasma proteins cause fluid to accumulate in the extravascular space because the osmotic pressure that normally keeps fluid in the lymphatic vessels and the veins is reduced. If the plasma protein level drops below the normal range of 6 g/dL to 8 g/dL or the plasma albumin levels fall below 3.3 g/dL to 5.7 g/dL, lymphedema is likely to result. A healthy diet and adequate protein absorption are required to keep plasma protein at an appropriate

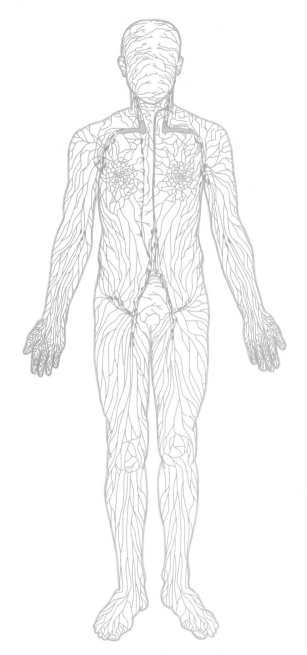

Figure 11-3. Lymphatic circulation.

lymphatic vessels, whereas secondary lymphedema is caused by some other disease or dysfunction. An example of primary lymphedema is Milroy's disease, in which the individual has hypoplastic, aplastic, or varicose and incompetent lymphatic vessels. Patients with primary lymphedema often have backflow in the lymphatic vessels, and the rate of protein reabsorption across the vessel walls is also usually slowed. In secondary lymphedema, lymphatic flow is impaired by blockage or insufficiency of the lymphatics. Inflammation, pregnancy, neoplasm, radiation therapy, trauma, surgery, and filariasis are all common causes of secondary lymphatic obstruction.[10-13] The most common cause of secondary lymphedema in the world is filariasis, a disease characterized by infestation of the lymphatics and obstruction of the lymph vessels and nodes by microscopic filarial worms. Although this disease is common in Asia, it is rarely seen in America, Australia, or Europe. In the United States, secondary lymphedema is usually the result of mechanical obstruction of the vessels by a tumor or inflammation, dysfunction of the valves due to degeneration, or removal of the lymph nodes as a component of the treatment of breast cancer.

Adverse consequences of edema

Edema of any origin can result in a variety of adverse clinical consequences, such as restrictions of range of motion (ROM), limitations of function, or pain. Reducing edema has also been shown to increase joint ROM and to decrease pain and joint stiffness.[14,15] Persistent chronic edema, particularly lymphedema that has a high level of protein, can also cause collagen to be laid down in the area, leading to subcutaneous tissue fibrosis and hard induration of the skin. This may eventually cause disfiguring and disabling contractures and deformities (Fig. 11-4). Chronic edema due to venous or lymphatic insufficiency also increases the risk of infection because tissue oxygenation is reduced; this risk is further elevated with lymphedema because of the presence of a protein-rich environment for bacterial growth.[13,16] Advanced chronic lymphatic or venous obstruction may result in cellulitis, ulceration, and, if unmanaged, partial limb amputation.[16] These more serious sequelae are most likely to occur if the pressure of the excess fluid accumulated in the interstitial extravascular spaces causes arterial obstruction. Chronic venous insufficiency also often causes itching, due to stasis dermatitis, and brown pigmentation of the skin due

level. When lymphedema is caused by hypoproteinemia, this underlying problem should be addressed first to prevent further edema formation and other adverse consequences.

Lymphedema can be primary or secondary, although most cases are secondary. Primary lymphedema is caused by a congenital disorder of the

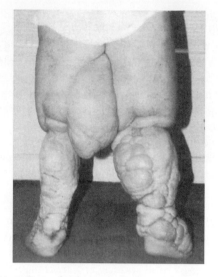

Figure 11-4. Lymphedema. (From *Living with lymphoedema*, Courtesy Michael Mason, Director, Adelaide Lymphoedema Clinic.)

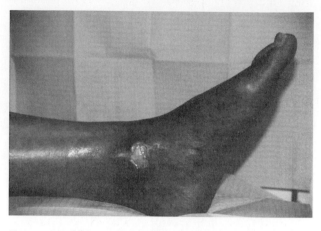

Figure 11-5. Venous stasis ulcer. Note the areas of darkened skin around the ulcer due to hemosiderin deposits. (Courtesy Jim Staicer, Beverly Manor Convalescent Hospital, Fresno, CA.)

to hemosiderin deposition. These signs are commonly seen on the medial lower leg (see Fig. 11-6). Early control of edema can help to prevent the progression and development of the signs and symptoms of chronic edema and its associated complications.

How compression reduces edema

Compression is effective in controlling edema due to venous insufficiency, lymphatic dysfunction, or any of the other previously mentioned causes because it increases extravascular hydrostatic pressure and circulation.[11,12,17-21] If the patient has other underlying causes of edema, such as infection, malnutrition, inadequate physical activity, or organ dysfunction, these must also be addressed to achieve an optimal outcome and to prevent recurrence of the edema.

Compression of a limb with a static or intermittent device increases the pressure surrounding the extremity to counterbalance any increased osmotic or hydrostatic pressure causing fluid to flow out of the vessels into the extravascular space. If sufficient pressure is applied, the hydrostatic pressure in the interstitial extravascular spaces becomes greater than that in the veins and lymphatic vessels, reducing outflow from the vessels and causing fluid in the interstitial spaces to return to the vessels.[22] Once fluid is in the vessels it can be circulated out of the periphery, preventing or reversing edema formation. In addition, if an inter-

mittent compression device is used, it may also help to move the fluid proximally through the vessels.

Prevention of Deep Venous Thrombosis

Deep venous thromboses (DVTs) are blood clots in the deep veins. They can occur when circulation is poor or when there is inflammation of the veins. If circulation is poor, the blood may move slowly enough to allow coagulation and the formation of a thrombus; thus, an intervention that increases the circulatory rate can reduce the risk of thrombus formation. DVT formation is most common in immobilized patients, particularly after surgery or when recovering from cardiac failure or stroke. Although thrombus formation in the peripheral venous system is not generally itself a medical hazard, it can pose a significant risk to a patient because any thrombus in the periphery may become dislodged and move to block the blood supply to vital organs or the brain. Such blockage may cause organ failure, a myocardial infarct, a stroke, or even death. Therefore preventing the formation of DVTs in at-risk patients is imperative.

The prophylactic application of external compression devices to the foot and calf has been shown to reduce the incidence of DVT formation in patients hospitalized for a variety of reasons including postoperative and postacute stroke care and after spinal cord injury[23,24-26] (Fig. 11-5). External compression devices may also protect against pulmonary embolism and reduce mortality. A recent review and metaanalysis of studies on graded compression stockings reported that, of 624 patients who used graded compression stockings, 81 (13%) developed DVTs, whereas in the control group of 581 patients, 154 (27%) developed DVTs.[27] This is approximately a 60% reduction in risk of DVT formation. This effect was even more pronounced when the stockings were used in combination with other prophylactic methods such as heparin. Metaanalyses have shown compression to be similarly, or possibly more, effective than heparin in reducing the risk of DVTs and pulmonary emboli.[28,29]

Compression is thought primarily to reduce thrombus formation by improving venous flow and thus reducing venous stasis and the opportunity for thrombus formation.[30,31] However, the intermittent compression may also inhibit tissue factor pathways that initiate blood coagulation or degrade thrombi by enhancing fibrinolytic activity.[32-35]

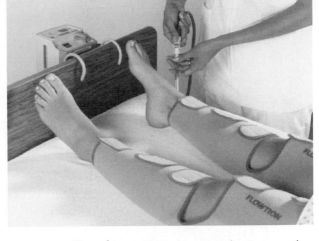

Figure 11-6. Use of intermittent pneumatic compression to prevent DVT formation in a bedridden patient. (Courtesy Huntleigh Healthcare, Manalapan, NJ.)

Venous Stasis Ulcers

Venous stasis ulcers are areas of tissue breakdown and necrosis that occur as the result of impaired venous circulation (Fig. 11-6). Impaired venous circulation, which may be the result of lack of muscle contraction, venous insufficiency, or mechanical obstruction, can result in poor tissue oxygenation and nutrition, reduced local immunological responses, and an accumulation of waste products, all of which can contribute to cell death and tissue necrosis.[36-37] Because compression can improve venous circulation, and because improving circulation may reduce these adverse effects, diminish the risk of vascular ulcer formation, and facilitate healing of previously formed ulcers, compression is the treatment of choice for venous stasis ulcers.

Compression has been shown to increase the rate of healing and reduce the rate of recurrence of venous stasis ulcers.[9,38,39] The addition of 4 hours of sequential intermittent compression daily to other regular ulcer care procedures has been demonstrated to accelerate healing by close to a factor of 10.[40] Compression therapy is considered to be the most important aspect of the treatment of venous stasis ulcers.[41]

It is proposed that compression facilitates the healing of venous stasis ulcers by improving venous circulation, increasing tissue oxygenation, altering white cell adhesion, and reducing edema.[42,43] Although compression may facilitate the healing of arterial ulcers when they result from excessive pressure on the arterial vessels due to chronic edema, in general compression is contraindicated in the presence of arterial insufficiency because compression of the arterial vessels may further impair arterial flow, aggravating rather than improving the condition.

Residual Limb Shaping After Amputation

Compression can be used for residual limb reduction and shaping after amputation in order to help prepare the limb for prosthetic fitting (Fig. 11-7). Both static and intermittent compression are used for this application, although intermittent compression has been shown to reduce the residual limb in approximately half of the time required by other techniques.[44] For this type of application, when intermittent compression is used, it is applied in conjunction with wrapping with an elastic bandage. Compression reduces residual limb size because it controls postsurgical edema and prevents stretching of the soft tissues by excessive fluid accumulation. Residual limb reduction and shaping is required in order to create appropriate areas for functional weight bearing on a prosthetic device. The residual limb must be shaped so that the prosthesis maintains its position and alignment and promotes weight bearing on the appropriate structures. Excessive pressure on unprotected bony

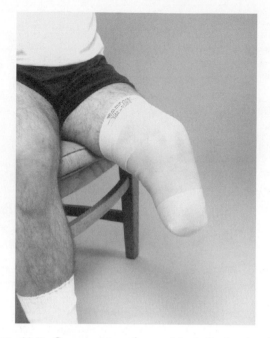

Figure 11-7. Compression for residual limb shaping. (Courtesy Silipos, New York, NY.)

prominences should be avoided to promote comfort and function and to limit the risk of tissue breakdown.

Control of Hypertrophic Scarring

Hypertrophic scarring is a common complication of deep burns and other extensive skin and soft tissue injuries.[45,46] While normal skin is pliable and aesthetically pleasing, and has clearly identifiable layers, hypertrophic scars are not pliable, have a raised and ridged appearance, and have loss of identity of the skin layers[47] (Fig. 11-8). Hypertrophic scars result in poor cosmesis and the development of contractures that may restrict ROM and function. The risk of hypertrophic scarring is increased when there is delayed healing, a deep wound, repeated trauma, infection, or a foreign body present and in individuals with a genetic predisposition. Hypertrophic scarring is most common in the areas of the sternum, upper back, and shoulders.[48]

Although many approaches, including surgery, pharmaceuticals, passive stretch with positioning, massage, and silicone gel, are used to control hypertrophic scar formation, compression is the most common.[48-51] Larson and colleagues first published a

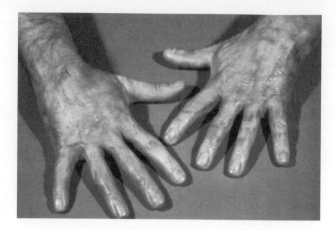

Figure 11-8. Hypertrophic scarring.

report in the United States of this application of compression in 1971. They demonstrated that compression garments decreased the height and vascularity of scar tissue and increased its pliability.[52]

Many mechanisms for the effect of compression on controlling hypertrophic scarring have been proposed. Compression may directly shape the scar tissue by acting as a mold for the new tissue, decreasing local edema formation, and facilitating improved collagen orientation. It has also been proposed that compression reduces scar formation by increasing collagenase activity, either due to the increased skin temperature or due to the increase in prostaglandin E2 release, both of which have been shown to be induced by compression.[8,49,53] Alternatively, compression may control scar formation by inducing local tissue hypoxia.[50]

When applying compression to control hypertrophic scar formation, treatment is generally initiated once the new epithelium has formed, and is then continued for 8 to 12 months or longer until the scar is no longer growing and has reached maturity. Compression can be applied with elastic bandages, self-adherent wraps, tubular elastic cotton supports, or elastic custom-fit garments. With any of these approaches, the compression pressure is maintained at approximately 20 mm Hg to 30 mm Hg. It is recommended that the compression device be worn 24 hours a day, except when bathing, in order to achieve maximum benefit. Common complications of this treatment include skin irritation, constriction of circulation, and restriction of joint motion.[48]

CONTRAINDICATIONS AND PRECAUTIONS FOR EXTERNAL COMPRESSION

There are few contraindications that apply to all types of compression devices; however, when compression is being used to treat edema or impaired circulation, the underlying cause of these problems should be ascertained, and addressed as well as possible, before compression therapy is initiated. Compression therapy will be ineffective and contraindicated in cases where edema is caused by a blockage of the circulation or when there is active infection or malignancy in the affected extremity. When peripheral edema is caused by cardiovascular disease, such as congestive heart failure or cardiomyopathy, one must also ascertain that the increased fluid load that could be placed on the heart by the shifting of fluid from the periphery in response to treatment with compression will not be detrimental to the patient. In such cases, the patient's physician should always be consulted before the initiation of compression therapy.

Particular care should be taken when donning and doffing compression bandages and garments in order to avoid trauma to healing tissue or fragile skin. Details of the contraindications and precautions for the use of compression pumps are provided following.

CONTRAINDICATIONS
for the Use of Intermittent or Sequential Compression Pumps

- Heart failure or pulmonary edema
- Recent or acute DVT, thrombophlebitis, or pulmonary embolism
- Obstructed lymphatic or venous return

- Severe peripheral arterial disease or ulcers due to arterial insufficiency
- Acute local skin infection
- Significant hypoproteinemia—protein levels less than 2 g/dL
- Acute fracture or other trauma

The use of intermittent or sequential compression pumps is contraindicated . . .

. . . in patients with heart failure or pulmonary edema

Although edema of the dependent parts of the body is a common consequence of congestive heart failure (CHF), compression pumps should not be used to treat edema of this etiology because the shift of fluid from the peripheral to the central circulation may increase the stress on the failing organ system. CHF is the result of a decrease in the ability or efficiency of cardiac muscle contraction that leads to decreased cardiac output. This stimulates an increase in venous pressure and increased sodium and water retention, which all act to cause edema. Treatment of CHF requires decreasing the load on the heart, whereas compression increases the cardiac load by increasing the fluid load of the veins. Thus compression tends to aggravate the underlying condition, resulting in worsening edema and potentially other, more serious side effects, such as pulmonary edema, as CHF progresses.

Peripheral edema due to CHF is usually bilateral and symmetrical.

Pulmonary edema occurs with prolonged or severe CHF. It is the result of elevated lung capillary pressure causing fluid to leave the circulation and accumulate in the alveolar air spaces in the lungs. Compression is contraindicated when pulmonary edema is present because it increases the fluid load of the vascular system and the pressure in the lung capillaries, potentially aggravating this serious medical condition.

ASK THE PATIENT:
- Do you have any heart or lung problems?
- Do you have difficulty breathing?
- Are you taking any medications for your heart or blood pressure?
- Do you have swelling in both legs?

ASSESS:
- Check for the presence of bilateral edema.
- Do not use compression to treat edema until you have ascertained that the edema is not due to CHF or pulmonary edema.

Continued

CONTRAINDICATIONS—cont'd

. . . in patients with recent or acute DVT, thrombophlebitis, or pulmonary embolism

Compression, particularly intermittent compression, should not be used when the patient is known to have a DVT, thrombophlebitis, or a pulmonary embolus because the thrombus may become dislodged or the embolus may travel. This can occur because of direct mechanical agitation of the clot by the compression or because of increased circulation produced by compression. If a thrombus or embolus becomes dislodged, it may travel in the bloodstream to a distant site and lodge in a location where it impairs blood flow to an organ sufficiently to cause organ damage, severe morbidity, or even death. For example, an embolus in the pulmonary arteries produces about a 30% mortality rate, while an embolus that lodges in the arteries supplying the brain may cause a stroke or death.[70] Compression can help prevent the formation of DVTs, but it should not be used when it is thought that a thrombus may already be present.

ASK THE PATIENT:
- Do you have pain in your calves?
- How long have you not been walking?

ASSESS:
- Check for Homan's sign (discomfort in the calf on forced dorsiflexion of the foot), a sign of thrombosis in the leg.

Request further evaluation by a physician if you suspect that there may be a thrombus in the deep veins of the leg. Delay the use of compression until the patient has been cleared for the presence of thromboses or thrombophlebitis in the area to be treated.

. . . when lymphatic or venous return is obstructed

- Compression is contraindicated when lymphatic or venous return is totally obstructed because, in such cases, increasing the fluid load of the vessels cannot reduce the edema until the obstruction has been removed. Lymphatic or venous return may be obstructed by a thrombus, radiation damage to the lymph nodes, an inguinal or abdominal tumor, or other masses. With partial obstruction of the ves-

sels or complete occlusion of only a few of the vessels, treatment with compression may enhance the functioning of the intact collateral vessels

ASK THE PATIENT:
- Do you know why you have swelling in your legs/arms?
- Is something obstructing your circulation?

If there is complete lymphatic or venous obstruction, compression should not be used. Such obstruction may need to be treated surgically. When there is partial obstruction, compression may be used in conjunction with careful monitoring of the patient's response to the treatment to ensure that the treatment is helping to resolve the edema rather than just shifting the fluid to a more proximal area of the affected limb.

. . . in patients with severe peripheral arterial disease or ulcers due to arterial insufficiency

Compression should not be used in patients with severe peripheral arterial disease or where there are ulcers due to arterial insufficiency because it can aggravate these conditions by closing down the diseased arteries and further impairing circulation into the area.

ASK THE PATIENT:
- Do you get pain in your calves when walking? This can be due to intermittent claudication, a sign of peripheral arterial disease.

If an ulcer is present: Have you had problems with your arteries; for example, heart bypass surgery or bypass surgery in your legs? A history of bypass surgeries suggests the presence of arterial disease in other areas.

ASSESS:
- If an ulcer is present, try to determine if it is due to arterial insufficiency. Ulcers due to arterial insufficiency are usually small and round, with definite borders, and painful. They occur most often on the interdigital spaces between the toes or on the lateral malleolus.

Request that an ankle-brachial index (ABI) be obtained. This is generally performed by vascular services and is a measure of the ratio of the systolic blood pressure in the lower extremity to the systolic blood pressure in the upper extremity. Compression should not be applied if the ABI is less than 0.8, indicating that the blood pressure at the ankle is less than 80% of that in the upper extremity.

. . . in patients with acute local skin infection

A local skin infection is likely to be aggravated by the application of compression because the sleeves and skin coverings used increase the moisture and temperature of the area, encouraging the growth of microorganisms. If a chronic skin infection is present, single-use sleeves that avoid cross-contamination from one patient to another, or reinfection of the same patient, may be used for the application of intermittent compression.

ASK THE PATIENT:
- Do you have any skin infections in the area to be treated?

ASSESS:
- Inspect the skin for rashes, redness, or skin breakdown indicating the possible presence of infection.

. . . in patients with significant hypoproteinemia (serum protein level less than 2 g/dL)

Although peripheral edema is a common symptom of severe hypoproteinemia, when the serum protein level is less than 2 g/dL, the resulting edema should not be treated with compression because returning fluid to the vessels will further lower the serum protein concentration, potentially resulting in severe adverse consequences, including cardiac and immunological dysfunction. Severe hypoproteinemia can occur due to inadequate food intake, increased nutrient losses, or increased nutrient requirements due to an underlying disease.

ASK THE PATIENT:
- Have you recently lost weight?
- Have you changed your diet?
- Do you have any other disease?

ASSESS:
- Check the lab values section of the chart for the serum protein level.

Delay the use of compression until the patient's serum protein level is above 2 g/dL.

. . . in patients with acute trauma or fracture

Intermittent compression is contraindicated immediately after an acute trauma because the motion caused by this intervention may cause excessive motion at the site of trauma, increasing bleeding, aggravating the acute inflammation, or destabilizing an acute fracture. Such effects can cause further damage at the site of injury and impair healing. Intermittent compression should be used for treating posttraumatic edema only after the initial acute inflammatory phase has passed, bleeding has stopped, and the area is mechanically stable. Static compression, as provided by stockings or wraps, may be used immediately after an acute trauma to prevent edema and reduce bleeding. Directly after an injury, static compression is frequently applied in conjunction with rest, ice, and elevation in order to optimize the control of pain, edema, and inflammation.

ASK THE PATIENT:
- When did your injury happen?
- Do you know if you broke a bone?

PRECAUTIONS
for the Use of Intermittent or Sequential Compression Pumps

- Impaired sensation or mentation
- Uncontrolled hypertension
- Cancer
- Stroke or significant vascular insufficiency
- Superficial peripheral nerves

PRECAUTIONS—cont'd

Apply compression with caution to . . .

. . . patients with impaired sensation or mentation

Compression should be applied with caution to patients with impaired sensation or mentation because such patients may be unable to recognize or communicate when pressure is excessive or painful.

ASK THE PATIENT:

- Do you have normal feeling in this area?

ASSESS:

- Sensation in the area
- Alertness and orientation

Compression garments or low levels of intermittent compression may be used if the patient has impaired sensation or mentation; however, such patients must be carefully monitored for adverse effects such as skin irritation or any aggravation of edema due to constriction of the garments in tight areas.

. . . patients with uncontrolled hypertension

Compression should be applied with caution to patients with uncontrolled hypertension because compression can further elevate blood pressure by increasing the vascular fluid load. Blood pressure should be monitored frequently during treatment of these patients, and treatment should be stopped if their blood pressure increases above the safe level determined by their physician.

ASK THE PATIENT:

- Do you have high blood pressure?
If so, is it well controlled with medication?

ASSESS:

- Resting blood pressure.
Check with the patient's physician for guidelines on blood pressure limits.

. . . patients with cancer

Compression can increase circulation, which may disturb or dislodge metastatic tissue, promoting metastasis, or may improve tissue nutrition, promoting tumor growth. Therefore although there have been no reports of metastasis or accelerated tumor growth due to the use of compression, it is generally recommended that compression not be applied where a tumor is present or when it is thought that an increase in circulation may cause a tumor to move or grow more rapidly. Compression is frequently used to control lymphedema that results from the treatment of breast cancer with mastectomy or radiation. Experts in this field vary in their opinions regarding the safety of this treatment and the precautions to be applied.[12,54,55] While some do not consider the presence or history of malignancy to be a contraindication to the use of compression, others recommend avoiding the use of compression in areas close to the malignancy and still others recommend not applying this type of treatment until the patient has been cancer-free for 5 years. In general, most agree that the use of compression need not be restricted during the time that patients are receiving chemotherapy, hormone therapy, or biological response modifiers for treatment of their cancer.

ASK THE PATIENT:

- If edema results from treatment of breast cancer, ask the patient if he or she is receiving chemotherapy, hormone therapy, or biological response modifiers for treatment of the cancer.

ASSESS:

- How recent was the diagnosis of cancer?

If the cause of edema is unknown and the patient has signs of cancer, such as recent unexplained changes in body weight or constant pain that does not change, treatment with compression should be deferred until a follow-up evaluation to rule out malignancy has been performed by a physician.

. . . patients with stroke or significant cerebrovascular insufficiency

Compression should be applied with caution to patients who have had a stroke or have signs of significant cerebrovascular insufficiency, such as a history of transient ischemic attacks. Caution is required because the hemodynamic changes caused by the compression may alter circulation to the brain.

Peroneal nerve palsy has been documented following the application of intermittent sequential compression.[56-58] Significant weight loss, resulting in loss of fat and muscle mass around the peroneal nerves, may predispose these nerves to injury from compression devices. When compression is applied over an area where there is a superficial nerve, particularly in a patient with significant weight loss, the clinician should monitor closely for symptoms of nerve compression, including changes in or loss of sensation or strength.

ADVERSE EFFECTS OF EXTERNAL COMPRESSION

The potentially adverse effects of compression generally relate to aggravating a condition that is causing edema or impairing rather than improving circulation if excessive pressure is used. When edema is the result of heart, kidney or liver failure or circulatory obstruction, as explained in detail above in the discussions of contraindications and precautions, compression may aggravate the underlying condition. Also, if too much pressure is used, the compression device may act as a tourniquet, impairing arterial circulation and causing ischemia and edema. If ischemia is prolonged, impaired healing or tissue death can occur. When compression is effective in reducing edema in an extremity, it is recommended that if this fluid accumulates at the proximal end of the extremity or where the extremity attaches to the trunk, it should be mobilized using massage.[16,59] In order to minimize the probability of adverse circulatory effects from treatment with compression, it is also recommended that the patient always be monitored closely for undesired changes in blood pressure or edema, particularly with the first application of the treatment or with changes in treatment parameters.

APPLICATION TECHNIQUES

Compression can be applied in a variety of ways, depending on the patient's clinical presentation and the goals of treatment. Static compression can be applied with bandages or garments, and intermittent compression can be applied with electric pneumatic pumps. Static compression can be used to help control edema due to venous or lymphatic dysfunction or inflammation, to form the shape of amputated residual limbs in preparation for the use of a prosthetic device, or to control scar formation after burn injury. Both static and intermittent compression, used either alone or together, can be applied to help prevent the development of DVT in bedridden patients (see Fig. 11-5). Intermittent compression is used primarily to prevent or reduce edema formation in limbs with poor venous or lymphatic drainage, with static compression being applied after this treatment to maintain the edema control.

Compression Bandaging

Compression bandages are generally applied by wrapping them around the limb in a figure 8 manner, starting distally and progressing proximally (Fig. 11-9). Circular circumferential or spiral wrapping are generally not recommended because these configurations can result in the uneven application of pressure and thus the uneven control of edema. The bandage should be applied tightly enough to apply moderate, comfortable compression without impairing circulation. To avoid slipping of the compression bandage on the skin, cohesive gauze or foam bandages are often applied under the compression bandages directly against the patient's skin. Soft cotton may also be used as an underwrapping to absorb sweat and to help distribute pressure more evenly.

Compression bandages with different amounts of elasticity and extensibility are available. These bandages provide varying amounts of resting or working pressure and can be applied in layers or individually. Resting pressure is pressure exerted by elastic when put on stretch. An elastic bandage exerts this pressure whether or not the patient is moving.

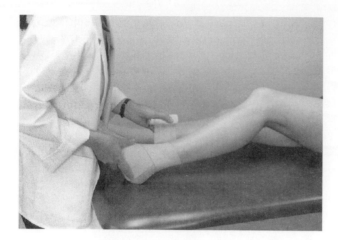

Figure 11-9. Elastic compression wrap of the foot, ankle, and leg. Note the figure 8 wrap at the ankle.

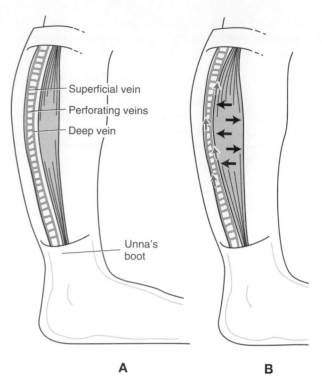

Figure 11-10. Development of working pressure. **A,** Muscle relaxed. **B,** Calf muscle contracting and pressing against the Unna's boot to compress the veins.

Highly extensible bandages, which can be extended by 100% to 200%, provide the greatest resting pressure because they exert the greatest restoring force. Working pressure is pressure produced by the muscles when they are active and push against an inelastic bandage (Fig. 11-10). Highly elastic bandages do not promote the development of working pressure because they stretch rather than provide resistance when the muscles expand. Inelastic bandages that are not extensible produce a low resting pressure but provide adequate resistance to allow for the development of high working pressure during muscle activity.

In general, it is recommended that if high-stretch bandages, such as a new Ace wrap, are used to control edema, they should be applied with only moderate tension to avoid excessive resting pressure, since, without activity, the high resting pressure provided by this type of bandage may impair circulation. Low-stretch bandages, with 30% to 90% extension, provide some degree of both resting and working pressure and can therefore be somewhat effective when the patient is either active or at rest. Inelastic bandages are optimal for use during exercise when the activity of the muscles results in high working pressure, but generally they do not control edema effectively or improve circulation in a flaccid or inactive limb.

A semirigid bandage formed of zinc oxide–impregnated gauze can also exert working pressure. When this type of bandage is applied to the lower extremity

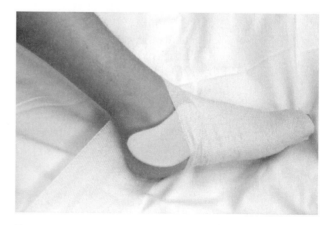

Figure 11-11. Foam padding around anatomical indentations.

it is known as an *Unna's boot*. This is typically used for the treatment of venous stasis ulcers.[60] Zinc oxide–impregnated gauze bandages become soft when wet, to allow molding around the involved limb, and then harden as they dry to form a semirigid boot. The boot is left on the patient for as long as 1 to 2 weeks, and is then removed and replaced. An Unna's boot is reported to provide a sustained compression force of 35 mm Hg to 40 mm Hg.[58]

For all types of bandages, it is recommended that tension, and thus compression, be greatest distally, and gradually decrease proximally in order to achieve an appropriate pressure gradient. In order to maintain consistency of pressure around anatomical indentations, such as the ankles, pieces of foam or cotton cut to size should be placed in these indentations before the bandage is applied (Fig. 11-11).

APPLICATION TECHNIQUE
Compression Bandage

Equipment Required
- Cohesive gauze, foam, or cotton under bandage
- Bandages of appropriate elasticity
- Cotton or foam for padding

PROCEDURE
1. Remove clothing and jewelry from the area to be treated.
2. Inspect the skin in the area.
3. Apply foam or cotton padding around anatomical indentations.
4. Dress and cover any wound according to the treatment regimen being used for that wound.
5. Apply a cohesive gauze, foam, or cotton under bandage to protect the skin from the compression bandage and minimize slipping of the compression bandage. Start distally and progress proximally.
6. Apply the compression bandage, starting distally and progressing proximally. When applying a bandage to the lower extremity, first apply it around the ankle to fix the bandage in place; then wrap the foot and then bandage the leg and thigh. Wrapping around the foot should be from medial to lateral when on the dorsum of the foot, in the direction of pronation.[61] When applying a bandage to the upper extremity, first apply it to the wrist to fix it in place; then wrap the hand and bandage the forearm and arm. For all areas, slightly more tension should be applied distally than proximally, and the bandage should be applied in a figure 8 manner.

ADVANTAGES
- Inexpensive.
- Quick to apply once skill is mastered.
- Readily available.
- Extremity can be used during treatment.
- Safe for acute conditions.

DISADVANTAGES
- When used alone, does not reverse edema.
- Effective only for controlling edema formation.
- Requires moderate skill, flexibility, and level of cognition to apply.
- Compression not readily quantifiable or replicable.
- Bulky and unattractive.
- Inelastic bandages are ineffective in controlling edema in a flaccid limb.

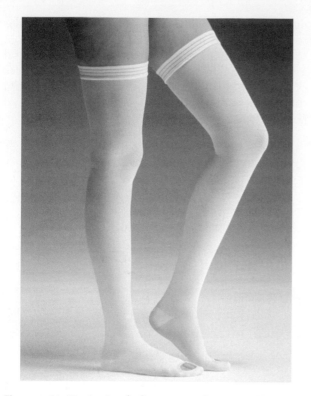

Figure 11-12. Antiembolism stockings. (Courtesy Beiersdorf-Jobst, Charlotte, NC.)

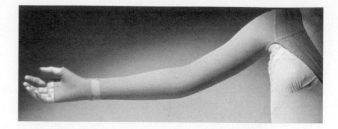

Figure 11-13. Upper extremity compression garment. (Courtesy Beiersdorf-Jobst, Charlotte, NC.)

Compression Garments

Compression garments can provide various degrees of compression, and are available in custom-fit sizes for all areas of the body and standard off-the-shelf sizes for the limbs. They are generally made of washable Lycra spandex and nylon and have moderate elasticity to provide a combination of moderate resting and working pressure. Inelastic or low-stretch garments, which provide more working pressure, are not made because these are too difficult to put on and take off.

Off-the-shelf stockings providing a low compression force of about 16 mm Hg to 18 mm Hg, known as *antiembolism stockings,* are used to prevent DVT in bedridden patients[62] (Fig. 11-12). These stockings are not intended to provide sufficient compression to prevent DVT formation or alter circulation when the lower extremities are in a dependent position. These stockings should fit snugly but comfortably around the lower extremities, and they should be worn by the patient 24 hours a day, except when bathing. Knee high and thigh high stockings are simi-

larly efficient at reducing venous stasis, and knee high stockings are more comfortable to wear and wrinkle less.[63]

Custom-fit and off-the-shelf compression garments, providing sufficient compression to control edema and counteract the effects of gravity on circulation in active patients or to modify scar formation after burns, are also available (Fig. 11-13). These garments are available in different thicknesses and with different degrees of pretensioning to provide pressure ranging from 10 mm Hg to 50 mm Hg.[62] A pressure of 20 mm Hg to 30 mm Hg is generally appropriate for the control of scar tissue formation, while 30 mm Hg to 40 mm Hg pressure will control edema in most ambulatory patients. Lower pressure may be sufficient in mild cases of edema, and higher pressure may be necessary in more severe cases. Some garments provide a pressure gradient such that the compression is greatest distally and decreases proximally. Although off-the-shelf stockings can improve venous circulation and control edema in most patients, custom-fit garments may be necessary in severe conditions or when an individual's limb contours do not match off-the-shelf sizing. Custom-fit garments may include options such as zippers and reinforced, padded areas to improve ease of use and fit, and are effective in normalizing venous flow in many cases where off-the-shelf garments are ineffective.[64] In order for sizing to be appropriate, both custom-fit and off-the-shelf compression garments should be fitted when edema is minimal. This is generally first thing in the morning or after treatment with an intermittent compression pump. Garments are available for both the upper and lower extremities, as well as for the trunk and head (see Fig. 11-13). They are also available in a number of colors for improved cosmesis.

APPLICATION TECHNIQUE
Compression Garment

Compression garments should be applied by gathering them up, placing them on the distal area first, and then gradually unfolding them proximally. Since the higher-compression garments have more pretensioning, some patients have difficulty putting them on. A number of devices have been developed to assist with donning these garments, or the patient may wear two sets of lower-compression garments to provide a total compression equal to the sum of both of them. For example, the patient could wear two pairs of 20 mm Hg compression stockings instead of one pair of 40 mm Hg stockings to achieve the same effect.

Compression garments need to be worn every day throughout the day, except for bathing, to control edema, improve circulation, or control scar formation most effectively. In general, with proper care, these garments last about 6 months, after which time they lose their elasticity and no longer exert the appropriate amount of pressure. Garments also need to be replaced if there is a significant change in limb size, as may occur with changes in edema or in body weight. In order for the compression device to be effective, and to avoid the expense of purchasing many sets of garments, it is recommended that a patient use bandages to treat edema initially, while limb size is still diminishing, and that compression garments be

ordered when the limb size appears to have stabilized.

ADVANTAGES
- Compression quantifiable (unlike bandaging).
- Extremity can be used during treatment (unlike a pump).
- Less expensive than intermittent compression devices for short-term use.
- Thin and attractive, available in various colors.
- Safe for acute condition.
- Can be used 24 hours/day, as for modification of scar formation.
- Preferred by patients to compression bandages.[43]

DISADVANTAGES
- When used alone, may not reverse edema that is already present.
- More expensive than most bandages.
- Need to be fitted appropriately.
- Require strength, flexibility, and dexterity to put on.
- Hot, particularly in warm weather.
- Expensive for long-term use, as they need to be replaced at least every 6 months and the patient requires at least two identical garments so that one is available when the other is being laundered.

Intermittent Pneumatic Compression Pump

Intermittent pneumatic compression pumps are used to provide the force for intermittent compression. The pump is attached, via a hose, to a chambered sleeve placed around the involved limb (Fig. 11-14). The specific methods of application for different pumps differ slightly, and specific instructions for the application of intermittent compression are provided with all pumps. General instructions that apply to the application of most pumps are given below. Although intermittent compression is suitable for home use, the patient should always begin the course of therapy under medical supervision.

Once satisfactory reduction of edema has been achieved with the pump, the clinician should determine if continued control will be maintained with

continued use of the pump or if better results would be obtained with a compression garment or bandaging. In general, since a compression pump is used for only a number of hours each day, the patient should use a static compression device between treatments with the pump in order to maintain the reversal of edema produced by the pump.[44] The use of intermittent compression in conjunction with static compression also generally improves the outcome if compression is being used to modify circulation. For example, intermittent compression pumping twice a week in conjunction with static compression with an Unna's boot was found to approximately double the rate of venous ulcer healing compared with the use of static compression with the Unna's boot alone.[65] Intermittent compression is not generally used for the control of scar tissue formation.

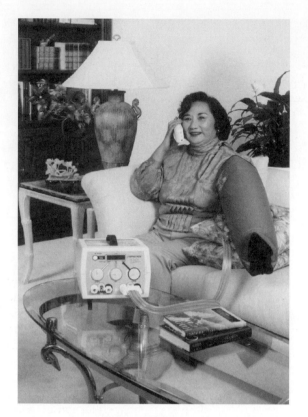

Figure 11-14. Intermittent pneumatic compression being applied for treatment of lymphedema. (Courtesy Huntleigh Healthcare, Manalapan, NJ.)

There is some controversy in the current literature with regard to the use of compression pumps for the treatment of lymphedema. Some authors state that compression pumps should not be used for the treatment of this type of edema due to the possibility of increasing proximal swelling and nonpitting, fibrotic edema.[66,67] These authors recommend that specific massage techniques be used to reduce proximal and then distal edema, and that bandages or compression garments be applied after the edema has been reduced by these techniques. Other authors continue to recommend the use of intermittent compression pumps for the treatment of lymphedema, stating that nonpitting, fibrotic edema is a common complication of chronic lymphedema and that its development is not related to the use of compression pumps.[68] At this time, the author of this book has been unable to find any published data in the peer-reviewed literature documenting complications from the use of compression pumps for the treatment of lymphedema.

APPLICATION TECHNIQUE
Intermittent Pneumatic Compression Pump

Equipment Required
- Intermittent pneumatic compression unit
- Inflatable sleeves for upper and lower extremities
- Stockinette
- Blood pressure cuff
- Stethoscope
- Tape measure

PROCEDURE

1. Determine that compression is not contraindicated for the patient or the condition. Be certain to check for signs of DVT, including calf pain or tenderness associated with swelling. Take the patient's history or check the chart for CHF, pulmonary edema, or other contraindications that may be the cause of the edema.

2. Remove jewelry and clothing from the treatment area and inspect the skin. Cover any open areas with gauze or an appropriate dressing.

3. Place the patient in a comfortable position, with the affected limb elevated. Limb elevation reduces both the pain and the edema caused by venous insufficiency, if applied soon after the development of these

symptoms, because elevation allows gravity to accelerate the flow of blood in the veins toward the heart. With chronic venous insufficiency or lymphatic dysfunction, elevation of the limbs is generally less effective in reducing edema because the fluid is trapped within fibrotic tissue and cannot return as readily to the venous or lymphatic capillaries, from where it can flow back to the central circulation.

4. Measure and record the patient's blood pressure.
5. Measure and record the limb circumference at a number of places with reference to bony landmarks[69] or take volumetric measurements by displacement of water from a graduated cylinder.
6. Place a stocking or stockinette over the area to be treated and smooth out all the wrinkles (Fig. 11-15).
7. Apply the sleeve from the unit (Fig. 11-16). Reusable sleeves made of washable Neoprene and nylon are generally used (Fig. 11-17), although vinyl sleeves intended for single use are also available for application when there is concern about cross-contamination. The Neoprene and nylon sleeves can

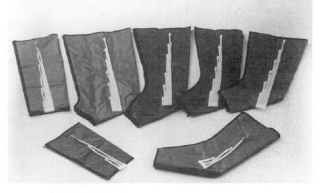

Figure 11-17. Compression sleeves. (Courtesy Chattanooga Group, Inc., Hixson, TN.)

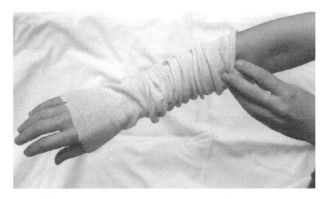

Figure 11-15. Application of stockinette before application of compression sleeve.

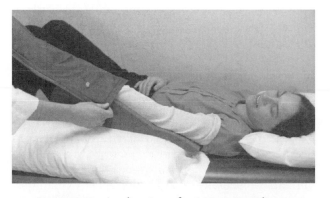

Figure 11-16. Application of compression sleeve.

be machine washed in warm water and air dried or dried at low heat in a drier. The sleeves provide intermittent or sequential compression, depending on their design. Single-chamber sleeves provide intermittent compression only, while sleeves composed of a series of overlapping chambers can inflate sequentially, starting distally and progressing proximally, to produce a milking effect on the extremity. As noted above, sequential compression has been shown to result in more complete emptying of the deep veins and a greater increase in fibrinolytic activity than single-chamber, intermittent compression and is therefore preferred for most applications,[31,43] although it has not been shown to result in greater acceleration of venous blood flow than single-chamber compression.[31]

Both single- and multi-chamber sleeves are available in a variety of lengths and widths for treatment of upper or lower extremities of various sizes. When using a compression pump for the treatment of edema, it is recommended that the sleeve be long enough to cover the entire involved limb so that fluid does not accumulate in areas of the limb proximal to the end of the sleeve. When using a compression pump for the prevention of DVT formation, either calf-high or thigh-high sleeves can be used since both have been found to be effective for this application.[24,30]

8. Attach the hose from the pneumatic compression pump to the sleeve. The pumps vary in size and complexity from small home units intended for the treatment of one extremity to larger clinical units that can be used to treat four extremities at different settings all at one time (Fig. 11-18).

Continued

APPLICATION TECHNIQUE—cont'd
Intermittent Pneumatic Compression Pump

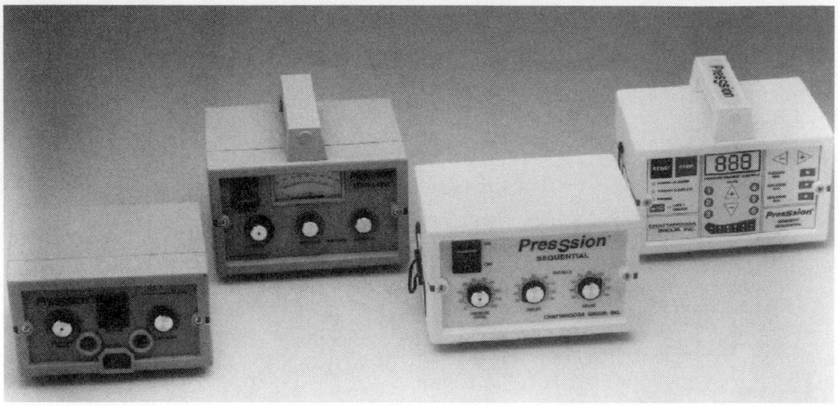

Figure 11-18. Intermittent compression units. (Courtesy Chattanooga Group, Inc., Hixson, TN.)

9. Set the appropriate compression parameters, including inflation and deflation times, inflation pressure, and total treatment time. At this time there are little research data to guide precise selection of any of these parameters. Thus, the parameters used clinically are derived from an understanding of the pathology being treated, measures of the patient's blood pressure, comfort, and observed efficacy in the individual patient. Most protocols use an inflation pressure slightly below the patient's diastolic blood pressure, although higher pressures can be used, and all units come with guidelines for treatment parameters based on their design and manufacture. The parameter ranges provided below, and listed in Table 11-1, cover the ranges suggested by most manufacturers for most pumps.

INFLATION AND DEFLATION TIMES

The inflation time is the period during which the compression sleeve is being inflated or is at the maximal inflation pressure, and the deflation time is the period during which the compression sleeve is being deflated or is fully deflated. For the treatment of edema or venous stasis ulcers or for DVT prevention, the inflation time is generally between 80 and 100 seconds, and the deflation time is generally between 25 and 50 seconds in order to allow for venous refilling after compression. For residual limb reduction, these periods are generally shorter, with inflation time being between 40 and 60 seconds, and deflation time being between 10 and 15 seconds. Usually, the

pressure is applied in approximately a 3:1 ratio of inflation to deflation time and then adjusted if necessary according to the patient's tolerance and response.

INFLATION PRESSURE

Inflation pressure is the maximum pressure during the inflation time and is measured in millimeters of mercury (mm Hg). Most units can deliver between 30 mm Hg and 120 mm Hg of inflation pressure. When a single-chamber sleeve is used to provide intermittent compression, the chamber inflates to the maximum pressure and then deflates. When a multichamber sleeve is used to provide sequential compression, the distal segment inflates first to the maximum pressure and then, as it deflates, the more proximal segments inflate sequentially, generally to slightly lower levels of pressure. Some recommend that inflation pressure not exceed diastolic blood pressure in the belief that higher pressures may impair arterial circulation; however, since the tissues of the body protect the arterial vessels from collapse, higher pressures may be used if this is necessary to achieve the desired clinical outcome and does not cause pain, although close patient supervision is recommended when higher pressures are used. For all indications, inflation pressure is generally between 30 mm Hg and 80 mm Hg and frequently just below the patient's diastolic blood pressure. Because venous pressure is usually lower in the upper extremities than in the lower extremities, the lower end of the pressure range, 30 mm Hg to 60 mm Hg, is generally used for the upper extremities, while the higher end of the range, 40 mm Hg to 80

TABLE 11-1   Recommended Parameters for the Application of Intermittent Compression

Problem	Inflation/deflation time (seconds) (ratio)	Inflation pressure (mm Hg)	Treatment time (hours)
Edema DVT prevention, venous stasis ulcer	80-100/25-35 (3:1)	30-60 UE 40-80 LE	2-3
Residual limb reduction	40-60/10-15	30-60 UE 40-80 LE	2-3

mm Hg, is generally used for the lower extremities. Lower pressures are generally recommended for residual limb reduction and shaping and for the treatment of posttraumatic edema rather than for the treatment of problems caused by venous insufficiency. Although high pressures have been recommended for the treatment of lymphedema, current guidelines indicate that lower pressures are safer and may still be effective for this condition.[68] Treatment with inflation pressures below 30 mm Hg is not likely to affect circulation or tissue form and is therefore not recommended for any condition.

TOTAL TREATMENT TIME

Total treatment time recommendations vary from 1 to 4 hours per treatment, with treatment frequency ranging from 3 times per week to 4 times per day. For most applications, treatments of 2 to 3 hours once or twice a day are recommended. The frequency and duration of treatment should be the minimum necessary to maintain good edema control or satisfactory progress toward the goals of treatment.

10. Provide the patient with a means to call you during the treatment. Measure and record the patient's blood pressure during the treatment, and discontinue treatment if either the systolic or diastolic pressure exceeds the limits set for the patient by the physician.
11. When the treatment is complete, turn off the unit, disconnect the tubing, and remove the sleeve and the stockinette.
12. Remeasure and record limb volume in the same manner as in step 5.
13. Reinspect the patient's skin.
14. Remeasure and document the patient's blood pressure.
15. Apply a compression garment or bandage to maintain the reduction in edema between treatments and after discontinuing the use of a compression pump. Maximum reduction of edema is usually achieved with use of the pump for 3 to 4 weeks.

ADVANTAGES
- Actively moves fluids and therefore may be more effective than static devices, particularly for a flaccid limb.
- Compression quantifiable.
- Can provide sequential compression.
- Requires less finger and hand dexterity to apply than compression bandages or garments.
- Can be used to reverse as well as control edema.
- Use can be supervised in a patient who is noncompliant with static compression.

DISADVANTAGES
- Used only for limited times during the day, and therefore not appropriate for modification of scar formation.
- Generally requires a static compression device to be used between treatments.
- Expensive to purchase unit or to pay for regular treatments in a clinic.
- Requires moderate comfort using machinery to apply.
- Requires electricity.
- Extremity cannot be used during treatment.
- Patient cannot move about during treatment.
- Pumping motion of device may aggravate an acute condition.

DOCUMENTATION

When applying external compression, document the type of compression device, the area of the body being treated, inflation and deflation times, compression or inflation pressure, the total treatment time as applicable to the treatment, and the patient's response to the treatment. Documentation is typically written in the SOAP note format. The following examples only summarize the modality component of treatment and are not intended to represent a comprehensive plan of care.

Examples

When applying a compression bandage to the left ankle after an acute sprain, document:

S: Pt c/o L ankle swelling that increases in the PM
O: High stretch elastic bandage to L ankle & leg, figure 8. Pt to keep LE elevated.
A: Pretreatment ankle girth R 9″, L 10 1/2″. 3 days later, L ankle girth 10″.

P: Instruct pt in wrapping ankle as above, independently.

When applying intermittent pneumatic compression to the right arm to treat lymphedema, document:

S: Pt reports decreasing R UE edema in the past 2 weeks and is now able to use a key with her R hand.
O: IPC R UE, 80 sec/30 sec, 50 mm Hg, 2 hr bid.
A: Pretreatment arm volume to elbow R 530 cc, L 410cc. After 1 treatment R 500 cc after 2 weeks of treatment R 450 cc. BP pretreatment 135/80, during and immediately after treatment 140/85. No overall change in pretreatment blood pressure during 2-week course of treatment.
P: Continue daily IPC as above.

When applying compression hose to prevent DVT formation, document:

S: Pt not oriented × 3.
O: Compression hose bilat. LE's, approx 20 mm Hg compression. To be worn 24 hr/day while pt in bed.
A: Negative Homan's sign. No other signs of DVT formation.
P: Instruct other caregivers in pt's compression hose program.

▶ Clinical Case Studies ◀

The following case studies summarize the concepts of compression discussed in this chapter. Based on the scenarios presented, an evaluation of the clinical findings and goals of treatment are proposed. These are followed by a discussion of the factors to be considered in selection of compression as the indicated treatment modality and in selection of the ideal compression device and treatment parameters to promote progress toward the goals.

Case 1

FR is a 40-year-old carpenter. She has chronic lymphedema of her right upper extremity and complains of pain and swelling in this extremity that worsens with use and is moderately alleviated by elevation and avoiding use of the extremity. She first noticed the swelling 2 or 3 years ago, but at that time it occurred only after extensive use of her upper extremity at work; the swelling was mild and resolved with a night's rest. Over the last year, the swelling has worsened. Now it never resolves fully and is easily aggravated by even light activity at work or by yard work. FR reports that 8 years ago she had a right mastectomy and 16 lymph nodes removed as part of her treatment for breast cancer. She was also treated with chemotherapy and radiation therapy at that time and has had no recurrence of the malignancy. FR has been advised by her physician to reduce the use of her right arm and elevate it when possible to control the swelling. At her request, she has been referred to therapy for further management of her lymphedema. The objective exam reveals moderate pitting edema of the right arm and forearm, with circumferential measurements of 7 inches at the right wrist compared with 6 inches at the left wrist, 9½ inches at the right elbow compared with 11 inches at the left elbow, and 14 inches at the right mid-biceps compared with 11 inches at the same level on the left. The swelling also causes moderate restriction of elbow, wrist, hand, and finger ROM. Passive elbow ROM was measured as 130° flexion and −10° extension on the right compared with 145° flexion and full extension on the left. The skin of the patient's right upper extremity appears thin, flaky, and red, and her blood pressure is 120/80. All other tests, including shoulder ROM and upper extremity sensation, are within normal limits.

EVALUATION OF THE CLINICAL FINDINGS

This patient presents with increased girth and loss of motion of the right upper extremity and a risk of skin breakdown of this extremity. These impairments limit her work and home activities.

PREFERRED PRACTICE PATTERN

Impaired Circulation and Anthropometric Dimensions Associated With Lymphatic Systems Disorders, (6H)

PLAN OF CARE

The goals of treatment at this time are to control and reduce edema and restore ROM in order to allow this patient to continue to work at her present job and to perform her usual home and recreational activities. Control of lymphedema is also indicated to minimize the risk of skin breakdown and infection associated with this condition.

ASSESSMENT REGARDING THE APPROPRIATENESS OF COMPRESSION AS THE OPTIMAL TREATMENT

Although experts in the field of lymphedema vary in their recommendations for treatment of this condition, most agree that some form of compression is indicated. Compression can provide working or resting pressure to control fluid flow out of the venous circulation and into the lymphatic circulation, and can also promote the movement of fluid through the lymphatic vessels. Some experts recommend the use of special massage techniques in conjunction with compression in order to promote lymphatic flow, particularly in proximal areas such as the axilla and the trunk, to aid or divert flow in areas where lymphatic function is compromised and where most compression devices are not effective. Without such additional treatment, compression alone may result in the accumulation of fluid proximal to the compression device, particularly if proximal lymphatic function is impaired.

Although the use of compression is generally not recommended in the presence of malignancy, since this patient has had no recurrence of her disease after more than 5 years, most experts agree that compression may be used. Although the lymphatic circulation in this patient is clearly impaired, the fact that the severity of her edema varies, resolving to some extent with rest and elevation, indicates that the lymphatic circulation in the right upper extremity is not completely blocked, and therefore compression is not contraindicated for this reason.

PROPOSED TREATMENT PLAN AND RATIONALE

Initially, it is recommended that compression be provided by using an intermittent sequential pneumatic pump. This form of compression is likely to produce the fastest and most effective reversal of edema because it provides both compression and the milking action of sequential distal to proximal compression. In order to control the formation of edema between treatments

with the pneumatic device, wrapping with an inelastic bandage during the day to provide a high working pressure is recommended. When the reduction of edema plateaus, which usually takes 2 to 3 weeks, pumping can be gradually discontinued. The patient should continue to use the bandages when working or exercising her upper extremity. If the patient is not compliant with long-term use of bandages, a compression garment may be used. However, since this type of garment is made of a moderately elastic material, which develops limited working pressure, it may not be as effective as an inelastic bandage in maintaining edema control during exercise or other heavy upper extremity activity. It is recommended that the patient not be measured for fitting of a compression garment at the initiation of treatment because a garment fitted at that time will soon be too big if any edema reversal is achieved with pumping or bandaging.

The recommended treatment parameters at the initiation of treatment, when the sequential intermittent pneumatic compression pump is being used, are 80 to 100 seconds of inflation and 25 to 35 seconds of deflation, with a maximum inflation pressure of 30 mm Hg to 60 mm Hg. The lowest inflation pressure that achieves reduction of edema should be used in order to minimize the risk of collapsing the superficial lymphatic or venous vessels. For most patients, treatment with the pump for 2 to 3 hours once or twice a day is sufficient. All parameters within these ranges should be adjusted to achieve optimal edema control without pain and with the least disruption of the patient's regular activities. Compression bandages or garments should be worn at all times, except for bathing, when the pump is not being used.

The appropriate use of massage, exercise, and activity modification should also be considered, in addition to treatment with compression, to achieve the optimal outcome for this patient. The patient's blood pressure should be monitored before, during, and after the use of the compression pump. If it becomes excessively elevated, the pressure, and if necessary the duration, of pumping should be reduced. During pumping, the patient's upper extremity should also be elevated above the level of her heart. This is most readily achieved if the patient lies supine and places her arm on a pillow.

Case 2

JU is a 65-year-old male. He has a full-thickness venous stasis ulcer on his distal medial left leg. He reports that the ulcer is minimally painful but requires frequent dressing changes because a large amount of fluid leaks from it. The ulcer has been present for 4 to 6 months and is gradually getting larger. The only treatment being

Continued

▶ Clinical Case Studies—cont'd ◀

provided for the ulcer at this time is the application of a gauze dressing, which the patient changes two or three times a day when he notices seepage. The objective exam reveals a shallow, flat ulcer with a red base fully covered with granulation tissue, approximately 5 cm by 10 cm in area, with darkening of the intact skin around the ulcer. Edema is also present in the left foot, ankle, and leg. Ankle girth measured at the medial malleolus is 9 inches on the right and 10 ½ inches on the left. There are no signs of edema in the right lower extremity. The patient's blood pressure is 140/100, and he is currently taking medications to control hypertension. He had coronary artery bypass surgery 2 years ago, at which time the left saphenous vein was removed to be used for the graft.

EVALUATION OF THE CLINICAL FINDINGS

This patient presents with loss of skin and subcutaneous tissue integrity requiring him to apply wound dressings frequently and placing him at risk for local infection and possible sepsis. He also has increased girth of the left distal lower extremity.

PLAN OF CARE

The goals of treatment are to achieve wound closure in order to eliminate the need for dressing changes and to reduce the risk of infection. Control of lower extremity edema is also desirable.

PREFERRED PRACTICE PATTERN

Impaired Integumentary Integrity Associated With Full-Thickness Skin Involvement and Scar Formation, (7D)

ASSESSMENT REGARDING THE APPROPRIATENESS OF COMPRESSION AS THE OPTIMAL TREATMENT

This patient's ulcer and edema of the distal lower extremity are probably due to poor venous circulation. Compression is an indicated intervention because it can improve venous circulation to facilitate wound healing and edema control. Specialized dressings that are more absorbent and less adherent than gauze are also recommended to reduce the required frequency of dressing changes and thus reduce the potential for wound trauma and inconvenience to the patient. Contraindications to the use of compression, including arterial insufficiency, heart failure, and DVT, should be ruled out before the initiation of treatment with compression. The patient's history of cardiac bypass surgery suggests the possibility of arterial insufficiency in the lower extremities, although the presence of edema and the conformation of the leg ulcer indicate that it is probably due to venous

rather than arterial insufficiency. In order to rule out arterial insufficiency, an ankle-brachial index (ABI) should be obtained and compression should be applied only if this is above 0.8. The presence of unilateral rather than bilateral edema indicates that this patient's edema is probably not due to cardiac failure. Assessment for Homan's sign should be performed to rule out a DVT before treatment with compression is initiated.

PROPOSED TREATMENT PLAN AND RATIONALE

Twice-a-week treatments with intermittent compression using an intermittent sequential pneumatic pump in conjunction with static compression with an Unna's boot between pumping treatments is recommended for this patient. This combination of compression treatments has been shown to promote the healing of venous stasis ulcers and to result in healing in half the time needed when static compression is provided with the Unna's boot alone.[66] It is thought that this combination of types of compression produces such rapid, complete wound healing and resolution of edema because it reduces edema by the milking action associated with sequential distal to proximal intermittent compression and then maintains edema control with the continuous compression of the rigid Unna's boot. The recommended treatment parameters for the sequential intermittent pneumatic compression pump to promote circulation and control edema are 80 to 100 seconds of inflation and 25 to 35 seconds of deflation, with a maximum inflation pressure of 30 mm Hg to 60 mm Hg and a treatment duration of 2 to 3 hours. Adjustments should be made within these ranges in order to achieve optimal edema control without pain and with the least disruption of the patient's regular activities. The Unna's boot should be worn at all times between intermittent compression treatments. If an Unna's boot is not available, then compression stockings providing 30 mm Hg to 40 mm Hg of pressure may be worn between pumping treatments. Since these stockings are easier to remove and reapply than the Unna's boot, the frequency of pumping may be increased to once or twice a day. The patient's blood pressure should be monitored before, during, and after use of the compression pump. If it becomes significantly elevated, the force, and if necessary the duration, of pumping should be reduced. An appropriate dressing should be placed on the ulcer site before the application of the compression sleeve, boot, or stocking. A single-use sleeve should be used for pumping, or an occlusive barrier should be placed over the ulcer during pumping in order to avoid cross-contamination.

It is essential that the patient continue to wear a compression stocking after the ulcer has healed since his circulatory compromise puts him at high risk for recurrence of edema and tissue breakdown in this extremity.

Case 3

ND is a 20-year-old male who sustained an inversion sprain of his right ankle within the last hour while playing football. He complains of ankle pain, stiffness, and swelling. The pain is primarily at the lateral ankle and increases when he bears weight on his right lower extremity when walking. He is unable to run because of the pain. The objective evaluation reveals mildly increased temperature, swelling, and restricted passive ROM of the right ankle. Ankle girth at the level of the medial malleolus is 12 inches on the right and 11 inches on the left. Passive ankle ROM was measured as 30° of inversion on the right, limited by pain, compared with 50° on the left, 20° of eversion on the right compared with 25° on the left, 0° of dorsiflexion on the right compared with 15° on the left, and 40° of plantar flexion on the right compared with 50° on the left. During ambulation, ND protected his right ankle by decreasing the duration of stance phase on the right, decreasing dorsiflexion of the right ankle during midstance, and decreasing plantar flexion of the right ankle during terminal stance.

EVALUATION OF THE CLINICAL FINDINGS

This patient presents with increased girth, temperature, pain, and restricted motion of his right ankle resulting in gait deviations, reduced ambulation tolerance, and an inability to run.

PREFERRED PRACTICE PATTERN

Impaired Joint Mobility, Motor Function, Muscle Performance, and Range of Motion Associated With Connective Tissue Dysfunction, (4D)

PLAN OF CARE

The goals of treatment at this time are to control inflammation and swelling and to prevent further injury or damage to the involved ankle or to other areas. The anticipated long-term goals of treatment include regaining normal girth and ROM of the right ankle so that the patient can return to his prior functional activities, including a normal gait for ambulation and running.

ASSESSMENT REGARDING THE APPROPRIATENESS OF COMPRESSION AS THE OPTIMAL TREATMENT

Compression is indicated as a component of this patient's intervention because this treatment can help to control the formation of edema; however, it will not be optimally effective in promoting the achievement of this or other goals of treatment if used alone. When edema is caused by acute inflammation, compression is likely to be most effective if it is applied in conjunction with rest, ice, and elevation. Local rest can be achieved by the appropriate use of crutches; ice may be applied as described in Chapter 6; and, for optimal benefit, the patient's ankle should be elevated above the level of his heart. The use of crutches will also reduce the risk of further injury to other areas due to stresses of an abnormal gait pattern. Although the use of compression is not contraindicated in this patient, the use of intermittent compression is not recommended because, with such an acute trauma, the motion produced by intermittent compression may aggravate bleeding or displace a fracture if one is present.

PROPOSED TREATMENT PLAN AND RATIONALE

Since the use of intermittent compression is not recommended, static compression should be used. This can be provided most readily by the use of an elastic compression bandage. This type of bandage is recommended because it provides high resting pressure during rest, is readily available, can easily be used by the patient at home, and is inexpensive. The bandage should be wrapped in a figure 8 manner to provide consistent and comfortable compression in all areas. It should be snug but not so tight that it limits circulation. For optimal control of edema, slightly more compression should be applied distally than proximally. To apply cryotherapy in conjunction with the compression, the bandage may be applied over or under an ice pack or cold pack. Since compression should be maintained at all times until the edema resolves, whereas cryotherapy should generally be applied for 15 minutes every 1 to 2 hours, placing the pack over the compression bandage may be more time efficient. The patient should also elevate his lower extremity above the level of his heart when possible to achieve the most rapid resolution of the edema. Compression should be applied at all times until the edema resolves. As the patient recovers and the edema is reduced, an elastic compression brace may be used in place of the compression bandage.

Chapter Review

Compression applies an inwardly directed force to the tissues, thereby increasing extravascular pressure and venous and lymphatic circulation. External compression can be used to control edema, prevent the formation of DVT, facilitate venous stasis ulcer healing, and shape residual limbs after amputation. Compression can be provided by a pneumatic pump or by special bandages or garments. Pneumatic pumps provide intermittent compression for limited periods of time, whereas bandages and garments provide static compression and can be worn throughout the day. The choice of compression device depends on the nature of the problem being treated and the ability of the patient to comply with the treatment. The use of traction and compression is contraindicated when they may aggravate any existing condition or when they may cause damage to other areas. The reader is referred to the Evolve website at http://evolve.elsevier.com/Cameron for study questions pertinent to this chapter.

References

1. Ramos R, Salem BI, DePawlikowski MP et al: The efficacy of pneumatic compression stockings in the prevention of pulmonary embolism after cardiac surgery, *Chest* 109(1):82-85, 1996.

2. Samson RH: Compression stockings and non-continuous use of polyurethane foam dressings for the treatment of venous ulceration: a pilot study, *J Dermatol Surg Oncol* 19(1):68-72, 1993.

3. Chen AH, Frangos SG, Kilaru S et al: Intermittent pneumatic compression devices—physiological mechanisms of action, *Eur J Vasc Endovasc Surg* May;21(5):383-392, 2001.

4. Whitelaw GP, Oladipo OJ, Shah BP et al: Evaluation of intermittent pneumatic compression devices, *Orthopedics* Mar;24(3):257-261, 2001.

5. Kamm RD: Bioengineering studies of periodic external compression as prophylaxis against deep venous thrombosis, part I: Numerical studies, *J Biomech Eng* 104:87-95, 1982.

6. Olson DA, Kamm RD, Shapiro AH: Bioengineering studies of periodic external compression as prophylaxis against deep venous thrombosis, part II: Experimental studies on a simulated leg, *J Biomech Eng* 104:96-104, 1982.

7. Wakim KG, Martin GM, Krusen FH: Influence of centripetal rhythmic compression on localized edema of an extremity, *Arch Phys Med Rehabil* 36:98-103, 1955.

8. Lee RC, Capelli-Schellpfeffer M, Astumian RD: *A review of thermoregulation of tissue repair and remodeling,* 1995, Abstract Soc Phys Reg Biol Med 15th Ann Mtg. Washington, DC.

9. Ganong WF: *Review of Medical Physiology,* Norwalk, CT, 1987, Appleton & Lange.

10. Nelson PA: Recent advances in treatment of lymphedema of the extremities, *Geriatrics* 21:162-173, 1966.

11. Jungi WF: The prevention and management of lymphoedema after treatment for breast cancer, *Int Rehabil Med* 3:129-134, 1981.

12. Swedborg I: Effects of treatment with an elastic sleeve and intermittent pneumatic compression in post-mastectomy patients with lymphoedema of the arm, *Scand J Rehabil Med* 26:35-41, 1984.

13. Zeissler RH, Rose GB, Nelson PA: Postmastectomy lymphedema: late results of treatment in 385 patients, *Arch Phys Med Rehabil* 53:159-166, 1972.

14. Airaksinen O: Changes in posttraumatic ankle joint mobility, pain, and edema following intermittent pneumatic compression therapy, *Arch Phys Med Rehabil* 70(4):341-344, 1989.

15. Chleboun GS, Howell JN, Baker HL et al: Intermittent pneumatic compression effect on eccentric exercise-induced swelling, stiffness and strength loss, *Arch Phys Med Rehabil* 76(8):744-749, 1995.

16. Boris M, Weindorf S, Lasinski B et al: Lymphedema reduction by noninvasive complex lymphedema therapy, *Oncology* 8(9):95-106, 1994.

17. Matsen FA, Krugmire RB: The effect of externally applied pressure on postfracture swelling, *J Bone Joint Surg* 56-A:1586-1591, 1974.

18. Airaksinen O, Kolari PJ, Herve R et al: Treatment of post-traumatic oedema in lower legs using intermittent pneumatic compression. *Scand J Rehabil Med* 20(1):25-28 1998.

19. Quillen WS, Roullier LH: Initial management of acute ankle sprains with rapid pulsed pneumatic compression and cold, *J Orthop Sports Phys Ther* 4:39-43, 1982.

20. Kolb P, Denegar C: Traumatic edema and the lymphatic system, *Athletic Training* 17:339-341, 1983.

21. Kraemer WJ, Bush JA, Wickham RB et al: Influence of compression therapy on symptoms following soft tissue injury from maximal eccentric exercise, *J Orthop Sports Phys Ther* 31:282-290, 2001.

22. Gilbart MK, Ogilivie-Harris DJ, Broadhurst C et al: Anterior tibial compartment pressures during intermittent sequential pneumatic compression therapy, *Am J Sports Med* 23(6):769-772, 1995.

23. Nicolaides AN, Fernandes JF, Pollock AV: Intermittent sequential pneumatic compression of the legs in the prevention of venous stasis and postoperative deep vein thrombosis, *Surgery* 87:69-76, 1980.

24. Caprini JA, Scurr JH, Hasty JH: The role of compression modalities in a prophylactic program for deep vein thrombosis, *Semin Thromb Hemostat* 14:77-87, 1988.

25. Handoll HH, Farrar MJ, McBirnie J et al: Heparin, low molecular-weight heparin, and physical methods for preventing deep vein thrombosis and pulmonary embolism following surgery for hip fractures, *Cochrane Database Syst Rev* (2):CD000305, 2000.

26. Muir KW, Watt A, Baxter G et al: Randomized trial of graded compression stockings for prevention of deep-vein thrombosis after acute stroke, *QJM* Jun;93(6): 359-364, 2000.

27. Amarigiri SV, Lees TA: Elastic compression stockings for prevention of deep vein thrombosis, *Cochrane Database Syst Rev* (3):CD001484, 2000.

28. Freedman KB, Brookenthal KR, Fitzgerald RH Jr et al: A meta-analysis of thromboembolic prophylaxis following elective total hip arthroplasty, *J Bone Joint Surg Am* Jul;82-A(7):929-938, 2000.

29. Westrich GH, Haas SB, Mosca P et al: Meta-analysis of thromboembolic prophylaxis after total knee arthroplasty, *J Bone Joint Surg Br* Aug;82(6):795-800, 2000.

30. Pidala MJ, Donovan DL, Kepley RF: A prospective study on intermittent pneumatic compression in the prevention of deep vein thrombosis in patients undergoing total hip or total knee replacement, *Surgery* 175:47-51, 1992.

31. Flam E, Berry S, Coyle A et al: Blood-flow augmentation of intermittent pneumatic compression systems used for the prevention of deep vein thrombosis before surgery, *Am J Surg* 171:312-315, 1996.

32. Tarnay TJ, Rohr PR, Davidson AG et al: Pneumatic calf compression, fibrinolysis, and the prevention of deep venous thrombosis, *Surgery* 88:489-495, 1980.

33. Knight MTN, Dawson R: Effect of intermittent compression of the arms on deep venous thrombosis in the legs, *Lancet* 2(7998):1265-1268, 1976.

34. Salzman EW, McManama GP, Shapiro AH et al: Effect of optimization of hemodynamics on fibrinolytic activity and antithrombotic efficacy of external calf compression, *Ann Surg* 206:636-641, 1987.

35. Chouhan VD, Comerota AJ, Sun L et al: Inhibition of tissue factor pathway during intermittent pneumatic compression: a possible mechanism for antithrombotic effect, *Arterioscler Thromb Vasc Biol* Nov;19(11): 2812-2817, 1999.

36. Homans J: The aetiology and treatment of varicose ulcers of the leg, *Surg Gynecol Obstet* 24:300-311, 1917.

37. Browse NL, Burnand KG: The cause of venous ulceration, *Lancet* 2:243-245, 1982.

38. McCulloch JM: Intermittent compression for the treatment of a chronic stasis ulceration, *Phys Ther* 61: 1452-1453, 1981.

39. Samson RH, Showalter DP: Stockings and the prevention of recurrent venous ulcers, *Dermatol Surg* Apr;22(4): 373-376, 1996.

40. Smith PC, Sarin S, Hasty J et al: Sequential gradient pneumatic compression enhances venous ulcer healing: a randomized trial, *Surgery* 108:871-875, 1990.

41. Kunimoto B, Cooling M, Gullinver W et al: Best practices for the prevention and treatment of venous leg ulcers, *Ostomy Wound Manage* Feb;47(2):34-46, 48-50, 2001.

42. Pekanmaki K, Kolari PJ, Kirstala U: Intermittent pneumatic compression treatment for post-thrombotic leg ulcers, *Clin Exp Dermatol* 12:350-353, 1987.

43. Coleridge Smith PD, Thomas PRS, Scurr JH et al: The aetiology of venous ulceration:a new hypothesis, *Br Med J* 296:1726-1728, 1988.

44. *The Jobst Extremity Pump: Clinical Applications with an Overview of the Pathophysiology of Edema.* Charlotte, NC, 1996, Beiersdorf-Jobst.

45. Deitch EA, Wheelahan TM, Rose MP et al: Hypertrophic burn scars: analysis of variables, *J Trauma* 23:895-898, 1983.

46. Hunt TK: Disorders of wound healing, *World J Surg* 4:271-277, 1980.

47. Sullivan T, Smith J, Kermode J et al: Rating the burn scar, *J Burn Care Rehabil* 11:256-260, 1990.

48. Ward RS: Pressure therapy for the control of hypertrophic scar formation after burn injury: a history and review, *J Burn Care Rehabil* 12:257-262, 1991.

49. Reno F, Grazianetti P, Cannas M: Effects of mechanical compression on hypertrophic scars: prostaglandin E2 release, *Burns* May;27(3):215-218, 2001.

50. Berman B, Flores F: The treatment of hypertrophic scars and keloids, *Eur J Dermatol* Dec;8(8):591-595, 1998.

51. Staley MJ, Richard RL. Use of pressure to treat hypertrophic burn scars, *Adv Wound Care* May-Jun;10(3):44-46, 1997.

52. Larson DL, Abston S, Evans EB et al: Techniques for decreasing scar formation and contractures in the burned patient, *J Trauma* 11:807-823, 1971.

53. Kircher CW, Shetlar MR, Shetlar CL: Alteration of hypertrophic scars induced by mechanical pressure, *Arch Dermatol* 111:60-64, 1975.

54. Brennan MJ, DePompolo RW, Garden FH: Focused review: postmastectomy lymphedema, *Arch Phys Med Rehabil* 77:S74-S80, 1996.

55. Reynolds JP: Lymphedema: an "orphan" disease, *PT Magazine* June:54-63, 1996.

56. McGrory BJ, Burke DW: Peroneal nerve palsy following intermittent sequential pneumatic compression, *Orthopedics* Oct;23(10):1103-1105, 2000.

57. Pittman GR: Peroneal nerve palsy following sequential pneumatic compression, *JAMA* 261:2201-2202, 1989.

58. Lachmann EA, Rook JL, Tunkel R et al: Complications associated with intermittent pneumatic compression, *Arch Phys Med Rehabil* 73(5):482-485, 1992.

59. Harris R: An introduction to manual lymphatic drainage: The Vodder Method, *Massage Ther J* 5:55-66, 1992.

60. Hiatt WR: Contemporary treatment of venous lower limb ulcers, *Angiology* 43(10):852-855, 1992.

61. Staudinger P: *Compression Step by Step*, Nuremberg, 1991, Beiersdorf Medical Bibliothek.
62. *The At-A-Glance Guide to Vascular Stockings*, Charlotte, NC, 1991, Jobst.
63. Benko T, Cooke EA, McNally MA et al: Graduated compression stockings: knee length or thigh length, *Clin Orthop* Feb;(383):197-203, 2001.
64. Samson RH: Compression stocking therapy for patients with chronic venous insufficiency, *J Cardiovasc Surg* 26:10, 1985.
65. McCulloch JM, Marler KC, Neal MB et al: Intermittent pneumatic compression improves venous ulcer healing, *Adv Wound Care* 7(4):22-24, 26, 1994.
66. Foldi M: Treatment of lymphedema, *NLN Newsletter* 7(3):1, 2, 6, 8, 1995.
67. Augustine E: *Lymphedema: the debate continues,* PT *Magazine* November:10-11, 1996.
68. Jacobs L: Lymphedema: the debate continues, *PT Magazine* November:11, 1996.
69. Swedborg I: Voluminometric estimation of the degree of lymphedema and its therapy by pneumatic compression, *Scand J Rehabil Med* 9:131-135, 1977.

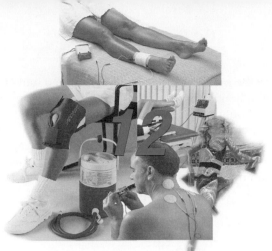

Electromagnetic Radiation

Michelle H. Cameron, PT, OCS, Diana Perez, BSc, PT, MSc, and
Suzana Otaño-Lata, MS

OBJECTIVES
Upon completion of this chapter, the reader will be able to:

1. Discuss the physical properties of electromagnetic radiation.
2. Classify the different ranges and types of electromagnetic radiation used therapeutically, including infrared, ultraviolet, cold lasers, shortwave, and microwave.
3. Identify the physiological effects of the different ranges of electromagnetic radiation.
4. Determine how the physical properties and physiological effects of electromagnetic radiation can promote particular treatment goals.
5. Assess the indications, contraindications, and precautions for the application of electromagnetic radiation of different frequency ranges with respect to different patient management situations.

6. Design methods for selecting the most appropriate electromagnetic radiation device and treatment parameters to produce desired physical and physiological effects.
7. Evaluate different electromagnetic radiation devices with respect to their potential to produce desired physical and physiological effects.

8. Presented with a clinical case, evaluate the clinical findings, propose goals of treatment, assess whether electromagnetic radiation would be the best treatment, and, if so, formulate an effective treatment plan including the appropriate device and treatment parameters for achieving the goals of treatment.

This chapter serves as an introduction to the application of electromagnetic radiation in rehabilitation. Physical agents that deliver energy in the form of electromagnetic radiation include various forms of visible and invisible light, and radiation in the shortwave and microwave ranges. There are a number of clinical devices that deliver electromagnetic energy, and a number of recommended or suggested applications for each; however, none of these devices are widely used by rehabilitation professionals in the United States.

Some are effective for the treatment of disorders not related to the musculoskeletal system and are therefore more commonly used by other health professionals. For example, ultraviolet radiation has proven beneficial in the treatment of many skin disorders and is therefore most frequently used by dermatologists. Others, such as cold lasers, have not yet received FDA approval for clinical application, and still others, such as diathermy, are unpopular due to the risks associated with their misuse and the lack of definitive information on their mechanisms of action.

Although electromagnetic agents are used in a limited manner at this time, since they all have been shown in the literature to have therapeutic benefits, they will be discussed in this chapter. It is valuable for the therapist to have a good understanding of these agents and their effects because they can be utilized to achieve improved clinical outcomes in appropriate patients. This chapter discusses the physical properties and physiological effects of electromagnetic radiation, and provides guidelines for clinical application and case studies describing the application of each type of electromagnetic radiation that may be used for rehabilitation in the United States.

PHYSICAL PROPERTIES OF ELECTROMAGNETIC RADIATION

Electromagnetic radiation is composed of electric and magnetic fields that vary over time and are oriented perpendicular to each other (Fig. 12-1). Electromagnetic radiation can propagate without the need of a medium. All living organisms are continuously exposed to electromagnetic radiation from both natural sources, such as the Earth's magnetic field and the ultraviolet radiation from the sun, and from manufactured sources such as domestic electrical appliances, computers, and power lines.

Electromagnetic radiation is categorized according to its frequency and wavelength, which are inversely proportional to each other (Fig. 12-2). Lower-frequency electromagnetic radiation, including extremely low

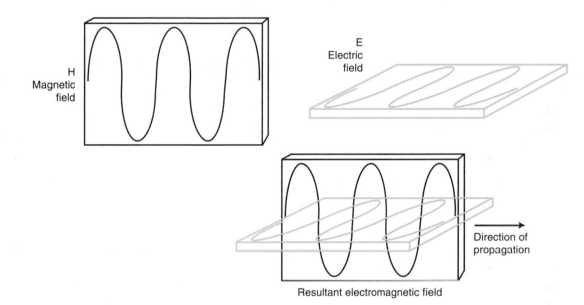

Figure 12-1. Perpendicular orientation of the electric and magnetic components of an electromagnetic field.

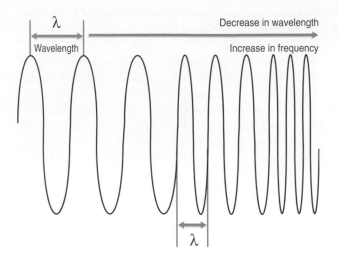

Figure 12-2. The frequency and wavelength of an electromagnetic wave are inversely related. As the frequency increases, the wavelength decreases.

frequency (ELF) waves, shortwaves, microwaves, infrared (IR) radiation, visible light, and ultraviolet A and B (UVA and UVB), is nonionizing and cannot break molecular bonds or produce ions, and can therefore be used for therapeutic medical applications. Higher-frequency electromagnetic radiation, such as x-rays and gamma rays, is ionizing and can break molecular bonds to form ions.[1,2] Ionizing radiation can also inhibit cell division and is therefore either not used clinically or used in very small doses for imaging or to destroy tissue. Approximate frequency ranges for the different types of radiation are shown in Fig. 12-3 and are stated in the sections concerning each type of radiation. Only approximate ranges are given because the reported values differ slightly among texts.[3] This chapter describes the basic physical properties, physiological effects, and clinical uses of ultraviolet radiation, lasers, continuous and pulsed shortwave diathermy, and microwave

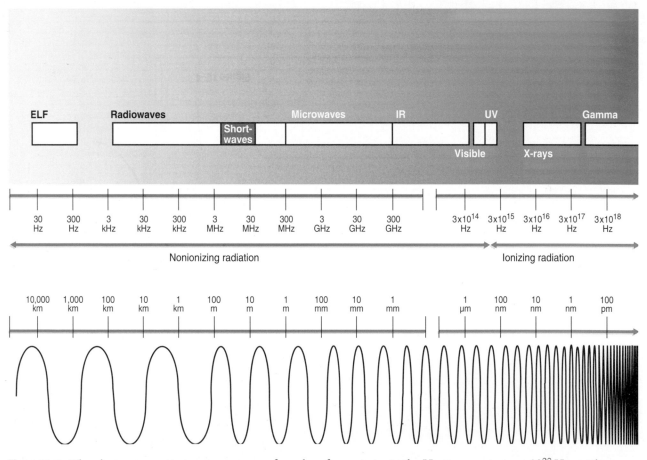

Figure 12-3. The electromagnetic spectrum ranges from low frequencies in the Hertz range to over 10^{23} Hz, with wavelengths varying from over 10,000 km to less than 1 picometer.

diathermy. Because IR radiation produces superficial heating, the clinical application of IR lamps is described in Chapter 6, together with other superficial heating agents.

The intensity of any type of electromagnetic radiation that reaches the patient from a radiation source, such as a UV lamp or a diathermy coil, is proportional to the energy output from the source, the inverse square of the distance of the source from the patient and to the cosine of the angle of incidence of the beam with the tissue. Thus the intensity reaching the skin is greatest when the radiation source is close to the patient and when the beam is perpendicular to the surface of the skin. As the distance from the skin or the angle with the surface increases, the intensity of the radiation reaching the skin will fall.

PHYSIOLOGICAL EFFECTS OF ELECTROMAGNETIC RADIATION

Electromagnetic radiation can affect biological systems via thermal and/or nonthermal mechanisms. Because IR radiation and both continuous shortwave and microwave diathermy can increase tissue temperature, they are thought to affect tissues primarily by thermal mechanisms. IR radiation heats superficial tissues, whereas shortwave and microwave continuous diathermy heat both superficial and deep tissues. The physiological and clinical effects of these thermal agents are generally the same as those of the superficial heating agents, as described in detail in Chapter 6, except that the tissues affected are different.

UV radiation and low levels of pulsed diathermy or laser light do not increase tissue temperature and are therefore thought to affect tissues by nonthermal mechanisms. It has been proposed that these types of electromagnetic energy cause changes at the cellular level by altering cell membrane function and permeability.[4] Nonthermal electromagnetic agents may promote binding of chemicals to the cell membrane to trigger complex sequences of cellular reactions. Because these agents could promote the initial steps in cellular function, this mechanism of action could explain the wide variety of stimulatory cellular effects that have been observed in response to the application of nonthermal levels of electromagnetic energy. Electromagnetic energy may also affect tissues by causing proteins to undergo conformational changes to promote active transport across cell membranes and to accelerate adenosine triphosphate (ATP) synthesis and use.[5]

Many have invoked the Arndt-Schulz law to explain the effects of low nonthermal levels of electromagnetic radiation (Fig. 12-4). According to this law, a certain minimum stimulus is needed to initiate a biological process. In addition, although a slightly stronger stimulus may produce greater effects, beyond a certain level, stronger stimuli will have a progressively less positive effect and at yet higher levels will become

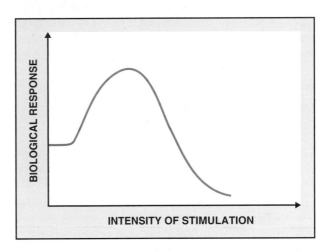

Figure 12-4. The Arndt-Schulz law.

inhibitory. This is demonstrated in many instances. For example, a low level of mechanical stress during childhood promotes normal bone growth; either too little or too much stress can result in abnormal growth or fractures. Similarly, with some forms of electromagnetic radiation such as diathermy, although too low a dose may not produce any effect, the optimal dose to achieve a desired physiological effect may be lower than that which produces heat. If excessive doses are used, tissue damage due to burning may result.

PHYSICAL PROPERTIES OF ULTRAVIOLET RADIATION

UV radiation is electromagnetic radiation with a frequency range of 7.5×10^{14} to over 10^{15} Hz and wavelengths from 400 nm to below 290 nm. UV radiation lies between x-ray and visible light (see Fig. 12-3). UV radiation is divided into three bands—*UVA, UVB,* and *UVC*—with wavelengths of 320 to 400, 290 to 320, and less than 290 nm, respectively. UVA, also known as long-wave UV, is nonionizing and produces fluorescence in many substances, while UVB, or middle-wave UV, which is also nonionizing, produces the most skin erythema. UVC, short-wave UV, is ionizing and germicidal. Because UV does not produce heat, it is thought to produce physiological effects by nonthermal mechanisms. The most significant source of UV radiation is the sun, which emits a broad spectrum of UV including UVA, UVB, and UVC. Both UVA and the UVB reach the earth from the sun; however, UVC is filtered out by the ozone layer.

The physiological effects of UV radiation are influenced not only by the wavelength of the radiation, but also by the intensity reaching the skin and the depth of penetration. The depth of penetration is affected by the intensity of radiation reaching the skin, the wavelength and power of the radiation source, the size of the area being treated, the thickness and pigmentation of the skin, and the duration of treatment. The intensity of UV radiation reaching the skin is proportional to the power of the output of the lamp, the inverse square of the distance of the lamp from the patient, and the cosine of the angle of incidence of the beam with the tissue. Thus the intensity reaching the skin is greatest when a high-power lamp is used, when the lamp is close to the patient, and when the radiation beam is perpendicular to the surface of the skin. Penetration is deepest for UV radiation with the highest intensity, longest wavelength, and lowest frequency. Thus UVA penetrates farthest and reaches through several millimeters of skin, while UVB and UVC penetrate less deeply and are almost entirely absorbed in the superficial epidermal layers. The penetration of UV radiation is also less deep if the skin is thicker or darker.[6,7]

EFFECTS OF ULTRAVIOLET RADIATION

Erythema production
   Tanning
   Epidermal hyperplasia
Vitamin D synthesis
   Other effects of ultraviolet radiation

UV radiation has been shown to cause skin erythema, tanning, epidermal hyperplasia, and vitamin D synthesis. It is thought that these effects are the result of absorption of electromagnetic energy by the cells of exposed tissue, causing chemical excitation and facilitation of photobiological processes.

Erythema Production

Erythema, or redness of the skin due to dilation of the superficial blood vessels caused by the release of histamines, is one of the most common and most obvious effects of exposure to UV radiation.[8] Erythema is produced primarily in response to UVB exposure or in response to UVA exposure after drug sensitization. Without drug sensitization, UVA is 100 to 1000 times less potent in inducing erythema than UVB. With sensitization, the erythemal efficacy of UVA is similar to that of UVB alone, with less risk of overexposure or burning. The precise mechanism of UV-induced erythema is unknown; however, it is known that this effect is mediated by prostaglandin release from the epidermis, and it may also be related to the DNA-damaging effects of UV radiation. The severity of erythema, which can produce blistering, tissue burning, and pain, and the risk of cell damage are the primary factors limiting the frequency and intensity of UV exposure used clinically.

Tanning

Tanning, a delayed pigmentation of the skin, also occurs in response to UV radiation exposure. This effect is the result of increased production and upward migration of melanin granules and oxidation of premelanin in the skin.[9,10] Because the darkening of skin pigmentation that occurs with tanning reduces the penetration of UV to deeper tissue layers, it is thought that tanning is a protective response of the body.

Epidermal hyperplasia

Epidermal hyperplasia, a thickening of the superficial layer of the skin, occurs approximately 72 hours after exposure to UV radiation and, with repeated exposure, eventually results in thickening of both the epidermis and the stratum corneum that persists for several weeks. This effect is thought to be caused by the release of prostaglandin precursors leading to increased DNA synthesis by epidermal cells, resulting in increased epithelial cell turnover and cellular hyperplasia.[11] Epidermal hyperplasia is most pronounced in response to UVB exposure. It is also thought to occur in order to protect the skin from excessive UV exposure.

Because tanning and epidermal hyperplasia impair UV penetration, progressively higher doses of UV radiation are generally required during a course of clinical treatment with UV.

Vitamin D synthesis

UV irradiation of the skin is necessary for the conversion of ingested provitamin D to vitamin D.[12,13] Because vitamin D acts to control calcium absorption and exchange, it is an essential vitamin for bone formation; it also influences brain, kidney, intestine, and endocrine function. Vitamin D deficiency can result in poor intestinal absorption of calcium and can cause rickets, a disease characterized by failure of bone mineralization. Rickets can be the result of inadequate exposure to UV radiation, inadequate intake of provitamins, or poor kidney function. Although for most individuals the exposure to UV in sunlight is sufficient to maintain adequate levels of vitamin D production, UV exposure may be inadequate in bedridden patients or in those who work for long hours in underground environments.

Other effects of ultraviolet radiation

UVB radiation has been shown to affect the immune system, causing depression of contact sensitivity, changes in the distribution of circulating lymphocytes, and suppression of mast cell-mediated whealing.[14-16] It is proposed that these effects are dose dependent, such that with low doses the immune response is suppressed and with higher doses the immune response is activated. Recently UVA has also been shown to inhibit cyclooxygenase 2 expression and prostaglandin E2 production.[17] This mechanism is thought to underlie the beneficial effects of psoralen with ultraviolet A (PUVA) in the treatment of scleroderma. It has also been reported that UVC, in adequate doses, is bactericidal.[18]

CLINICAL INDICATIONS FOR THE USE OF ULTRAVIOLET RADIATION

Psoriasis
Wound healing

The earliest modern clinical use of UV radiation, for which Neils Finsen was awarded the Nobel Prize in 1903, was for the treatment of cutaneous tuberculosis. In the 1920s and 1930s the use of UV radiation for the treatment of skin disorders, including psoriasis, acne, and alopecia, was very popular; however, with the advent of antibiotics and other medications, the role of UV radiation in dermatological medicine has been reduced. At this time, UV radiation is used primarily in the treatment of psoriasis, and there are also recent reports of UV therapy being used for the treatment of scleroderma, eczema, atopic dermatitis, mycosis fungoides and vitiligo.[17,19] These treatments may be applied in conjunction with the use of photosensitizing drugs. UV is also used occasionally as a component of the treatment of chronic open wounds.[19-22] Although the clinical application of UV radiation for the treatment of skin disorders is within the scope of physical therapy, such treatments are generally provided by dermatologists or their assistants. Treatment of chronic wounds with UV radiation, however, generally is performed by a physical therapist.

UVB alone, or UVA in conjunction with psoralen sensitization, known as *PUVA,* may be used for the treatment of psoriasis and other skin disorders, including eczema, acne, pityriasis lichenoides, pruritus, and polymorphic light eruption.[23-25] PUVA or UVA radiation alone is also used for the treatment of vitiligo, eczema, urticaria, lichen planus, graft-versus-host disease, cutaneous T-cell lymphoma, urticaria pigmentosa, and a variety of photosensitive disorders.[26,27] Clinical recommendations for the treatment of psoriasis are given below, and recommendations for the treatment of other skin disorders are available in the literature.[28,29] Clinical protocols for the treatment of other disorders should be developed and agreed upon in conjunction with the referring physician.

Psoriasis

Psoriasis is a common benign, acute, or chronic inflammatory skin disease that appears to be based on genetic predisposition. It is characterized by bright red plaques with silvery scales, usually on the knees, elbows, and scalp, and is associated with mild itching (Fig. 12-5). These dermatological symptoms may also be associated with arthritic symptoms known as *psoriatic arthritis.*

There are numerous reports of successful treatment of psoriasis with UV radiation alone or in conjunction with sensitizing drugs.[25,30-34] Phototherapy of psoriasis with UV has a history of more than 75 years: in 1925, Goeckerman introduced a combination of topical crude coal tar and subsequent UV irradiation. This treatment became a standard therapy for psoriasis for half a century. The therapeutic efficacy of UV radiation in the treatment of this condition is thought to be due to its ability to inactivate cell division and inhibit the DNA synthesis and mitosis of hyperproliferating epidermal cells that are characteristic of psoriasis.[25] Other proposed mechanisms

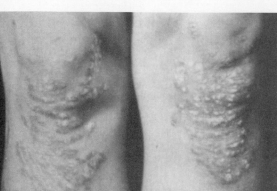

Figure 12-5. Psoriatic plaques. (From Arndt KA et al: *Cutaneous Medicine and Surgery: An Integrated Program in Dermatology,* vol 1, Philadelphia, 1996, WB Saunders. Used with permission.)

include altered leukocyte behavior and immunological activity, altered prostaglandin and cytokine release, as well as effects on cell metabolic function. The precise cellular targets and effector mechanisms of phototherapy have not yet been determined.

Psoriasis is most responsive to UVA administered in conjunction with oral or topical psoralen sensitization (PUVA) and is almost as responsive to narrow band UVB alone, at a wavelength of 311 ± 2 nm.[23,35,36] Psoriasis is not responsive to UVC radiation and is minimally responsive to UVA radiation without drug sensitization. Use of UVA alone is also not recommended because the dose that does effectively clear psoriatic plaques also causes severe erythema, pigmentation, and an increased risk of melanoma.[37]

The use of UV sensitizers in conjunction with UV radiation for treatment of psoriasis has been studied extensively. The most commonly used sensitizers were tar-based topicals and psoralen-derived drugs. However, since studies on the use of tar-based derivatives in conjunction with UV radiation in the management of psoriasis have yielded mixed results, with some reporting that these products are valuable adjuncts to treatment and others reporting that tar-based products are no more effective than simple oil-based ointments, the use of tar-based products has lapsed and psoralen-derived drugs are now the product of choice for this application.[38,39] The fact that tar-based products are messy and expensive also limits their popularity.

In recent years, the use of psoralen-based topical and systemic drugs in conjunction with UVA (PUVA)

for the treatment of psoriasis has grown in popularity. This treatment combination was first described by Tronnier and Schule in 1972 and has since been shown to be effective by a number of other researchers.[40] It is thought that psoralen reduces appearance of psoriatic plaques because, when activated by UVA, it causes cross-links to form between adjacent strands of DNA, thus interfering with cell replication and preventing the excessive cell proliferation characteristic of psoriasis.

PUVA treatment has a number of side effects, including epidermal pigmentation and hyperplasia, immune suppression, and the release of free radicals. Free radicals can damage cell membranes and cytoplasmic structures. Psoralens alone have also been found to be carcinogenic. Therefore, work is in progress to search for safer alternative sensitizers. Although acitretin, corticosteroids, and fish oil have been evaluated for this application, there is insufficient evidence at this time to support the use of these UV sensitizers for the treatment of psoriasis.[41-43]

Refer to specific information on contraindications and precautions in the boxes that follow.

Wound Healing

UV is only occasionally used as a component of the treatment of chronic wounds. However, unlike ultrasound and electrical stimulation, most authors state that UV does not have sufficient evidence at this time to support its use for this application.[44] When UV is used for wound treatment, UVC is the frequency band most commonly chosen.[20,21] This frequency band is selected because it enhances epithelialization, destroys bacteria, causes minimal erythema or tanning, has a low carcinogenic effect, and is absorbed almost equally by all skin colors.[45] UV radiation is thought to facilitate wound healing by increasing epithelial cell turnover, causing epidermal cell hyperplasia,[20] accelerating granulation tissue formation, increasing blood flow,[46] killing bacteria,[18] increasing vitamin D production by the skin, and promoting sloughing of necrotic tissue.[47] Although the data on the efficacy of UVC for this application are mixed, with some studies reporting faster or more complete healing with the addition of UVC to their treatment protocol for wounds and others reporting no significant benefit, since this physical agent has proven to be beneficial in some cases, it may be appropriate to consider adding UVC to the treatment of wounds that have not responded to, or are inappropriate for, other types of treatment.[48]

CONTRAINDICATIONS
for the Use of Ultraviolet Radiation

- Irradiation of the eyes
- Skin cancer
- Pulmonary tuberculosis

- Cardiac, kidney, or liver disease
- Systemic lupus erythematosus
- Fever

The application of ultraviolet radiation is contraindicated . . .

. . . to the eyes

UV irradiation of the eyes should be avoided because it can damage the cornea, the eyelids, or the lens. Exposure of the eyes can be avoided by having the patient wear UV-opaque goggles throughout treatment and by having the therapist wear UV opaque goggles when at risk of irradiation, such as when turning the UV lamp on or off. Patients taking UV sensitizing drugs such as psoralens should continue to wear UV opaque eye protection for 12 hours after taking these drugs.

. . . with patients with skin cancer; pulmonary tuberculosis; cardiac, kidney, or liver disease; systemic lupus erythematosus; or fever

UV radiation should not be applied to areas where skin cancer is present because it is known to be carcinogenic.[49] For details of the carcinogenic effects of UV radiation, please see the section below on adverse effects. It is generally recommended that UV radiation not be used in patients with pulmonary tuberculosis; cardiac, kidney, or liver disease; systemic lupus erythematosus; or fever, because these conditions may be exacerbated by exposure to UV radiation.

PRECAUTIONS
for the Use of Ultraviolet Radiation

- Photosensitizing medication use
- Photosensitivity

- Recent x-ray therapy
- No dose of UV radiation should be repeated until the effects of the previous dose have disappeared

Use ultraviolet radiation with caution . . .

. . . with patients using photosensitizing medication

Care should be taken when applying UV radiation to patients who are taking photosensitizing medications. These medications include sulfonamide, tetracycline, and quinolone antibiotics; gold-based medications used for the treatment of rheumatoid arthritis; amiodarone hydrochloride and quinidines used for the treatment of cardiac arrhythmias; phenothiazines used for the treatment of anxiety; and psoralens used for the treatment of psoriasis. While patients are taking these medications, they have increased sensitivity to UV radiation, resulting in a decrease in the minimal erythemal dose and an increased risk of burning if too high a dose is used. A patient's minimal erythemal dose must also be remeasured if the patient starts to take a photosensitizing medication during a course of UV treatment.

. . . with photosensitive patients

Some individuals, particularly those with fair skin and hair coloring and those with red hair, are particularly sensitive to UV exposure. Because these individuals have an accelerated and exaggerated skin response to UV radiation, low levels of UV radiation should be used both when determining the minimal erythemal dose and for treatment.

Continued

PRECAUTIONS—cont'd

. . . with patients who have had recent x-ray radiation treatment

It is recommended that UV radiation be applied with caution to areas that have had recent x-ray radiation exposure because the skin in these areas may be more susceptible to the development of malignancies.

. . . until the effects of the prior dose have disappeared

In order to minimize the risk of burns or an excessive erythemal response, UV irradiation should not be repeated until the erythemal effects of the previous dose have disappeared.

ADVERSE EFFECTS OF ULTRAVIOLET RADIATION[25,50]

Burning
Premature aging of skin
Carcinogenesis
Eye damage
Adverse effects of PUVA

Burning

Burning by UV radiation will occur if too high a dose is used. Burning can usually be avoided by careful assessment of the minimal erythemal dose prior to initiating treatment and by avoiding further exposure when signs of erythema from a prior dose are still present.

Premature Aging of Skin

Chronic exposure to UV radiation, including sunlight, is associated with premature aging of the skin. This effect, known as *actinic damage,* causes the skin to have a dry, coarse, leathery appearance with wrinkling and pigment abnormalities. It is thought that these changes are primarily due to the collagen degeneration that accompanies long-term exposure to UV radiation.

Carcinogenesis

Most of the information regarding the carcinogenic effect of UV radiation concerns the effect of prolonged and/or intense sunlight exposure. Prolonged exposure to UV radiation, as occurs with excessive exposure to sunlight, is considered to be a major risk factor for the development of basal cell and squamous cell carcinoma and malignant melanoma. A recent review of the literature on the carcinogenicity of UV phototherapy, with and without psoralens, concluded that the therapeutic use of UVB has a low risk of producing cutaneous cancers, except possibly on the skin of the male genitals; however, there is a definite cutaneous carcinogenic risk from PUVA treatment when oral systemic psoralens medications are used.[51,52] The increased cancer risk with PUVA may be due to the carcinogenicity of the psoralens or may be a response specific to the wavelength of UV radiation used for this treatment application. PUVA treatments may also exacerbate the effects of previous exposure to carcinogens.[49]

Because of the potential cumulative adverse effects of repeated low-level exposure to UV radiation, it is recommended that clinicians avoid frequent or excessive exposure during treatment. This can be achieved by wearing UV-opaque goggles and UV opaque clothing.

Eye Damage

UV irradiation of the eyes can cause a number of eye problems including photokeratitis, conjunctivitis, and possibly some forms of cataracts.[53] Photokeratitis and conjunctivitis can occur acutely after exposure to UVB or UVC. The symptoms of photokeratitis, an inflammation of the cornea that can be extremely painful, generally appear 6 to 12 hours after UV exposure and resolve fully within 2 days, without permanent or long-term damage. Conjunctivitis, an inflammation of the insides of the eyelids and the membrane that covers the cornea, results in a sensation of gritty eyes and varying degrees of photophobia, tearing, and blepharospasm. Chronic UVA and UVB exposure have been associated with the development of cataracts, characterized by a loss of transparency of the lens or lens capsule of the eye. This association is even stronger for PUVA because psoralens are deposited in the lens of the eye.

Because of the risks of eye irritation or damage, UV opaque eye protection should always be worn by the patient and the clinician during UV treatment. Patients should also wear UV-opaque eye protection for 12 hours after psoralen administration in order to protect their eyes from sunlight exposure.

Adverse Effects of PUVA

PUVA is associated with all the adverse effects of UV radiation, as described previously. It is also associated with short-term nausea and vomiting, which lasts for 1 to 4 hours after ingestion of the psoralen. Prolonged high-dose PUVA therapy can also result in skin damage, including small, hyperpigmented, nonmalignant lesions, keratotic lesions that may have premalignant histological characteristics, and squamous cell carcinomas.[54]

APPLICATION TECHNIQUES

When applying UV radiation for therapeutic purposes, one must first determine the individual patient's sensitivity to UV radiation.[55] This varies widely among individuals and can be affected by skin pigmentation, age, prior exposure to UV radiation, and use of sensitizing medications. For example, even for Caucasians, there can be a four- to sixfold variation in minimal erythemal dose.[7] Sensitivity to UV radiation is assessed using the dosimetry procedure described below.

Because the response to UV radiation can vary significantly with even slightly different frequencies of radiation, the same lamp must be used for assessing an individual's sensitivity and for all subsequent treatments. For example, the skin is 100 times more sensitive to UV with a wavelength of 300 nm than to UV with a wavelength of 320 nm. If the lamp must be changed, the individual's response to the new lamp must be assessed before it is used for treatment. Reassessment is also necessary if there is a long gap between treatments because lamp output intensity decreases with prolonged use and skin tanning and hyperplasia decreases over prolonged periods.

Once the individual's responsiveness to a particular UV lamp has been determined, the treatment dose can be selected to produce the desired erythemal response.

Dose-Response Assessment

The UV dose is graded according to the individual's erythemal response and is categorized as *suberythemal, minimal erythemal,* or *first-, second-,* or *third-degree erythemal,* as described following.[56]

- *Suberythemal dose* (SED): No change in skin redness occurs in the 24 hours following UV exposure.
- *Minimal erythemal dose* (MED): The smallest dose producing erythema within 8 hours after exposure that disappears within 24 hours after exposure.
- *First-degree erythema* (E_1): Definite redness with some mild desquamation appears within 6 hours after exposure and lasts for 1 to 3 days. This dose is generally about 2½ times the MED.
- *Second-degree erythema* (E_2): Intense erythema with edema, peeling, and pigmentation appears within 2 hours or less after treatment and is like a severe sunburn. This dose is generally about 5 times the MED.
- *Third-degree erythema* (E_3): Erythema with severe blistering, peeling, and exudation. This dose is generally about 10 times the MED.

In general, treatment time is selected as a proportion of the MED. The MED for an individual is determined in the manner described below. Because repeated exposure to UV radiation generally decreases sensitivity to UV, prior exposure should also be taken into account when determining UV treatment dosage parameters.

Since people build up a tolerance to UV radiation with repeated exposure due to darkening of the skin with tanning and thickening of the skin by epidermal hyperplasia, their MED will also increase. Thus to maintain effective treatment with a consistent proportion of the MED, either the exposure time should be increased or the distance of the lamp from the skin should be decreased with repeated treatments. Exposure time should be increased between 35% and 50% at each treatment, with a maximum of 5 minutes total exposure if possible. If exposure for more than 5 minutes is needed to produce an MED, since the intensity of the radiation reaching the patient increases as the lamp gets closer to the patient, the effective dose can be increased by moving the lamp rather than by increasing the treatment time. For example, the distance of the lamp from the patient can be halved to increase the intensity of radiation reaching the patient by a factor of 4. If the patient is receiving whole body exposure in a cabinet, where the distance between the lamps and the patient cannot be changed, then the treatment time must be adjusted to produce the desired erythemal response.

Once an individual's MED for a particular lamp has been determined, the treatment dose is set according to the disease being treated and the protocol being used. Guidelines for treatment of psoriasis with UVB or with PUVA are given in the following section. Guidelines for the treatment of other problems with UV can be obtained from the lamp manufacturers or from some texts focusing on the treatment of the particular problem or disease.

APPLICATION TECHNIQUE
How to Determine the MED of UV for an Individual

1. Place UV-opaque goggles on the patient and the clinician.
2. Remove all clothing and jewelry from, and wash, an area of the body least exposed to natural sunlight. The areas usually used are the volar forearm, the abdomen, or the buttocks.
3. Take a piece of cardboard approximately 4 by 20 cm and cut four square holes 2 by 2 cm in it.
4. Place the cardboard on the test area and drape the area around the cardboard so that the surrounding skin will not be exposed to the radiation.
5. Set up the lamp 60 to 80 cm away from, and perpendicular to, the area to be exposed. Measure and record the distance of the lamp from the area to be exposed.
6. Cover all but one of the holes in the cardboard.
7. Turn on the lamp. If using an arc lamp, allow the lamp to warm up for 5 to 10 minutes to reach full power before turning it toward the patient. A fluorescent lamp will reach full power and can be used within 1 minute of being turned on.
8. Once the lamp has reached full power, direct the beam directly toward the area to be exposed and start the timer.
9. After 120 seconds, uncover the second hole.
10. After another 60 seconds, uncover the third hole.
11. After another 30 seconds, uncover the fourth hole.
12. After another 30 seconds, turn off the lamp.
    According to this protocol, the first window will have been exposed for 240 seconds, the sec-

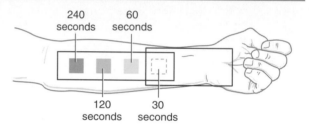

Figure 12-6. Setup for UV sensitivity assessment.

ond for 120 seconds, the third for 60 seconds, and the fourth for 30 seconds (Fig. 12-6). This protocol can be adjusted according to the individual's self-reported tanning and burning response to sunlight. For individuals who tan but never or rarely burn, longer exposures can be used, whereas for those who burn easily but do not tan, or for those taking photosensitizing drugs, shorter exposures are recommended. More holes with shorter time differences between exposures can also be used to increase the accuracy of the dose sensitivity assessment. For example, there could be eight holes in the cardboard, and one hole could be exposed every 10 seconds.

13. The patient should observe the area for the 24 hours following exposure. The area that shows mild reddening of the skin within 8 hours that disappears within 24 hours was treated with the MED.

APPLICATION TECHNIQUE
Treatment Setup for UVB or PUVA Treatment

The treatment setups for UVB and PUVA treatment are the same, except that for PUVA treatment the radiation is applied after psoralen sensitization.

1. Place UV opaque goggles on the patient and the clinician.
2. Remove clothing and jewelry from the area to be treated.
3. Wash and dry the area to be treated.
4. Cover all areas *not* needing treatment, which may otherwise be exposed to the radiation, with a UV-opaque material such as a cloth or paper towel.
5. Position the area to be exposed comfortably. Adjust the position of the lamp and/or the patient so that the distance between the lamp and the area to be exposed is the same as it was when the MED was determined. Also adjust the lamp to have the UV beam as perpendicular to the treatment area as possible. Measure and record the distance of the lamp from the patient.
6. Warm up the lamp if necessary. If using an arc lamp, allow the lamp to warm up for several minutes so that it reaches full power before being used. A fluorescent lamp will reach full power within 1 minute of being switched on. If there is a glass filter on the lamp, the lamp should be run for about 20 minutes before being used for treatment in order for the filter to reach thermal equilibrium.
7. Stay close to the patient, or give the patient a bell to call you and a means to turn off the lamp. Also, provide the patient with a means to open the cabinet if whole body treatment is being given.
8. Set the timer.
9. When the treatment is complete, observe the treated area, and document the treatment given and any observable response to the treatment.

Dosimetry for the Treatment of Psoriasis with UV Radiation

Using UVB

Initial dose recommendations for the treatment of psoriasis vary from 50% of the MED to an E_1 dose (about 2½ times the MED), with increases of 10% to 40% at each treatment, depending on the skin response.[25,57] Treatment is given once or twice a day, once the erythema from the prior dose resolves, and is terminated when the plaques clear. Plaque clearance may take several weeks. Treatment may be continued for a few sessions after complete clearance of the plaques in order to increase the period of remission, and some clinicians continue with less frequent maintenance therapy with the goal of keeping the patient symptom free.[58] If severe, painful erythema with blistering develops at any time, the treatment should be stopped until these signs clear and a lower UV dose should be used when treatment is resumed.

Using PUVA

When providing PUVA treatments using oral psoralens, the UV irradiation is usually applied 2 hours after ingestion of the drug. When the psoralen is delivered topically, the UV exposure is provided immediately after the patient has soaked in a bath of weak psoralen solution for 15 minutes. Topical delivery of psoralens is less common than oral administration, although this route of drug delivery is associated with fewer acute side effects and may result in a longer period of remission after therapy.[59] Erythema in response to PUVA has a delayed onset compared with UVB-induced erythema and at first usually appears 24 to 48 hours after the exposure and peaks 72 hours after the exposure. PUVA-induced erythema also differs from erythema induced by UV alone in that even 2 to 3 times the MED causes only a slightly greater effect. PUVA treatments are usually given 2 or 3 times a week to allow time for the erythema of one treatment to resolve before the next treatment is applied. The treatment dose is determined by assessing the MED after the patient has taken the psoralen. Treatment is generally applied to the whole body, and is usually started at 40% to 70% of the MED and increased by 10% to 40% each week in order to maintain the response. Complete clearance usually takes about 6 weeks, although there is much variation among individuals.

DOCUMENTATION

Document the area of the body treated, the type of UV radiation used, the serial number of the lamp, the distance of the lamp from the patient, the treatment duration, and the response to treatment.

Example

UV-B to R forearm, lamp #6555, 60 cm from pt, 4 minutes.
Outcome: Mild erythema 6 hours after exposure lasted for 24 hours. Psoriatic plaques 50% resolved.

SELECTING A UV LAMP

A number of different lamps that output UV radiation at different ranges in the UV spectrum and use different technology to produce the radiation are currently available in the United States (Fig. 12-7). The output ranges include broad-spectrum UVA with wavelengths of 320 to 400 nm, wide band (250 to 320 nm) and narrow band (311 to 312 nm) UVB, and UVC with wavelengths of 200 to 290 nm with a peak at 250 nm. The lamps can be of the arc or fluorescent type. Arc lamps are generally small and emit radiation of a consistent intensity, whereas fluorescent lamps are long and emit higher-intensity radiation in the middle than at the ends.[60] Single arc lamps are recommended for treating small areas such as the hand, and units incorporating an array of arc lamps are recommended for treatment of larger areas. Fluorescent tubes are generally not recommended because of the variability of intensity along their length. Ideally, a lamp that produces a narrow band of radiation and provides uniform treatment of the area within a reasonable amount of time should be selected.

UV Lamp Maintenance

Lamp surfaces should be cleaned regularly to remove dust, which will attenuate the radiation. Lamps

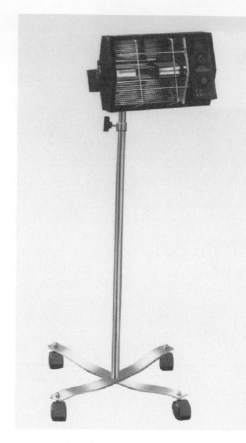

Figure 12-7. A UV lamp. (Courtesy Brandt Industries, Inc., Bronx, NY.)

should be replaced when their intensity decreases to the point where treatment times become unacceptably long. The useful lifetime of most UV lamps is between 500 and 1000 hours; afterward, the output falls by about 20% compared with the initial output.

▶ *Clinical Case Study* ◀

The following case study summarizes some of the concepts of ultraviolet radiation discussed in this chapter. Based on the scenario presented, an evaluation of the clinical findings and goals of treatment are proposed. These are followed by a discussion of the factors to be considered in treatment selection.

FR is a 25-year-old female with psoriasis. She has had this disease for about 8 years and has been successfully treated with PUVA in the past. Prior courses of treatment have generally taken about 6 weeks and have resulted in clearance of plaques for 6 months, with a gradual recurrence thereafter. Her last course of PUVA treatments was completed 1 year ago, and she now has plaques covering areas approximately 4 by 8 cm on the dorsal aspects of both elbows and covering areas approximately 5 by 7 cm on the anterior aspects of both knees. She complains that these areas itch and are unsightly, and that she therefore always wears clothing that covers her elbows and knees when in public.

EVALUATION OF THE CLINICAL FINDINGS

This patient presents with impairments of skin integrity and cosmesis, as well as the abnormal, uncomfortable sensation of itching. The poor cosmesis has resulted in her always wearing clothing that covers her elbows and knees.

PREFERRED PRACTICE PATTERN

Impaired Integumentary Integrity Associated With Superficial Skin Involvement, (7B)

PLAN OF CARE

The goals of treatment at this time include complete clearing of the psoriatic plaques and a return to a feeling of comfort when wearing clothes that expose the patient's elbows and/or knees.

ASSESSMENT REGARDING THE APPROPRIATENESS OF UV RADIATION AS THE OPTIMAL TREATMENT

UVB and UVA in conjunction with psoralen sensitization are indicated treatments for psoriasis and have been shown to result in the temporary clearance of psoriatic plaques.

PROPOSED TREATMENT PLAN AND RATIONALE

Although both UVB and PUVA have been found to be effective for the treatment of psoriasis, the use of PUVA is recommended for this patient because this treatment has produced good results for her in the past and because the risk of burning with PUVA treatment is less than that with UVB. The use of UVB may be considered because of the carcinogenic nature of psoralens and treatment with PUVA.

In order to provide treatment with PUVA, FR's skin sensitivity to UV radiation should first be assessed. Sensitivity testing should be carried out approximately 2 hours after the patient has taken oral psoralen and should be conducted using the same lamp that will be used for treatment. Because FR has a number of areas with plaques, treatment should be provided in a UV cabinet and the areas without plaques should be covered. Alternatively, a single lamp could be used to treat each of the four involved areas sequentially. Once FR's sensitivity to UV radiation while taking psoralen has been determined, treatment with 40% to 70% of her MED, increasing by 10% to 40% each week, applied 2 or 3 times per week, is recommended. This treatment regimen should be continued until complete clearance has been achieved, and possibly for a few more sessions in order to increase the period of remission. After treatment with PUVA has been completed, the patient should be encouraged to wear clothes that expose her elbows and knees because the UV radiation in sunlight may help to control her psoriasis; however, she should try to avoid exposing her skin to sunlight during the period of PUVA treatment since this would increase her UV exposure and thus increase her risk of burning.

PHYSICAL PROPERTIES OF LASERS

The term *laser* is an acronym for light amplification by stimulated emission of radiation (LASER). Although Albert Einstein originally outlined the principles underlying the production of laser light at the beginning of this century, the first laser was produced by Theodore Maiman in 1960. Laser light is produced when an electron of an active medium undergoes a stimulated quantum jump from a higher to a lower energy state, causing the emission of photons. The emitted photons collide with other excited electrons, causing more photon emission. This chain reaction produces laser light with a frequency characteristic of the active medium. For example, a helium-neon (He-Ne) laser emits visible red light with a wavelength of 633 nm, whereas a gallium-arsenide (Ga-As) laser emits IR radiation with a wavelength of 830 nm.

The difference between laser light and other light is that laser light is *monochromatic, coherent,* and *directional*. Monochromatic light is all of the same frequency; thus, if it is within the visible range, it is all of one color. Because it is coherent, all the waves are in phase with each other (Fig. 12-8), and because it is directional, a laser beam exhibits minimal divergence (Fig. 12-9).

The frequency of the laser light, as well as the type of tissue being irradiated, determines the depth to which the light penetrates. Laser light with wavelengths of between 600 and 1300 nm optimizes the depth of penetration in human tissue, at 1 to 4 mm, and is therefore most commonly used in the clinical setting.[61,62] For example, almost 99% of laser light with wavelengths of 300 to 1000 nm is absorbed in the superficial 3.6 mm of tissue, which is usually composed of skin.[63,64] Laser light with a longer

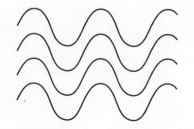

Figure 12-8. Coherent waves produced by a laser.

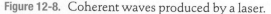

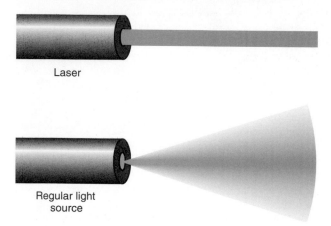

Figure 12-9. Directional light produced by a laser, in contrast to the divergent light produced by other sources.

wavelength and lower frequency, such as the IR produced by the Ga-As laser, penetrates deeper, whereas laser light with a shorter wavelength and higher frequency, such as the red light produced by the HeNe laser, penetrates less deeply. Although all frequencies of laser light penetrate only a few millimeters, deeper physiological effects are thought to occur because the energy may promote chemical reactions that mediate processes distant from the site of application.

Laser intensity can be expressed in terms of power, measured in Watts; power density, measured in watts per centimeter squared (W/cm²); or energy density, measured in Joules per centimeter squared (J/cm²).

$$\text{Power density (W/cm}^2\text{)} = \frac{\text{Power (W)}}{\text{Area of irradiation (cm}^2\text{)}}$$

$$\text{Energy density (J/cm}^2\text{)} = \frac{\text{Power (W)} \times \text{Time (s)}}{\text{Area of irradiation (cm}^2\text{)}}$$

The intensity of the laser alters its clinical effects. High-intensity "hot" lasers heat and destroy tissue, and, since the laser light is absorbed selectively by chromophores (light-absorbing materials) within the skin, it generates heat in and destroys only the selected tissue directly in the beam while avoiding damage to surrounding tissues.[65] Hot lasers are used clinically to make incisions and to cauterize during surgical procedures. They have a number of advantages over traditional surgical implements: the beam is sterile, allows fine control, cauterizes as it cuts, and results in less scarring. Because hot lasers destroy tissue, they are not used for rehabilitation.

Low-intensity "cold" lasers (Fig. 12-10), which output laser light with less than 500 mW power, generally at around 50 mW/cm² power density and with an energy density of less than 35 J/cm², have been studied and recommended for use in rehabilitation because there is evidence that this form of electromagnetic energy may be biostimulative and facilitate healing.[66,67] In general, lower-energy density ranges of between 0.05 and 1 J/cm² have been recommended for the treatment of acute conditions, whereas higher dosages of up to 40 J/cm² have been recommended for the treatment of chronic conditions.[66] Some studies have also found that the effects of the laser are more pronounced with short-duration, high-power doses than with long-duration, low-power doses delivering the same total amount of energy.[68]

The use of cold lasers as a component of rehabilitation first became popular in Eastern Europe[69] and Asia and has since also become common in Europe and Canada; however, the FDA has not yet approved the use of cold laser therapy because of insufficient validation of its clinical efficacy. The FDA considers the animal and cell culture studies to be inconclusive and the controlled clinical studies to be too few and not adequately replicated. The FDA, however, has granted an investigational device exemption for the gallium-aluminum-arsenide (GaAlAs) low-level laser for treating soft tissue injuries and, should further research support the efficacy of cold lasers, it is possible that the FDA will approve their clinical application for rehabilitation. Given the restrictions on the clinical application of cold lasers at this time, only their physiological effects and clinical indications and contraindications are discussed in this book. For a more complete discussion on the clinical application of cold lasers, including specific application techniques, case studies, and directions for selecting a device, the reader should consult a Canadian or European text that covers this subject or read the materials provided by the manufacturers of these devices.[70,71]

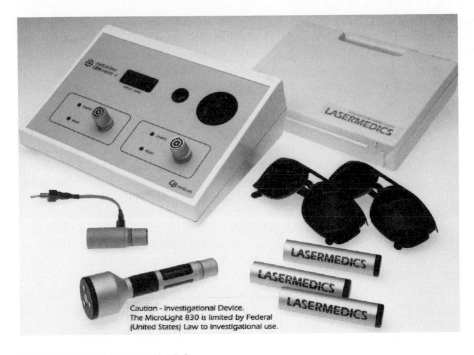

Figure 12-10. A low-level laser device limited by federal law to investigational use. (Courtesy Lasermedics, Inc., Sugar Land, TX.)

EFFECTS OF COLD LASERS

Cellular effects
Increased ATP and nucleic acid production
Stimulation of macrophages
Stimulation of fibroblasts to increase collagen production
Altered nerve conduction and regeneration
Vasodilation

No mechanism of action has yet been established for the possible biostimulative effects of the cold laser; however, given the limited depth of penetration and heating provided by this type of radiation, and the fact that electromagnetic radiation in the IR to UVB range of the spectrum is nonionizing, it is most likely that any physiological effects of cold lasers occur at the cellular level and are produced by photochemical means.[72,73] It has been proposed that cold lasers stimulate or inhibit biochemical, physiological, and/or proliferative activities by altering intercellular communication.[70,74]

Cellular Effects

In vitro cell studies have demonstrated short-term activation of the electron transport chain, increased ATP synthesis, and a reduction in cellular pH with the application of cold lasers.[75,76] It has also been proposed that low-level laser irradiation can initiate reactions at the cell membrane level via photophysical effects on calcium channels.[77] These biochemical and cell membrane changes are believed to cause the increases in macrophage, fibroblast, and lymphocyte activity observed with low-level laser irradiation.[78-82] These cellular reactions are thought to form the basis for the clinical benefits of low-level laser therapy.

It has been suggested that laser light, which is of a single wavelength, may be more clinically effective than other forms of light because specific cell types may respond optimally to specific wavelengths of light; however, this theory has been criticized because it is known that laser light loses coherence in the tissues due to diffraction and scattering.[83] Thus some authors have proposed that both noncoherent light sources and cold lasers may have similar biostimulative effects.[84]

Nerve Conduction and Regeneration

A number of studies have attempted to determine the impact of low-level laser irradiation on nerve conduction and regeneration; however, these studies have yielded conflicting results. Some studies have shown increased rates of nerve conduction, increased frequency of action potentials, decreased distal sensory latencies, and accelerated nerve regeneration in response to laser stimulation, all of which indicate increased activation of the nervous tissue.[85-88] In contrast, other studies have shown decreased rates of nerve conduction and increased distal conduction latencies, indicating decreased activation of the nervous tissue.[89,90] Still other studies, attempting to replicate prior results, have failed to demonstrate any change in nerve conduction in response to cold laser irradiation.[91-94] Given the conflicting nature of these findings, further research is necessary to clarify the effects of lasers on nerve conduction and to determine the specific parameters required to achieve these effects.

Vasodilation

Some authors claim that cold laser irradiation can induce vasodilation, particularly of the microcirculation.[95,67] Although this effect has not been thoroughly researched, should vasodilation occur in response to the clinical application of laser therapy, this could accelerate tissue healing by increasing the availability of oxygen and other nutrients and by speeding the removal of waste products from the irradiated area.

CLINICAL INDICATIONS FOR THE USE OF COLD LASERS

Wound and fracture healing
Musculoskeletal disorders
Pain management

Wound and Fracture Healing

A number of studies have been published concerning the use of cold lasers to promote the healing of chronic and acute surgical wounds in both humans and animals.[77,96-106] Some of these studies have reported acceleration of wound healing, increased tensile strength of the wound, and increased collagen content of the wound tissue after the application of low-level lasers. In addition, it has been shown that laser therapy can be delivered through a variety of wound dressings.[107] It is proposed that laser energy facilitates wound healing by stimulating leukocytic phagocytosis and fibroblast proliferation, increasing collagen synthesis and procollagen RNA levels, improving circulation, and inhibiting bacterial growth. Although many of the studies examining the effect of lasers on wound healing report positive results, the lack of adequate controls and the variation in, or poor reporting of, treatment parameters limit the ability to develop clear guidelines for the clinical application of cold lasers for the treatment of wounds in patients. A further limitation to the application of lasers for tissue healing is that a number of studies have failed to show improved wound healing with the use of this physical agent.[21,96,108-110] A recent metaanalysis of the studies on low-level laser therapy on venous leg ulcer healing reported finding no evidence of any benefit associated with this specific application of laser therapy.[111] At this time, systematic, well-documented clinical trials are still needed to ascertain if, when, and how the use of low-intensity lasers may facilitate soft tissue healing.

Studies on the effect of lasers on the healing of bone have also yielded mixed results, with some showing acceleration of fracture healing, some showing no effect on bone healing, and others reporting delayed postfracture ossification after laser irradiation.[112-116] It is thought that low-level laser accelerates bone healing because this type of energy may increase the rate of hematoma absorption, bone remodeling, blood vessel formation, and calcium deposition, as well as macrophage, fibroblast, and chondrocyte activity.[108] In addition, low-level laser energy produces a heat shock response and increases intracellular calcium in osteoblastic cells.[117] As with soft tissue healing, further systematic studies are needed to delineate the criteria that determine whether low-level laser irradiation enhances bone healing.

Musculoskeletal Disorders

A number of studies have been published regarding the application of low-level laser therapy for the management of pain and dysfunction associated with a wide range of musculoskeletal disorders. Although these studies have yielded mixed results, a metaanalysis reported that, on average, low-level laser therapy was more effective than placebo for the treatment of musculoskeletal disorders.[118]

Studies concerning the treatment of musculoskeletal disorders with low-level lasers have focused on arthritic and soft tissue conditions. Some studies have reported that low-level laser therapy can benefit patients with arthritis, resulting in increased hand grip strength and flexibility and decreased pain and swelling in patients with rheumatoid arthritis, decreased pain and increased grip strength in patients with osteoarthritis affecting the hands, and decreased pain and improved function in patients with cervical osteoarthritis.[119-123] In contrast, a number of blinded, controlled studies using low-intensity lasers for the treatment for osteoarthritis reported that this intervention did not relieve pain in the subjects studied.[124,125] A recent metaanalysis and reviews of the studies concerning the effects of low-level laser therapy on rheumatoid arthritis (RA) and osteoarthritis (OA) concluded that there is sufficient evidence to recommend consideration of low-level laser therapy for short-term relief of pain and morning stiffness in RA, but that for OA, the results are conflicting in different studies.[126-129] Different outcomes may be due to different laser doses and different methods of application. It is proposed that improvements in arthritic conditions are the result of reduced inflammation due to changes in the activity of inflammatory mediators or the result of reduced pain due to changes in nerve conduction or activation. More studies are needed in this area to elucidate both the nature and the mechanism for the effects of low-level laser therapy on arthritic conditions. For these studies to be most useful in directing care, the characteristics of the laser device and the application techniques used, including wavelength, treatment duration, dosage and site of application over nerves instead of joints, should be clearly and consistently documented.

Pain Management

A number of studies have found that low-level laser therapy can reduce the pain and dysfunction associated with musculoskeletal conditions other than arthritis, including lateral epicondylitis, low back and neck pain, trigger points, and chronic pain.[130-135] However, other studies have found no significant difference in subjective or objective treatment outcomes when comparing the treatment with the low-level laser with alternative sham treatments.[136-138]

Given the limitations of the published research on the efficacy of low-level laser therapy and the lack of definitive information regarding the mechanisms of action of this type of electromagnetic radiation or the ideal treatment parameters, it is difficult to make definitive recommendations for the clinical application of cold lasers in rehabilitation.

CONTRAINDICATIONS AND PRECAUTIONS FOR LASERS

CONTRAINDICATIONS
for the Use of Lasers

- Direct irradiation of the eyes
- Within 4 to 6 months after radiotherapy
- Hemorrhaging regions
- Locally to the endocrine glands

The application of lasers is contraindicated . . .

. . . directly to the eyes

Because lasers can damage the eyes, all patients treated with lasers should wear goggles opaque to the wavelength of the light emitted from the laser being used throughout treatment.[63] The clinician applying the laser should also wear goggles that reduce the wavelength of the device used to a nonhazardous level. Goggles should be marked with the wavelength range they attenuate and their optical density within that band. The greater the optical density, the greater the attenuation of the light. Safety goggles suitable for one wavelength should not be assumed to be safe at any other wave length. Particular care should be taken with IR lasers since their radiation is invisible but can easily damage the retina. The laser beam should never be directed at the eyes, and one should never look directly along the axis of the laser light beam.

. . . within 4 to 6 months after radiotherapy

It is recommended that lasers not be used after recent radiotherapy, because radiotherapy increases tissue susceptibility to malignancy and burns.

. . . over hemorrhaging regions

Laser therapy is contraindicated in hemorrhaging regions because the laser may cause vasodilation and thus increase bleeding.

. . . locally to the endocrine glands

Given the wide variety of reported cellular-level effects of laser therapy, there is concern that such treatment may alter endocrine gland function. Therefore the application of cold lasers to the endocrine glands is contraindicated.

PRECAUTIONS
for the Use of Lasers[95,142]

- Epilepsy
- Fever
- Malignancy
- To the low back or abdomen during pregnancy or menstruation

- Embryo or fetus
- Over the gonads
- Epiphyseal lines in children
- Confused or disoriented patient
- Areas of decreased sensation
- Infected tissue
- Sympathetic ganglia, vagus nerves, or cardiac region in patients with heart disease

Although there are no published reports of adverse effects in treating patients with these conditions, it is recommended that laser therapy not be applied to patients with epilepsy, fever, or malignancy for fear of worsening these conditions. Because the effects of low-level laser therapy on fetal development and fertility are not known, it is also recommended that this type of treatment not be applied to the abdomen or low back during pregnancy or menstruation or over the gonads at any time. Application over the epiphyseal plates prior to their closure is also not recommended.

Caution is recommended when treating patients who are disoriented or confused and when treating areas with impaired sensation since the patient may not be able to report discomfort during the treatment. Caution also is recommended in treating areas of infection due to the possible adverse effects of increasing circulation in the area, and in the areas of the sympathetic ganglia, vagus nerves, and cardiac region in patients with heart disease, should nerve conduction be altered in these structures.

Adverse Effects of Lasers

Although most reports concerning the use of cold lasers report no adverse effects in the treatment area from the application of this physical agent, there have been reports of transient tingling, mild erythema, a burning sensation, and increased pain, numbness, and skin rash in response to the application of low-level lasers.[13,122,139-141]

The primary hazards of laser irradiation are the adverse effects that can occur with irradiation of the eyes. Laser devices are classified on a 1 to 4 scale according to their intensity and associated risk of adverse effects to unprotected skin and eyes. The low-level lasers used in clinical and experimental applications are generally of class 3b, which means that although they are harmless to unprotected skin, they do pose a potential hazard to the eyes if viewed along the beam. Exposure of the eyes can cause retinal damage due to the limited attenuation of the beam intensity by the outer structures of the eye.

PHYSICAL PROPERTIES OF DIATHERMY— THERMAL AND NONTHERMAL

Diathermy, from the Greek meaning "through heating," is the application of shortwave (10 to 100 MHz frequency and 3 to 30 m wavelength) or microwave (300 MHz to 300 GHz frequency and 1 mm to 1 m wavelength) electromagnetic energy to produce heat within tissues (see Fig. 12-3). Shortwave radiation is within the radiofrequency range (3 kHz to 300 MHz and wavelengths of 1 m to 100 km), which is between ELF and microwave radiation. Microwave radiation has a frequency between that of radiofrequency and IR radiation. Both shortwave and microwave radiation are nonionizing.

In order to avoid interference with other radiofrequency signals used for communications, the Federal Communications Commission (FCC) determines which frequencies of shortwave and microwave radiation can be used for medical applications. Shortwave diathermy (SWD) devices have been allocated the three frequency bands centered on 13.56, 27.12, and 40.68 MHz, with ranges of ±6.78, 160, and 20 kHz, respectively.[2] The 27.12 MHz band is most commonly used for SWD devices because it has the widest bandwidth and is therefore the easiest and least expensive to generate. Microwave diathermy (MWD) devices for medical application have been allocated the frequency of 2450 MHz. The different frequency ranges are used to achieve clinical effects in different tissue types and at different depths (Table 12-1).

Both SWD and MWD can be delivered in a continuous or pulsed mode and, when delivered at a sufficient average intensity, can generate heat in the body.[143-145] When delivered in a pulsed mode at low average intensities, heat is dissipated before it can accumulate; however, pulsed low-intensity electromagnetic energy in the shortwave or microwave frequency range is also thought to produce a number of physiological effects by nonthermal mechanisms. Pulsed SWD, when applied at nonthermal levels, is generally referred to as *pulsed shortwave diathermy (PSWD)*; however, the terms *pulsed electromagnetic field (PEMF)*, *pulsed radiofrequency (PRF)*, or *pulsed electromagnetic energy (PEME)* have also been used to describe this type of radiation. The term *PSWD* is used in this text.

The key factor that determines whether or not a diathermy device will increase tissue temperature is the amount of energy absorbed by the tissue. This is determined by the intensity of the electromagnetic field produced by the device and the type of tissue to which the field is applied. A pulsed signal can allow heat to dissipate during the off cycle of the pulse. Previously published literature has categorized devices with an average power driving the applicator of less than 38 W as nonthermal;[146] however, this is misleading because the strength of the output field delivered to the tissue is only a fraction of this average power. The strength of the incident magnetic field delivered to the tissue is the important factor to consider. In clinical practice, one must rely on the patient's report and on the data provided by the device's manufacturer to ascertain whether or not the device increases tissue temperature.

When applied at sufficient power to increase tissue temperature, diathermy has a number of advantages over other thermal agents. It can heat deeper tissues than superficial thermal agents such as hot packs, and it can heat larger areas than ultrasound. SWD is not reflected by bones and therefore does not concentrate at the periosteum or pose a risk of periosteal burning, as does ultrasound; however, MWD is reflected at tissue interfaces, including those between air and skin, between skin and subcutaneous fat, and between soft tissue and superficial bones, and therefore does produce more heat in the areas close to these interfaces. The reflection of microwaves can also lead to the formation of standing waves, resulting in hot spots in other areas. Both SWD and MWD treatments generally need little time for application and do not require the clinician to be in direct contact with the patient throughout the treatment period.

TYPES OF DIATHERMY APPLICATORS

There are three different types of diathermy applicators: inductive coils, capacitive plates, and a magnetron.[146] Inductive coils or capacitive plates can be used to apply SWD, while a magnetron is used to apply MWD. All PSWD devices available at this time use inductive coil applicators in a drum form. PSWD devices deliver very short pulses of energy to avoid any cumulative increase in temperature within the tissues.

Inductive Coil Applicators

An inductive applicator is made up of a coil through which an alternating electric current flows (Fig. 12-11). The alternating current in the coil produces a magnetic field perpendicular to the coil, which, in turn, induces electric eddy currents in the tissues (Fig. 12-12). These induced electric currents cause charged particles in the tissue to oscillate. The friction produced by this oscillation causes an elevation in tissue temperature.

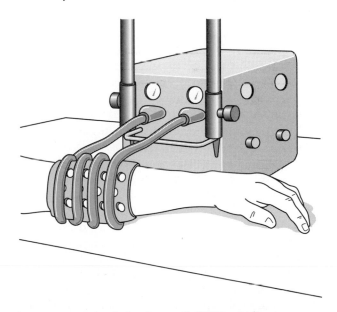

Figure 12-11. An inductive coil SWD applicator setup with cables around the patient's limb. This type of applicator produces a uniform, incident electromagnetic field that induces an electric field and current within the target tissue.

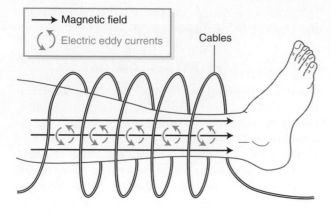

Figure 12-12. Generation of magnetic fields and induction of electric fields by an inductive coil.

Heating with an inductive coil is known as heating by the magnetic field method because the electric current that generates the heat is induced in the tissues by a magnetic field. The amount of heat generated in an area of tissue is affected by the strength of the magnetic field that reaches the tissue and by the strength and density of the induced eddy currents. The strength of the magnetic field is determined by the distance of the tissue from the applicator, and decreases in proportion to the square of the distance of the tissue from the applicator, according to the inverse square law, but does not vary with tissue type (Fig. 12-13). The strength of the induced eddy currents is determined by the strength of the magnetic field in the area and by the electrical conductivity of the tissue in the area. The electrical conductivity of tissue depends primarily on the tissue type and the frequency of the signal being applied. Metals and tissues with a high water and electrolyte content, such as muscle or synovial fluid, have high electrical conductivity, whereas tissues with a low water content, such as fat, bone, and collagen, have low electrical conductivity (Tables 12-1 and 12-2). Thus, inductive coils can heat both deep and superficial tissues, but they produce the most heat in tissues closest to the applicator and in tissues with the highest electrical conductivity.

Inductive coil applicators are available in two basic forms, cables and drums. The cables are bundles of plastic-coated wires that are applied by wrapping them around the patient's limb. When an alternating electric current flows through these wires, eddy currents are induced inside the limb. A drum applicator is made of a flat spiral coil inside a plastic housing (Fig. 12-14). The drum is placed directly over the area being treated, and the flow of alternating electric current

TABLE 12-1	Conductivity of Muscle at Different Frequencies
Frequency (MHz)	**Conductivity (siemens/meter)**
13.56	0.62
27.12	0.60
40.68	0.68
200	1.00
2450	2.17

From Durney CH, Massoudi H, Iskander MF: Radiofrequency Radiation Dosimetry Handbook. USAFSAM-TR-85-73. University of Utah, 1985, Electrical Engineering Department.

TABLE 12-2	Conductivity of Different Tissues at 25 MHz
Tissue	**Conductivity (siemens/meter)**
Liver	0.48–0.54
Kidney	0.83
Brain	0.46
Muscle	0.7–0.9
Fat	0.04–0.06
Bone	0.01

From Durney CH, Massoudi H, Iskander MF: Radiofrequency Radiation Dosimetry Handbook. USAFSAM-TR-85-73. University of Utah, 1985, Electrical Engineering Department.

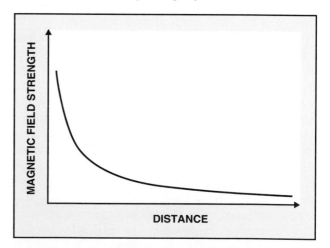

Figure 12-13. The typical behavior of magnetic field strength delivered by an SWD device as the distance from the applicator increases. Note that this is an inverse square relationship.

in the coil produces a magnetic field, which in turn induces eddy currents within the tissues (Fig. 12-15). Diathermy devices with drum applicators may have one or two drums or a single drum that can be bent to conform to the area being treated.

Capacitive Plates

Capacitive plate applicators are made of metal encased in a plastic housing. A high-frequency alternating electric current flows from one plate to the other through the patient, producing an electric field and a flow of current in the body tissue that is between the plates (Figs. 12-16 and 12-17). Thus the patient becomes a part of the electrical circuit connecting the two plates. As current flows through the tissue, it causes oscillation of charged particles and thus an increase in tissue temperature.

Heating with capacitive plate applicators is known as heating by the electric field method because the electric current that generates the heat is produced directly by an electric field. As with the inductive coils, the amount of heat generated in an area of tissue depends

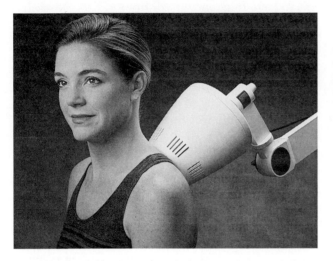

Figure 12-14. An inductive coil SWD applicator in drum form. (Courtesy Mettler Electronics Corporation, Anaheim, CA.)

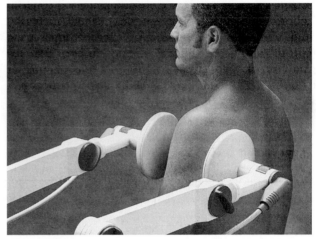

Figure 12-16. Capacitive plate SWD applicators placed around the target to produce an electric field directly. (Courtesy Mettler Electronics Corporation, Anaheim, CA.)

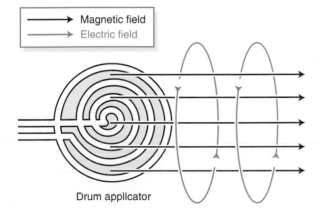

Figure 12-15. Magnetic field generated by an inductive drum SWD applicator and the resultant induced electric field.

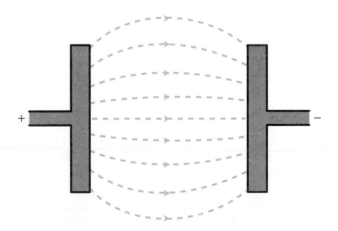

Figure 12-17. Electric field distribution between capacitive SWD plates.

on the strength and density of the current, with most heating occurring in tissues with the highest conductivity. Because current will always take the path of least resistance, when a capacitive plate type of applicator is used, the current will generally concentrate in the superficial tissues and will not penetrate as effectively to deeper tissues if there are poorly conductive tissues, such as fat, that is superficial to them. Thus capacitive plates generally produce most heat in skin and less heat in deeper structures, in contrast to inductive applicators, which heat the deeper structures more effectively because the incident magnetic field can achieve greater penetration to induce the electric field and current within the targeted tissue[147-150] (Fig. 10-18).

Magnetron

A magnetron, which produces a high-frequency alternating current in an antenna, is used to deliver MWD. The alternating current in the antenna produces an electromagnetic field that is directed toward the tissue by a curved reflecting director surrounding the antenna (Fig. 12-19). The presence of a director and the short wavelength of microwave radiation allow this type of diathermy to be focused and applied to small, defined areas. Therefore these devices can be useful during rehabilitation when only small areas of tissue are involved; they are also popular for the treat-

ment of malignant tumors by hyperthermia. The magnetrons used clinically are similar to those used in microwave ovens intended for cooking food.

The microwaves produced by a magnetron generate the most heat in tissues with high electrical conductivity; however, this high-frequency, short-wavelength radiation penetrates less deeply than SWD. Microwaves usually generate the most heat in the superficial skin, although some authors have also reported significant temperature increases in muscles and joint cavities in response to microwave application.[144,151,152] These differences in reported depth of heating appear to be related to variations in the microwave frequency used, from 915 to 2450 MHz, and to variability in tissue deposition among different areas of the body and among different species.[153] The shallow depth of microwave penetration, the reflection at tissue interfaces, and the potential for standing waves all contribute to an increased risk of excessive heating and burning of the superficial skin or fat with this type of diathermy device.

EFFECTS OF DIATHERMY

Thermal Effects

If applied at sufficient intensity, both SWD and MWD increase tissue temperature. The physiological

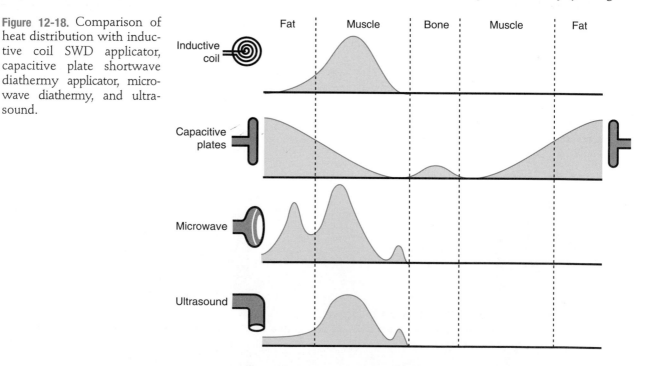

Figure 12-18. Comparison of heat distribution with inductive coil SWD applicator, capacitive plate shortwave diathermy applicator, microwave diathermy, and ultrasound.

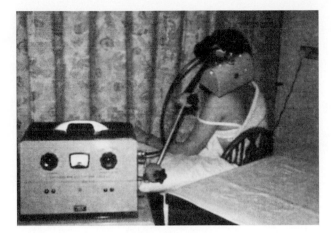

Figure 12-19. Microwave diathermy applicator. (From Kitchen S, Bazin S: *Clayton's Electrotherapy,* ed 10, London, 1996, WB Saunders. Used with permission.)

effects of increasing tissue temperature are described in detail in Chapter 6 and include vasodilation, increased rate of nerve conduction, elevation of the pain threshold, alteration of muscle strength, acceleration of enzymatic activity, and increased soft tissue extensibility. All of these effects have been observed in response to the application of diathermy.[154-158] The mechanisms underlying these physiological effects of increasing tissue temperature are also described in detail in Chapter 6.

The difference between the effects of superficial heating agents and diathermy is that superficial heating agents increase the temperature of only the superficial first few millimeters of tissue, while diathermy heats the deeper tissues. Therefore the physiological effects of superficial heating agents occur primarily in the superficial tissues, whereas diathermy also produces thermal effects in deeper tissues. For example, superficial heating agents primarily increase cutaneous circulation, while both SWD and MWD significantly increase muscular circulation.[154,159,160]

Nonthermal Effects

When applied at a low average intensity, with a short pulse duration and a low duty cycle, diathermy does not produce any maintained increase in tissue temperature because any transient heating of tissues that may occur is dissipated by the blood perfusing the area during the off time of the pulse. SWD, when applied at such nonthermal levels, is also thought to

have a variety of physiological effects.[161] Although the mechanisms by which PSWD achieves these effects are unknown, it has been proposed that they are due to modification of ion binding and cellular function by the incident electromagnetic fields and the resulting electric currents.[162,163]

Increased microvascular perfusion

The application of PSWD for 40 to 45 minutes at the maximum settings of 600 pulses per second (pps) at a generator power setting of 6 has been shown to increase local microvascular perfusion in healthy subjects and around the ulcer site in patients with diabetic ulcers.[164,165] Increasing microvascular perfusion, and thus local circulation, can increase local tissue oxygenation, nutrient availability, and phagocytosis. It has been proposed that the clinical benefits of treatment with PSWD are in part the result of increased microvascular perfusion.

Altered cell membrane function and cellular activity

It has been reported that electromagnetic fields can affect ion binding to the cell membrane, which can trigger a cascade of biological processes including growth factor activation in fibroblasts and nerve cells, macrophage activation, and changes in myosin phosphorylation.[166-171] PSWD is also thought to affect the regulation of the cell cycle by altering calcium ion binding, and it has been shown that exposure to electric fields can accelerate cell growth and division when it is too slow and inhibit it when it is too fast.[172,173] It has been proposed that alteration of cellular activity and stimulation of ATP and protein synthesis may underlie the observed clinical benefits of PSWD.[174]

CLINICAL INDICATIONS FOR THE USE OF DIATHERMY

History

The use of diathermy dates back to 1892, when d'Arsonval used electromagnetic fields with 10 kHz frequency to produce a sensation of warmth without the muscular contractions that occur at lower frequencies. SWD was introduced to the medical field in the early 20th century, and it was frequently used in the United States in the 1930s for the treatment of infections. However, despite a number of reports indicating that SWD can be an effective treatment modality, its use declined by the 1950s with the advent of antibiotics and with concerns regarding potential hazards to the patient and the operator if the equipment was applied inappropriately. Diathermy also lost popularity because, by its nature, the electromagnetic field cannot be readily contained to eliminate interference with other electronic equipment and because most diathermy devices are large, expensive, and cumbersome to use. In recent years there has been some resurgence of interest in this technology, particularly in specialized wound care practices, in response to the publication of a number of studies regarding the nonthermal effects of pulsed diathermy and the production of some smaller treatment devices; however, the clinical application of diathermy, whether for thermal or nonthermal effects, is still limited due to the paucity of well-substantiated treatment guidelines and information regarding the physiological mechanism of action of this type of intervention, the poor historical record of these devices, and the high cost of the devices. It is probable that, with further research regarding dosage and mechanism of action, and with technological advances to improve the shielding of these devices, the use of diathermy may regain popularity in the United States for certain clinical applications.

Thermal-Level Diathermy

The clinical benefits of applying diathermy at a sufficient intensity to increase tissue temperature are the same as those of applying other thermal agents, as described in detail in Chapter 6. These benefits include pain control, accelerated healing, decreased joint stiffness, and, if applied in conjunction with stretching, increased joint range of motion (ROM).[175,176] Because diathermy can increase the temperature of large areas of deep tissue, its use is indicated when trying to control pain, accelerate healing, or decrease joint stiffness in large, deep structures such as the hip joint or diffuse areas of the spine.

Nonthermal Pulsed Shortwave Diathermy

The first documented clinical application of diathermy at a nonthermal level in the United States was in the 1930s, when Ginsberg used a pulsed form of SWD to fight infection without producing a significant temperature rise in tissue.[177] He reported successfully treating a variety of acute and chronic infections with

this type of electromagnetic radiation and stated that this was the most effective treatment he had ever used. However, at this time, antibiotics were not commonly available or used. In 1965, A.S. Milinowski patented a device designed to deliver electrotherapy without heat generation. He stated that this device produced good clinical results while eliminating the factors of patient heat tolerance and contraindications when treating with heat.[178] Such nonthermal levels of PSWD have been evaluated and used clinically, primarily to control pain and edema and to promote wound, nerve, and fracture healing.

Clinical indications for the use of nonthermal PSWD

Control of pain and edema
Pain control
Wound healing
Nerve healing
Bone healing

Control of pain and edema

A number of studies concerning the effects of PSWD on recovery from soft tissue injury have shown improved edema resolution and/or reduction of pain in response to the application of this type of electromagnetic energy.[179-182] Two double-blind studies on the effects of nonthermal PSWD on acute ankle sprains found a significant decrease in edema, pain, and/or disability in the treated group compared with a placebo-treated group, and a double-blind study assessing the effects of PSWD treatment found that it decreased pain, erythema, and edema after foot surgery.[179-182] Maximum power and pulse frequency were used in all of these studies. It should be noted, however, that not all studies on the use of PSWD have shown such improvements. Both Barker et al. and McGill found no significant differences in pain, swelling, or gait between patients treated with PSWD and those treated with a placebo after acute ankle injuries.[183,184]

Pain control

A number of studies have evaluated the effect of PSWD on pain. Double-blind studies on the effects of using a home PSWD device placed in a soft cervical collar on patients with persistent neck pain or acute cervical injuries found significantly greater decreases in pain and increases in ROM in patients using this device for 3 weeks than in patients treated with a sham device.[185,186] The authors of these studies suggested that these effects could be due to modification of cell membrane function by the electromagnetic field. Studies without double-blind controls have also reported that PSWD can decrease low back and post-operative pain.[187,188]

Wound healing

Nonthermal PSWD has been shown to increase the rate of wound healing in both animal and human subjects.[189-192] This effect has been found with incisional wounds,[189] pressure ulcers,[190,192] and burn-related injuries.[191] Surgical wound sites in animals demonstrated increased collagen formation, white blood cell infiltration, and phagocytosis after treatment with PSWD. It was proposed that these were the result of increased circulation and improved tissue oxygenation.

Nerve healing

Acceleration of peripheral nerve regeneration in rats and cats, and spinal cord regeneration in cats, in response to the application of PSWD have been reported;[193-195] however, the authors of this book are not aware of any published clinical studies regarding the effect of PSWD on the recovery or regeneration of human nerves at this time.

Bone healing

Animal studies have shown acceleration of bone healing with the application of PSWD. A study in 1971 reported acceleration of osteogenesis by PSWD after tooth extraction wounds in dogs,[196] and a recent study found that PSWD accelerated the healing of the rabbit fibula after osteotomy.[197] The authors of this book are not aware of any published clinical studies regarding the effect of PSWD on human bone healing at this time.

Other applications

It has been suggested that nonthermal PSWD may also have therapeutic benefits when applied in the treatment of various forms of neuropathy, ischemic skin flaps, cerebral diseases, and myocardial diseases.[162] There is also one report on the use of PSWD in the management of head injuries.[198]

CONTRAINDICATIONS AND PRECAUTIONS FOR DIATHERMY

Although diathermy is a safe treatment modality when applied appropriately, in order to avoid adverse effects, it should not be used when contraindicated, and appropriate precautions should be taken when necessary.[199,200] When applying any form of diathermy at an intensity that may increase tissue temperature, all the contraindications and precautions that apply to the use of thermotherapy, as described in detail in Chapter 6, apply. In addition, there are a number of other contraindications and precautions that apply uniquely to this type of physical agent and some unique reasons for these restrictions. These are described in detail in the related boxes that follow.

Precautions for the Therapist Applying Diathermy

There is concern regarding potential hazards to therapists applying diathermy due to the greater exposure as a result of treating multiple patients throughout the day. These devices produce diffuse radiation and can thus irradiate the therapist if she or he is standing close to the machine.[209,210] It is therefore recommended that therapists stay at least 1 to 2 m away from all continuous diathermy applicators, at least 30 to 50 cm away from all PSWD applicators, and out of the direct beam of any MWD device during patient treatment.[65,214,215]

Some reports have noted above-average rates of spontaneous abortion and abnormal fetal development in therapists following the use of SWD equipment; however, other studies have failed to demonstrate a statistically significant correlation between SWD exposure and either congenital malformation or spontaneous abortion.[216,217] One comparison of SWD and MWD exposure of therapists found that only MWD increased the risk of miscarriage.[218] However, a recent study found that shortwaves have potentially harmful effects on pregnancy outcome and are specifically associated with low birth weight. This effect increased in a dose-related manner.[219] On balance, given the current research findings, it is recommended that therapists avoid SWD and MWD exposure during pregnancy.[220]

Malignancy and Electromagnetic Fields

Substantial controversy exists regarding the effects of electromagnetic fields on malignancy. The literature on this topic is primarily concerned with the risks associated with living near and working with power lines. While some reports suggest that the electromagnetic fields generated from power lines may be linked to childhood cancers and leukemia, others have failed to show such an association.[221,222] In 1995, the Council of the American Physical Society determined that "The scientific literature and the reports of reviews by other panels show no consistent, significant link between cancer and power line fields. . . . No plausible biophysical mechanisms for the systematic initiation or promotion of cancer by these power line fields have been identified."

The electromagnetic fields associated with power lines are of much lower frequency (50 to 60 Hz) than those used in pulsed or continuous SWD devices (27.12 MHz); thus, the application of the data from the studies on power lines to the effects of SWD are limited. At this time there are no recommendations against using PSWD in the area of a malignancy, and there are no indications that PSWD is carcinogenic.

CONTRAINDICATIONS
for All Forms of Diathermy

- Implanted or transcutaneous neural stimulators

All forms of diathermy are contraindicated . . .

. . . in patients with implanted or transcutaneous neural stimulators

Diathermy of any sort should not be used in patients with implanted or transcutaneous neural stimulators because the electromagnetic energy of the diathermy may interfere with the functioning of the device. Cases of coma and death have been reported when diathermy has been applied to patients with implanted deep brain stimulators. Also, burns can occur if diathermy is applied to patients with electrical stimulation wires or metal containing electrodes on their skin.

CONTRAINDICATIONS
for Thermal-Level Diathermy

- Metal implants or pacemakers
- Malignancy
- Pregnancy
- Eyes
- Testes
- Growing epiphyses

Thermal-level diathermy is contraindicated . . .

. . . in patients with metal implants or pacemakers

Metal is highly conductive electrically and therefore can become very hot with the application of diathermy, leading to potentially hazardous temperature increases in adjacent tissues. The risk of extreme temperature increases is greatest when there is metal in the superficial tissues, as can occur with pieces of shrapnel; however, it is recommended that diathermy not be used in any areas containing or close to metal. This contraindication applies to metal both inside and outside the patient. Therefore all jewelry should be removed before diathermy is applied, and care should be taken that there is no metal in the furniture or other objects close to the patient being treated.

Diathermy should not be used on patients with pacemakers because these devices have metal components that can become overheated in response to the application of diathermy and because the electromagnetic fields produced by diathermy devices may interfere directly with the performance of pacemakers, particularly those of the demand type. Although the risk of adverse effects is greatest if the thorax is being treated, it is generally recommended that diathermy not be used to treat any area of the body if a patient has a pacemaker, although some authors state that the extremities may be treated in patients with pacemakers.[201]

. . . in areas of malignancy

The use of diathermy in an area of malignancy is contraindicated unless the treatment is for the tumor itself. Diathermy is occasionally used to treat tumors by hyperthermia; however, such treatments require fine control of tissue temperature and are outside the realm of the rehabilitation professional. Fine temperature control is required because certain cancer cells have been shown to die at temperatures of 42° to 43° C but to proliferate at temperatures of 40° to 41° C.[202]

. . . in pregnant patients

The application of diathermy during pregnancy is contraindicated due to concerns regarding both the effects of deep heat and the effects of electromagnetic fields on fetal development. Maternal hyperthermia has been shown to increase the risk of abnormal fetal development, and SWD has been shown to be linked to increased rates of spontaneous abortion and abnormal fetal development in animals.[203-206] Diathermy exposure, particularly of the lower abdominal and pelvic regions, should be avoided during pregnancy, and since the distribution of an electromagnetic field is not predictably constrained in the body, it is recommended that diathermy exposure of any other part of the body also be avoided. A discussion of the risks and precautions for pregnant therapists applying diathermy to patients follows the section on precautions for applying diathermy to patients.

. . . over the eyes

The eyes should not be treated with diathermy because increasing the temperature of intraocular fluid may damage the internal structures of the eyes.

. . . over the testes

It is recommended that diathermy not be applied over the testes due to the risk of adversely affecting fertility by increasing local tissue temperature.

. . . over growing epiphyses

The effects of diathermy on growing epiphyses is unknown; however, its use is not recommended in these areas due to the concern that diathermy may alter the rate of epiphyseal closure.

CONTRAINDICATIONS
for Nonthermal Pulsed Shortwave Diathermy

- Deep tissue
- Substitute for conventional therapy for edema and pain

- Pacemakers, electronic devices, or metal implants (warning)

Nonthermal pulsed shortwave diathermy is contraindicated . . .

. . . for the treatment of deep tissues such as internal organs

Although contraindicated for the treatment of internal organs, nonthermal PSWD can be used to treat soft tissue overlying an organ.

ASSESS:

- Check the patient's chart for any record of organ disease. Check with the patient's physician before applying PSWD in an area with organ disease present.

. . . as a substitute for conventional therapy for edema and pain

PSWD should not be used as a substitute for conventional therapy for edema and pain. It is intended to be

Continued

CONTRAINDICATIONS—cont'd

an adjunctive modality for application in conjunction with conventional methods including compression, immobilization, and medications.

. . . in the presence of pacemakers, electronic devices, or metal implants

The electromagnetic radiation of PSWD may interfere with the functioning of a cardiac pacemaker and thus may adversely affect patients with cardiac pacemakers. The EMF emitted by nonthermal PSWD devices can also interfere with other electromedical and electronic devices. Therefore PSWD should not be used over or near medical electronic devices, including pacemakers, and should be used with caution with and around patients with other external or implanted medical electronic devices.

Nonthermal PSWD devices can be used to treat soft tissue adjacent to most metal implants without significantly heating the metal; however, when the metal forms closed loops, as occurs with the wires used for fixating rods and plates in surgical fracture repairs, heating may occur because current can flow in the wire loops. Therefore if a patient has a metal implant, the clinician should determine the type of implant before applying PSWD.

ASK THE PATIENT:

- Do you have a pacemaker or any other metal in your body?

ASSESS:

- Check the patient's chart for any information regarding a pacemaker or other metal implants. If the patient has a pacemaker or is using other medical electronic devices, PSWD should not be used except in extreme circumstances, such as when trying to save a limb from amputation. When considering the use of PSWD in such circumstances, the patient's physician should be consulted, and the clinician should try to shield all medical electronic devices from the electromagnetic field. In the presence of metal implants, request an x-ray and do not treat with PSWD if the metal forms loops. If the patient has nonlooping metal implants, PSWD may be applied with caution.

PRECAUTIONS
for All Forms of Diathermy

- Electronic or magnetic equipment in the vicinity
- Obesity
- Copper-bearing intrauterine contraceptive devices

Use all forms of diathermy with caution . . .

. . . in the presence of electronic or magnetic equipment

A number of studies and reports have demonstrated the presence of unwanted electrical and magnetic radiation around diathermy applicators.[207-210] Because the treatment field may interfere with any electronic or magnetic equipment, such as computers or computer-controlled medical devices, it is recommended that the leads and applicators of diathermy devices be at least 3 m, and preferably 5 m, from other equipment. Precise guidelines are not available because interference depends on the exact arrangement and the shielding of both the diathermy device and the other equipment being used. If interference occurs, then the two types of equipment should be used at different times.

. . . with obese patients

Diathermy should be used with caution in obese patients because it may heat fat excessively. Capacitive plate applicators, which generally result in greater increases in the temperature of fat than other types of applicators, should not be used with obese patients.[146,211]

. . . with patients using copper-bearing intrauterine contraceptive devices

Although copper-bearing intrauterine contraceptive devices do contain a small amount of metal, calculations and in vivo measurements have shown that these devices and the surrounding tissue increase only slightly in temperature when exposed to therapeutic levels of diathermy.[212,213] Therefore diathermy may be used by both therapists and patients with such devices.

PRECAUTIONS
for Nonthermal Pulsed Shortwave Diathermy

- Pregnancy
- Skeletal immaturity

Use nonthermal PSWD with caution . . .

. . . with pregnant or skeletally immature patients

The use of thermal-level diathermy is contraindicated during pregnancy. In addition, since the effects of electromagnetic energy on fetal or child development are not known, nonthermal PSWD should also be used with caution during pregnancy and in skeletally immature patients.

ADVERSE EFFECTS OF DIATHERMY

Burns

Diathermy can cause soft tissue burns when used at normal or excessive doses, and because the distribution of this type of energy varies significantly with the type of tissue, it can burn some layers of tissue while sparing others.[223] Fat layers are at the greatest risk of burning, particularly when capacitive plate applicators are used, because they are more effectively heated by this type of device and because fat is less well-vascularized than muscle or skin and therefore is not cooled as effectively by vasodilation. Because water is preferentially heated by all forms of diathermy, the patient's skin should be kept dry by wrapping with towels to avoid scalding from hot perspiration.

APPLICATION TECHNIQUES

Thermal-level diathermy is the most effective modality for increasing the temperature of large areas of deep tissue. Therefore treatment with this physical agent is most appropriate when the goal(s) of treatment can be achieved by increasing the temperature of large areas of deep tissue.

Nonthermal PSWD can reduce pain and edema and may accelerate tissue healing. It can be used at the acute, subacute, and chronic stages of an injury; however, the literature and anecdotal reports suggest that better results are achieved when acute conditions are treated. Although not documented in the literature, favorable results have also been reported anecdotally for patients with lymphedema, cerebrovascular accidents, and reflex sympathetic dystrophy (RSD).

APPLICATION TECHNIQUE
Diathermy

1. Evaluate the patient's problem and determine the goals of treatment.
2. Determine that diathermy is the most appropriate treatment.

    Because diathermy induces an electrical current in the tissues without touching the patient's body, the use of this physical agent may be particularly appropriate in cases where direct contact with the patient is not possible or desirable—for example, if infection control is an issue, if the patient cannot tolerate direct contact with the skin, or if the area is in a cast. Because no heat accumulates with the application of nonthermal PSWD and since little or no sensation is associated with its use, nonthermal PSWD can be used where heat is contraindicated or potentially hazardous, and it can be applied to insensate patients or to those who cannot tolerate the sensations associated with other physical agents, such as cryotherapy or electrical stimulation.

3. Determine that diathermy is not contraindicated.

    Ask the appropriate questions and make the necessary assessments, as described in detail in the section on contraindications and precautions, to determine if treatment with diathermy is safe.

4. Select the most appropriate diathermy device.

    Choose between a thermal and a nonthermal device according to the desired effects of the treatment, and between the different types of applicators (inductive coil, capacitive plate, or magnetron) according to the desired depth of penetration and the tissue to be treated.

5. Explain the procedure and the reason for applying diathermy to the patient and the sensations the patient can expect to feel.

    During the application of thermal-level diathermy, the patient should feel a comfortable sensation of mild warmth without any increase in pain or discomfort.

    The application of PSWD is not generally associated with any change in patient sensation, although some patients report feeling slight tingling and/or mild warmth. This sensation may be the result of increased local circulation in response to the treatment.

6. Remove all metal jewelry and clothing from the area to be treated.

    All clothing with metal fastenings or components, such as buttons, zippers, or clips, must be removed from the treatment area. Nonmetal clothing, bandages, or casts do not need to be removed prior to treatment with diathermy because magnetic fields penetrate these materials unaltered; however, when thermal-level diathermy is used, it is recommended that clothing be removed from the area so that towels can be applied to absorb local sweating.

7. Clean and dry the skin and inspect it if necessary.
8. Position the patient comfortably on a chair or plinth with no metal components. Position the patient so that the area to be treated is readily accessible.
9. If applying thermal-level diathermy, wrap the area to be treated with toweling to absorb local perspiration. If applying PSWD, it is not necessary to place towels between the applicator and the body, but a disposable cloth or plastic covering can be used over the applicator when treating conditions in which there is a risk of cross-contamination or infection.
10. Position the device and the applicator(s) for effective and safe treatment application.

For an Inductive Applicator

With cables, wrap the cable around the towel-covered limb to be treated, spacing the turns of the cable at least 3 cm apart. Use rubber or wooden spacers to ensure that adjacent turns of the cable do not come into contact with each other.

Alternatively, coil the cable into a flat spiral approximately the size of the area to be treated. Use spacers to separate adjacent pieces of cable to ensure that adjacent turns of the cable do not come into contact with each other. Place the coil over the area to be treated separated by six to eight layers of towels (Fig. 12-20).

With a drum applicator, place the drum directly over and close to the skin or tissues to be treated, keeping a slight air gap to allow for heat dissipation. Contact should be avoided when infection control is an issue. Position the center of the applicator over the area to be treated. The treatment surface of the applicator should be placed facing and as parallel to the tissues being treated as possible.

The patient should be advised to move as little as possible during the treatment because the strength of the field will change if the distance between the applicator and the treatment area changes, decreasing in proportion to the square of the distance between the treatment surface of the applicator and the tissues being treated (see Fig. 12-13). For example, if the distance doubles, the strength of the magnetic field will decrease by a factor of 4. Thus, maintaining the applicator at a constant distance from the patient is important for consistent treatment.

For a Capacitive Applicator

Place the two plates at an equal distance on either side of the area to be treated, approximately 2 to 10 cm (1 to 3 inches) from the skin surface (see Fig. 12-16). Equal placement at a slight distance from the body is recommended for even field distribution in the treatment area because the field is most concentrated near the plates. Unequal placement will result in uneven heating, with the areas closest to the plate becoming hotter than those farther from the plate (Fig. 12-21).

For a Magnetron Microwave Applicator

Place the applicator a few inches from the area to be treated. Direct the applicator toward the area, with the beam perpendicular to the patient's skin.

11. Tune the device.

SWD devices allow tuning of the applicator to each particular load. Tuning adjusts the precise frequency of the device, within the accepted range, to optimize coupling between the device and the load. Most modern diathermy devices tune automatically. To tune a device that requires manual tuning, first turn it on and allow it to warm up according to the manufacturer's directions; then turn up the intensity to a low level and adjust the tuning dial until a maximal reading on the power/intensity indicator is obtained.

12. Select the appropriate treatment parameters.

When applying thermal-level diathermy, the intensity should be adjusted to produce a sensation of mild warmth in the patient. The gauge of heating used in clinical practice is the patient's reported sensation because calculations of energy delivery and temperature increases are not reliable.[224] The pattern of energy and heat distribution by both SWD and MWD is difficult to predict because it is influenced by the amount of reflection, the electrical properties of different types of tissue in the field, the tissue size and composition, the frequency of the field, and the type, size, geometry, and orientation of the applicator. This issue is further complicated by evidence that the thermal sensation threshold may be affected by the frequency of radiation applied.[224] Thermal-level diathermy is generally applied for about 20 minutes.

When applying nonthermal PSWD, most clinicians select the intensity, pulse frequency, and total treatment time based on the manufacturer's recommendations and on their individual experience because the clinical research using these devices does not indicate clearly which parameters are most effective. Most manufacturers and studies recommend using the

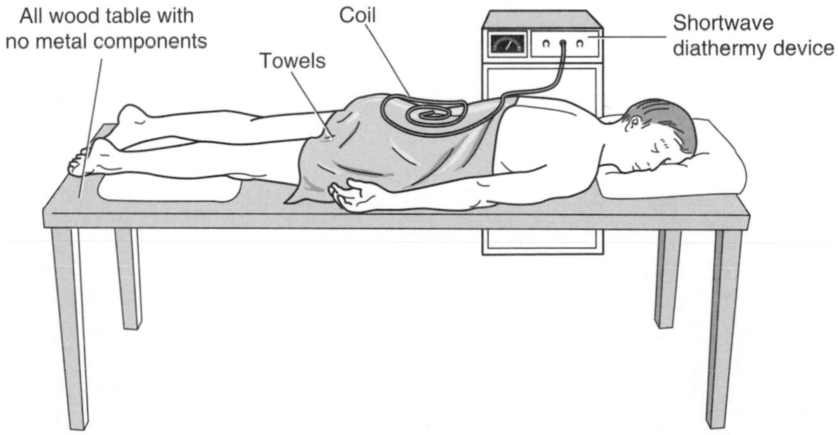

Figure 12-20. Inductive coil applicator for SWD. Setup with "pancake" coil on the patient's back. Note the layer of towels.

Continued

APPLICATION TECHNIQUE—cont'd
Diathermy

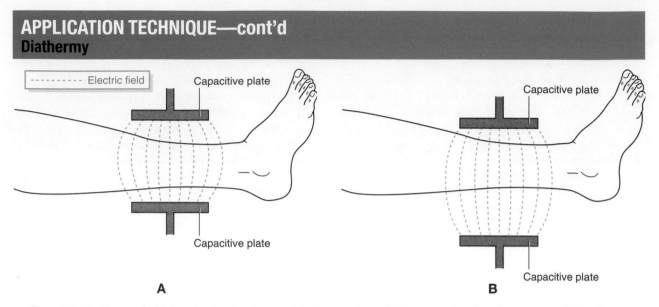

Figure 12-21. Electric field distribution in tissue with **(A)** evenly and **(B)** unevenly placed capacitive SWD plates.

maximum strength and frequency available on the device for all conditions and, if the patient reports any discomfort, reducing the pulse rate until the discomfort resolves. Most PSWD treatments are administered for 30 to 60 minutes once or twice a day, 5 to 7 times a week.

Both of the nonthermal PSWD devices manufactured in the United States have six intensity settings, to provide various field strengths, and six pulse frequency settings, to provide between 80 and 600 pulses, of 65 microsecond duration, per second.[225,226]

13. Provide the patient with a bell or other means to call for assistance during treatment and a means to turn off the diathermy device. Instruct the patient to turn off the device and call immediately if he or she experiences excessive heating or an increase in pain or discomfort.

14. After 5 minutes, check to be certain that the patient is not too hot or is experiencing any increase in symptoms.

15. When the treatment is complete, turn off the device, remove the applicator and towels, and inspect the treatment area. It is normal for the area to appear slightly red, and it may also feel warm to the touch.

16. Assess the outcome of treatment.
    Reassess the patient, checking particularly for any signs of burning and for progress toward the goals of treatment. Remeasure quantifiable subjective complaints and objective impairments and disabilities.

17. Document the treatment.

DOCUMENTATION

Document the area of the body treated, the frequency range, average power or power setting, pulse rate, time of irradiation, type of applicator, treatment duration, patient positioning, distance of the applicator from the patient, and the patient's response to the treatment. Documentation is typically written in the SOAP note format. The following examples summarize only the modality component of treatment and are not intended to represent a comprehensive plan of care.

Examples

When applying shortwave diathermy to low back, document:

S: Pt c/o low back pain at level 7/10.
O: 27.12 MHz continuous SWD, power level 3, to low back, drum applicator 3" from patient, patient prone, 20 min.
A: Report of mild warmth, pain decreased to 4/10.
P: Continue SWD as above before ther ex program.

When applying microwave diathermy to posterior left knee, document:

S: *Pt c/o stiffness and pain with L knee extension.*

O: *2450 MHz continuous MWD to posterior knee, 3" from skin surface, power level 4, 15 minutes. Patient prone with 3 lb cuff weight at ankle.*

A: *Extension ROM increased from −40° to −30°.*

P: *Continue MWD as above followed by active ROM exercises into extension.*

When applying pulsed shortwave diathermy to ulcer on the lateral aspect of the right distal leg, document:

S: *Pt reports he is scheduled to have a cardiac pacemaker implanted in 2 weeks.*

O: *PSWD intensity 6, pulse rate 600 pps, to R distal leg in area of venous insufficiency ulcer, applicator 3" from lateral leg., 45 minutes.*

A: *Ulcer dimensions decreased from 9 × 5 cm to 7 × 4 cm over last week.*

P: *Continue PSWD as above 1× per day. Discharge PSWD component of care after pacemaker is implanted.*

SELECTING A DIATHERMY DEVICE

When considering purchasing a diathermy device, the first consideration should be whether it outputs a thermal or nonthermal level of energy (Table 12-3). This is particularly important with devices for which manufacturers make both thermal and nonthermal claims. There are diathermy devices manufactured in Europe, and available in the United States, that can be adjusted to be used for either thermal or nonthermal application; by contrast, the diathermy devices currently manufactured in the United States can be used either for thermal or for nonthermal application but

not for both. The FDA differentiates between diathermy devices according to their thermal or nonthermal mechanism of action. Specifically, the FDA separates diathermy devices into "diathermy for use in applying therapeutic deep heat for selected medical conditions" and "diathermy intended for the treatment of medical conditions by means other than the generation of deep heat."[226]

When purchasing a device intended for thermal treatments, one should consider the type of applicator (plates, coils, or drum), the frequency band of the energy (shortwave or microwave), and whether the device is self-tuning. In general, drums are the easiest to apply, although coils may provide deeper penetration when applied to the limbs. SWD is generally preferred over MWD since it has a more predictable distribution pattern, and self-tuning devices provide greater ease of use.

The two nonthermal PSWD devices currently manufactured in the United States are very similar. They both have six intensity settings, produce 65-microsecond pulses, and allow adjustment of the pulse frequency to a maximum of 600 pps. At this maximum frequency, these devices deliver energy for 3.9% of the total treatment time. For example, during a 30-minute treatment at maximum frequency, the electromagnetic field is on for 70.2 seconds and is off for the remaining 28 minutes and 49.8 seconds. It is this high proportion of off time to on time, and the resulting low average power, that allow any heating that may occur during the on time to be dissipated by the circulating blood during the off time between pulses.

TABLE 12-3 **Comparison of Different Types of Diathermy Devices**

Type	Thermal			Nonthermal
	Shortwave		*Microwave*	*Pulsed Shortwave*
Frequency	27.12 MHz*		2450 MHz	27.12 MHz
Applicator	Inductive coil	Capacitive plate	Magnetron	Inductive coil drum
Incident field	Electromagnetic	Electric	Electromagnetic	Electromagnetic
Tissues most affected	Deep and superficial	Superficial	Small areas	Deep and superficial

*SWD can also have a frequency of 13.56 or 40.68 MHz; however, the most commonly used frequency is 27.12 MHz.

▶ *Clinical Case Studies* ◀

The following case studies summarize the concepts of diathermy discussed in this chapter. Based on the scenario presented, an evaluation of the clinical findings and goals of treatment are proposed. These are followed by a discussion of the factors to be considered in the selection of diathermy as the indicated treatment modality, and in the selection of the ideal diathermy device and parameters to promote progress toward the goals.

Case 1

SJ is a 45-year-old female physical therapist. She has been diagnosed with adhesive capsulitis of the right shoulder and has been referred to physical therapy. She complains of shoulder stiffness, with a tight sensation at the end of range. Although she is able to perform most of her work functions, she has difficulty reaching overhead, which interferes with placing objects on high shelves and with serving when playing tennis, and she has difficulty reaching behind her to fasten clothing. The objective exam reveals restricted right shoulder active and passive range of motion (ROM) (see the following information) and restricted passive glenohumeral joint inferior and posterior gliding. All other tests, including cervical and elbow ROM and upper extremity strength and sensation, are within normal limits.

Shoulder ROM

AROM	R	L
Flexion	120°	170°
Abduction	100°	170°
Hand behind back	R 5″ below L	

PROM		
Flexion	130°	175°
Abduction	110°	175°
Internal rotation	50°	80°
External rotation	10°	80°

EVALUATION OF THE CLINICAL FINDINGS

This patient presents with the impairments of restricted right shoulder active and passive ROM and restricted glenohumeral joint passive mobility in a capsular pattern. These impairments have limited her ability to participate in sports and to perform normal activities of daily living, including dressing and lifting over her head.

PREFERRED PRACTICE PATTERN

Impaired Joint Mobility, Motor Function, Muscle Performance, and Range of Motion Associated With Connective Tissue Dysfunction, (4D)

PLAN OF CARE

The goals of treatment at this time are to regain full active and passive ROM of the right shoulder and to return to full sports participation and daily living activities.

ASSESSMENT REGARDING THE APPROPRIATENESS OF DIATHERMY AS THE OPTIMAL TREATMENT

The loss of active and passive joint motion associated with adhesive capsulitis is thought to be due to adhesion and loss of length of the anterior inferior joint capsule. Thus effective treatment should attempt to increase the length of the joint capsule. Increasing tissue temperature prior to stretching will increase the extensibility of soft tissue, allowing the greatest increase in soft tissue length with the least force while minimizing the risk of tissue damage. Diathermy is the optimal modality for heating the shoulder capsule because this thermal agent can reach large areas of deep tissue. A superficial heating agent such as a hot pack would not be as effective because it does not increase the temperature of tissue at the depth of the joint capsule, and ultrasound would not generally be as effective because its heating is limited by the effective radiating area of the sound head.

PROPOSED TREATMENT PLAN AND RATIONALE

A continuous diathermy device must be used in order to increase tissue temperature. An SWD device with an inductive coil applicator in a drum form is recommended since this mode of application provides deep, even heat distribution and is easy to apply. The device should be applied to the right shoulder, ideally with the shoulder positioned at end of range flexion and abduction so as to apply a gentle stretch to the anterior inferior capsule. The diathermy device should be set to produce a sensation of mild, comfortable warmth, and the treatment should be applied for approximately 20 minutes. This diathermy treatment should be followed immediately by a low-load, prolonged stretch in order to maximize ROM gains.

Case 2

MB is a 24-year-old female recreational soccer player who sustained a grade II left ankle inversion sprain approximately 48 hours ago. She has been applying ice and a compression bandage to the ankle, resting and elevating the ankle as much as possible, and using a cane to reduce weight bearing when walking. She has been referred to physical therapy in order to attain a pain-free return to sports as rapidly as possible. She complains of moderate pain at the lateral ankle that is aggravated by weight bearing and of ankle swelling that is aggravated when her ankle is in a dependent position. The objective exam reveals a mild increase in superficial skin temperature at the left lateral ankle and edema of the left ankle, with a girth of 25½ cm (10 inches) on the left compared with 21½ cm (8½ inches) on the right. Left ankle ROM is restricted in all planes, with 0° of dorsiflexion on the left and 10° on the right, 20° of plantar flexion on the left and 45° on the right, 10° of inversion on the left, with pain at the lateral ankle at the end of range, and 30° on the right, and 20° of eversion on the left and 30° on the right. Isometric testing of muscle strength against manual resistance at midrange revealed no abnormalities.

EVALUATION OF THE CLINICAL FINDINGS

This patient presents with the impairments of left ankle pain, increased temperature, swelling, and restricted ROM. These have resulted in the functional limitations of decreased weight-bearing tolerance and limited ambulation.

PREFERRED PRACTICE PATTERN

Impaired Joint Mobility, Motor Function, Muscle Performance, and Range of Motion Associated With Connective Tissue Dysfunction, (4D)

PLAN OF CARE

The goals of treatment at this time are to control pain, resolve edema, and restore normal ROM in order for the patient to return to full sports participation. The diagnosis of a grade II ankle sprain indicates that there has been some damage to the ankle ligaments; therefore, the goals of treatment should also include healing of these soft tissues.

ASSESSMENT REGARDING THE APPROPRIATENESS OF DIATHERMY AS THE OPTIMAL TREATMENT

Nonthermal PSWD is an indicated adjunctive treatment for pain and edema and has also been shown to accelerate soft tissue healing. Because this patient is already applying rest, ice, compression, and elevation to her ankle at home and desires a rapid return to full sports participation, the addition of PSWD treatment may help maximize her rate of recovery. Thermal-level diathermy should not be applied to this patient since the use of all thermal agents is contraindicated in the presence of acute injury or inflammation.

PROPOSED TREATMENT PLAN AND RATIONALE

It is proposed that treatment with nonthermal PSWD be started immediately following the evaluation in order to reduce pain and swelling. The patient's limb should be placed in a comfortable elevated position in order to optimize the reduction of swelling. The PSWD applicator should be positioned over the lateral aspect of the ankle, as close to the skin as possible, with the center of the applicator over the area of the ankle presenting with the most marked swelling, and as parallel as possible to the damaged tissues.

Daily application of PSWD for 30 minutes, with power and pulse rate settings of 6, is generally used for treatment of this type of acute injury. If the patient complains of any increase in discomfort, the pulse rate should be decreased until the discomfort resolves. The PSWD treatment can be followed by the application of ice, after which the ankle should be wrapped in a compression bandage. The patient should continue with rest, ice, elevation, and compression and should be instructed in appropriate ambulation, weight bearing, and ROM exercises. She may also need to wear a splint if the ankle is unstable.

Case 3

FG is an 85-year-old male with a stage IV sacral pressure ulcer. He is bedridden, minimally responsive, and dependent for all bed mobility and feeding activities. He is able to swallow but eats poorly. The pressure ulcer is 15 by 8 cm and 3 cm deep in the deepest area. There is no tunneling or undermining. Approximately 70% of the wound bed is red and granulating, and 30% is covered with yellow slough. Treatment until this time has consisted of sharp debridement and hydrocolloid dressings. Although this treatment has resulted in a reduction of the yellow slough, there has been little change in wound area over the last month.

EVALUATION OF THE CLINICAL FINDINGS

This patient presents with impaired soft tissue integrity and reduced strength. The impairment of tissue integrity places him at risk for infection and increases his need for medical care. His limited strength has made him dependent for functional movement, including bed mobility.

PREFERRED PRACTICE PATTERN

Impaired Integumentary Integrity Associated With Skin Involvement Extending Into Fascia, Muscle, or Bone and Scar Formation, (7E)

PLAN OF CARE

The short-term goals of treatment include achieving a completely red wound base and preventing infection. Long-term goals may include reduction of wound size and, ideally, wound closure; however, given this patient's impaired nutritional and mobility status, wound closure may not be achievable.

Continued

> **Clinical Case Studies—cont'd** ◀

ASSESSMENT REGARDING THE APPROPRIATENESS OF DIATHERMY AS THE OPTIMAL TREATMENT

Nonthermal PSWD has been shown to accelerate the healing of chronic open wounds, including pressure ulcers. One advantage of this treatment modality over other adjunctive treatments is that it can be applied without removing the dressing, thus limiting the mechanical and temperature disturbance to the wound and reducing the time required to set up the treatment. Also, since PSWD produces no sensation, it can be applied even if the patient is insensate or cognitively incapable of giving sensory feedback about the treatment. Limiting the mechanical disruption of the wound is particularly important in this case since 70% of the wound bed is covered with red granulation tissue that is fragile but does have the potential to heal.

PROPOSED TREATMENT PLAN AND RATIONALE

A comprehensive wound care program that addresses pressure relief, dressings, the nutritional status of the patient, and debridement, when necessary, is required to optimize the healing of this patient's wound. Nonthermal PSWD may be used as an adjunct to these interventions to facilitate wound healing and closure. The patient should be positioned with the wound exposed and with the treatment surface of the applicator as close and as parallel to the tissues to be treated as possible, with the center of the applicator over the deepest part of the wound. If tunneling were present, the center of the applicator should be positioned over the deepest portion of the tunnel in order to promote closure of the tunnel before the more superficial wound site closes. The treatment surface of the applicator head can be covered with a plastic bag or surgical covering if infection control is an issue. It is recommended that this wound be treated either twice a day for 30 minutes or once a day for 45 to 60 minutes at power and pulse rate settings of 6. If the patient appears to have any discomfort, the pulse rate should be lowered to 5 or 4. The pulse rate setting should also be reduced if the surface of the wound appears to be closing before the depth of the wound has completely filled.

Chapter Review

Electromagnetic radiation can be applied to a patient to achieve a wide variety of clinical effects. The nature of these effects is determined primarily by the frequency and wavelength of the radiation and, to some degree, by the intensity of the radiation. The frequencies of electromagnetic radiation used clinically can be in the IR, visible light, UV, shortwave, or microwave range. IR radiation produces superficial heating and can be used for the same purposes as other superficial heating agents. It has the advantage over other superficial heating agents of not requiring direct contact with the body. UV radiation produces erythema and tanning of the skin and epidermal hyperplasia and is essential for vitamin D synthesis. It is used primarily for the treatment of psoriasis. Low-intensity lasers in the visible, IR, and UV frequency ranges are used outside of the United States for a wide variety of clinical applications; however, they are not approved by the FDA for general clinical application at this time. Shortwave and microwave energy can produce heat in deep tissues and, when applied at a low average intensity using a pulsed signal, may decrease pain and edema and facilitate tissue healing by nonthermal mechanisms. Although none of these electromagnetic agents are now in widespread use in the United States, most are commonly used in other countries. Additional supportive literature will most likely increase their use in the United States. The reader is referred to the Evolve website at http://evolve.elsevier.com/Cameron for study questions pertinent to this chapter.

References

1. Sears FW, Zemansky MW, Young HD: *College Physics*, Reading, MA, 1987, Addison-Wesley.
2. Hitchcock RT, Patterson RM: *Radio-frequency and ELF Electromagnetic Energies: A Handbook for Health Professionals*, New York, 1995, Van Nostrand Reinhold.
3. Thomas CL: *Taber's Cyclopedic Medical Dictionary*, Philadelphia, 1993, FA Davis.
4. Adley WR: Physiological signalling across cell membranes and cooperative influences of extremely low frequency electromagnetic fields. In Frohlich H, ed: *Biological Coherence and Response to External Stimuli*, Heidelberg, 1988, Springer-Verlag.

5. Tsong TY: Deciphering the language of cells, *TIBS* 14: 89-92, 1989.

6. Anderson RR, Parrish JA: The optics of human skin, *J Invest Dermatol* 77:13-19, 1981.

7. Kaidbey K, Agin P, Sayre R et al: Photoprotection by melanin: a comparison of black and Caucasian skin, *Am Acad Dermatol* 1:249-260, 1979.

8. Farr P, Diffey B: The erythemal response of human skin to ultraviolet radiation, *Br J Dermatol* 113:65-76, 1985.

9. Faber M: Ultraviolet radiation. In Suess M, Benwell-Morrison D, eds: *Non-ionising Radiation Protection*, ed 2, WHO Regional Publications, European Series No. 25. Geneva, 1989, World Health Organization.

10. Murphy T: Nucleic acids: interaction with solar UV radiation, *Curr Top Radiat Res Q* 10:199, 1975.

11. Eaglestein W, Weinstein G: Prostaglandin and DNA synthesis in human skin: possible relationship to ultraviolet light effects, *J Invest Dermatol* 64:386-396, 1975.

12. Ganong WF: *Review of Medical Physiology*, ed 13, East Norwalk, CT, 1987, Appleton & Lange.

13. Holick MF: The cutaneous photosynthesis of previtamin D: a unique photoendocrine system, *J Invest Dermatol* 76:51-58, 1981.

14. Rasanen L, Reunala T, Lehto M et al: Immediate decrease in antigen-presenting function and delayed enhancement of interleukin-I production in human epidermal cells after in vivo UV-B irradiation, *Br J Dermatol* 120:589-596, 1989.

15. Horkay I, Bodolay E, Koda A: Immunologic aspects of prophylactic UV-B and PUVA therapy in polymorphic light eruption, *Photodermatology* 3:47-49, 1986.

16. Gollhausen R, Kaidbey K, Schechter N: UV suppression of mast cell mediated whealing in human skin, *Photodermatology* 2:58-67, 1985.

17. Kanekura T, Higashi Y, Kanzaki T: Cyclooxygenase-2 expression and prostaglandin E2 biosynthesis are enhanced in scleroderma fibroblasts and inhibited by UVA irradiation, *J Rheumatol* Jul;28(7):1568-1572, 2001.

18. High AS, High JP: Treatment of infected skin wounds using ultra-violet radiation: an in-vitro study, *Physiotherapy* 69(10):359-360, 1983.

19. Reynolds NJ, Franklin V, Gray JC et al: Narrow-band ultraviolet B and broad-band ultraviolet A phototherapy in adult atopic eczema: a randomised controlled trial, *Lancet* Jun 23;357(9273):2012-2016, 2001.

20. Freytes H, Fernandez B, Fleming W: Ultraviolet light in the treatment of indolent ulcers, *South Med J* 223-226, 1965.

21. Nussbaum EL, Biemann I, Mustard B: Comparison of ultrasound/ultraviolet-C and laser for treatment of pressure ulcers in patients with spinal cord injury, *Phys Ther* 74:812-823, 1994.

22. Scott BO: Ultraviolet application. In Stillwell K, ed: *Therapeutic Electricity and Ultraviolet Radiation*, ed 3, Baltimore, 1983, Williams & Wilkins.

23. Sjovall P, Moller H: The influence of locally administered ultraviolet light (UV-B) on allergic contact dermatitis in the mouse, *Acta Dermatol Venereol* 65:465-471, 1985.

24. Sjovall P, Christensen O: Local and systemic effect of UV-B irradiation in patients with chronic hand eczema, *Acta Dermatol Venereol* 67:538-541, 1987.

25. Epstein JH: *Phototherapy and photochemotherapy*, N Engl J Med 322:1149-1151, 1990.

26. Wolska H, Kleniewaska D, Kowalski J: Successful desensitization in a case of solar urticaria with sensitivity to UV-A and positive passive transfer test, *Dermatosensitivity* 30:84-86, 1982.

27. Norris PG, Hawk JLM, Baker C et al: British photodermatology group guidelines for PUVA, *Br J Dermatol* 130:246-255, 1994.

28. Honig B, Morison WL, Karp D, Photochemotherapy beyond psoriasis, *J Am Acad Dermatol* 31:775-790, 1994.

29. Fitch DH, Soderstrom RM, Kinzie S: PUVA therapy in the treatment of psoriasis, *Clin Manage* 7:24:26-27, 1987.

30. Fusco RJ, Jordon PA, Kelly A et al: PUVA treatment for psoriasis, *Physiotherapy* 66:40, 1980.

31. Klaber MR: Ultra-violet light for psoriasis, *Physiotherapy* 66:36-38, 1980.

32. Shurr DG, Zuehlke RL: Photochemotherapy treatment for psoriasis, *Phys Ther* 62:33-36, 1981.

33. Fotaides J, Lim HW, Jiang SB et al: Efficacy of ultraviolet B phototherapy for psoriasis in patients infected with human immunodeficiency virus, *Photodermatol Photoimmunol Photomed* 11(3):107-111, 1995.

34. Honigsmann H. Phototherapy for psoriasis, *Clin Exp Dermatol* Jun;26(4):343-350, 2001.

35. Ortel B, Perl S, Kinciyan T et al: Comparison of narrow-band (331 nm) UVB and broad band UVA after oral or bath-water 8-methoxypsoralen in the treatment of psoriasis, *J Am Acad Dermatol* 29(5 pt 1):736-740, 1993.

36. Tanew A, Radakovic-Fijan S, Schemper M et al: Paired comparison study on narrow-band (TL-01) UVB phototherapy versus photochemotherapy (PUVA) in the treatment of chronic plaque type psoriasis, *Arch Dermatol* 135: 519-524, 1999.

37. Fisher T, Alsisns J, Berne B: Ultraviolet action spectrum and evaluation of ultraviolet lamps for psoriasis healing, *Int J Dermatol* 23:633-637, 1984.

38. Lowe NJ, Wortzman MS, Breeding J et al: Coal tar phototherapy for psoriasis reevaluated: erythemogenic versus suberythemogenic ultraviolet with a tar extract in oil and crude coal tar, *J Am Acad Dermatol* 8:781-789, 1983.

39. Stern RS, Gange RW, Parrish JA et al: Contribution of topical tar oil to ultraviolet B phototherapy for psoriasis, *J Am Acad Dermatol* 14(5):742-747, 1986.

40. Tronnier H, Schule D: *First results of therapy with long wave UV-A after photosensitization of the skin.* Abstracts of the Sixth International Congress of Photobiology, Germany, 1972.

41. Iest J, Boer J: Combined treatment of psoriasis with acitretin and UV-B phototherapy compared with acitretin alone and UV-B alone, *Br J Dermatol* 120: 665-670, 1989.

42. Dover JS, McEvoy MT, Rosen CF et al: Are topical corticosteroids useful in phototherapy for psoriasis? *J Am Acad Dermatol* 21(3):592-593, 1989.

43. Gupta AK, Ellis CN, Tellner DC et al: Double blind placebo controlled study to evaluate the efficacy of fish oil and low dose UV-B in the treatment of psoriasis, *Br J Dermatol* 120:801-807, 1989.

44. Houghton PE, Campbell KE: Choosing an adjunctive therapy for the treatment of chronic wounds, *Ostomy Wound Manage* Aug;45(8):43-52, 1999.

45. Parrish J, Zaynoun S, Anderson R: Cumulative effect of repeated subthreshold doses of ultraviolet radiation, *J Invest Dermatol* 76:356-358, 1981.

46. Ramsay C, Challoner A: Vascular changes in human skin after ultraviolet irradiation, *Br J Dermatol* 94: 487-493, 1976.

47. Kloth LC: Physical modalities in wound management: UVC, therapeutic heating and electrical stimulation, *Ostomy Wound Manage* 41(5):18-20, 22-24, 26-27, 1995.

48. Wills EE, Anderson TW, Beatie LB et al: A randomised placebo controlled trial of ultraviolet in the treatment of superficial pressure sores, *J Am Geriatr Soc* 31:131-133, 1983.

49. Burns F: Cancer risks associated with therapeutic irradiation of the skin, *Arch Dermatol* 125:979-981, 1989.

50. Swanbeck G: To UV-B or not to UV-B? *Photodermatology* 1:2-4, 1984.

51. Studniberg HM, Weller P: PUVA, UVB, psoriasis, and nonmelanoma skin cancer, *J Am Acad Dermatol* 29(6):1013-1022, 1993.

52. Stern RS & Laird N: The carcinogenic risk of treatments for severe psoriasis, *Cancer* 73: 2759-2764, 1994.

53. Taylor HR: The biological effects of ultraviolet-B on the eye, *Photochem Photobiol* 50(4):489-492, 1989.

54. Stern RS, Liebman EJ, Vakeva L: Oral psoralen and ultraviolet-A light (PUVA) treatment of psoriasis and persistent risk of nonmelanoma skin cancer: PUVA follow-up study, *J Natl Cancer Inst* 90:1278-1284, 1998.

55. Tromovitch TA, Thompson LR, Jacobs PH: Testing for photosensitivity, *J Am Phys Ther Assoc* 143:348-349, 1963.

56. Low J: Quantifying the erythema due to UVR, *Physiotherapy* 72:60-64, 1986.

57. Levine M, Parrish JA: Out-patient phototherapy of psoriasis, *Arch Dermatol* 116:552-554, 1980.

58. Stern RS, Armstrong RB, Anderson TF et al: Effect of continued ultraviolet B phototherapy on the duration of remission of psoriasis: a randomised study, *J Am Acad Dermatol* 15(3):546-556, 1986.

59. Karrer S, Eholzer C, Ackermann G: Phototherapy of psoriasis: comparative experience of different phototherapeutic approaches, *Dermatology* 202(2):108-115, 2001.

60. Chue B, Borok M, Lowe NJ: Phototherapy units: comparison of fluorescent ultraviolet B and ultraviolet A units with high-pressure mercury system, *J Am Acad Dermatol* 18:641-645, 1998.

61. Kolari PJ: Penetration of unfocused laser light into the skin, *Arch Dermatol Res* 277:342-344, 1985.

62. King PR: Low level laser therapy—a review, *Lasers Med Sci* 4:141-150, 1989.

63. Goldman L, Michaelson SM, Rockwell RJ et al: Optical radiation with particular reference to lasers. In Suess M, Benwell-Morrison D, eds: *Nonionizing Radiation Protection*, ed 2, WHO Regional Publication, European Series No. 25. Geneva, 1989, World Health Organization.

64. Goldman L, Rockwell JR: *Lasers in Medicine*, New York, 1971, Gordon & Breach.

65. Alster TS, Kauvar AN, Geronemus RG: Histology of high-energy pulsed CO_2 laser resurfacing, *Semin Cutan Med Surg* 15(3):189-193, 1996.

66. Oshiro T, Calderhead RG: *Low Level Laser Therapy: A Practical Introduction*, Chichester, United Kingdom, 1988, Wiley.

67. Basford JR: Low energy laser therapy: controversies and new research findings, *Lasers Surg Med* 9:1-5, 1989.

68. Trelles MA, Mayayo E, Miro L: The action of low reactive laser therapy on mast cells, *Laser Ther* 1:1, 27-30, 1989.

69. Mester E, Ludany G, Vagda G et al: Effect of laser on bacteria phagocytosis of the leukocytes, *Orv Hetil* 108:1546-1550, 1967.

70. Baxter D: Low intensity laser therapy. In Kitchen S, Bazin S, eds: *Clayton's Electrotherapy*, ed 10, London, 1996, WB Saunders.

71. Castel MF: *A Clinical Guide to Low Power Laser Therapy*, Downsview, Ontario, Canada, 1985, Educational Division, Physio Technology Ltd.

72. Belkin M, Schwartz M: New biological phenomena associated with laser radiation, *Health Phys* 56:687-690, 1989.

73. Karu T: Photobiology of low-power laser effects, *Health Phys* 56:691-704, 1989.

74. Kitchen SS, Partridge CJ: A review of low level laser therapy, *Physiotherapy* 77:161-168, 1991.

75. Passarella S, Casamassima E, Molinari S et al: Increase of proton electrochemical potential and ATP synthesis in rat liver mitochondria irradiated in vitro by Helium-Neon laser, *FEBS Lett* 175:95-99, 1984.

76. Karu TI: Molecular mechanisms of the therapeutic effects of low intensity laser radiation, *Lasers Life Sci* 2:53-74, 1989.

77. Smith KC: The photobiological basis of low level laser radiation therapy, *Laser Ther* 3:19-24, 1991.

78. Young S, Bolton P, Dyson M et al: Macrophage responsiveness to light therapy, *Lasers Surg Med* 9:497-505, 1989.

79. Lam TS, Abergel RP, Castel JC et al: Laser stimulation of collagen synthesis in human skin fibroblast cultures, *Laser Life Sci* 1:61-77, 1986.

80. Lyons RF, Abergel RP, White RA et al: Biostimulation of wound healing in vivo by a helium-neon laser, *Ann Plast Surg* 18(1):47-50, 1987.

81. Kupin IV, Bykov VS, Ivanov AV et al: Potentiating effects of laser radiation on some immunologic traits, *Neoplasma* 29:403-406, 1982.

82. Passarella S, Casamassima E, Quagliariello E et al: Quantitative analysis of lymphocyte-Salmonella interaction and effects of lymphocyte irradiation by He-Ne laser, *Biochem Biophys Res Commun* 130:546-552, 1985.

83. Spector WS: *Handbook of Biological Data*, Philadelphia, 1956, WB Saunders.

84. Basford JR: The clinical and experimental status of low energy laser therapy, *Crit Rev Phys Med Rehabil* 1(1):1-9, 1989.

85. Nissan M, Rochkind S, Razon N et al: Ne-He laser irradiation delivered transcutaneously: its effects on the sciatic nerve of the rat, *Lasers Surg Med* 6:435-438, 1986.

86. Schwartz M, Doron A, Erlich M et al: Effects of low energy He-Ne laser irradiation on posttraumatic degeneration of adult rabbit optic nerve, *Lasers Surg Med* 7(1):51-55, 1987.

87. Rochkind S, Nissan M, Lubar R et al: The in-vivo nerve response to direct low energy laser irradiation, *Acta Neurochir* 94:74-77, 1988.

88. Walker JB, Akhanjee LK: Laser induced somatosensory evoked potentials: evidence of photosensitivity in peripheral nerves, *Brain Res* 344(2):281-285, 1985.

89. Snyder-Mackler L, Cork C: Effect of helium neon laser irradiation on peripheral sensory nerve latency, *Phys Ther* 68:223-225, 1988.

90. Baxter D, Bell AJ, Allen JM: *Laser mediated increase in median nerve conduction velocities.* Presented at the Fourth International Biotherapy Laser Association Seminar, London, 1990, Guy's Hospital.

91. Basford JR, Daube JR, Hallman HO et al: Does low intensity helium neon laser irradiation alter sensory nerve action potentials or distal latencies? *Lasers Surg Med* 10:35-39, 1990.

92. Lundeberg T, Haker E, Thomas M: Effects of laser versus placebo in tennis elbow, *Scand J Rehabil Med* 19:135-138, 1987.

93. Wu WH, Ponnudurai R, Katz J et al: Failure to confirm report of light-evoked response of peripheral nerve to low power helium neon laser light stimulus, *Brain Res* 401(2):407-408, 1987.

94. Jarvis D, MacIver MB, Tanelian DL: Electrophysiologic recording and thermodynamic modeling demonstrate that helium-neon laser irradiation does not affect peripheral A-delta or C-fiber nociceptors, *Pain* 43(2):235-242, 1990.

95. Moolenar H: *Endolaser 476 Therapy Protocol*, Delft, the Netherlands, 1990, Enraf-Nonius Delft.

96. Surchinak JS, Alago ML, Bellamy RF et al: Effects of low level energy lasers on the healing of full thickness skin defects, *Laser Surg Med* 2:267-274, 1983.

97. Mester E, Spiry T, Szende B et al: Effects of laser rays on wound healing, *Am J Surg* 122:532-535, 1971.

98. Mester E, Ludany G, Sellyei M et al: The stimulating effects of low power laser rays on biological systems, *Laser Rev* 1:3, 1968.

99. Ma SY, Hou H: Effect of He-Ne laser irradiation on healing skin wounds in mice, *Laser* 7:146, 1981.

100. Mester AF, Mester A: Wound healing, *Laser Ther* 1:7-15, 1989.

101. Dyson M, Young S: Effect of laser therapy on wound contraction and cellularity in mice, *Lasers Med Sci* 1:125-130, 1986.

102. Gogia PP, Hurt BS, Zirn TT: Wound management with whirlpool and infrared cold laser treatment: a clinical report, *Phys Ther* 68(8):1239-1242, 1988.

103. Mester AF, Mester A: Clinical data of laser biostimulation in wound healing, *Lasers Surg Med* 7:78, 1987.

104. Kahn J: Case reports: open wound management with the HeNe cold laser, *J Orthop Sport Phys* 6(3):203-204, 1984.

105. Reddy GK, Stehno-Bittel D, Enwemeka CS: Laser photostimulation accelerates wound healing in diabetic rats, *Wound Repair Regen* May-Jun;9(3):248-255, 2001.

106. Schindl A, Schindl M, Schon H et al: Low-intensity laser irradiation improves skin circulation in patients with diabetic microangiopathy, *Diabetes Care* 21:580-584, 1998.

107. Lilge L, Tierney K, Nussbaum E: Low-level laser therapy for wound healing: feasibility of wound dressing transillumination, *J Clin Laser Med Surg* Oct;18(5):235-240, 2000.

108. Cambier DC, Vanderstraeten GG, Mussen MJ et al: Low power laser and healing of burns: a preliminary assay, *Plast Reconstr Surg* 97(3):555-558, 1996.

109. McCaughan JS Jr, Bethel BH, Johnson T et al: Effect of low dose argon irradiation on rate of wound closure, *Lasers Surg Med* 5(6):607-614, 1985.

110. Basford JR, Hallman HO, Sheffield SG et al: Comparisons of cold-quartz ultraviolet, low-energy laser, and occlusion in wound healing in a swine model, *Arch Phys Med Rehabil* 106(6):358-363, 1986.

111. Flemming K, Cullum N: Laser therapy for venous leg ulcers, *Cochrane Database Syst Rev* (2):CD001182, 2000.

112. Trelles MA, Mayayo E: Bone fracture consolidates faster with low-power laser, *Lasers Surg Med* 7:36-45, 1987.

113. Chen JW, Zhou YC: Effect of low level carbon dioxide laser irradiation on biochemical metabolism of rabbit mandibular bone callus, *Laser Ther* 1:83-87, 1989.

114. Tang XM, Chai BP: Effect of CO_2 laser irradiation on experimental fracture healing: a transmission electron microscopy study, *Lasers Surg Med* 7:36-45, 1987.

115. Niccoli-Filho W, Okamoto T: The effect of exposure to continuous Nd: YAG laser radiation on the wound healing process after removal of the teeth (a histological study on rats), *Stomatologiia* 74(5):26-29, 1995.

116. Kucerova H, Dostalova T, Himmlova L et al: Low-Level laser therapy after molar extraction, *J Clin Laser Med Surg* Dec;18(6):309-315, 2000.

117. Coombe AR, Ho CT, Darendeliler MA et al: The effects of low level laser irradiation on osteoblastic cells, *Clin Orthod Res* 4(1):3-14, 2001.

118. Beckerman H, Bde Bie RA, Bouter LM et al: The efficacy of laser therapy for musculoskeletal and skin disorders: a criteria-based meta-analysis of randomized clinical trials, *Phys Ther* 72(7):483-491, 1992.

119. Goldman JA, Chiarpella J, Casey H et al: Laser therapy of rheumatoid arthritis, *Lasers Surg Med* 1:93-101, 1980.

120. Palmgren N, Jensen GF, Kaae K et al: Low power laser therapy in rheumatoid arthritis, *Lasers Med Sci* 4:193-195, 1989.

121. Asada K, Yutani Y, Shimazu A: Diode laser therapy for rheumatoid arthritis: a clinical evaluation of 102 joints treated with low level laser therapy, *Laser Ther* 1:147-151, 1989.

122. Lonauer G: Controlled double blind study on the efficacy of He-Ne laser beams v He-Ne + infrared laser beams in therapy of activated OA of the finger joint, *Lasers Surg Med* 6:172, 1986.

123. Ozdemis F, Birtane M, Kokino S: The clinical efficacy of low-power laser therapy on pain and function in cervical osteoarthritis, *Clin Rheumatol* 20(3):181-184, 2001.

124. Basford JR, Sheffield CG, Mair SD et al: Low energy helium neon laser treatment of thumb osteoarthritis, *Arch Phys Med Rehabil* 68(11):794-797, 1987.

125. McAuley R, Ysala R: Soft laser: A treatment for osteoarthritis of the knee? *Arch Phys Med Rehabil* 66:553-554, 1985.

126. Brosseau L, Welch V, Wells G et al: Low level laser therapy for osteoarthritis and rheumatoid arthritis: a metaanalysis: *J Rheumatol* 27(8):1961-1969, 2000.

127. Brosseau L, Welch V, Wells G et al: Low level laser therapy (classes I, II and III) in the treatment of rheumatoid arthritis, *Cochrane Database Syst Rev* (2):CD002049, 2000.

128. Brosseau L, Welch V, Wells G et al: Low level laser therapy (classes I, II and III) for the treatment of osteoarthritis, *Cochrane Database Syst Rev* (2):CD002046, 2000.

129. Marks R, de Palma F: Clinical efficacy of low power laser therapy in osteoarthritis, *Physiother Res Int*, 4(2):141-157, 1999.

130. Haker E, Lundeberg T: Is low-energy laser treatment effective in lateral epicondylalgia? *J Pain Symptom Manage* 6(4):241-246, 1991.

131. Vasseljen O, Hoeg N, Kjelstad B et al: Low level laser versus placebo in the treatment of tennis elbow, *Scand J Rehabil Med* 24(1):37-42, 1992.

132. Snyder-Mackler L, Barry AJ, Perkins AI et al: Effects of helium-neon laser irradiation on skin resistance and pain in patients with trigger points in the neck or back, *Phys Ther* 69(5):336-341, 1989.

133. Snyder-Mackler L, Bork C, Bourbon B et al: Effect of helium-neon laser on musculoskeletal trigger points, *Phys Ther* 66(7):1087-1090, 1986.

134. Walker J: Relief from chronic pain by low power laser irradiation, *Neurosci Lett* 43:339-344, 1983.

135. Basford JR, Sheffield CG, Harmsen WS: Laser therapy: a randomized, controlled trial of the effects of low-intensity Nd:YAG laser irradiation on musculoskeletal back pain, *Arch Phys Med Rehabil* Jun;80(6):647-652, 1999.

136. Moore KC, Hira N, Kumar PS et al: A double blind crossover trial of low level laser therapy in the treatment of post-herpetic neuralgia, *Laser Ther* Pilot Issue:7-9, 1989.

137. Siebert W, Seichert N, Siebert B et al: What is the efficacy of soft and mid lasers in therapy of tendinopathies? *Arch Orthop Trauma Surg* 106:358-363, 1987.

138. Haker EH, Lundeberg TC: Lateral epicondylalgia: report of noneffective midlaser treatment, *Arch Phys Med Rehabil* 72(12):984-988, 1991.

139. Chartered Society of Physiotherapy, Safety of Electrotherapy Equipment Working Group: *Guidelines for the Safe Use of Lasers in Physiotherapy*, London, 1991, Chartered Society of Physiotherapy.

140. Moholkar R, Zukowski S, Turbill H et al: The safety and efficacy of low level laser therapy in soft tissue

injuries: a double-blind randomized study, *Phys Ther* 81(5):A49, 2001.

141. Blidall H, Hellesen C, Ditlevesen P et al: Soft laser therapy of rheumatoid arthritis, *Scand J Rheumatol* 16: 225-228, 1987.

142. Waylonis GW, Wilke S, O'Toole DO et al: Chronic myofascial pain: management by low output helium-neon laser therapy, *Arch Phys Med Rehabil* 69: 1017-1020, 1988.

143. Silverman DR, Pendleton LA: A comparison of the effects of continuous and pulsed shortwave diathermy on peripheral circulation, *Arch Phys Med Rehabil* 49:429-436, 1968.

144. Conradi E, Pages IH: Effects of continuous and pulsed microwave irradiation on distribution of heat in the gluteal region of minipigs, *Scand J Rehabil Med* 21: 59-62, 1989.

145. Draper DO, Knight K, Fujiwara T et al: Temperature change in human muscle during and after pulsed short-wave diathermy, *J Orthop Sports Phys Ther* Jan;29(1):13-8; discussion 19-22, 1999.

146. Kloth LC, Zisken MC: Diathermy and pulsed radio frequency radiation. In Michlovitz SL, ed: *Thermal Agents in Rehabilitation*, Philadelphia, 1996, FA Davis.

147. Verrier M, Falconer K, Crawford SJ: A comparison of tissue temperature following two shortwave diathermy techniques, *Physiotherapy Canada* 29(1): 21-25, 1977.

148. Guy AW, Lehmann JF, Stonebridge JB: Therapeutic applications of electromagnetic power, *Proc IEEE* 62:55-75, 1974.

149. Van der Esch M, Hoogland R: *Pulsed Shortwave Diathermy with the Curapuls 419*, Delft, the Netherlands, 1990, Delft Instruments Physical Medicine BV.

150. Hand JW: Biophysics and technology of electromagnetic hyperthermia. In Guthrie M, ed: *Methods of External Hyperthermic Heating*, Berlin, 1990, Springer-Verlag.

151. McMeeken JM, Bell C: Effects of selective blood and tissue heating on blood flow in the dog hind limb, *Exp Physiol* 75:359-366, 1990.

152. Fadilah R, Pinkas J, Weinberger A et al: Heating rabbit joint by microwave applicator, *Arch Phys Med Rehabil* 68(10):710-712, 1987.

153. Scott RS, Chou CK, McCumber M et al: Complications resulting from spurious fields produced by a microwave applicator used for hyperthermia, *Int J Radiat Oncol Biol Phys* 12(10):1883-1886, 1986.

154. McNiven DR, Wyper DJ: Microwave therapy and muscle blood flow in man, *J Microwave Power* 11:168, 1976.

155. McMeeken JM, Bell C: Microwave irradiation of the human forearm and hand, *Physiother Theory Practice* 75:359-366, 1990.

156. Wyper DJ, McNiven DR: Effects of some physiotherapeutic agents on skeletal muscle blood flow, *Physiotherapy* 60(10):309-310, 1976.

157. Benson TB, Copp EP: The effect of therapeutic forms of heat and ice on the pain threshold of the normal shoulder, *Rheumatol Rehabil* 13:101-104, 1974.

158. Abramson DL, Chu LSW, Tuck S et al: Effect of tissue temperature and blood flow on motor nerve conduction velocity, *J Am Med Soc* 198:1082-1088, 1966.

159. Chastain PB: The effect of deep heat on isometric strength, *Phys Ther* 58(5):543-546, 1978.

160. McMeeken JM, Bell C: Effects of microwave irradiation on blood flow in the dog hind limb, *Exp Physiol* 75:367-374, 1990.

161. Hayne CR: Pulsed high frequency energy:its place in physiotherapy, *Physiotherapy* 70(12):459-466, 1984.

162. Markov MS: Electric current electromagnetic field effects on soft tissue: implications for wound healing, *Wounds* 7(3):94-110, 1995.

163. Pilla AA, Markov MS: Bioeffects of weak electromagnetic fields, *Rev Environ Health* 10(3-4):155-169, 1994.

164. Mayrovitz HN, Larsen PB: A preliminary study to evaluate the effect of pulsed radio frequency field treatment on lower extremity peri-ulcer skin microcirculation of diabetic patients, *Wounds* 7(3):90-93, 1995.

165. Mayrovitz HN, Larsen PB: Effects of pulsed electromagnetic fields on skin microvascular blood perfusion, *Wounds* 4(5):197-202, 1992.

166. Rozengurt E, Mendoza S: Monovalent ion fluxes and the control of cell proliferation in cultured fibroblasts, *Ann NY Acad Sci* 339:175-190, 1980.

167. Boonstra J, Skper SD, Varons SJ: Regulation of Na^+, K^+ pump activity by nerve growth factor in chick embryo dorsal root ganglia cells, *J Cell Physiol* 113:452-455, 1982.

168. Gemsa D, Seitz M, Kramer W et al: Ionophore A 23187 rasis cyclic AMP levels in macrophages by stimulation of prostaglandin E formation: *Exp Cell Res* 118:55-62, 1979.

169. Pilla A: *Electrochemical information and energy transfer in vivo*, Proc 7th IECEC, Washington, DC, 1972, American Chemical Society.

170. Markov MS, Muechsam DJ, Pilla AA: Modulation of cell-free myosin phosphorylation with pulsed radio frequency electromagnetic fields. In Allen MJ, Cleary SF, Sowers AE, eds: *Charge and Field Effects in Biosystems*, ed 4, Singapore, 1995, World Scientific. Publishing Co.

171. Markov MS, Pilla AA: Modulation of cell-free myosin light chain phosphorylation with weak low frequency and static magnetic fields, In Frey AH, ed: *On the Nature of Electromagnetic Field Interactions with Bioilogical Systems*, Austin/New York, 1995, RG Landes/Springer.

172. Whitfield JF, Boynton AL, McManus JP et al: The roles of calcium and cyclic AMP in cell proliferation, *Ann NY Acad Sci* 339:216-240, 1981.

173. Canaday DJ, Lee RC: Scientific basis for clinical application of electric fields in soft tissue repair. In Brighton CT, Pollack SR, eds: *Electromagnetics in Biology Medicine,* San Francisco, 1991, San Francisco Press.

174. Markov MS, Pilla AA: Electromagnetic field stimulation of soft tissues: pulsed radio frequency treatment of post-operative pain and edema, *Wounds* 7(4): 143-151, 1995.

175. Vance AR, Hayes SH, Spielholz NI: Microwave diathermy treatment for primary dysmenorrhea, *Phys Ther* 76(9):1003-1008, 1996.

176. Goats GC: Continuous short-wave (radio-frequency) diathermy, *Br J Sports Med* 23:123-127, 1989.

177. Ginsberg AJ: Ultrasound radiowaves as a therapeutic agent, *Med Rec* 19:1-8, 1934.

178. Milinowski AS: *Athermapeutic device,* United States Patent #3181535, 1965.

179. Pilla AA, Martin DE, Schuett AM et al: Effect of PRF therapy on edema from grades I and II ankle sprains: a placebo controlled randomized, multi-site, double-blind clinical study, *J Athletic Training* 31:S53, 1996.

180. Wilson DH: Treatment of soft tissue injuries by pulsed electrical energy, *Br Med J* 2:269-270, 1972.

181. Pennington GM, Danley DL, Sumko MH: Pulsed, non-thermal, high frequency electromagnetic field (Diapulse) in the treatment of Grade I and Grade II ankle sprains, *Milit Med* 153:101-104, 1993.

182. Kaplan EG, Weinstock RE: Clinical evaluation of Diapulse as adjunctive therapy following foot surgery, *J Am Podiatr Assoc* 58(5):218-221, 1968.

183. Barker AT, Barlow PS, Porter J et al: A double blind clinical trial of low power pulsed shortwave therapy in the treatment of soft tissue injury, *Physiotherapy* 71(12):500-504, 1985.

184. McGill SN: The effects of pulsed shortwave therapy on lateral ankle sprains, *N Z J Physiother* 51:21-24, 1988.

185. Foley-Nolan D, Barry C, Coughlan RJ et al: Pulsed high frequency (27 MHz) electromagnetic therapy for persistent neck pain: a double blind placebo-controlled study of 20 patients, *Orthopedics* 13: 445-451, 1990.

186. Foley-Nolan D, Moore K, Codd M et al: Low energy, high frequency, pulsed electromagnetic therapy for acute whiplash injuries, *Scand J Rehabil Med* 24:51-59, 1992.

187. Wagstaff P, Wagstaff S, Downey M: A pilot study to compare the efficacy of continuous and pulsed magnetic energy (shortwave diathermy) on the relief of low back pain, *Physiotherapy* 72(1):563-566, 1986.

188. Santiesteban AJ, Grant C: Post-surgical effect of pulsed shortwave therapy, *J Am Podiatr Assoc* 75(6):306-309, 1985.

189. Cameron BM: Experimental acceleration of wound healing, *Am J Orthop* 3(12):336-343, 1961.

190. Itoh M, Montemayor JS, Matsumoto E et al: Accelerated wound healing of pressure ulcers by pulsed high peak power electromagnetic energy (Diapulse), *Decubitus* 2:24-28, 1991.

191. Ionescu A, Ionescu D, Milinescu S et al: *Study of efficiency of Diapulse therapy on the dynamics of enzymes in burned wound.* Proceedings of the Sixth International Congress on Burns, 6:25-26, 1982.

192. Salzberg CA, Cooper-Vastola SA, Perez FJ et al: The effect of non-thermal pulsed electromagnetic energy (Diapulse) on wound healing of pressure ulcers in spinal cord injured patients: a randomized, double-blind study, *Wounds* 7(1):11-16, 1995.

193. Raji ARM, Bowden REM: Effects of high peak pulsed electromagnetic fields on the degeneration and regeneration of the common peroneal nerve in rats, *J Bone Joint Surg* 65:478-492, 1983.

194. Wilson DH, Jagadeesh P, Newman PP et al: The effects of pulsed electromagnetic energy on peripheral nerve regeneration, *Ann NY Acad Sci* 238:575-580, 1974.

195. Wilson DH, Jagadeesh P: Experimental regeneration in peripheral nerves and the spinal cord in laboratory animals exposed to a pulsed electromagnetic field, *Paraplegia* 14:12-20, 1976.

196. Cook HH, Narendan NS, Montogomery JC: The effects of pulsed, high-frequency waves on the rate of osteogenesis in the healing of extraction wounds in dogs, *Oral Surg* 32(6):1008-1016, 1971.

197. Pilla AA: *27.12 MHz pulsed radiofrequency electromagnetic fields accelerate bone repair in a rabbit fibula osteotomy model.* Presented at the Bioelectromagnetics Society meeting, Boston, 1995.

198. Sambasivan M: Pulsed electromagnetic field in management of head injuries, *Neurol India* 41(Suppl):56, 1993.

199. Hayward L, Statham A: Microwave, *Physiotherapy* (South Africa) 37(1):7-9, 1981.

200. Low J, Reed A: *Electrotherapy Explained: Principles and Practice,* London, 1990, Butterworth-Heinemann.

201. Health Notice (Hazard) 80(10): *Implantable Cardiac Pacemakers–Interference Generated by Diathermy Equipment.* Washington, DC, 1980, Department of Health and Human Services.

202. Burr B: *Heat as a therapeutic modality against cancer.* Report 16. Bethesda, MA, 1974, U.S. National Cancer Institute.

203. Mcmurray RG, Katz VL: Thermoregulation in pregnancy: implications for exercise, *Sports Med* 10(3): 146-158, 1990.

204. Edwards MJ: Congenital defects in guinea pigs following induced hyperthermia during gestation, *Arch Pathol Lab Med* 84:42-48, 1967.

205. Edwards MJ: Congenital defects due to hyperthermia, *Adv Vet Sci Comp Med* 22:29-52, 1978.

206. Brown-Woodman PD, Hadley JA, Waterhouse J et al: Teratogenic effects of exposure to radiofrequency radiation (27.12 MHz) from a short wave diathermy unit, *Ind Health* 26(1):1-10, 1988.

207. Tofani S, Agnesod G: The assessment of unwanted radiation around diathermy RF capacitive applicators, *Health Phys* 47(2):235-241, 1984.

208. Lau RW, Dunscombe PB: Some observations on stray magnetic fields and power outputs from shortwave diathermy equipment, *Health Phys* 46(4):939-943, 1984.

209. Lerman Y, Caner A, Jacubovich R et al: Electromagnetic fields from shortwave diathermy equipment in physiotherapy departments, *Physiotherapy* 82(8):456-458, 1996.

210. Martin JC, McCallum HM, Strelley S et al: Electromagnetic fields from therapeutic diathermy equipment: a review of hazards and precautions, *Physiotherapy* 77(1):3-7, 1991.

211. Christensen DA, Durney CH: Hyperthermia production for cancer therapy: a review of fundamentals and methods, *J Microwave Power* 16:89-105, 1981.

212. Nielson NC, Hansen R, Larsen T: Heat induction in copper bearing IUDs during short wave diathermy, *Acta Obstet Gynecol Scand* 58(5):495, 1979.

213. Heick A, Espesen T, Pedersen HL et al: Is diathermy safe in women with copper-bearing IUDs? *Acta Obstet Gynecol Scand* 70(2):153-155, 1991.

214. Delpizzo V, Joyner KH: On the safe use of microwave and shortwave diathermy units, *Aust J Physiother* 33:152-161, 1987.

215. Chartered Society of Physiotherapy: *Guidelines for Safe Use of Microwave Therapy Equipment*, London, 1994, Chartered Society of Physiotherapy.

216. Kallen B, Malmquist G, Moritz U: Delivery outcome among physiotherapists in Sweden: is non-ionising radiation a fetal hazard? *Arch Environ Health* 37:81-84, 1982. Reprinted in *Physiotherapy* 78(1):15-18, 1992.

217. Larsen A, Olsen J, Svane O: Gender specific reproductive outcome and exposure to high frequency electromagnetic radiation among physiotherapists, *Scand J Work Environ Health* 17:318-323, 1991.

218. Ouellet-Hellstrom R, Stewart WF: Miscarriages among female physical therapists who report using radio and microwave frequency electromagnetic radiation, *Am J Epidemiol* 10:775-785, 1993.

219. Lerman Y, Jacubovich R, Green MS: Pregnancy outcome following exposure to shortwaves among female physiotherapists in Israel, *Am J Ind Med* May;39(5):499-504, 2001.

220. Takininen H, Kyyronene P, Hemminki K: The effects of ultrasound, shortwaves and physical exertion on pregnancy outcomes in physiotherapists, *J Epidemiol Commun Health* 44:196-201, 1990.

221. Werheimer N, Leeper E: Electrical wiring configurations and childhood cancer, *Am J Epidemiol* 109:273-284, 1979.

222. Milham S Jr: Mortality from leukemia in workers exposed to electrical and magnetic fields (letter), *N Engl J Med* 307:249, 1982.

223. Surrell JA, Alexander RC, Cohle SD: Effects of microwave radiation on living tissues, *J Trauma* 27:935-939, 1987.

224. Justesen D, Adair ER, Stevens J et al: Human sensory thresholds of microwave and infra-red radiation, *Bioelectromagnetics* 3.117, 1982.

225. sofPulse™: Pompano Beach, FL: Electropharmacology, Inc.

226. Diapulse®: Great Neck, NY: Diapulse Corporation of America.

Section Three

Integrating Physical Agents into Present and Future Practice

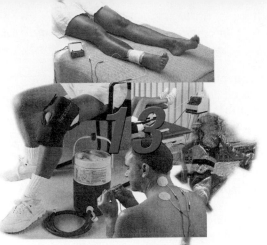

Integrating Physical Agents into Patient Care

OBJECTIVES

Upon completion of this chapter, the reader will be able to:

1. Summarize the attributes to be considered in the selection of physical agents.
2. Design treatment plans for a variety of patient problems that integrate the use of physical agents within a complete rehabilitation program.
3. Evaluate clinical findings to determine when to use specific physical agents and when to change agents or treatment parameters.
4. Make decisions regarding the application of physical agents under different health care delivery systems.

During rehabilitation, patients frequently have problems that may benefit from several interventions, including treatments using a number of physical agents. In such circumstances the clinician must select the optimal intervention, or combination of interventions. Selection is based on an evaluation of the clinical findings from the initial patient examination, the goals of treatment, and the expected effects of the various available treatment options.

Physical agents have direct effects primarily at the level of impairment and, when appropriately selected, can accelerate and enhance resolution of functional limitations and disabilities. In order to select and use physical agents most effectively, the therapist must understand the physical and physiological processes underlying the patient's problems, the kinds of changes that would promote resolution of these problems, and the nature of the effects of available physical agents.

The first section of this book discussed the types of problems most commonly treated with physical agents in rehabilitation, and the second section discussed the nature of the effects of the available physical agents, particularly as they relate to these problems and their underlying physiological processes. This chapter integrates and summarizes the information from these earlier sections. Additional guidelines are provided to aide in the selection of treatment options in order to achieve optimal patient outcome within the constraints of the health care delivery system. Three clinical case studies demonstrating the application of these guidelines are provided at the end of the chapter.

ATTRIBUTES TO BE CONSIDERED IN THE SELECTION OF PHYSICAL AGENTS

When selecting a physical agent for use in patient treatment, a number of attributes of the agent should be considered, the first two being the goals of treatment and the physiological effects required to achieve these goals (Fig. 13-1). Having determined which physical agents can promote progress toward the goals of treatment, the clinician should then decide which of the potentially effective interventions would be most appropriate for the particular patient and the current clinical presentation. Attending to the rule of "do no harm," all interventions that are contraindicated should be rejected and all precautions

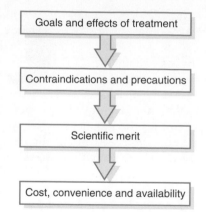

Figure 13-1. Attributes to be considered in the selection of physical agents.

should be adhered to. If a number of methods would be effective and could be applied safely, the scientific merit of the treatment approach, the ease and cost of application, and the availability of necessary resources should also be considered. Having selected the ideal physical agent(s), the clinician must then also select the ideal treatment parameters and means of application and appropriately integrate the use of the chosen physical agent(s) into a complete treatment program.

Goals and Effects of Treatment

Reducing impairments by affecting:
  Inflammation and tissue healing
  Pain
  Muscle tone
  Motion restrictions

The immediate goals of treatment that can be met with physical agents generally relate to reducing impairments by affecting inflammation and tissue healing, pain, muscle tone, or motion restrictions. By reducing impairments, interventions with physical agents contribute to reducing functional limitations and disabilities. Guidelines for treatment selection based on the direct effects of physical agents are presented below in a narrative form and are summarized in Tables 13-1 to 13-4. Should the patient present with more than one problem, and thus have a number of goals for treatment, a limited number of these goals may need to be addressed at any one time. It is generally recommended that the primary problems, those underlying the other problems, and those most likely to respond to the available interventions be addressed first; however, the ideal intervention will facilitate progress in a number of areas (Fig. 13-2). For example, if a patient has knee pain due to acute joint inflammation, treatment should first be directed at resolving the inflammation; however, the ideal intervention would also help to relieve pain. When the primary underlying problem, such as a malignancy, cannot benefit directly from an intervention with a physical agent, treatment with physical agents may still be used to help alleviate the sequelae of these problems, such as pain or swelling.

Effects of different physical agents on inflammation and healing

Many physical agents affect inflammation and healing and, when appropriately applied, can accelerate progress, limit adverse consequences of the healing process, and optimize the final patient outcome (Table 13-1). However, when poorly selected or misapplied, physical agents may impair or potentially prevent complete healing. After any injury, physiological tissues proceed through three stages—inflammation, proliferation, and maturation—in order to heal. At each of these stages, the goals of treatment, and thus the appropriate interventions, will change.

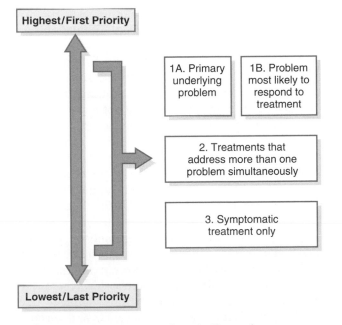

Figure 13-2. Prioritizing goals and effects of treatment.

Initial injury

Immediately after an injury or trauma, the goals of treatment are to prevent further injury or bleeding and to clean away any wound contaminants if the skin has been broken. Immobilization of the injured area with the aid of a static compression device such as an elastic wrap or with the use of assistive devices such as crutches, a cast, or a brace, can limit further injury and bleeding. Motion of the injured area, whether active, electrically stimulated, or passive, is contraindicated at this stage due to the risk of causing further tissue damage and bleeding. Cryotherapy will also contribute to the control of bleeding by limiting blood flow to the injured area as a result of vasoconstriction and increased blood viscosity.[1,2] Thermotherapy is contraindicated at this early stage because it can increase bleeding at the site of injury by increasing blood flow or reopening vascular lesions due to vasodilation.[3-5] Hydrotherapy, involving immersion or nonimmersion techniques, can be used to cleanse the injured area if the skin has been broken and the wound has become contaminated; however, since thermotherapy is contraindicated, only neutral warmth or cooler water should be used.[6]

Acute Inflammation

During the acute inflammatory stage of healing, the goals of treatment are to control pain, edema, bleeding, and the release and activity of inflammatory mediators and to facilitate progression to the proliferation stage. A number of physical agents, including cryotherapy, hydrotherapy, electrical stimulation, and pulsed shortwave diathermy (PSWD), can be used to control pain; however, the use of thermotherapy, intermittent traction, and motor-level electrical stimulation is not appropriate.[7-11] The use of thermotherapy is not recommended because it causes vasodilation, which may aggravate edema, and it increases the metabolic rate, which may aggravate the inflammatory response. Intermittent traction and motor-level electrical stimulation should be used with caution because the movement produced by these physical agents may cause further tissue irritation and thereby aggravate the inflammatory response. A number of physical agents, including cryotherapy, compression, sensory-level electrical stimulation, PSWD, and contrast baths, may be used to control or reduce edema.[12-15] Cryotherapy and compression can also help to control bleeding; furthermore, cryotherapy will inhibit the activity and release

TABLE 13-1   Physical Agents for Promoting Tissue Healing

Stage of tissue healing	Goals of treatment	Effective agents	Contraindicated
Initial injury	Prevent further injury or bleeding	Static compression Cryotherapy	Local motion due to exercise, intermittent traction or motor-level electrical stimulation Thermotherapy
	Clean open wound	Hydrotherapy (immersion or nonimmersion)	
Chronic inflammation	Prevent/decrease joint stiffness	Thermotherapy, motor e.s., whirlpool, Fluidotherapy	Cryotherapy
	Control pain	Thermotherapy, e.s.	
	Increase circulation	Thermotherapy, e.s., compression, hydrotherapy (immersion or exercise)	Cryotherapy
	Progress to proliferation stage	Pulsed ultrasound, e.s., PSWD	
Remodeling	Regain or maintain strength	Motor e.s., water exercise	Immobilization
	Regain or maintain flexibility	Thermotherapy, brief ice massage	Immobilization
	Control scar tissue formation	Compression	

e.s. = electrical stimulation.

of inflammatory mediators. Should healing be delayed due to the inhibition of inflammation, as may occur in the patient who is on high-dose catabolic corticosteroids, cryotherapy should not be used because it may further impair the process of inflammation and thus potentially delay tissue healing. There is also evidence to indicate that pulsed ultrasound and PSWD may promote progression from the inflammatory stage of healing to the proliferative stage.

Chronic inflammation

Should the inflammatory response persist and become chronic, the goals, and thus the selection of interventions, will change. During this stage of healing the goals of treatment are to prevent or decrease joint stiffness, control pain, increase circulation, and promote progression to the proliferation stage. The most effective interventions for reducing joint stiffness are thermotherapy and motion.[16,17] Superficial structures such as the skin and subcutaneous fascia may be heated by superficial heating agents such as hot packs or paraffin; however, in order to heat deeper structures such as the shoulder or hip joint capsules, deep heating agents such as ultrasound or diathermy must be used.[18-20] Motion may be produced by active exercise or electrical stimulation, and motion can be combined with heat by having the patient exercise in warm water or Fluidotherapy. Thermotherapy and electrical stimulation can be used to relieve pain during the chronic inflammatory stage; however, cryotherapy is generally not recommended during this stage because it can increase the joint stiffness frequently associated with chronic inflammation. Selection between thermotherapy and electrical stimulation will generally depend on the need for the additional benefits of each modality and the other selection factors discussed below. Circulation may be increased by the use of thermotherapy, electrical stimulation, compression, water immersion, or exercise, and possibly by the use of contrast baths.[3,21-25] A final goal of treatment at the chronic inflammatory phase of tissue healing is to promote progression to the proliferative phase. Some studies indicate that pulsed ultrasound, electrical currents, and electromagnetic fields may promote this transition.

Proliferation

Once the injured tissue moves beyond the inflammatory stage to the proliferative stage of healing, the primary goals of treatment become controlling scar tissue formation, ensuring adequate circulation, maintaining strength and flexibility, and promoting progression to the remodeling stage. Static compression garments can control superficial scar tissue formation, thereby promoting enhanced cosmesis and reducing the severity and incidence of contractures.[26-28] Adequate circulation is required to provide oxygen and nutrients to the newly forming tissue. Circulation may be enhanced by the use of thermotherapy, electrotherapy, compression, water immersion, or exercise and possibly by the use of contrast baths. Although active exercise can increase or maintain strength and flexibility during the proliferative stage of healing, the addition of motor-level electrical stimulation or water exercise may accelerate recovery and provide additional benefits. The water environment reduces loading, and thus the potential for trauma to weight-bearing structures, and may thereby decrease the risk of regression to the inflammatory stage.[29] The support provided by the water may also assist motion should the muscles be very weak, and water-based exercise and thermotherapy may promote circulation and help to maintain or increase flexibility.[30,31]

Maturation

During the final stage of tissue healing, maturation, the goals of treatment are to regain or maintain strength and flexibility and to control scar tissue formation. At this point in the healing process, the injured tissues are approaching their final form. The focus of treatment should therefore be on reversing any adverse effects of the earlier stages of healing, such as weakening of muscles or loss of flexibility. Strengthening and stretching exercises most effectively address these problems. Strengthening may be more effective with the addition of motor-level electrical stimulation or water exercise, while stretching may be more effective with the prior application of thermotherapy or brief ice massage.[16,32] Should the injury be of a type that is particularly prone to excessive scar formation, such as a burn, control of scar formation with compression garments should be continued throughout the remodeling stage.

Effects of different physical agents on pain

In addition to modifying the signs and symptoms associated with inflammation and tissue healing, and promoting the progression of these processes, physical agents can be used to relieve pain (see Table 13-2). Different physical agents are indicated or contraindicated for treating different types of pain and for treating pain of differing etiologies.

TABLE 13-2   Physical Agents for the Treatment of Pain

Type of pain	Goals of treatment	Effective agents	Contraindicated
Acute	Control pain	Sensory e.s., cryotherapy	
	Control inflammation	Cryotherapy	Thermotherapy
	Prevent aggravation of pain	Immobilization Low-load static traction	Local exercise, motor e.s.
Referred	Control pain	e.s., cryotherapy, thermotherapy	
Spinal radicular	Decrease nerve root inflammation	Traction	
	Decrease nerve root compression		
Pain due to malignancy	Control pain	e.s., cryotherapy, superficial thermotherapy	

e.s. = electrical stimulation.

Acute pain

When treating acute pain, the goals of treatment are to control the pain and any associated inflammation and to prevent aggravation of the pain or its cause. Many physical agents, including sensory-level electrical stimulation and cryotherapy, can relieve or at least reduce the severity of acute pain.[7,8] Thermotherapy may reduce the severity of acute pain; however, since acute pain is frequently associated with acute inflammation, which is aggravated by thermotherapy, thermotherapy is generally not recommended for the treatment of acute pain.[33] Cryotherapy is thought to control acute pain by modulating transmission at the spinal cord, by slowing or blocking nerve conduction, and by controlling inflammation and its associated signs and symptoms.[7] Sensory-level electrical stimulation also relieves acute pain by modulating transmission at the spinal cord or by stimulating the release of endorphins. Briefly limiting motion of a painful area with the aid of a static compression device, an assistive device, or bed rest can prevent aggravation of the symptom or cause of acute pain. Very low-load, prolonged static traction may be used for a number of hours or even a few days to immobilize a symptomatic spinal area temporarily, thereby relieving the spinal pain and inflammation that would be aggravated by lumbar spine motion.[34,35] Because excessive movement or muscle contraction in the area of acute pain is generally contraindicated, exercise or motor-level electrical stimulation of this area should be avoided or restricted to a level that does not exacerbate pain. As acute pain starts to resolve, controlled reactivation of the patient may accelerate pain resolution. The water environment may be used to facilitate such activity.

Chronic pain

Pain that does not resolve in the normal recovery time expected for an injury or disease is known as chronic pain.[36] The goals of treatment for chronic pain shift from resolution of the underlying pathology and control of symptoms to promotion of function, enhancement of strength, and improvement of coping skills. Although psychological interventions are the mainstay of improving coping skills in patients with chronic pain, exercise should be used to regain strength and function. The water environment may be used to promote the development of the functional abilities and the capacity of certain patients with chronic pain, and both motor-level electrical stimula-tion and water exercise may be used to increase muscle strength in weak or deconditioned patients. Bed rest, which can result in weakness and further reduce function, should be discouraged in this patient population, and since passive physical agent treatments provided by a clinician can encourage dependence on the clinician rather than improving the patient's own coping skills, such interventions are generally not recommended for the treatment of chronic pain. The judicious use of pain-controlling physical agents by patients themselves may be indicated when this helps to improve the patient's ability to cope with pain on a long-term basis; however, it is important that such interventions do not excessively disrupt the patient's functional activities. For example, TENS applied by a patient to relieve or reduce his chronic back pain may promote function by allowing him to participate in work-related activities; however, a hot pack applied by the patient for 20 minutes every few hours would interfere with his ability to perform normal functional activities and would therefore not be recommended.

Referred pain

If the patient's pain is referred to a musculoskeletal area from an internal organ or from another musculoskeletal area, physical agents may be used to control it; however, the source of the pain should also be treated if possible. Pain-relieving physical agents such as thermotherapy, cryotherapy, or electrical stimulation may control referred pain and may be particularly beneficial if complete resolution of the problem is prolonged or cannot be achieved. For example, although surgery may be needed to fully relieve pain caused by endometriosis, should the disease not place the patient at risk, pain-controlling interventions such as physical or pharmacological agents may be used to control the associated pain.

Radicular pain in the extremities caused by spinal nerve root dysfunction may be effectively treated by the application of spinal traction or by the use of physical agents that cause sensory stimulation of the involved dermatome, such as thermotherapy, cryotherapy, or electrical stimulation.[37,38] Spinal traction is effective in such circumstances because it can reduce nerve root compression, addressing the source of the pain, while sensory stimulation may modulate the transmission of pain at the spinal cord level.[39]

Pain due to malignancy

The treatment of pain due to malignancy may differ from the treatment of pain of other etiologies because particular care must be taken to avoid using agents that can promote the growth or metastasis of malignant tissue. Because the growth of some malignancies can be accelerated by increasing local circulation, agents such as ultrasound and diathermy, which are known to increase deep tissue temperature and circulation, should generally not be used in an area of malignancy.[40,41] However, in patients with end-stage malignancies, pain-relieving interventions that can improve the patient's quality of life but may adversely affect disease progression may be used with the patient's informed consent.

Complex regional pain syndrome

Physical agents can be used to control the pain of complex regional pain syndromes with sympathetic nervous system involvement. In general, low-level sensory stimulation of the involved area, as can be provided by neutral warmth, mild cold, water immersion, or gentle agitation of Fluidotherapy, may be effective, while more aggressive stimulation, as can be provided by very hot water, ice, or aggressive agitation of water or Fluidotherapy, will probably not be tolerated and may aggravate this type of pain.

Effects of different physical agents on muscle tone

Physical agents can temporarily modify muscle hypertonicity, hypotonicity, or fluctuating tone (Table 13-3). Hypertonicity may be reduced directly by the application of neutral warmth or prolonged cryotherapy to the hypertonic muscles, or it may be reduced indirectly by the stimulation of antagonist muscle contraction with motor-level electrical stimulation or quick icing. Stimulation of antagonist muscles indirectly reduces hypertonicity because the

stimulated activity in these muscles causes reflex relaxation and tone reduction in opposing muscles.[42] Stimulation of hypertonic muscles with motor-level electrical stimulation or quick icing has generally not been recommended because this can increase muscle tone; however, recent reports indicate that electrical stimulation of hypertonic muscles improves patient function by increasing the strength and voluntary control of these muscles.[43,44]

In patients with muscle hypotonicity, where the goal of treatment is to increase tone, quick icing or motor-level electrical stimulation of the hypotonic muscle(s) may be beneficial. In contrast, the application of heat to these muscles should generally be avoided since this may further reduce muscle tone. In patients with fluctuating tone, where the goal of treatment is to normalize tone, functional electrical stimulation may be applied to cause a muscle, or muscles, to contract at the appropriate time during functional activities. For example, if a patient cannot maintain a functional grasp because he cannot contract the wrist extensors while contracting the finger flexors, contraction of the wrist extensors could be produced by electrical stimulation at the appropriate time during active grasping.

Effects of different physical agents on motion restrictions

Physical agents can be effective adjuncts to the treatment of motion restrictions caused by muscle weakness, pain, soft tissue shortening, or a bony block; however, the appropriate interventions for these different sources of motion restriction vary (Table 13-4). When active motion is restricted by muscle weakness, the treatment should be aimed at increasing muscle strength. This can be achieved by repeated

---

TABLE 13-3 Physical Agents for the Treatment of Tone Abnormalities

Tone abnormality	Goals of treatment	Effective agents	Contraindicated
Hypertonicity	Decrease tone	Neutral warmth or prolonged cryotherapy to hypertonic muscles Motor e.s. or quick ice of antagonists	Quick ice of agonist
Hypotonicity	Increase tone	Quick ice or motor e.s. of agonists	Thermotherapy
Fluctuating tone	Normalize tone	Functional e.s.	

e.s. = electrical stimulation.

overload muscle contraction through active exercise and may be further facilitated by the use of water exercise or motor-level electrical stimulation. Water can provide support to allow weaker muscles to move joints through greater range and can provide resistance for stronger muscles to work against. Motor-level electrical stimulation can provide preferential training of larger muscle fibers, isolation of specific muscle contraction, and precise control of the timing and number of muscle contractions. When range of motion (ROM) is limited by muscle weakness alone, rest and immobilization of the area are contraindicated because restricting the active use of weakened muscles will further reduce their strength and thus exacerbate the existing motion restriction.

When motion is restricted by pain, treatment selection will depend on whether the pain occurs at rest and with all motion or if it occurs in response to active or passive motion only. When motion is restricted by pain that is present at rest and with all motion, the first goal of treatment is to reduce the severity of the pain. This can be achieved, as described above, with the use of electrical stimulation, cryotherapy, thermotherapy, or PSWD. If the pain and motion restriction are related to a compressive spinal dysfunction,

spinal traction may also be used to alleviate the pain and promote increased motion. When active motion is restricted by pain with active motion only, this indicates an injury of contractile tissue such as muscle or tendon, without complete rupture.[45] When active and passive motion are both restricted by pain, this indicates that noncontractile tissue such as ligament or meniscus is involved. Physical agents may help restore motion after an injury to contractile or noncontractile tissue by promoting tissue healing or by controlling pain, as described previously.

When active and passive motion are restricted by soft tissue shortening or a bony block, the restriction is generally not accompanied by pain. Soft tissue shortening may be reversed by stretching, and thermal agents may be used prior to, or in conjunction with, stretching in order to increase soft tissue extensibility and thus promote a safer, more effective stretch.[30,31,46] The ideal thermal agent depends upon the depth, size, and contouring of the tissue to be treated. Deep heating agents such as ultrasound or diathermy should be used when motion is restricted by shortening of deep tissues such as the shoulder joint capsule, while superficial heating agents, such as hot packs, paraffin, warm whirlpools, or infrared (IR)

TABLE 13-4 Physical Agents for the Treatment of Motion Restrictions

Source of motion restriction	Goals of treatment	Effective agents	Contraindicated
Muscle weakness	Increase muscle strength	Water exercise, motor e.s.	Immobilization
Pain			
At rest and with motion	Control pain	e.s., cryotherapy, thermotherapy, PSWD, spinal traction	Exercise
With motion only	Control pain	e.s., cryotherapy, thermotherapy, PSWD	Exercise into pain
	Promote tissue healing	Depends on stage of healing (see Table 13-1)	
Soft tissue shortening	Increase tissue extensibility	Thermotherapy	Prolonged cryotherapy
	Increase tissue length	Thermotherapy or brief ice massage and stretch	
Bony block	Remove block	None	Stretching blocked joint
	Compensate	Exercise Thermotherapy or brief ice massage and stretch	

e.s. = electrical stimulation.

lamps, should be used when motion is restricted by shortening of superficial tissues such as the skin or subcutaneous fascia. Ultrasound should be used for treating small areas of deep tissue, while diathermy is more appropriate for larger areas. Hot packs can be used to treat large or small areas of superficial tissue with little or moderate contouring, while paraffin or a whirlpool are more appropriate for treating small areas with greater contouring. IR lamps can be used to heat large or small areas, but they provide consistent heating only to relatively flat surfaces. Because increasing tissue extensibility alone will not decrease soft tissue shortening, thermal agents must be used in conjunction with stretching techniques in order to increase soft tissue length and reverse motion restrictions caused by soft tissue shortening. Brief forms of cryotherapy such as brief ice massage or vapocoolant sprays may also be used prior to stretching to facilitate greater increases in muscle length by reducing the discomfort of stretching; however, prolonged cryotherapy should not be used prior to stretching because cooling soft tissue decreases its extensibility.[47,48]

When a bony block restricts motion, the goals of treatment are to remove the block or to compensate for the loss of motion. While physical agents cannot remove a bony block, they may help with compensation for the loss of motion by facilitating increased motion at other joints. Motion may be increased at other joints by the judicious use of thermotherapy or brief cryotherapy with stretching, as described directly above. Such treatment should be applied with caution to avoid causing injury, hypermobility, or other dysfunctions in previously normal joints. Applying a stretching force to a joint that is blocked by a bony obstruction is not recommended because this force will not increase ROM at that joint and may cause inflammation by traumatizing the intraarticular structures.

Addressing multiple problems and goals

When patients present with multiple problems and thus have multiple treatment goals, physical agents that have multiple effects, or a variety of physical agents with different effects, may be applied either simultaneously or sequentially. For example, the patient with chronic tendonitis and tendon shortening may benefit from the application of a thermal agent because this type of physical agent can increase soft tissue extensibility to promote more effective

stretching, and can also increase blood flow and circulation to facilitate healing. Both of these effects would facilitate progress toward the goals of treatment. Ideally, those physical agents that produce the effect or effects that most closely match the processes needed for resolution of the patient's problem(s) should be selected. Further discussion of the sequential or simultaneous application of different physical agents is provided in the section on combining treatment options.

Contraindications and Precautions

Once the goals of treatment, and the treatment interventions that may promote progress toward these goals, have been determined, treatment selection may be guided further by evaluation of the contraindications and precautions for the application of these treatment options. In all cases, physical agents that are contraindicated for the presenting condition or for the specific patient should not be used, and appropriate precautions must be taken when indicated. Since all physical agents have some conditions for which they are contraindicated and since all should be applied with caution in certain circumstances, a consideration of contraindications and precautions may eliminate some treatment options.

Although a number of conditions, including pregnancy, malignancy, the presence of a pacemaker, impaired sensation, and impaired mentation, indicate the need for caution with the use of most physical agents, the specific contraindications and precautions for the specific agent being considered and the specific patient situation must be evaluated before a treatment may be used or should be rejected. For example, although the application of ultrasound to a pregnant patient is contraindicated in any area where the ultrasound may reach the fetus, this physical agent may be applied to the distal extremities of a pregnant patient because ultrasound penetration is limited to the area close to the applicator. In contrast, it is recommended that diathermy not be applied to any area of a pregnant patient because the electromagnetic radiation produced by this type of agent reaches areas distant from the applicator. Contraindications and precautions for the application of specific physical agents are included in section two of this book within the chapter concerning each type of physical agent.

Since physical agents have differing levels of associated risk, when all other factors are equal, those with a lower level of risk should be selected. Physical agents with a low level of associated risk have a potentially harmful dose that is difficult to achieve or is much greater than the effective therapeutic dose and have contraindications that are easy to detect. In contrast, physical agents with a high level of associated risk have an effective therapeutic dose that is close to the potentially harmful dose and have contraindications that are difficult to detect. For example, hot packs that are heated in hot water have a low associated risk because although they can heat superficial tissues to a therapeutic level in 15 to 20 minutes, they are unlikely to cause a burn if applied for a longer period, provided that sufficient insulation is used, because they start to cool as soon as they are removed from the hot water. In contrast, ultraviolet (UV) radiation has a high associated risk because a slight increase in the treatment duration, for example, from 5 to 10 minutes, or using the same treatment duration for patients with different skin sensitivity may change the effect of the treatment from a therapeutic level of erythema to a severe burn. Diathermy also has a high associated risk because it preferentially heats metal, which may have been previously undetected, and can burn tissue that is near any metal object(s) in the treatment field. It is generally recommended that agents with higher associated risk be used only if those with lower risks would not be as effective and, when used, that special care be taken to minimize these risks.

Scientific Merit

If several agents may promote progress toward the goals of treatment, are not contraindicated, and can be applied with the appropriate precautions, selection should be based on the scientific merit of the treatment approach. Six criteria of scientific merit have been proposed for guidance in treatment selection.[49] Treatment approaches that meet these criteria are considered to have a high degree of scientific merit. The proposed criteria for determination of scientific merit are as follows:

1. The theories underlying the treatment approach are supported by valid anatomical and physiological evidence.
2. The treatment approach is designed for a specific patient population.
3. Potential side effects of the treatment are presented.

4. Studies from peer-reviewed journals support the treatment's efficacy.
5. Peer-reviewed studies include well-designed, randomized, controlled clinical trials or well-designed single-subject experimental studies.
6. The proponents of the treatment approach are willing to discuss its limitations.

The more of these criteria that are met, the better the quality of support for a treatment and therefore the more appropriate the treatment selection. For example, it is recommended that ultrasound or SWD, at intensities sufficient to raise the temperature of the shoulder capsule by 3° to 5° C, followed by stretching, be used to treat a restriction in shoulder joint ROM when the motion is restricted by capsular shortening because this approach meets most of the above criteria. There is valid evidence that increasing tissue temperature increases tissue extensibility, that increasing soft tissue extensibility promotes greater increases in tissue length in response to stretching, and that both ultrasound and diathermy can increase deep tissue temperature.[16,30,31,45,50-52] This treatment approach is designed for patients with specific problems related to loss of soft tissue length. Precautions and contraindications for the use of ultrasound, diathermy, and stretching have been well documented, and there are studies showing that the application of deep heating agents prior to stretching can promote ROM gains. The authors of these studies are also open to discussing the limitations of their findings.[30] Although this treatment approach does not fully meet the fifth criterion for scientific merit, because there are no well-designed, randomized, controlled clinical trials or well-designed single-subject experimental studies specifically supporting the use of these deep-heating agents prior to stretching of the shoulder capsule, selection of this treatment approach is recommended, given no effective and safe alternative meets all of the other criteria for scientific merit. Commonly, even the best treatments currently available meet most but not all of the criteria for scientific merit, and given the absence of better alternatives, these should be used; however, treatment approaches that meet few or none of the above criteria should generally be avoided.

Treatment approaches that meet few or none of the criteria for scientific merit are also often characterized by the following properties:[53]

1. Treatments are based on theories that are incongruent with anatomical or physiological function.

2. Treatment is said to be effective for a broad range of diagnoses.
3. Treatments cannot cause harm.
4. There are no adequately controlled studies in peer-reviewed journals.
5. The therapies have an emotional appeal, and studies that fail to confirm their effectiveness are attacked.
6. Treatment is advocated by those selling or manufacturing the necessary equipment when other treatments or equipment are more effective.

Treatments that fail to meet many of the criteria for high-quality support or that have many of the characteristics of treatments with poor support ideally should not be used. For example, the use of magnets to control pain and accelerate healing is recommended by some publications and practitioners;[54] however, the evidence to support their use does not have great scientific merit at this time. Treatment with magnets has been recommended for a wide range of diagnoses, and it is claimed that magnets have no adverse effects. Although the poor quality of support for this and other treatment approaches should guide clinicians away from their application at this time, clinicians should keep informed of new findings in order to integrate the use of innovative treatment approaches into clinical care should sufficient high-quality evidence be presented to support their use.

In general, the treatments with physical agents presented in this book have sufficient scientific merit to strongly support their use; however, the scientific merit of the support for different applications of each physical agent varies. In addition, further research is frequently needed to validate the efficacy of commonly used treatments and to determine the ideal treatment parameters and patient characteristics for optimal effect. During treatment selection, both the overall scientific merit of an approach and the scientific merit of the specific application should be considered.

Cost, Convenience, and Availability

Frequently, cost, convenience, and availability influence the selection of a physical agent treatment. Although ideally these should not be the limiting factors in treatment selection, when all other factors are equal, cost efficiency should be considered and, in any situation, cost or lack of equipment may prevent the application of certain treatments. When determining the cost of a treatment, the cost of the required materials and equipment, as well as the associated labor and time costs, should all be considered. Because, in general, the materials used for applying physical agents are reusable or inexpensive, the cost of materials rarely limits treatment selection; however, since the cost of equipment or labor may be high, particularly if a high level of skill is required, these may limit or guide the selection. For example, when considering applying ultrasound, the cost of the ultrasound gel is not likely to limit the selection of this treatment; however, the cost of an ultrasound unit and the amount of skilled clinician time required to apply it may lead to the choice of a different course of treatment.

Convenience can be an important consideration when using a physical agent in the clinical setting and even more so when considering recommending a physical agent for home use by a patient. In general, the easier an agent is to use, the more readily its application can be delegated to less well-trained and less costly personnel, or to the patient, and the less likely the agent will be used inappropriately or unsafely. However, it is important that physical agents that are convenient to use not be substituted for those that would be more effective. For example, although hot packs, which heat superficial tissues, are easier to apply than ultrasound, which heats both deep and superficial tissues, hot packs should not be used when the goals of treatment require deep heating.

The availability of a physical agent may also influence treatment selection. Most rehabilitation facilities in the United States have hot packs, paraffin, cold packs or ice packs, ultrasound, electrical current stimulation devices, and mechanical traction units available, and many facilities also have compression devices and whirlpool(s); however, few have swimming pools, IR lamps, UV lamps, or other electromagnetic field devices. Even when a specific physical agent is available, the device may not allow selection of the ideal treatment parameters or setup and therefore should not be used. For example, the traction device may not have the appropriate halter for applying cervical traction without compression of the temporomandibular joints, or the ultrasound unit may not have pulsed duty cycles to allow for ultrasound application without heating. Clinics outside the United States may have and use different physical agents than those commonly used in the United

States. For example, since the FDA approves low-intensity lasers only as investigational devices at this time, they are not commonly used in the United States. However, they are commonly used in Canada and Europe. SWD is also rarely available in the United States at this time because of its associated risks and its interference with other electronic devices; however, it is still commonly available elsewhere. When treating patients in their homes, the limited availability of physical agents generally restricts treatment to the application of hot packs, ice packs, or water.

USING PHYSICAL AGENTS IN COMBINATION WITH EACH OTHER OR WITH OTHER INTERVENTIONS

In order to promote progress toward the goals of treatment, a number of physical agents may be used simultaneously, sequentially, or in conjunction with other interventions. Treatments are generally combined when they have similar effects or when they address different aspects of a common array of symptoms. For example, splinting, ice, pulsed ultrasound, PSWD, and phonophoresis or iontophoresis may be used during the acute inflammatory phase of healing. Splinting can limit further injury; ice may control pain and limit circulation; pulsed ultrasound and PSWD may promote progress to the proliferative stage; and phonophoresis and iontophoresis may limit the inflammatory response. During the proliferative stage, heat, motor-level electrical stimulation, and exercise may all be used, while ice or other inflammation-controlling interventions may continue to be applied after activity in order to reduce the risk of recurring inflammation.

Rest, ice, compression, and elevation (RICE) are frequently combined for the treatment of inflammation and edema because all of these interventions can contribute to inflammation and edema control or reduction. Rest limits and prevents further injury; ice reduces circulation and inflammation; compression elevates hydrostatic pressure outside the blood vessels; and elevation reduces hydrostatic pressure within the blood vessels of the elevated area to decrease capillary filtration pressure at the arterial end and facilitate venous and lymphatic outflow from the limb. [55-58] Electrical stimulation may also be added to this combination to further control inflammation and the formation of edema by repelling negatively charged blood cells and ions associated with inflammation.

When the goal of treatment is to control pain, a number of physical agents may be used to impact different mechanisms of pain control. For example, cryotherapy or thermotherapy may be used to modulate pain transmission at the spinal cord, while motor-level electrical stimulation may be used to modulate pain through stimulation of endorphin release. These physical agents may be combined with other pain-controlling interventions, such as medications, and may also be used in conjunction with treatments such as joint mobilization and dynamic stabilization exercise, which are intended to address the underlying impairment causing the pain.

When the goal of treatment is to alter muscle tone, a number of tone-modifying physical agents or other interventions may be applied during or prior to activity in order to promote more normal movement and to increase the efficacy of other aspects of treatment. For example, ice may be applied for 30 to 40 minutes to the leg of a patient with hypertonicity of the ankle plantar flexors due to a stroke in order to control the hypertonicity of these muscles temporarily and thereby promote a more normal gait pattern during gait training. Because practicing normal movement is thought to facilitate the recovery of more normal movement patterns, such treatment may promote a superior treatment outcome.

When the goal of treatment is to reverse soft tissue shortening, the application of thermal agents before or during stretching or mobilization is recommended in order to promote relaxation and increase soft tissue extensibility, thereby increasing the efficacy and safety of the treatment. For example, hot packs are often applied in conjunction with mechanical traction in order to promote relaxation of the paraspinal muscles and increase the extensibility of the superficial soft tissues in the area to which the traction is being applied.

Physical agents are generally used more extensively during the initial treatment sessions in rehabilitation when inflammation and pain control are a priority, with progression over time to more active or aggressive treatments, such as exercise or passive mobilization. Progression from one physical agent to another, or from the use of a physical agent to another form of treatment, should be based on the progression of the patient's problem. For example, hydrotherapy may be applied to cleanse and debride an open wound during the initial treatment sessions; however, once the wound is clean, this treatment should be stopped, while the use of electrical stimulation may be initiated to promote collagen deposition.

USING PHYSICAL AGENTS WITHIN DIFFERENT HEALTH CARE DELIVERY SYSTEMS

Clinicians may be called upon to treat patients within different health care delivery systems both in the United States and abroad. These systems may vary in both the quantity and nature of available health care resources. Some systems provide high levels of resources, in the forms of skilled clinicians and costly equipment, while others do not. At the present time, the health care delivery system in the United States is undergoing change due to the need and desire to contain the growing costs of medical care. Utilizing available resources of both personnel and equipment in the most cost-effective manner is being emphasized, resulting in new systems of reimbursement and increased monitoring of treatment outcomes. Reimbursement has moved from fee-for-service, where third-party insurance companies pay individual service providers according to the nature and quantity of service provided, to capitated payment systems, where insurance companies pay a set rate per treatment, or per case, independent of the type of treatment provided. There has also been a growth of health maintenance organizations that collect premiums from insured individuals and provide health care services by employing health care providers.

In order to improve the efficiency and efficacy of health care as it relates to patient function, both health care providers and those paying for treatment are attempting to assess functional outcome in response to different treatment options. These changes in reimbursement and outcome assessment are pressuring both service providers and third-party payers to find the most cost-efficient means to provide rehabilitation services and to demonstrate the efficacy of their interventions in improving patient function and reducing disability.

Some payers are attempting to improve the cost effectiveness of care by denying or reducing reimbursement for certain physical agent treatments or by including the cost of physical agent treatments in the reimbursement for other services. For example, prior to January 1995, many third-party payers provided a higher level of reimbursement for treatments involving physical agents than for other interventions;

however, since that time, reimbursement for these services has been reduced to reflect the lower perceived level of skill required to apply these agents. In January 1997, Medicare changed its reimbursement schedule, bundling the payment for hot pack and cold pack treatments into the payment for all other services rather than reimbursing separately for these treatments.[59] The rationale proposed for this change was that (1) hot packs are easily self-administered; (2) these packs are commonly used in the home and thus require minimal professional attention; and (3) the application of hot packs is usually a precursor to other interventions.

Although there is a growing emphasis on the cost effectiveness of care, the goals of treatment continue to be, as they always have been, to obtain the best outcome for the patient within the constraints of the health care delivery system. Although it has been suggested that the need for cost efficiency may eliminate the use of physical agents, this is not so. Rather, this requirement pushes the clinician to find and use the most efficient ways to provide those treatments that can be expected to help the patient progress toward the goals of treatment, whether this does or does not include the use of physical agents. In order to use physical agents in this manner, the clinician must be able to assess the presenting problem and know when physical agents can be an effective component of treatment. The clinician must also know when and how to use physical agents most effectively and know which ones can be used by patients to treat themselves (Table 13-5). To achieve the most cost-effective treatment, the clinician should also optimize the use of the varied skill levels of different practitioners and the use of home programs when appropriate. In many cases, the licensed therapist may not need to apply the physical agent but instead may assess and analyze the presenting clinical findings, determine the treatment plan, provide those aspects of care requiring the skills of the licensed therapist, and then train the patient or supervised unlicensed personnel to apply those treatments requiring a lower level of skill. The therapist can then reassess the patient regularly to determine the efficacy of the treatments provided and the patient's progress toward the goals of treatment, and adjust the plan of care accordingly. Aides may then provide many treatments with physical agents, such as hot packs and cold packs, to patients in the clinic and teach patients how, when, and why to apply these agents safely and

TABLE	**13-5** Requirements for Cost-Effective Use of Physical Agents

- Assess and analyze the presenting problem.
- Know when physical agents can be an effective component of treatment.
- Know when and how to use physical agents most effectively.
- Know the skill level required for the application of different physical agents.
- Optimize the use of the skill levels of different practitioners.
- Use home programs when appropriate.
- Treat in groups when appropriate.
- Reassess patients regularly to determine the efficacy of the treatments provided.
- Adjust the plan of care according to the findings of reassessments.

independently at home. In this situation, the time with the clinician could then be spent providing treatment that the patient cannot perform.

Cost efficiency may also be increased by providing treatment to groups of patients, such as group water exercise programs for patients recovering from total joint arthroplasty or for those with osteoarthritis.

Such programs may be designed to facilitate the transition to a community-based exercise program when the patient reaches the appropriate level of function and recovery. Used in this manner, physical agents can provide cost-effective care and involve the patient in promoting recovery and achieving the goals of treatment.

▶ *Clinical Case Studies* ◀

The following six case studies demonstrate the processes involved in the selection of physical agents for the treatment of patients with a variety of problems that progress and change as their treatment progresses. These studies focus on the decision-making process involved in the selection of physical agents. Details of application techniques, including specific treatment parameters and duration of treatment, are not included since these are provided in the chapters regarding the specific physical agents recommended.

Case 1

TJ is a 78-year-old female who sustained a stroke 2 weeks ago. Upon evaluation, TJ has a right hemiparesis with decreased tone of her right upper and lower extremities. Her right humeral head is inferiorly subluxed from the glenoid fossa, and she has minimal active movement of her right upper extremity. TJ's right hand is also mildly edematous and pale. During gait she has a foot drop on the right and uses a steppage gait with circumduction on the right to clear her toes during swing phase. She also hyperextends her knee on the right during stance phase. TJ ambulates at a slow pace but with good balance on a level surface without an assistive device. She has poor balance when attempting to walk on an uneven surface. Passive range of all major joints is within normal limits. TJ does not complain of any pain.

EVALUATION OF THE CLINICAL FINDINGS

This patient presents with impairments of restricted active range of motion (ROM), decreased strength and hypotonicity of the right extremities, subluxation of the right glenohumeral joint, and edema of the right hand. These impairments have resulted in functional limitations in the use of her right upper extremity and have interfered with her gait pattern and speed. She also has poor balance, and thus impaired safety, when walking on uneven surfaces.

PREFERRED PRACTICE PATTERN

Impaired Motor Function and Sensory Integrity Associated with Nonprogressive Disorders of the Central Nervous System-Acquired in Adolescence or Adulthood, (5D)

PLAN OF CARE

The goals of treatment at this time are to reduce the shoulder subluxation, improve functional use of the right upper extremity, control the right hand edema, and optimize the pattern, speed, and safety of TJ's gait.

ASSESSMENT REGARDING THE OPTIMAL PHYSICAL AGENT INTERVENTION(S)

Electrical stimulation may be effective for reducing the shoulder glenohumeral subluxation, the edema of the right hand, and the foot drop and knee hyperextension on the right. An intermittent pneumatic compression pump could be used in place of electrical stimulation for reducing the hand edema, and, once the edema is reduced, a compression sleeve may be effective for maintaining normal volume and fluid balance. Orthotic bracing may be used in place of electrical stimulation for the shoulder subluxation, or for the foot drop and knee hyperextension. Selection among these options depends on their effectiveness for this particular patient, their availability, patient and clinician comfort with their use, and their cost. Water- or land-based exercise should also be integrated into the treatment in order to improve the patient's balance and her other functional activities and to maintain active and passive ROM of the joints of the right upper and lower extremities.

PROPOSED TREATMENT PLAN AND RATIONALE

The physical agents that could promote progression toward the goals of treatment at this time, and that are not contraindicated, include electrical stimulation, compression, and water exercise. Because using electrical stimulation for multiple purposes on different parts of the body is not generally practical, it is recommended that electrical stimulation be reserved at this time for the application for which it is most likely to be effective and for which other options are not as effective. Therefore it is recommended that electrical stimulation be used to reduce the shoulder subluxation. Intermittent pneumatic compression can then be used for limited periods to reduce the upper extremity edema, and a compression glove or sleeve can be worn to maintain the edema control. The right foot-drop and knee hyperextension can be controlled by use of an ankle foot orthosis (AFO). In addition to these interventions, exercise and functional activities should be incorporated in the treatment plan in order to optimize functional recovery.

FOLLOW-UP

One month later, after therapy sessions twice a week, the tone in TJ's right upper and lower extremities has increased. She now has mild spasticity of the right upper extremity flexors, and the shoulder subluxation and right hand edema have resolved. Her gait has improved such that she has only mild knee hyperextension during stance phase and a mild foot-drop during swing phase. The lower extremity steppage and circumduction have resolved with use of an ankle foot orthosis (AFO), and TJ is now able to walk up and down stairs safely holding on to one hand rail.

EVALUATION OF THE CLINICAL FINDINGS

At this time, TJ continues to have impairments of tone and functional limitations in her gait; however, her tone has changed from hypotonic to hypertonic, the edema in her right hand has resolved, and her gait is much improved.

PLAN OF CARE

The goals of treatment at this time are to optimize functional use of the right upper extremity by normalizing tone and motor control, and to optimize TJ's gait pattern, speed, and safety.

ASSESSMENT REGARDING THE OPTIMAL PHYSICAL AGENT INTERVENTION(S)

The application of electrical stimulation to the right shoulder and the compression to the right hand can be decreased and probably discontinued. The use of these interventions should be tapered with close monitoring for recurrence of the problems they were intended to control. Should the impairments recur, treatment should be resumed, and a trial of discontinuation may be considered again at a later date. Because TJ continues to have a foot drop and knee hyperextension during gait, it is recommended that use of the AFO be continued. Alternatively, this may be replaced with motor- level electrical stimulation with use of a foot switch to produce ankle dorsiflexion during swing phase by stimulating the tibialis anterior and to control knee hyperextension during stance phase by stimulating the gastrocnemius-soleus muscles. At this time, thermal agents, including prolonged icing or gentle heat, may be considered for reducing spasticity of the right upper extremity, particularly prior to exercise and functional activities.

PROPOSED TREATMENT PLAN AND RATIONALE

The physical agents that could promote progression toward the goals of treatment at this time, and that are not contraindicated, include electrical stimulation, cryotherapy, and thermotherapy. It is proposed that at this time motor-level electrical stimulation be tried to control the right foot drop and knee hyperextension during gait. This is recommended in place of the AFO because the active contractions produced by the electrical stimulation more closely simulate the motor activity required for normal gait. Therefore this may

Continued

promote greater long-term recovery than the passive orthosis. It is also proposed that gentle heat be used to reduce the hypertonicity of the right upper extremity prior to exercise and functional activities. This is recommended over prolonged icing as it is better tolerated by most patients and is often as effective. Motor-level electrical stimulation to the antagonist extensors of the right upper extremity may also be considered to reduce tone in the agonist flexors.

Case 2

FS is a 23-year-old male who fell and twisted his right knee while playing football and immediately limped off the field. Upon evaluation within a few minutes of his injury, FS complained of medial right knee pain that increased with weight bearing on his right lower extremity. Objective testing of his right knee revealed tenderness over the medial joint line, with some redness and heat in the same area. Some edema was noted on palpation; however, knee girth was equal bilaterally. Passive right knee flexion and extension were limited to 90° and 30°, respectively, with complaints of medial knee pain and tightness at the limit of both motions. Active motion and strength testing are deferred due to the acute nature of the injury.

EVALUATION OF THE CLINICAL FINDINGS

This patient presents with impairments of restricted ROM, edema, and pain in his right knee. The injury is in the acute inflammatory stage of healing, as indicated by the presence of the cardinal signs of pain, heat, redness, and edema; the pain is acute; and the restriction of motion is due to the pain and edema. The functional limitation of limping is likely to be due to the restriction of knee ROM and pain, and may also be influenced by reflex inhibition of contraction of the muscles controlling knee extension.

PREFERRED PRACTICE PATTERN

Impaired Joint Mobility, Motor Function, Muscle Performance, and Range of Motion Associated With Connective Tissue Dysfunction, (4D)

PLAN OF CARE

The goals of treatment at this time are to control pain and limit edema formation, bleeding, and the release of inflammatory mediators associated with the acute inflammatory stage of healing. Treatment should also promote progression to the proliferation stage of healing and prevent aggravation of the pain or injury. Although regaining normal ROM is a long-term goal for this patient, it is recommended that the focus of treatment at this stage be on controlling the pain and inflammation.

ASSESSMENT REGARDING THE OPTIMAL PHYSICAL AGENT INTERVENTION(S)

Cryotherapy, compression, electrical stimulation, or PSWD can safely be used to control edema at this time, and all of these, except compression, may also contribute to relieving pain. Although thermotherapy can also be used to relieve pain, its use is not recommended for this patient at this time because it may aggravate the edema and bleeding and increase the release of inflammatory mediators associated with acute inflammation. Cryotherapy should be included in the treatment, because decreasing tissue temperature will also control the release of inflammatory mediators, and pulsed ultrasound or PSWD may be included to promote progression to the proliferation stage of healing. Motion of the injured area should be restricted at this time to avoid aggravation of the pain or injury.

PROPOSED TREATMENT PLAN AND RATIONALE

The physical agents that could promote progression toward the goals of treatment at this time, and that are not contraindicated, include cryotherapy, compression, electrical stimulation, pulsed ultrasound, and PSWD. Because it is not practical to apply all of these agents, the therapist should select those that can be expected to have the greatest beneficial effect on the greatest number of the patient's problems and that could be applied together. Selection should also take into account the scientific merit of the proposed intervention(s) and the cost efficiency and convenience of providing the treatment. Considering all of these criteria, it is proposed that the patient be treated with the physical agents of ice and compression, with the possible addition of electrical stimulation. It is proposed that PSWD and ultrasound not be used, although they may also be beneficial, because these physical agents cannot be applied by the patient at home, are more costly to provide, and may not provide significant additional benefit. It is recommended that the ice and compression be applied in conjunction with rest and elevation to optimize the control of edema and inflammation, completing the classical combination of RICE. This combination, with the addition of electrical stimulation, could be applied in the clinic and repeated by the patient at home. Cryotherapy and compression could be provided by a controlled cold compression unit; however, since this device is costly and not available in most settings, it is recommended that cryotherapy be provided with an ice pack or cold pack and that compression be provided by an elastic compression bandage. The area should be rested between treatments, with the patient using crutches and limiting ambulation. Electrical stimulation could be provided by a portable stimulation device. It is proposed that this combination of interventions be applied by the patient at home until the warmth and redness of his medial knee resolve, indicating progression from the inflammatory to the proliferative stage of healing.

FOLLOW-UP

FS is evaluated by a physician 3 days after his initial injury and is diagnosed with a sprained medial collateral ligament of the right knee. He returns for therapy 2 weeks after the injury and reports that he applied ice, compression, and electrical stimulation to his right knee, with his right leg elevated, for 15 minutes every 2 hours for the first 2 days after the injury and then twice a day for another week. He also used crutches for ambulation for the first week after his injury. He discontinued self-treatment and the use of crutches after 1 week because the heat and redness of his knee had fully resolved, and he is now taking an oral NSAID twice a day in compliance with his physician's instructions.

At this time, FS complains of soreness of the right medial knee that increases with turning to the left and worsens at the end of the day. He also reports that his knee is stiff in the morning or after prolonged sitting. He is able to walk for about 20 to 30 minutes without an assistive device and is then limited by pain and increased swelling of his knee. He has been able to return to work in a manufacturing plant, on limited duty, restricted to sitting and no walking for longer than 5 minutes. It is now 4 p.m., and FS was at work for 7 hours prior to this physical therapy appointment.

The objective evaluation is significant for swelling and mild warmth of the right knee. Knee girth is 15 inches on the left and 16 ½ inches on the right. Knee ROM is as follows:

	Left	**Right**
Active ROM	Full extension, 130° flexion	15° extension, 90° flexion
Passive ROM	Full extension, 140° flexion	−10° extension, 100° flexion

Passive motion of the right knee has a firm end feel, with pain in the medial knee at the end of both flexion and extension range. Medial knee pain is also produced with the application of a valgus stress to the right knee.

Although FS can ambulate without an assistive device, he has a shortened stance phase on the right with reduced right knee extension during midstance. He uses a step to gait for ascending and descending stairs.

EVALUATION OF THE CLINICAL FINDINGS

At this time, this patient continues to have restricted ROM, edema, and pain in his right knee; however, the ROM has increased since the initial injury, and the pain has decreased in both severity and frequency. The injury is progressing from the acute inflammatory stage of healing to the proliferative stage, as indicated by the reduced pain, heat, and redness. The pain continues to be acute since it is associated with the normal duration of healing for this type of injury. The restriction of motion may be due to edema, shortening of the knee capsule, or adhesion of the medial collateral ligament. FS continues to have an abnormal gait, which has resulted in an inability to perform his usual job-related activities.

PLAN OF CARE

The goals of treatment at this time continue to include controlling pain and edema and preventing aggravation of the pain or injury; however, since this injury is now progressing to the proliferation stage of healing, the current goals of treatment also include increasing ROM by controlling scar tissue formation, increasing soft tissue extensibility, and decreasing edema. It is also important to maintain strength and flexibility and to ensure adequate circulation in order to promote tissue healing and progression to the remodeling stage of healing.

ASSESSMENT REGARDING THE OPTIMAL PHYSICAL AGENT INTERVENTION(S)

Because this patient continues to have pain and edema after 20 to 30 minutes of walking, it is recommended that he continue to rest and apply ice and compression, with his knee elevated, when this occurs. Pulsed ultrasound or PSWD may be used to promote progression to the remodeling phase of healing. The physical agents of thermotherapy or hydrotherapy may be used to promote circulation, while motor-level electrical stimulation and water exercise may be used to maintain strength and flexibility. Thermotherapy to increase soft tissue extensibility, or brief icing to distract from discomfort, may also be used prior to stretching to optimize increases in soft tissue length and ROM.

PROPOSED TREATMENT PLAN AND RATIONALE

The physical agents that could promote progress toward the goals of treatment at this time, and that are not contraindicated, include cryotherapy, sensory-level and motor-level electrical stimulation, compression, pulsed

Continued

▶ *Clinical Case Studies—cont'd* ◀

ultrasound, PSWD, thermotherapy, and hydrotherapy. The optimal treatment for this patient would be to use flexibility- and strength-promoting agents such as heat, hydrotherapy, and motor-level electrical stimulation at the beginning of the treatment sessions and to use pain- and inflammation-controlling agents such as cryotherapy, compression, sensory-level stimulation, and PSWD after activity. These physical agents should be integrated with other interventions, including stretching or joint mobilization after thermotherapy, to increase soft tissue length and thus increase ROM and strengthening exercises on dry land or in water or motor-level electrical stimulation to maintain or increase strength. After these interventions, rest and elevation may be combined with ice, compression, and sensory-level electrical stimulation in order to control any pain or inflammation produced by the activity. These interventions may be performed by the patient at home as well as in the clinic. This combination of interventions would be appropriate until all signs of inflammation have fully resolved. When this has been achieved, the inflammation-controlling interventions should be discontinued and the other interventions continued until the patient's ROM and function have returned to normal. Depending on the availability of resources, much of this patient's treatment may be performed independently, although skilled intervention will be needed to guide the progression of his treatment as healing progresses.

Case 3

GH is a 45-year-old male diagnosed with a low back strain. He reports that his pain started 3 weeks ago after lifting a heavy box from the floor at work. When lifting the box, he immediately felt a brief, sharp pain in his right low back, followed by a dull ache in the same area that increased in severity and spread to his right buttock and posterior thigh over the following few hours. He stopped working immediately after the injury and was evaluated and treated by a physician on the same day. The physician prescribed an NSAID and a muscle relaxant and instructed the patient to use ice, to stay out of work for 1 week, to rest at home, and to avoid lifting. After 1 week the pain had subsided slightly but had not fully resolved. The physician recommended that GH stay out of work for another 3 weeks and referred him to physical therapy. GH reports having had a similar incident 5 years ago that kept him out of work for over a year, after which he returned to a job with fewer lifting demands and continued to have intermittent, moderate low back pain. He is concerned that he may not be able to return to this job, which involves occasional lifting of

up to 70 lb. At this time GH complains of constant low back pain on the right side that is deep and aching, with occasional sharp twinges. Although the pain is constant, it varies in intensity from 6/10 to 8/10 on a visual analog scale, worsening with forward bending and after prolonged sitting and occasionally disturbing the patient's sleep. GH denies having any lower extremity symptoms at this time. The objective evaluation is significant for restricted active lumbar ROM as follows:

- Forward bending: Fingertips to midthigh, limited by right low back pain
- Backward bending: 50% of normal, limited by stiffness
- Side bending to the right: 30% of normal, limited by right low back pain
- Side bending to the left: 50% of normal, limited by stiffness
- Straight leg raise is 45 degrees bilaterally, limited by hamstring tightness

There is increased tone of the lower lumbar paraspinal muscles and tenderness of the low back to palpation on the right, with decreased passive intervertebral motion of all lumbar spinal levels on central posterior-anterior testing.

EVALUATION OF THE CLINICAL FINDINGS

This patient presents with impairments of pain, decreased lumbar spine ROM, lumbar joint stiffness, decreased hamstring length, and lumbar paraspinal muscle hypertonicity. He has functional limitations of reduced sitting and lifting tolerance and disabilities of not working at this time. These problems are combined with preexisting low back pain, reduced lifting capacity, and limited work performance due to a previous low back injury. The current impairments, the absence of heat and swelling, and the fact that the initial injury occurred 3 weeks ago all indicate that this injury has progressed from the acute inflammatory stage. There are now signs of both chronic inflammation, including restriction of motion by pain and joint stiffness, and proliferation, including restriction of motion by weakness and loss of soft tissue length and extensibility. Lumbar ROM may be restricted by shortening of the paraspinal muscles or by pain from the facet joints or posterior ligamentous structures. There may also be spinal disc involvement. Straight leg raising is probably restricted by shortness of the hamstring muscles. The present complaints of pain may still be classified as acute because 3 weeks is within the usual time frame for pain due to a low back strain to resolve; however, this patient also has long-term low back pain from his prior injury. The hypertonicity of the left lower paraspinals is most likely a muscle spasm in response to local pain.

PREFERRED PRACTICE PATTERN
Impaired Joint Mobility, Motor Function, Muscle Performance, Range of Motion, and Reflex Integrity Associated With Spinal Disorders, (4F)

PLAN OF CARE
The goals of treatment at this time include decreasing pain and lumbar joint stiffness, increasing lumbar motion and straight leg raising, and increasing the patient's sitting and lifting tolerance so that he can return to work. Treatments that increase circulation are also recommended since they may accelerate progression of healing at this time. Controlling scar tissue formation, normalizing muscle tone, and maintaining strength and flexibility should also be promoted since these will promote a more complete and rapid resolution of disability.

ASSESSMENT REGARDING THE OPTIMAL PHYSICAL AGENT INTERVENTION(S)
Thermotherapy can be used to relieve pain, decrease joint stiffness, increase soft tissue extensibility, and increase circulation. Neutral warmth may be used to decrease muscle hypertonicity, or more aggressive heating may be used to control pain and thereby reduce hypertonicity by interrupting the pain-spasm-pain cycle. Given the probable deep location of the injury, the use of deep heating agents such as ultrasound or diathermy would be more appropriate than the use of superficial heating agents such as hot packs or paraffin. Although cryotherapy can also relieve pain, this form of treatment would not be indicated because it can increase joint stiffness, decrease soft tissue extensibility, and reduce circulation. Spinal traction may also be used to increase spinal joint mobility and decrease symptoms associated with spinal disc, muscle, or facet joint involvement, while water-based exercise and motor-level electrical stimulation may be used to enhance muscle strength.

PROPOSED TREATMENT PLAN AND RATIONALE
It is proposed that a deep heating agent such as ultrasound or diathermy be used to decrease pain and stiffness and enhance healing and circulation in the deep tissues of the low back. This may be followed by lumbar traction or manual joint mobilization. These passive interventions should be combined with an active exercise program involving stretching and strengthening exercises, either on land or in water, as well as posture and body mechanics training. GH's history of a lengthy and only partial recovery from a prior work-related back injury places him at increased risk of developing chronic pain; therefore, interventions that focus on functional activities, reactivation, and enhancing the patient's ability to help himself should be used. Because the deep heating agents, ultrasound and diathermy, cannot be applied by the patient himself, the therapist will have to choose between using these agents to optimize tissue healing and using only those treatments that the patient can perform himself, such as exercise, self-traction, and hot packs, in order to reduce the risk of dependence on passive intervention by the therapist.

FOLLOW-UP
After 3 weeks of treatment with diathermy to the low back, mechanical lumbar traction, lumbar flexion and hamstring stretching exercises, and posture and body mechanics training in the clinic, combined with instruction in a home exercise program, GH reports that his pain has decreased slightly, now varying in intensity from 5/10 to 7/10. He reports no improvement in his sleep, his sitting tolerance, or his lifting ability, and he has not returned to work. Lumbar active ROM has increased by approximately 10% in all planes, but straight leg raising has remained unchanged at 45 degrees bilaterally. Lumbar muscle tone is now normal. GH's recall of his home exercises is poor.

EVALUATION OF THE CLINICAL FINDINGS
At this time, GH continues to have impairments of pain, decreased lumbar ROM, lumbar joint stiffness, and decreased hamstring length. He also continues to have the functional limitations of reduced sitting and lifting tolerance and the disability of being unable to work. Six weeks after the initial injury, healing has probably progressed to the proliferation or possibly the remodeling stage, and pain has begun to progress to the chronic type rather than resolving. The ongoing pain, beyond the usual duration for resolution of a low back strain, the minimal change in the severity of the pain, limitations in activities, and sleep disturbances all indicate that chronic pain is developing. Motion restrictions are probably due primarily to soft tissue shortening and may be resolving poorly due to poor patient compliance with his home treatment program.

PLAN OF CARE
The primary goals of treatment at this time would be to address the impairments and disabilities related to the patient's chronic pain. These include promoting function, including sleep and return to work, increasing strength, and improving coping skills. Treatment should also address the goals of regaining strength, flexibility, and soft tissue length.

Continued

▶ *Clinical Case Studies—cont'd* ◀

ASSESSMENT REGARDING THE OPTIMAL PHYSICAL AGENT INTERVENTION(S)

Due to the importance of active patient involvement with his treatment at this time, it is recommended that the focus of treatment be on active exercise and that the use of passive physical agents, particularly those that cannot be applied by the patient himself, be minimized. Therefore the use of diathermy should be discontinued, and the use of hot packs, cold packs, home or self-traction, or electrical stimulation may be considered. Water-based exercise may be used to complement GH's land-based exercise program, and superficial heat or electrical stimulation may be applied by GH to control his pain, promoting increased participation in exercise and functional activities. Superficial heating agents may be applied by the patient because although such agents do not affect deep tissue temperature, they can cause some increase in deep tissue circulation and can alleviate pain originating in deeper structures.

PROPOSED TREATMENT PLAN AND RATIONALE

It is proposed that GH use superficial heat, cryotherapy, or electrical stimulation to control his pain and that he participate in a well-monitored active exercise program that may include land- and water-based exercises. This patient's history of prolonged low back pain and his presently slow recovery indicate that he is developing chronic pain. This, in conjunction with the indications of poor compliance with his home program, indicates a poor prognosis for a rapid recovery with physical intervention alone. Psychological evaluation and treatment may be needed to address psychosocial issues that may be contributing to his symptoms and disabilities and to provide this patient with improved skills for coping with these problems.

Case 4

CC is a 2½-year-old previously healthy boy with second- and third-degree burns to 30% of his total body surface area. He sustained these burns 2 days ago when a pot was knocked off the stove, pouring hot oil onto his abdomen and legs. He was wearing only diapers at the time. Upon evaluation CC had skin loss over his lower abdomen and the anterior surfaces of both lower extremities. Most of the skin loss was partial thickness, with some full thickness loss in patches in the central part of the burn. Most of the subcutaneous tissue is intact. There is necrotic skin present in the burned areas. The perineal area was spared due to protection by the diaper. CC complains of pain at rest that worsens with movement or with contact of the burned areas. Active

ROM and testing of passive ROM and strength of the lower extremities are limited by pain. CC tries to avoid moving to minimize his pain and therefore spends most of his day lying in bed.

EVALUATION OF THE CLINICAL FINDINGS

This patient presents with impairments of loss of integumentary integrity, pain, and restricted ROM. The injury is in the acute inflammatory stage of healing, the pain is acute, and the ROM restrictions are due to the pain. This patient's pain has also resulted in functional limitations in all activities.

PREFERRED PRACTICE PATTERN

Impaired Integumentary Integrity Associated with Full-Thickness Skin Involvement and Scar Formation, (7D)

PLAN OF CARE

The proposed goals of treatment at this time are to remove necrotic tissue, optimize the environment for tissue healing and control pain. Hydrotherapy can be used to remove necrotic tissue, electrical stimulation and ultrasound can be used to enhance tissue healing and cryotherapy, and thermotherapy and electrical stimulation can be used to control pain.

ASSESSMENT REGARDING THE OPTIMAL PHYSICAL AGENT INTERVENTION(S)

In this patient, it is recommended that hydrotherapy be used to assist with the removal of necrotic tissue. Water can soften the necrotic tissue and can also apply force to help remove it. In addition, soaking in warm water at a temperature close to body heat can help to control the pain of debridement to some degree. Because this patient is young and does not have other health problems, it is not likely that physical agents will be needed to enhance the environment for tissue healing. In addition, the area to be treated is too large for the application of electrical stimulation or ultrasound, and the use of therapeutic ultrasound is contraindicated in this skeletally immature child.

PROPOSED TREATMENT PLAN AND RATIONALE

The physical agent most likely to promote progression toward the goals of treatment at this time, and that is not contraindicated, is hydrotherapy. Nonimmersion hydrotherapy with a shower, or immersion in a whirlpool followed by a shower, is recommended. Hydrotherapy softens and helps to remove necrotic tissue, although it is likely that tools will also need to be used to ensure that all necrotic tissue is removed. Ending the treatment with nonimmersion hydrotherapy reduces the risk of wound infection by washing off contaminated water. Although a number of physical agents can effectively control pain, they are generally only effective for moderate pain in a limited area. Because this patient's pain is coming from such a large area of tissue damage and is likely to be severe much of the time, particularly during debridement, primarily pharmacologic approaches to pain management are recommended.

FOLLOW-UP
Three months later, CC's burns have closed. The newly formed skin is thin, red, and smooth and his pain is much reduced. CC only complains of pain from stretching when moving toward the end of his available ROM.

EVALUATION OF THE CLINICAL FINDINGS
Although the burned areas have closed, healing is not yet complete. If proliferation continues at this time, as it frequently does after burns, hypertrophic scars and contractures may form. The risk for contractures is increased by the fact that CC experiences pain with movements at the end of his available ROM and that he therefore probably avoids or limits these movements.

PLAN OF CARE
The goals of treatment at this time are to prevent hypertrophic scar and contracture formation and to maximize functional recovery.

ASSESSMENT REGARDING THE OPTIMAL PHYSICAL AGENT INTERVENTION(S)
Compression garments have been shown to reduce the formation of hypertrophic scars after burns, and these garments are generally well-tolerated. CC should also perform ROM exercises to minimize the risk of contracture formation. These exercises can be performed on dry land or in water. Exercise in water has the advantages of warming the tissues during the exercise, if warm water is used, and of being comfortable. However, with this young child, particular precautions for safety in the water should be observed, including continual supervision by a clinician in the water and the use of flotation devices.

PROPOSED TREATMENT PLAN AND RATIONALE
It is proposed that CC be fitted for custom-made compression garments for his lower extremities and trunk. These should be worn at all times, except when bathing, for the following 8 to 12 months. CC will need at least two sets of garments at any one time so that he can wear one while the other is being washed. It is likely that he will need to be fitted for at least three or four double sets

of garments as he is at an age where he is growing rapidly, and compression garments must fit closely to be effective. Water-based exercise, focusing on ROM, may be considered if CC does not tolerate or cooperate with land-based exercises. Water-based exercise is likely to be more comfortable and fun, and therefore better tolerated, but is likely to be more difficult to provide due to the need for special facilities, and special attention to safety with this young child.

Case 5
MP is a 40-year-old female diagnosed with adhesive capsulitis of the left shoulder. She reports that her shoulder first began to hurt about 6 months ago without any apparent cause. Although the pain has almost completely resolved since that time, her shoulder has also gradually become more stiff, preventing her from reaching up to brush her hair and from reaching behind to zip up her skirts. The objective evaluation is significant for restricted ROM of the left shoulder as follows:

	Right	**Left**
Active ROM		
Flexion	170°	100°
Abduction	170°	100°
Hand behind back	Central thoracolumbar junction	Left sacroiliac joint
Passive ROM		
Internal rotation	90°	50°
External rotation	80°	10°

Glenohumeral passive inferior and posterior glide are both restricted on the left. MP has had no prior treatment for this problem.

EVALUATION OF THE CLINICAL FINDINGS
This patient presents with impairments of restricted active and passive motion of her left shoulder. These have resulted in a reduced ability to perform activities of daily living, including grooming and dressing. This patient's signs and symptoms, and the duration of her problem, indicate that the condition has probably progressed to the remodeling stage of healing, with some possibility of chronic inflammation. She does not report significant pain at this time, and it appears that her left shoulder motion is restricted by shortening of the anterior inferior glenohumeral joint capsule. No tone abnormalities are noted.

PREFERRED PRACTICE PATTERN
Impaired Joint Mobility, Motor Function, Muscle Performance, and Range of Motion Associated With Connective Tissue Dysfunction, (4D)

Continued

▶ *Clinical Case Studies—cont'd* ◀

PLAN OF CARE

The goals of treatment at this time are to restore normal active and passive motion of the left shoulder and to allow MP to perform all activities of daily living in her prior manner using both upper extremities. Because her shoulder ROM is probably restricted by soft tissue shortening, the treatment should be directed at increasing the extensibility and length of the shortened tissue, the anterior inferior capsule of the glenohumeral joint. Appropriate goals for this late stage of healing would also be to control scar tissue formation and ensure adequate circulation. Although no strength abnormalities were noted on this initial evaluation, the patient's strength should be reevaluated as she regains ROM since she may have strength deficits at the end ranges due to disuse. Should strength deficits become apparent, an additional goal of treatment would be to restore normal strength to the left shoulder muscles.

ASSESSMENT REGARDING THE OPTIMAL PHYSICAL AGENT INTERVENTION(S)

Thermotherapy would be the most appropriate physical agent to use to increase soft tissue extensibility and promote circulation. Because the tissue restricting the ROM is the joint capsule, which is deep, a deep heating agent such as ultrasound or diathermy, rather than a superficial heating agent such as a hot pack, should be used. A deep heating agent applied to the anterior inferior aspect of the shoulder will increase capsular extensibility by elevating the tissue temperature and, since tissue extensibility will be increased only while the tissue is warm, the capsule should be stretched during or immediately after the application of this agent. Motor-level electrical stimulation and water-based exercise may also be used as components of an active stretching or strengthening program for this patient.

PROPOSED TREATMENT PLAN AND RATIONALE

The most appropriate physical agent for heating the anterior inferior capsule is thermal-level ultrasound. Although diathermy could be used for this application, it would be less appropriate because most forms of diathermy cannot be directed to such a small area and because diathermy devices are not readily available in most clinics at this time. Ultrasound should be applied to the anterior inferior aspect of the glenohumeral joint, with the shoulder in a position that places tension on the anterior inferior joint capsule, which would be at the limit of range for combined flexion, abduction, and external rotation. Manual joint mobilization and active and passive stretching should be applied during and immediately after the application of ultrasound in order

to optimize gains in ROM, and the patient should be instructed in a home program of stretching exercises in order to maintain and progress in gaining ROM. This program of deep heat and stretching techniques should be continued until the patient regains her full range of active, passive, and accessory motions. Strengthening exercises should be added if weakness is noted at the end of the range as ROM is regained.

Case 6

LM is an 84-year-old male with a stage IV pressure ulcer over his right greater trochanter. LM has suffered 3 strokes over the last 10 years. At this time he is bedbound, has flexion contractures of both upper and lower extremities, is cachectic and is being fed via a nasogastric tube. The pressure ulcer was first noticed 2 weeks ago, when it was a stage II, and its area was 4 cm by 3 cm. At this time LM's turning schedule was increased from every 4 hours to every 2 hours, and his bed was changed from a regular mattress to an air mattress. however, in the last 2 weeks the wound has worsened. It is now a stage IV, and its area has increased to 6 cm by 5 cm. Approximately 50% of the wound bed is black and 50% is yellow. There is no undermining present.

EVALUATION OF THE CLINICAL FINDINGS

This patient presents with impairments of loss of tissue integrity, decreased active and passive range of motion, and decreased strength. The tissue is not demonstrating healing at this time. Tissue healing must be initiated at the inflammatory stage.

PREFERRED PRACTICE PATTERN

Impaired Integumentary Integrity Associated with Skin Involvement Extending into Fascia, Muscle, or Bone and Scar Formation, (7E)

PLAN OF CARE

The proposed goals of treatment at this time are to remove necrotic tissue and optimize the environment for tissue healing. It is also hoped that wound closure can be achieved; however, with this patient's poor general state of health, wound closure may not be possible. If it is not possible, the goals of treatment would be to minimize wound progression and reduce the risk of wound and systemic infection.

ASSESSMENT REGARDING THE OPTIMAL PHYSICAL AGENT INTERVENTION(S)

Hydrotherapy or sharp tools can be used to debride necrotic tissue from the wound. Debridement will enhance wound healing and reduce the risk of infection. Dead tissue cannot heal and can act as a mechanical barrier to tissue growth and as a nidus for infection. Electrical stimulation or ultrasound may also be used to facilitate healing.

PROPOSED TREATMENT PLAN AND RATIONALE

The physical agents that could promote progression toward the goals of treatment at this time, and that are not contraindicated, include hydrotherapy, electrical stimulation, and ultrasound. Nonimmersion hydrotherapy, such as pulsed lavage, is safest and most effective to use for wound debridement because this allows control of the water pressure and avoids soaking the wound in contaminated water. Although both electrical stimulation and ultrasound have both been shown to enhance pressure ulcer healing, since the evidence for the effectiveness of electrical stimulation for this application is stronger, electrical stimulation is recommended for treatment of this patient. It is recommended that sensory-level high-volt pulsed current electrical stimulation be used since most studies have shown this to promote wound healing. In addition to interventions using physical agents, a frequent turning schedule avoiding the right side, positioning to minimize pressure on the right lateral hip, and transfer techniques that minimize shear and friction are recommended. A wound dressing that keeps the wound bed moist, keeps the surrounding skin dry, and does not require frequent changes should be used. A support surface that optimizes pressure distribution and moisture control should also be used.

FOLLOW-UP

Two months later the wound on LM's right lateral hip, in the area of the greater trochanter, is still open. However, there is no longer any necrotic tissue present, and the wound base is now red. The area of the wound has also decreased from 7 cm by 5 cm to 3 cm by 2 cm.

EVALUATION OF THE CLINICAL FINDINGS

The absence of necrotic tissue and the red wound base, which is most likely granulation tissue, indicates that this wound has progressed from the inflammatory stage of healing to the proliferative stage of healing.

PLAN OF CARE

The primary goals of treatment at this time are to continue to optimize the environment for wound healing and to protect the wound. Removal of necrotic tissue is not needed since none is present.

ASSESSMENT REGARDING THE OPTIMAL PHYSICAL AGENT INTERVENTION(S)

Debridement with hydrotherapy should be discontinued at this time as there is no longer necrotic tissue in the wound and the granulation tissue that is present may easily be damaged by the hydrotherapy. Electrical stimulation may be continued to enhance tissue healing.

PROPOSED TREATMENT PLAN AND RATIONALE

It is proposed that hydrotherapy be discontinued. Although electrical stimulation may be continued to promote tissue healing, a trial without this intervention is recommended so that disturbance of the fragile granulation tissue is minimized. Tissue healing should be carefully monitored and electrical stimulation resumed if healing plateaus or regresses.

Chapter Review

It is recommended that physical agents be selected for patient treatment when they can be expected to promote progression toward the goals of treatment, can be applied safely, and when the support for their use has high scientific merit. When appropriately selected and applied, physical agents can accelerate tissue healing, control pain, reduce motion restrictions, and modify muscle tone. However, for their application to be safe, physical agents must not be applied when contraindicated, and all recommended precautions must be adhered to. Although there are specific contraindications and precautions to the application of different physical agents, pregnancy, malignancy, the presence of a pacemaker, impaired sensation, and impaired mentation generally indicate the need for caution when considering the use of any physical agent. A treatment can be considered to have high scientific merit if its use is supported by valid theories, if it is designed for specific types of patients, if its potentially adverse effects are presented, and if its efficacy is supported by well-designed studies published in peer-reviewed journals. If the application of a physical agent is expected to promote achievement of the goals of treatment, to be safe, and to have high scientific merit, the cost, convenience, and availability of that agent should also be considered in treatment selection. Although the application of a physical agent may be the only intervention used with a patient, generally physical agents are used in conjunction with each other or in conjunction with other interventions, such as active exercise, passive mobilization, or functional activities, in order to optimize patient outcome.

The selection and application of physical agents may vary under different health care delivery systems due to differences in practical and financial constraints. Although under all systems the clinician should seek to provide the best possible care for patients, current health care delivery systems frequently require that such care also be provided in the most cost-effective manner. Costs may be controlled by having patients or practitioners with lower skill levels apply treatments under the direction of a therapist, when this can be done correctly and safely and when effectiveness can be maximized by evaluating the effects of specific interventions on patient functional outcome and selecting those that are shown to produce the greatest benefit; however, the potential for conflict between minimizing cost and maximizing benefit can make treatment selection a complex and difficult process. The reader is referred to the Evolve website at http://evolve.elsevier.com/Cameron for study questions pertinent to this chapter.

References

1. Weston M, Taber C, Casgranda L et al: Changes in local blood volume during cold gel pack application to traumatized ankles, *J Orthop Sport Phys Ther* 19(4):197-199, 1994.
2. Wolf SL: Contralateral upper extremity cooling from a specific cold stimulus, *Phys Ther* 51:158-165, 1971.
3. Bickford RH, Duff RS: Influence of ultrasonic irradiation on temperature and blood flow in human skeletal muscle, *Circ Res* 1:534-538, 1953.
4. Fox HH, Hilton SM: Bradykinin formation in human skin as a factor in heat vasodilation, *J Physiol* 142:219, 1958.
5. Schmidt KL: Heat, cold and inflammation, *Rheumatology* 38:391-404, 1979.
6. McCulloch J: Physical modalities in wound management: ultrasound, vasopneumatic devices and hydrotherapy, *Ostomy Wound Manage* 41(5):30-32, 35-37, 1995.
7. Ernst E, Fialka V: Ice freezes pain? A review of the clinical effectiveness of analgesic cold therapy, *J Pain Symptom Manage* 9(1):56-59, 1994.
8. Benson TB, Copp EP: The effects of therapeutic forms of heat and ice on the pain threshold of the normal shoulder, *Rheumatol Rehabil* 13:101-104, 1974.
9. Wilson DH: Treatment of soft tissue injuries by pulsed electrical energy, *Br Med J* 2:269-270, 1972.
10. Pennington GM, Danley DL, Sumko MH: Pulsed, nonthermal, high frequency electromagnetic field (Diapulse) in the treatment of Grade I and Grade II ankle sprains, *Milit Med* 153:101-104, 1993.
11. Kaplan EG, Weinstock RE: Clinical evaluation of Diapulse as adjunctive therapy following foot surgery, *J Am Podiatr Assoc* 58(5):218-221, 1968.
12. Cote DJ, Prentice WE, Hooker DN et al: Comparison of three treatment procedures for minimizing ankle sprain swelling, *Phys Ther* 68(7):1072-1076, 1988.
13. Wilkerson GB: Treatment of inversion ankle sprain through synchronous application of focal compression and cold, *Athletic Training* 26:220-225, 1991.
14. Quillen WS, Roullier LH: Initial management of acute ankle sprains with rapid pulsed pneumatic compression and cold, *J Orthop Sports Phys Ther* 4:39-43, 1982.
15. Pilla AA, Martin DE, Schuett AM et al: Effect of PRF therapy on edema from grades I and II ankle sprains: a placebo controlled randomized, multi-site, double-blind clinical study, *J Athletic Training* 31:S53, 1996.
16. Lehmann J, Masock A, Warren C et al: Effect of therapeutic temperatures on tendon extensibility, *Arch Phys Med Rehabil* 51:481-487, 1970.
17. Lehmann JF, DeLateur BJ: Application of Heat and Cold in the Clinical Setting. In Lehmann JF, (ed): *Therapeutic Heat and Cold,* ed 4, Baltimore, 1990, Williams & Wilkins.
18. Lehmann JF, DeLateur BJ: *Therapeutic Heat and Cold,* ed 4, Baltimore, 1990, Williams & Wilkins.
19. Lehmann JF, DeLateur BJ, Stonebridge JB et al: Therapeutic temperature distribution produced by ultrasound as modified by dosage and volume of tissue exposed, *Arch Phys Med Rehabil* 48:662-666, 1967.
20. Lehmann JF, DeLateur BJ, Warren G et al: Bone and soft tissue heating produced by ultrasound, *Arch Phys Med Rehabil* 48:397-401, 1967.
21. Kamm RD: Bioengineering studies of periodic external compression as prophylaxis against deep venous thrombosis: Part I: Numerical studies, *J Biomech Eng* 104:87-95, 1982.
22. Olson DA, Kamm RD, Shapiro AH: Bioengineering studies of periodic external compression as prophylaxis against deep venous thrombosis:Part II: Experimental studies on a simulated leg, *J Biomech Eng* 104:96-104, 1982.
23. Risch WD, Koubenec HJ, Beckmann U et al: The effect of graded immersion on heart volume, central venous pressure, pulmonary blood distribution and heart rate in man, *Pfluegers Arch* 374:117, 1978.
24. Haffor AA, Mohler JG, Harrison AAC: Effects of water immersion on cardiac output of lean and fat male subjects at rest and during exercise, *Aviat Space Environ Med* 62:125, 1991.

25. Balldin UI, Lundgren CEG, Lundvall J et al: Changes in the elimination of 133 Xenon from the anterior tibial muscle in man induced by immersion in water and by shifts in body position, *Aerospace Med* 42(5):489, 1971.

26. Ward RS: Pressure therapy for the control of hypertrophic scar formation after burn injury: a history and review, *J Burn Care Rehabil* 12:257-262, 1991.

27. Larson DL, Abston S, Evans EB et al: Techniques for decreasing scar formation and contractures in the burned patient, *J Trauma* 11:807-823, 1971.

28. Kircher CW, Shetlar MR, Shetlar CL: Alteration of hypertrophic scars induced by mechanical pressure, *Arch Dermatol* 111:60-64, 1975.

29. Wade J: Sports splash, *Rehabil Manage* 10(4):64-70, 1997.

30. Warren C, Lehmann J, Koblanski J: Elongation of rat tail tendon: effect of load and temperature, *Arch Phys Med Rehabil* 52:465-474, 484, 1971.

31. Warren C, Lehmann J, Koblanski J: Heat and stretch procedures: an evaluation using rat tail tendon, *Arch Phys Med Rehabil* 57:122-126, 1976.

32. Gersten JW: Effect of ultrasound on tendon extensibility, *Am J Phys Med* 34:362-369, 1955.

33. Lehmann JF, Brunner GD, Stow RW: Pain threshold measurements after therapeutic application of ultrasound, microwaves and infrared, *Arch Phys Med Rehabil* 39:560-565, 1958.

34. Judovich B: Lumbar traction therapy, *JAMA* 159:549, 1955.

35. Cheatle MD, Esterhai JL: Pelvic traction as treatment for acute back pain, *Spine* 16:1379-1381, 1991.

36. Bonica JJ: *The Management of Pain,* ed 2, Philadelphia, 1990, Lea & Febiger.

37. Hood LB, Chrisman D: Intermittent pelvic traction in the treatment of the ruptured intervertebral disc, *Phys Ther* 48:21-30, 1968.

38. Mathews JA, Mills SB, Jenkins VM et al: Back pain and sciatica: controlled trials of manipulation, traction, sclerosant, and epidural injections, *Br J Rheumatol* 26:416-423, 1987.

39. Lidstrom A, Zachrisson M: Physical therapy on low back pain and sciatica: an attempt at evaluation, *Scand J Rehabil Med* 2:37-42, 1970.

40. Sicard-Rosenbaum L, Lord D, Danoff JV et al: Effects of continuous therapeutic ultrasound on growth and metastasis of subcutaneous murine tumors, *Phys Ther* 75(1):3-11, 1995.

41. Burr B: *Heat as a therapeutic modality against cancer.* Report 16. Bethesda, MD, 1974, U.S. National Cancer Institute.

42. Baker LL, McNeal DR, Benton LA et al: *Neuromuscular Electrical Stimulation: A Practical Guide,* ed 3, Downey, CA, 1993, Rancho Los Amigos Medical Center.

43. Carmick J: Clinical use of neuromuscular electrical stimulation for children with cerebral palsy, *Phys Ther* 73:505-513, 1993.

44. Carmick J: Use of neuromuscular electrical stimulation and a dorsal wrist splint to improve hand function of a child with spastic hemiparesis, *Phys Ther* 77(6):661-671, 1997.

45. Cyriax J: *Textbook of Orthopedic Medicine, Volume I: Diagnosis of Soft Tissue Lesions,* London, 1982, Bailliere Tindall.

46. Lentell G, Hetherington T, Eagan J et al: The use of thermal agents to influence the effectiveness of low load prolonged stretch, *J Orthop Sport Phys Ther* 16(5):200-207, 1992.

47. Travell JG, Simons DG: *Myofascial Pain and Dysfunction: The Trigger Point Manual,* Baltimore, 1983, Williams & Wilkins.

48. Simons DG, Travell JG: Myofascial origins of low back pain. 1: Principles of diagnosis and treatment, *Postgrad Med* 73(2):70-77, 1983.

49. Harris SR: How should treatments be critiqued for scientific merit? *Phys Ther* 76(2):175-181, 1996.

50. Verrier M, Falconer K, Crawford SJ: A comparison of tissue temperature following two shortwave diathermy techniques, *Physiother Canada* 29(1):21-25, 1977.

51. Hand JW: Biophysics and technology of electromagnetic hyperthermia. In Guthrie M, ed: *Methods of External Hyperthermic Heating,* Berlin, 1990, Springer-Verlag.

52. Conradi E, Pages IH: Effects of continuous and pulsed microwave irradiation on distribution of heat in the gluteal region of minipigs, *Scand J Rehabil Med* 21:59-62, 1989.

53. Golden GS: Nonstandard therapies in developmental disabilities, *Am J Dis Child* 134:487-491, 1980.

54. Weinberger A, Nyaska A, Giler S: Treatment of experimental inflammatory synovitis with continuous magnetic field, *Isr J Med Sci* 32(12):1197-1201, 1996.

55. Abramson DI: Physiological basis for the use of physical agents in peripheral vascular disorders, *Arch Phys Med Rehabil* 46:216-244, 1965.

56. Stillwell GK: Physiatric management of postmastectomy lymphedema, *Med Clin North Am* 46:1051-1063, 1962.

57. Rucinski TJ, Hooker D, Prentice W: The effects of intermittent compression on edema in post acute ankle sprains, *JOSPT* 14(2):65-69, 1991.

58. Sims D: Effects of positioning on ankle edema, *JOSPT* 8:30-35, 1986.

59. PT Bulletin, 12/20/1997, p 11.

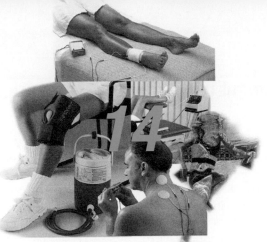

Directions for Future Research and Application

OBJECTIVES

Upon completion of this chapter, the reader will be able to:

1. Explain why there is a need for further research on the use of physical agents in rehabilitation.
2. Identify the areas in which further research on the effects of physical agents is needed.

3. Summarize the methodological characteristics required for research on physical agents to guide progress in clinical practice.

WHY FURTHER RESEARCH ON THE USE OF PHYSICAL AGENTS IN REHABILITATION IS NEEDED

Although, as demonstrated throughout this book, there is research to support the use of physical agents in rehabilitation, further research is needed in most areas because, as with most medical treatments, the available scientific evidence is generally insufficient to prove conclusively that current clinical practice is effective or that it is delivered in the optimal manner. Due to these limitations, the current practice of applying physical agents is based on the available research findings in conjunction with prior practice patterns and the personal experience of the provider. This has resulted in variability in practice among practitioners with different training and personal experience and from different locations, and has probably also resulted in lack of optimal care and suboptimal outcomes for some patients.

For example, although shortwave diathermy is commonly used in Europe, with reportedly good results, it is rarely used in the United States. Because this physical agent is unlikely to produce different effects in these different regions, it is probable that either some patients in Europe are receiving treatments that are not effective or that some patients in the United States are not receiving treatments that could benefit them. Further research will help to ascertain which interventions are effective and which are not, which methods and treatment parameters to use for optimal results, the benefits that can be expected from these interventions, and who will receive the greatest benefit from them. This will enhance clinical practice by improving patient outcomes, increasing the consistency and efficiency of care, and supporting reimbursement for treatments using physical agents.

It is recommended that future research on physical agents focus on applications where empirical clinical evidence, prior studies, and anecdotal reports suggest, but do not definitively prove, that certain interventions are effective. Future research should attempt to determine if current practice is effective, and if so, how it can be optimized, and if not, which alternative interventions would be effective. As further research is performed, it is expected that the findings will support many current applications of physical agents; however, it is also likely that future research will direct modifications in the application of some physical agents and fail to support the continued use of others. Studies may fail to support present practice if an intervention is found to be ineffective or to be less effective than other available treatment options. It is also expected that future research will promote the development of new applications of physical agents.

Once appropriate areas for research are selected, it is also essential that future studies be designed to permit ready interpretation and application of their findings. In many areas, more research is needed because flaws in the available studies, such as inappropriate design, the use of inappropriate types or numbers of subjects, lack of or poor controls, the use of measures that have not been shown to be valid or reliable, limited assessment of outcome, or poor reporting of the precise intervention used, restrict the application of their findings. For example, if the effects of an intervention have been monitored without comparison with a control group who did not receive that intervention, it cannot be determined whether the observed effects were caused by the intervention, thereby supporting its use, or whether they were due to chance or normal progression of the problem being treated, thus not supporting its use. Appropriately designed studies on the use of physical agents in rehabilitation will demonstrate whether or not specific interventions with physical agents can promote progression toward the goals of treatment for specific problems and how such benefits can be optimized.

High-quality research in the appropriate areas will improve the quality of patient care and provide support for reimbursement for treatments using physical agents based on proven positive functional outcomes. In the absence of such studies it is possible that patients will not receive optimal care, and it is likely that, over time, payers will not continue to reimburse for interventions that have not been proven to be effective.

AREAS FOR FUTURE RESEARCH ON PHYSICAL AGENTS

Physical properties and effects of physical agents
Physiological effects of physical agents
Clinical applications of physical agents
Contraindications, precautions, and adverse effects of physical agents

There are many areas where further research on physical agents could promote improvements in patient care. These include the physical properties and effects of physical agents, their physiological effects, their clinical applications, the contraindications and precautions to their use, and their potential adverse effects. Although for most physical agents there is some research in all of these areas, more research is needed in order to optimize clinical applications in rehabilitation.

In general, the physical properties and effects of physical agents are well understood, but their interactions with, and their effects on, physiological processes are less clear. In most areas, even less is known about the specific effects of physical agents on patient function. While further understanding of the physical properties and effects of physical agents may prove valuable in the development of treatment applications, studies regarding the changes produced in physiological processes and the resultant clinical outcomes are likely to provide the most guidance for advancing and improving clinical practice.

Physical Properties and Effects of Physical Agents

Although the physical properties of most physical agents are generally well understood and have been clearly described, further research is needed to clarify the nature and magnitude of their physical effects on the body. For example, although it is known that thermal energy is produced by friction between particles, that the amount of thermal energy increases in proportion to the relative rate of motion of these particles, and that the amount of thermal energy required to produce a given change in temperature in a material varies with the specific heat of that material, without further research the temperature increase and the distribution of heat in a patient's body when different thermal agents are applied cannot be readily or accurately predicted. Taking the specific examples of short wave diathermy and microwave diathermy, both of which produce thermal energy and have physical properties which are well understood, current research has produced conflicting findings regarding the distribution of the heat produced by these different wavelengths of electromagnetic radiation in different types of tissue and by the different applicators used to deliver these types of electromagnetic radiation.[1-3] Further research could clarify the factors impacting the distribution of the heat produced by these different forms of diathermy and thus increase the safety and effectiveness of their clinical application.

Another area where research on the physical properties and effects of physical agents has been valuable is in the development of new physical agents. Most devices developed in recent years deliver the same or similar types of energy as that delivered by previously available physical agents. However, these newer devices take advantage of technological and theoretical advances to provide greater ranges and control of the energy intensity or frequency as well as improved safety and convenience. Research using these newer devices is needed to gain a better understanding of their physical properties, potential applications in rehabilitation, and possible advantages over older devices. In addition, further basic science and engineering studies may yield other physical agents and further device improvements.

The low-energy cold laser is an example of a physical agent that was developed in recent years and that is now being applied clinically in rehabilitation in some settings. A laser produces a beam of electromagnetic energy that has the unique physical properties of being monochromatic, coherent, and directional. At this time, low-energy laser devices produce electromagnetic radiation with frequencies and wavelengths that penetrate through only a few millimeters of human tissue.[4,5] Further research on the physical properties of low-energy lasers may promote the development of devices that can penetrate more deeply.

Longwave ultrasound is another physical agent that was recently developed for application in rehabilitation. This type of ultrasound has a much lower frequency and a longer wavelength than traditionally used ultrasound, resulting in deeper penetration. This type of ultrasound was designed to be used for treatment of deep tissues; however, at this time, there is controversy in the literature concerning the distribution of the energy when such low frequencies are used.[6,7] Although initial reports indicated that the deeper penetration of ultrasound with this frequency could be beneficial for some clinical applications, later reports note that, since beam divergence increases at this lower frequency, the intensity of the ultrasound reaching deeper tissues is very much reduced, possibly to levels that are too low to produce the desired physiological effects. Further research on the physical properties of this frequency range of ultrasound is needed to ascertain how the energy is distributed and what clinical effects it has. Further technical developments may also allow focusing of the beam while maintaining the deeper penetration.

Another newer device, composed of a thermostatically controlled heating plate placed inside a wound dressing, has recently been developed specifically for the superficial delivery of heat by conduction to the site of an open wound. This device keeps the wound environment within a limited temperature range at all times and is thus thought to promote wound healing. Further research on the physical properties of this device, such as its range of operating temperature and its effect on local moisture, is needed to direct its clinical application.

It is likely that in the future other physical agents and devices that offer further control of energy delivery to patients will be developed. For example, devices that deliver heat for set amounts of time or at controlled but varying temperatures, devices that deliver electromagnetic energy with different pulse durations and duty cycles or with different types of applicators, devices that apply stationary magnetic fields, or devices that apply compression with different pressures or pressure gradients or with alternative application devices, may be developed. As new devices become available, research will be needed to determine their physical properties and effects and to ascertain whether they promote physiological changes that produce clinical benefits.

Physiological Effects of Physical Agents

Although further research on the physical properties of physical agents may facilitate progress in clinical practice, in order to optimize care, research on the physiological effects and clinical uses of physical agents whose physical properties are already well understood is also needed. Studies should examine the effects of physical agents on the physical properties of tissue, such as muscle or tendon extensibility and cell membrane permeability, their effects on physiological processes such as tissue healing and nerve conduction, and their effects on pathological states such as bacterial infection. Further research in these areas may delineate the magnitude of the effects produced by physical agents and the ideal treatment parameters to use to achieve these effects. Such research will also guide specific clinical applica-

tions such as the use of ultrasound or electrical currents to facilitate transdermal drug delivery and accelerate tissue healing or the use of thermotherapy, cryotherapy, or electrotherapy to control pain. Studies concerning the effects of physical agents on bacterial infection may be particularly valuable at this time since many bacteria are becoming resistant to available antibiotics, necessitating the development of alternative treatment approaches. Progress in these areas will require examination of the physiological processes involved in both normal and abnormal function and the changes produced in these processes by the application of physical agents.

In order to provide clinicians with information that allows them to apply physical agents with more predictable results, future studies should seek to determine both the nature and the magnitude of the effects of physical agents on physiological processes and attempt to determine how these effects vary with tissue type and pathology. While prior research generally evaluated the effects of physical agents at a macroscopic level, such as the effects of heat on soft tissue extensibility or on arterial circulation, since current technology also permits examination at the microscopic levels of the cell, cellular components, and molecules, future research should also evaluate the physiological effects of physical agents at these levels. This will lead to an improved understanding of the mechanisms underlying the macroscopic effects of physical agents, thereby providing guidelines for predicting and controlling the effects of physical agents on physiological processes with greater precision.

Clinical Application of Physical Agents

Although research on the physical properties and physiological effects of physical agents will indicate which interventions may be effective and may clarify the mechanisms of interventions that are known to be effective, clinical studies are needed to ascertain if interventions with physical agents actually promote progress toward treatment goals. Clinical studies should also examine the effects of different treatment parameters, such as method of application, treatment duration, intensity, and frequency. For example, when studying the effects of electrical stimulation on muscle strengthening, a range of parameters must be evaluated, including current waveform and parameters, electrode placement, and treatment duration. In addition, the effects of applying physical agents to patients of various ages with different pathologies and with symptoms of varied acuity should also be evaluated. These types of studies are needed to optimize the application of physical agents and maximize the accuracy of predictions concerning the nature and extent of the benefits of such interventions.

It is recommended that clinical studies examine applications of physical agents that are in frequent use at this time but in which the data regarding treatment efficacy and optimal treatment parameters are inconclusive. Novel applications of commonly used physical agents and possible applications of recently developed physical agents should also be evaluated. For example, clinical studies on the effects of phonophoresis and traction should be performed because, although these interventions are commonly used to treat local inflammatory conditions and symptoms related to spinal disc bulges or herniation, respectively, the benefit of these interventions has not yet been conclusively proven, and the optimal treatment parameters and patient presentations for their application have not yet been determined. Taking the example of phonophoresis, studies should first attempt to ascertain whether, when using the common current application techniques, phonophoresis reduces the impairments and functional limitations associated with inflammation. If phonophoresis is found to be effective, one should then evaluate whether changing any of the treatment parameters, such as the ultrasound duty cycle, intensity and frequency, drug type and vehicle, or treatment duration and frequency, alters the effects. Studies should also evaluate if the treatment is more effective during certain stages of inflammation or for certain types and depths of tissue. In the case of traction, studies should determine whether the common current applications are effective, and if so, whether changing treatment parameters such as the hold and relax times, traction force, or treatment duration alter the effects, or if the treatment is more effective when used for patients with symptoms of different etiology, duration, nature, or distribution.

Studies on the effects of specific physical agents will provide information to guide clinicians in selecting physical agent interventions and treatment parameters for different patients and in predicting more accurately and reliably the outcome of such interventions. However, in order to direct the selection of the ideal treatment, studies comparing the effectiveness of different treatment options are also needed. For example, although current studies indicate that ultrasound and electrical stimulation may facilitate the closure of open wounds, and that electrical stimulation, cryotherapy, and thermotherapy can reduce pain, until studies comparing the effectiveness of these interventions are performed, it will not be clear which treatments are most effective and should therefore be chosen for clinical application in patient care.

Contraindications, Precautions, and Adverse Effects of Physical Agents

Although more research on the benefits of applying physical agents in rehabilitation will help to guide treatment selection, studies on the specific contraindications, precautions, and adverse effects of physical agents are also needed to determine whether current precautions are appropriate and to ensure that treatments with physical agents are applied safely. At this time, restrictions on the use of physical agents are frequently based on expectations of possible adverse effects and prior common practice rather than on research-based evidence of the properties and effects of physical agents. This may fail to prevent some unsafe applications and may unnecessarily restrict the use of safe and effective interventions. For example, in the absence of research to rule out detrimental effects, and due to concern that the integrity of bone may be disrupted in some way by ultrasound, some authors recommend that ultrasound be applied with particular caution to patients with osteoporosis.[8] Although this may reduce the risk of harm to patients with osteoporosis, it may also prevent them from receiving treatment that may be beneficial.

Although research on the contraindications, precautions, and adverse effects of physical agents is necessary, it is difficult to perform studies in these areas that provide definitive data applicable to clinical practice. This is because it is not ethical to place human subjects at avoidable risk by applying treatments thought to be unsafe in order to determine if treatment warnings are justified. Therefore, in vitro studies, studies using animal subjects, and case reports on adverse effects are needed to clarify the potential risks associated with the application of physical agents.

A number of conditions, including pregnancy and malignancy, have generally been considered to be contraindications for the application of physical agents. Although there is little information on the effects of physical agents on these conditions, the potential adverse effects, such as fetal abnormalities or accelerated growth or metastasis of malignant tissue, can be so detrimental that, without evidence to demonstrate that such applications are safe, their risk is considered to be excessive for clinical application or for research using human subjects. Further information regarding the safety of applying physical agents to patients with these conditions may be particularly beneficial in clarifying when physical agents may be used, particularly to control pain. However, in order to protect patients and clinicians, until research demonstrates definitively that applying physical agents in the presence of these and other traditionally accepted contraindications is safe, clinicians must continue to practice within current restrictions and warnings.

Studies on the risks associated with the application of physical agents may promote improvements in practice by making applications previously thought unsafe available for clinical use. For example, in the past, the presence of metal in an area was considered to be a contraindication or a cause for caution to the application of ultrasound. The reason was that, lacking specific research, it was thought that this agent may produce excessive temperature increases in metal, as does diathermy, a previously available deep heating agent. There were also concerns that therapeutic ultrasound may loosen metal implants. However, since studies have shown that ultrasound is reflected by, but does not heat, metal and that it does not loosen metal implants, ultrasound may now be applied in areas where metal is present. For example, ultrasound may be applied to promote increased range of motion (ROM) in areas where there is soft tissue shortening after the implantation of metal plates and screws after a fracture.[9]

METHODOLOGICAL CHARACTERISTICS OF FUTURE RESEARCH ON PHYSICAL AGENTS

Study Design

Case report
Single-subject design
Group design

The goal of most research is to determine the effect, or effects, of specific interventions as precisely, definitively, and clearly as possible. Although this may appear to be a simple task, it is fraught with both theoretical and practical difficulties. Theoretically, it can be difficult to determine the effects of an intervention because, even if that intervention is consistently followed by a change in the subjects, one cannot be certain that the intervention actually caused that change. For example, if the application of traction is followed by a reduction in low back pain, one cannot be certain that the traction reduced the pain since, in many individuals, low back pain resolves with or without the application of any treatment. Practically, it is particularly difficult to ascertain cause and effect in clinical care because different individuals may respond differently to the same intervention, most interventions involve a number of components, and many patients progress, either toward or away from the goals of treatment, independently of the application of any intervention. Studies may be designed in various ways to attempt to overcome these problems and thus to determine, correctly and accurately, the effects of interventions with physical agents to appropriately guide future clinical practice.

Case report

The simplest form of research is a case report. A case report is a detailed description of an individual patient's clinical presentation, the course of treatment, and the changes in clinical presentation that occur during and generally after that course of treatment. A case report should include a thorough and complete description of all aspects of the patient's care and status, including which treatments were applied, when and how often they were applied, as well as the patient's age, gender, diagnosis, impairments, functional limitations and disabilities before, during, and after treatment.

A case report is generally the first type of formal evaluation of a treatment approach that is performed. It is most valuable for describing successful methods for treating various conditions when little other information is available. A case report generally concerns the application of a novel intervention for a common problem or the use of a common intervention for a novel application. The advantages of case reports are that, when well written, they provide information about all aspects of the patient's presentation and care in detail, and they require the investigator only to describe an individual's course of treatment and presentation. Case reports do not require the treatment to be changed in any way. The primary disadvantage of case reports is that they only provide information about what was done to a particular patient and what happened to that patient, without clearly indicating what caused the observed changes. Therefore one cannot be certain which, if any, of the intervention(s) in question caused the observed changes or if these changes occurred independently of the interventions. Caution should also be observed when considering applying the findings of a case report to other individuals since the changes that occurred in the subject of the report may have been unique to that individual.

Single case reports can provide valuable information to guide clinical practice and further research. When a number of case reports describe similar outcomes after the application of a specific intervention, this increases the likelihood that the intervention caused the observed changes and that it would cause similar changes in other individuals. This increases the confidence with which the findings can be applied to clinical practice. Single case studies where treatment is applied and then withdrawn, and studies involving groups of subjects, some of whom receive the intervention and some of whom do not, further strengthen the proof of an association between the treatment and proposed effect and improve the quality of evidence to justify application in clinical practice.

Single-subject design

A controlled study using one subject, whose status when an intervention is applied for a period of time is compared with the status when the intervention is not applied, provides more definitive information about the effects of an intervention than a case report. In general, for studies using single subjects, the intervention is applied and withdrawn a number of times, and the subject's status during or immediately following the periods of application is compared with the status during the periods when the intervention was not applied.

In contrast to case reports, single-subject studies can differentiate the effects of time alone from the effects of the intervention under investigation without the time and expense of studies involving groups of subjects. Single-subject studies also eliminate the differences in initial status or individual characteristics that can confound the interpretation of studies involving groups of subjects. In a single-subject study, since all outcome measurements are taken from one subject, any differences in status found between applying and not applying the intervention are likely to be due to the intervention. However, although single-subject studies have a number of advantages over case reports, since they only evaluate the response of a single individual to an intervention, caution should be applied in generalizing the findings of such studies to other subjects.

Studies using single subjects are particularly suitable for investigating the effects of interventions on uncommon problems where large groups of subjects may not be available and for analyzing the effects of interventions on problems whose normal progression is so variable as to obscure any effects of an intervention using a group design. However, in most situations, comparing the effects of providing an intervention to one group of subjects and withholding it from another group of subjects more clearly demonstrates the effects of that intervention and provides stronger evidence to support its application to other individuals in clinical practice.

Group design

When well-designed, studies involving groups of subjects usually provide the strongest evidence for the effectiveness of an intervention. In general, the size and homogeneity of the groups will have the greatest impact on the quality of the findings of a group study. Large, homogeneous groups of subjects should be used whenever possible in order to minimize the risk of failing to detect the effects of an intervention. When small, heterogeneous groups are used, differences between groups produced by an intervention may be masked by variability within the groups.

For example, if ultrasound is applied to a few patients with tendonitis of varying degrees of acuity and of varying tendons and, after the treatment, no differences in pain or dysfunction are found between these patients and others who did not receive ultrasound, the failure to detect a treatment effect could be due to the fact that (1) ultrasound does not reduce the pain or dysfunction associated with tendonitis, or that (2) the range of pain and dysfunction within the groups was greater than the range between the groups, or that (3) ultrasound is effective for treating tendonitis only at certain depths or at certain stages of acuity. If this study was performed with a large group of subjects who all had tendonitis of the extensor carpi radialis brevis tendon in the acute inflammatory stage, if the treatment was effective, its effect will not be obscured by variations within the groups of subjects.

Unfortunately, because large groups of individuals with similar characteristics are difficult to recruit, many studies, particularly those involving human subjects, use small, heterogeneous samples and may thus erroneously conclude that treatments are ineffective. Therefore when studies with small, heterogeneous groups of subjects fail to find treatment effects, while case reports and single-subject studies indicate that an intervention is effective, it is recommended that future research replicate these group studies using larger, more homogeneous samples.

Although studies using large, homogeneous groups of subjects optimize the probability of detecting small, statistically significant treatment effects, the clinical significance of these effects must also be taken into account when considering applying the findings to clinical practice. For example, although a study may find that applying heat before stretching the knees of patients who have had a total knee arthroplasty results in a statistically significantly greater gain in flexion ROM than stretching without prior heating, if the difference in ROM gains is only a few degrees, this may not be clinically significant if it does not affect patient function. A slight acceleration of recovery may also be statistically significant while not justifying the use of an intervention in general clinical care. For example, even if applying traction is found to decrease the recovery time from a low back injury from 40 days to 39 days, in most cases the cost of applying this treatment will not be justified by this small effect.

Subjects

In vitro (materials, tissue, cells)
Animals (normal, disease model, true disease)
Humans (normal, patients)

Having selected the appropriate study design, based on the nature of the effect being studied and the quality and availability of prior studies, an investigator must also select suitable research subjects. Subject selection will depend on the nature of the effect being studied, the type of outcome data desired, and the availability of different types of subjects.

In vitro (materials, tissue, cells)

The term *in vitro*, meaning "within glass," is used to describe studies that are carried out in a container or in a test tube rather than within a living organism. In vitro studies use various nonliving materials or cell cultures as subjects and can be used to evaluate many of the physical properties and effects of physical agents, including the penetration and absorption of different types of energy by different materials and the effects of these types of energy on these materials. In vitro studies using biological materials can also yield information about the effects of physical agents on the physical or physiological properties of these materials, such as skin or cell membrane permeability, tissue extensibility, or cell viability.

The advantages of in vitro studies are that they can generally be replicated accurately and they permit close control of subject and intervention variability. However, although in vitro studies may provide information regarding the effects of physical agents on the physical properties of tissue, caution should be exercised in applying findings of these studies directly to the more complex situation of a patient. For example, although a cell grown in agar in a Petri dish may be killed or may grow more rapidly when an electrical current is applied, because of differences in temperature, pH, tissue resistance, current density, chemical environment, or other factors, this same type of cell may not respond in the same manner if an electrical current is applied to it when it exists in an open wound in a patient. Some of these limitations of in vitro studies may be overcome by using animals as research subjects.

Animals (normal, disease model, true disease)

The term *in vivo* is used to describe studies that are carried out within a living body. In vivo studies using animals as subjects allow examination of the effects of physical agents on the physical properties of tissue within a normal physiological environment. This is necessary because normal physiological processes may alter the effects of physical agents. For example, a thermal agent applied to live tissue with an intact, responsive circulation will have less impact on tissue temperature than the same thermal agent applied to the same type of tissue in vitro, with no circulation. The circulatory system will bring blood from other areas to cool the heated tissue. This response will be exaggerated as the tissue warms up and vasodilation occurs. The effects of physical agents on physiological process such as circulation, heart rate, or temperature, may also be evaluated by in vivo studies with animal subjects.

Normal, healthy animals may be used to study the effects of physical agents on normal processes or characteristics such as temperature or circulatory rate, while animals with pathology can be used to study the effect(s) of physical agents on pathology or impairments such as muscle shortening, soft tissue injury, circulatory impairment, or pain. In addition to allowing for evaluation within the context of a complete physiological system, studies using animals allow the investigators to perform procedures and take risks that may not be ethical with human subjects. Studies can also use relatively large sample sizes at less expense than with human subjects and control many potentially confounding variables such as subject activity level, age, gender, and diet. Nonetheless, the results of animal studies should be applied to human patients with caution because differences in human characteristics, such as body size, body composition, skin thickness, or normal temperature, may alter the effects. Studies using animals also generally cannot provide information concerning the effect of interventions on the subjects' functional limitations or disabilities.

Humans (normal, patients)

Studies using human subjects can yield information regarding the physiological effects of interventions within the human body and their effects on the sequelae of pathology including impairments, functional limitations, and disabilities. The human subjects used in research may either be patients with pathology or subjects without pathology. Using individuals with pathology is generally preferred because this provides information that is more readily applicable to other patients. However, since there may be limited access to subjects with problems of similar types and severity, as well as financial and ethical constraints to applying or withholding potentially effective care from patients, many studies on humans are performed using normal subjects.

Studies using normal human subjects can provide information about the physical and physiological effects of interventions, such as their impact on tissue temperature, tissue length, muscle strength, or blood circulation, and may be used to investigate the effects of interventions on experimentally induced dysfunction such as pain; however, caution must be used in applying the findings of such studies to patients with pathology because the effects may be different in the presence of pathology.

For example, although electrical stimulation may not increase muscle strength more effectively than exercise in normal subjects, it has been found to augment strengthening when applied to patients after knee surgery. Studies using patients can provide information concerning the effects of interventions within the context of pathology, and can also provide information about changes in subjective complaints and objective impairments, functional limitations, and disabilities.

Studies using human subjects have a number of limitations, including the difficulty of recruiting adequate numbers of subjects; having limited control over variability in subject characteristics such as problem severity and duration, subject age, and subject gender; and having limited control over subject behaviors such as activity level, diet, and other medical interventions. There are also ethical constraints limiting the nature of the procedures that can be performed on human subjects. In general, procedures that may cause harm or discomfort, such as a tissue biopsy or the application of a physical agent in a circumstance previously contraindicated, may not be performed on human subjects, and informed consent must be obtained from all human subjects before their inclusion in a research study. These restrictions may limit the ability to determine the mechanism of an observed effect and prevent application of an intervention in a blinded fashion.

Controls

Because changes in subjects can occur whether or not any intervention has been applied, in order to determine whether observed changes are caused by an intervention, the outcome of subjects who have received that intervention should be compared with the outcome of subjects who have not received that intervention. The subjects who do not receive the intervention being evaluated are known as *controls*.

When appropriately selected and treated, control subjects can control for the effects of chance, normal progression of the outcome variable, and nonspecific effects of treatment. It is particularly important to control for these effects when evaluating the impact of physical agents in rehabilitation because many of the problems treated in rehabilitation may vary without any intervention and tend to resolve over time, and because most of the treatments provided by rehabilitation clinicians have a variety of nonspecific effects. For example, low back pain can vary in location from one day to the next, with no clear cause, and can vary in severity among individuals; however, for most individuals, acute low back pain resolves within 6 weeks whether or not any treatment is provided. Nonspecific effects of treatment include paying attention to the patient, which may increase the patient's motivation; monitoring progress, which may improve the patient's compliance; and touching the patient, either directly or with a device, which may provide a sensory stimulus to block pain transmission, whether or not any type of energy is being delivered.

Without the use of appropriate controls it is difficult, if not impossible, to determine if the changes observed in subjects who received an intervention were caused by that intervention. For example, if it is found that, in a group, most subjects' low back pain resolves within 6 weeks when a treatment such as traction has been applied, it cannot be concluded that their progress was due to the application of the treatment rather than being the normal recovery pattern for this problem unless a similar group of individuals with similar symptoms and no treatment took significantly longer to recover. A treatment can be considered effective only if subjects who received the treatment show greater or more rapid improvement than control subjects who did not receive the treatment.

There are many different ways to treat control subjects who are not receiving the intervention being evaluated. Although it may be simplest and most convenient to provide these subjects with no treatment, this is not recommended. If the control subjects are not provided with the attention and sensations associated with the active treatment, then only the effects of chance and normal progression, not the nonspecific effects of treatment, will be controlled for. Treatments with interventions that have no direct physiological effects can yield as much as forty percent improvement in outcome, particularly when subjective outcome measures such as pain are used. Therefore if the effects of the intervention group are compared with those of an untreated control group,

the intervention will probably appear to have been effective even when the effects may have not been specific to that intervention.

In order to control for nonspecific effects of an intervention, it is recommended that control subjects receive an alternative intervention that appears as similar as possible to the intervention being assessed but that is known, or thought, not to affect the outcome being evaluated. Such alternative interventions are known as *placebos*. When researching the effects of physical agents, it is recommended that placebos consist of applying the treatment in the normal manner, but without delivery of energy by the device.

For example, a placebo ultrasound treatment may be given by applying a transmission medium to the treatment area and then placing the ultrasound transducer on the area and moving it within that area for the same amount of time used for the active treatment group. The difference would be that, for the active treatment, ultrasound was delivered to the subject, whereas for the placebo treatment, no ultrasound was applied. Similarly, a placebo hot pack treatment could be applied by using a pack at body temperature instead of a heated pack. In both of these examples, the active and placebo treatments are similar with regard to the preparation for application of the treatment, the amount of attention from the person applying the intervention, and the amount of time the subject received care. Thus if a difference in outcome is found between those receiving the placebo treatment and those receiving the active treatment, it is likely that this difference is due to the intervention being studied rather than being a nonspecific effect of providing treatment.

In order to determine the effects of an intervention most accurately, it is recommended that neither the subjects of the study nor the individuals applying the intervention know whether an active or a placebo treatment is being applied. This is known as *double-blind application*. A physical agent may be applied with a double-blind placebo control if it does not produce any identifiable sensation in the subject and if the device providing the treatment appears to be delivering energy even when it is not. For example, low-intensity ultrasound may be applied with a double-blind placebo control if a device that operates normally is used for the active treatment and another device modified to produce no output, although it appears to operate normally, is used for the placebo treatment. The two devices should be marked for differentiation; however, the key to their identity should be concealed from the investigators until all intervention and data collection have been completed. Because this prevents both the subjects and the investigators from knowing which device is active and which is inactive, it will eliminate bias during application of the intervention and data collection.

If the physical agent being evaluated produces a distinct sensation in the subjects, such as the sensation of heat from a hot pack or the sensation of a pull from traction, or if deactivated devices to prevent knowledge of the person applying them are not available, then the intervention may be applied only in a single-blind manner. For example, if only one device is available, low intensities of ultrasound or short-wave diathermy (SWD) that do not produce a sensation of heat may be applied in a single-blind fashion, with blinding of the subjects only, by setting the device to the desired intensity for the active treatment group and not turning it on for the placebo treatment group. Hot packs, which produce a sensation of heat in the subject, may be applied in a single-blind fashion, with blinding of the investigators, if hot packs are used for the active treatment group and unheated packs similar in appearance are used for the placebo treatment group, and if the investigators wear heat-proof gloves so that they cannot feel the temperature of the packs.

Interventions that produce distinct sensations and that require specific behaviors by the individuals applying them, such as compression, traction, most forms of electrical stimulation, or ultrasound or diathermy at intensities that produce a sensation of heat, cannot be delivered in a blinded manner. When attempting to assess the effects of these types of physical agents, lower energy levels of the same intervention or other interventions recommended for the same problem may be applied to the control group for comparison. Ideally, in such circumstances, in order to control for confounding effects of changing multiple variables, the intervention applied to the control subjects should feel as similar as possible to the active treatment, require a similar frequency and duration of application, and involve a similar degree of personal attention from the individual applying it.

In order to avoid, or at least minimize, confounding effects when using human subjects, double-blind placebo controls should be used when possible; when this is not possible, single-blind placebo controls should be used. Only if neither double- nor single-blind application is possible should placebo or active alternative treatments be applied without blinding. When using animal subjects or performing in vitro studies, blinding of the subjects is not necessary; however, blinding of the investigators applying the intervention and collecting the outcome data is recommended.

Because, unlike most other rehabilitation interventions such as exercise, or joint or soft tissue mobilization, many physical agents can be applied readily with double-blind placebo controls, future research on the effects of physical agents should use double-blind controls whenever possible. This will support the conclusion that differences in outcome between subjects receiving an active treatment and controls are due to the treatment rather than to some other aspect of care and will allow therapists to apply the findings of such studies with confidence. In contrast, if appropriate controls are not used, although much time, effort, and expense may be expended, the study results will not readily improve patient care. It will not be known whether the treatments being evaluated are effective and should be used with patients, or whether any observed changes in subject status were the result of chance, normal progression, or nonspecific effects of the intervention.

Outcome Measures

Reliability

Once the investigator has selected the appropriate study design and controls for evaluating the effects of an intervention using a physical agent, appropriate measures of the outcome must also be chosen. The outcome measures selected should be reliable, valid, and clinically relevant. A measure is considered to be reliable if the same or a similar result is produced when the measure is repeated. For example, goniometric measurement of active knee flexion ROM may be considered reliable if the same or a similar angle is reported when active knee flexion ROM is measured repeatedly.

The reliability of a measure may vary for different applications or populations and with application by the same or another individual. For example, a numeric visual analog scale completed by the subject may be reliable for the assessment of pain severity in adults but unreliable when used for the assessment of pain in infants or young children or for the assessment of knee ROM in subjects. Since most measures produce more similar results when reapplied by the same individual (known as *intrarater reliability*) than when reapplied by different people (known as *interrater reliability*) it is recommended that measurements be performed by only one individual, or by as few as possible, during the course of a research study. Future research should only use measures whose reliability in the population being tested has been proven, and the measures' reliability should be clearly documented in all research reports.

Validity

In contrast to reliability, which relates to the reproducibility of a measure, validity relates to its usefulness and the degree to which it represents the property it claims to measure. For example, for a questionnaire to be a valid measure of disability in a population, it must actually measure the reduced ability of this population to perform normal activities. Various forms of validity are assessed in different ways, such as correlation with other measures of the same characteristic, logical analysis of how the content of a measure relates to the characteristic it claims to measure, or evaluation of how accurately the measure predicts what it claims to predict. Measures may be valid by one standard but not by another. For example, although measures of abdominal strength and lumbar flexibility may have high content validity as measures of low back pain, because it appears logical that they would be related to low back pain and may be predictors of future low back pain, they are not considered to have good criterion-related or predictive validity because it has been found that abdominal strength and trunk flexibility do not correlate with self-reports of low back pain and do not predict who will have low back pain in the future.[10]

Clinical relevance

As well as being reliable and valid, outcome measures used in future research concerning the effects of physical agents should relate directly to the goal(s) of treatment and should include measures of the effects of interventions on impairment, functional limitations, and disability. In contrast to prior research, which focused primarily on the effects of physical agents on impairment, examining, for example, the effect of thermotherapy on soft tissue length and extensibility or the effects of traction or electrical stimulation on pain, future studies should also evaluate the effects of these interventions on functional outcomes such as walking speed, lifting capacity, or sitting tolerance.

Future research should also evaluate whether these interventions reduce functional limitations. For example, research should evaluate whether spinal traction facilitates the subjects' return to work, promotes their ability to shop independently, or accelerates their return to sporting activity. Examples of possible studies on the effects of physical agents on functional limitations and disability include evaluating the effect of thermotherapy on ambulation distance, ambulation velocity, and the time required to return to functional independence after total knee arthroplasty or evaluating the effect of traction on the time required to return to work and the level of work returned to in patients with low back pain and radiculopathy. Data from such studies will allow prediction of functional outcome in response to treatment, and may be used to guide future practice and to support reimbursement for treatment.

In order to provide further support for using physical agents in rehabilitation, future studies should demonstrate not only that physical agents optimize the achievement of patient goals but also that they do so in the shortest amount of time and for the lowest cost. In order to achieve this, research evaluating the cost effectiveness of using physical agents to achieve specific functional outcomes is required. In order to evaluate the potential costs and benefits of an intervention realistically, the costs of providing the intervention should be compared with the potential savings associated with reducing the duration and severity of a patient's disability and handicap. Potential savings may include reducing loss of income to the patient, reducing costs to the employer associated with replacing a member of the workforce, and avoiding costs associated with providing further care to the patient. For example, providing traction to patients with low back pain for 10 visits may cost $500; however, if it is shown that this accelerates their return to work by an average of 1 week, this treatment can be considered cost effective if the costs to those patients, their employers, and their insurance carriers associated with not working for 1 week are greater than $500. Studies demonstrating the cost effectiveness of interventions can provide strong support to justify reimbursement for those interventions.

Reporting

In recent years there has been a growing interest and support for the practice of evidence-based medicine. In this context, a number of systematic reviews of the literature and metaanalyses have been carried out and published. These types of reports attempt to evaluate and synthesize the findings of prior direct studies in a particular area. A systematic review of the literature is comprised of a systematic search for published studies concerning a specific question, evaluation of the quality of the studies found, and a summary of their findings. A metaanalysis generally also combines data from all randomized controlled trials to determine the efficacy of an intervention. For example, there are recent metaanalyses of the studies concerning the use of spinal traction for the treatment of low back pain and of the studies concerning the use of low-level laser therapy for the treatment of osteoarthritis and rheumatoid arthritis.

Systematic reviews of the literature and meta-analyses concerning the efficacy of physical agents for various rehabilitation applications generally report that the evidence does support current practice. However, in almost all areas the research is criticized for insufficient numbers of subjects studied and poor descriptions of the interventions used. This limits the conclusions that can be drawn.

Ideally, future studies will include larger numbers of subjects. Also, it is essential that future studies describe fully all aspects of the subjects and of the intervention being evaluated. Subject descriptions should include the number of subjects, their average age and age range, their sex distribution, the types of problem being treated, severity and acuity or duration of the problem, and any other features thought to be pertinent to the specific question at hand. Descriptions of the interventions should include the nature of the physical agent used and all treatment parameters. For example, in studies of the effect of ultrasound on wound healing, the subjects' average age and age range and sex distribution should be given. Information about wound etiology, size, and stage should also be provided, and the ultrasound frequency, intensity, duty cycle, effective radiating area and treatment time, as well as the treatment area, should be clearly noted. This type of reporting will allow one to draw clearer conclusions regarding the efficacy of physical agents and the necessary or optimal treatment parameters to produce the best clinical effect.

CONCLUSION

Given the advantages and limitations of different study designs, subjects, controls, and outcome measures, various types of research are needed to gain a full understanding of the effects of physical agents and to optimize their clinical application in rehabilitation. If future research follows the guidelines provided in this chapter, the effects of physical agents, the mechanisms underlying these effects, and the critical variables for producing them will be more thoroughly understood, increasing the effectiveness and predictability of applying physical agents while potentially decreasing the costs of patient care. It is also expected that, although further research will provide many answers, it will also produce many more questions, particularly with regard to optimizing the effectiveness of treatment. It is likely that, as particular interventions are found to be effective, further research will be needed to determine when, to whom, and how these interventions should be applied to obtain the best results; if these interventions are more effective than available alternatives; and if they are more effective when used in conjunction with other interventions.

Similarly, if studies show that an intervention is not effective for a particular application, further studies to investigate if it would be effective if applied in a different manner, with different treatment parameters, or to subjects with different characteristics or problems, may still be valuable. Therefore although the clinical application of physical agents in rehabilitation at any time should be guided by the available research, in order to continually improve the quality of care provided to patients, it is essential that further research be performed and that clinicians stay informed of the findings of these studies and modify their practice accordingly.

Chapter Review

Further research concerning the use of physical agents in rehabilitation is needed to increase the development of evidence-based clinical practice. This will improve the outcomes of treatment and support continued reimbursement for such treatment. Research concerning the physical properties, physiological effects, clinical applications, and adverse effects of physical agents will help to elucidate the mechanisms by which physical agents exert their effects, clarify the nature of these effects, and determine the conditions under which these effects are optimized. Different study designs with varying degrees of complexity are needed to evaluate different applications of physical agents. Case reports and single-subject, controlled studies are needed to describe and evaluate treatments that appear to be clinically effective. These studies should be followed by controlled studies with groups of subjects in order to ascertain whether their findings can be applied to other individuals, to clarify the nature and magnitude of the specific effects of different interventions, and to identify ideal treatment parameters.

In order to provide information about the microscopic, macroscopic, and functional impacts of physical agents, future research will also need to use various types of subjects. Studies using patients as subjects will provide information that may be most readily applied to other patients; however, due to the practical and ethical limitations of performing research on people, particularly when using patients, in vitro studies, animal research, and studies using normal human subjects will be needed to evaluate the effects of physical agents where there may be risk to a patient from receiving the intervention being evaluated or from undergoing the assessment procedures being used. Future research will also need to use appropriate, and ideally double-blind, controls in order to produce results from which conclusions regarding ideal treatments can be drawn. This research will also need to evaluate the effects of interventions with reliable, valid, and functionally relevant outcome measures. Future research will identify who will benefit from treatments with particular physical agents, how these treatments should be applied to optimize their effectiveness, and what the nature and magnitude of the benefits of such interventions

on patients' functional outcome will be. The reader is referred to the Evolve website at http://evolve. elsevier.com/Cameron for study questions pertinent to this chapter.

References

1. Conradi E, Pages IH: Effects of continuous and pulsed microwave irradiation on distribution of heat in the gluteal region of minipigs, *Scand J Rehabil Med* 21:59-62, 1989.
2. Verrier M, Falconer K, Crawford SJ: A comparison of tissue temperature following two shortwave diathermy techniques, *Physiother Canada* 29(1):21-25, 1977.
3. Fadilah R, Pinkas J, Weinberger A et al: Heating rabbit joint by microwave applicator, *Arch Phys Med Rehabil* 68(10):710-712, 1987.
4. Kolari PJ: Penetration of unfocused laser light into the skin, *Arch Dermatol Res* 277:342-344, 1985.
5. King PR: Low level laser therapy: a review, *Lasers Med Sci* 4:141-150, 1989.
6. Bradnock B, Law HT, Roscoe K: A quantitative comparative assessment of the immediate response to high frequency and low frequency ultrasound ("longwave therapy") in the treatment of acute ankle sprains, *Physiotherapy* 81(7):78-84, 1995.
7. Ward AR, Robertson VJ: Comparison of heating of nonliving soft tissue produced by 45 kHz and 1 MHz frequency ultrasound machines, *J Orthop Sport Phys Ther* 23(4):258-266, 1996.
8. Sweitzer RW: Ultrasound. In Hecox B, Mehrteab TA, Weisberg J, eds: *Physical Agents: A Comprehensive Text for Physical Therapists,* East Norwalk, CT, 1993, Appleton & Lange.
9. Skoubo-Kristensen E, Sommer J: Ultrasound influence on internal fixation with rigid plate in dogs, *Arch Phys Med Rehabil* 63:371-373, 1982.
10. Jackson AW, Morrow JR, Brill PA et al: Relations of sit-up and sit-and-reach tests to low back pain in adults, *J Orthop Sport Phys Ther* 27(1):22-26, 1998.

Appendix A

Glossary of Commonly Used Terms

abscess: A localized collection of pus

absolute refractory period: Time after an action potential during which another action potential cannot occur

absorption: Conversion of energy into heat

accessory motion: The motion that occurs between joint surfaces during normal physiological motion

action potential: Depolarization of the nerve membrane; reversal of the transmembrane potential

active motion: The movement produced by contraction of the muscles crossing a joint

acute pain: A combination of unpleasant sensory, perceptual, and emotional experiences that occur in response to a noxious stimulus provoked by acute injury and/or disease

adhesion: Abnormal joining of parts to each other

adverse effect: Any result of a treatment that is undesirable

adverse neural tension: The presence of abnormal responses produced by peripheral nervous system structures when their range of motion and stretch capabilities are tested

alternating current: A continuous flow of charged particles in alternating directions

amplitude: Electrical current amplitude. This may be a measure of the current or the voltage

analgesia: Absence of sensibility to pain

anode: Positively charged electrode

atrophy: Wasting or decrease in the size of a muscle or an organ

attenuation: Decrease in energy as radiation passes through a material

buoyancy: A force experienced as an upward thrust on the body in the opposite direction to the force of gravity

capacitance: The ability to store charge; generally measured in Farads

capsular pattern: The specific combination of motion loss that is caused by shortening of the joint capsule surrounding a joint

carotid sinus: The dilated portion of the internal carotid artery that contains the pressoreceptors that are stimulated by and stimulate changes in blood pressure; located in the anterior neck

cathode: Negatively charged electrode

cavitation: The formation, growth, and pulsation of gas or vapor-filled bubbles caused by ultrasound

chemotaxis: Movement in response to a chemical concentration gradient

455

chronaxie: The minimum pulse duration that will excite a nerve fiber when a stimulus with an amplitude of twice rheobase is applied

chronic pain: Pain that does not resolve in the usual time it takes for a disorder to heal or that continues beyond the duration of noxious stimulation

collagen: The main supportive protein of skin, tendon, bone, cartilage, and connective tissue

compression: The application of a mechanical force that increases the external pressure on the body or a body part

conductivity: A material's ability to propagate current; conductivity is inversely proportional to resistivity

connective tissue: Tissue that binds together and supports the various structures of the body; made up of fibroblasts, fibroglia, collagen, and elastin

consensual response: A reflex occurring on the opposite side of the body from the point of stimulation

contracture: Shortening of soft tissue

contraindication: Any condition that renders a particular form of treatment undesirable or improper

convection: Heat transfer by circulation of a medium of a different temperature

cryotherapy: The therapeutic use of cold

current: The rate of flow of charged particles; generally measured in amperes

debridement: The removal of foreign matter and devitalized tissue from a lesion

diathermy: (Greek for "through heating") The application of shortware or microwave frequency electromagnetic energy to heat tissues

direct current: An uninterrupted flow of charged particles in one direction

disability: Inability to perform a task or the obligations of usual roles and typical daily activities as the result of impairment

disc herniation: Disruption of the annular fibers of the spinal disc

duty cycle: The proportion of the total treatment time that energy is being delivered; generally expressed as a percentage or ratio

edema: The presence of abnormal amounts of fluid in the extracellular tissue spaces of the body

elastic deformation: The elongation produced under loading that reverses after the load is removed

electric field: The force field between electric charges

electrode: The medium or object used to conduct an electrical current to an object or a person

electromagnetic radiation: Perpendicularly oriented electric and magnetic fields that vary over time

embolus: A clot or other plug brought by the blood from one vessel to another smaller one to obstruct the circulation

end-feel: The quality of the resistance felt by the clinician at the limit of passive motion

endogenous: Originating from the body

epiphysis: The end part of a long bone that is formed from a secondary center of ossification and that is separated from the main portion of the bone by cartilage until skeletal maturity is reached

erythema: Redness of the skin caused by capillary congestion

exogenous: Originating outside the body

extravascular: Outside the vessels

exudate: Fluid that has escaped from blood vessels and been deposited in tissues or on tissue surfaces; has a high concentration of protein, cells, or solid material derived from cells

fibroblast: Cell that produces connective tissue

flaccidity: An extreme type of muscle hypotonicity in which no muscle tone is detectable; usually associated with paralysis

frequency: The number of events per unit of time

functional limitation: The inability to perform the tasks or behaviors recognized as essential components of daily life

galvanic current: Direct current

galvanotaxis: Movement in response to an electrical charge

gate control theory of pain: The hypothesis that pain may be relieved due to modulation of nociceptor transmission at the spinal cord by large-diameter sensory fiber activation

handicap: The social disadvantage of a disability

hematoma: A confined effusion of blood

hemorrhage: Copious escape of blood from the vessels

histamine: An endogenous amine that causes vasodilation

hydrostatic pressure: The pressure exerted by a fluid on an immersed body

hydrotherapy: The therapeutic application of water

hypertonicity: Abnormally increased levels of muscle tone that are not readily decreased by voluntary relaxation

hypotonicity: Abnormally decreased levels of muscle tone that are not readily increased by voluntary tensing

impairment: Any loss or abnormality of anatomical, physiological, or psychological structure or function

impedance: The sum of resistance and capacitance

inflammation: Initial tissue reaction to tissue injury

infrared radiation: Electromagnetic radiation with a frequency of 10^{11} to 10^{14} cycles per second

intensity: Amount of power per unit area; usually expressed in Watts/cm^2

intravascular: Within the blood vessels

in vitro: "In glass"; study performed outside of a living organism

in vivo: "In life"; study performed on a living organism

ionizing radiation: Electromagnetic radiation that can break molecular bonds to form ions (e.g., X rays, gamma rays)

iontophoresis: The transcutaneous delivery of ions into the body for therapeutic purpose using an electrical current

ischemia: Deficiency of blood in a part due to constriction or obstruction of a blood vessel

laser: Acronym for Light Amplification by Stimulated Emission of Radiation; monochromatic, coherent, directional light

leukocyte: White blood cell; include a variety of cell types—neutrophils, basophils, eosinophils, lymphocytes, and monocytes

lymph: Transparent fluid found in lymph vessels; consists of liquid and a few cells that are mostly lymphocytes

lymphedema: Swelling of subcutaneous tissues due to the presence of excessive lymph

magnetic field: The force field between magnetic poles

margination: Adhesion of leukocytes to blood vessel walls during an early inflammation

modality: A physical agent

monochromatic: Of one color

muscle tone: The amount of resistance to passive stretch of a muscle; underlying tension in a muscle that serves as the background for contraction

myelin: A fatty insulating covering present at intervals along most nerve fibers

nerve conduction velocity: The speed at which action potentials travel along a nerve

nociceptor: Specific nerve ending that responds to painful stimuli

nonionizing radiation: Electromagnetic radiation that cannot break molecular bonds to form ions (e.g., microwave, shortwave, infrared, visible light, ultraviolet A and B)

Ohm's law: voltage = current $\times$ resistance

oncotic pressure: The osmotic pressure of colloids in a colloidal system

opiopeptins: Group of endogenous neurotransmitters that have effects similar to those of exogenous opiates

osmotic pressure: The pressure that brings about diffusion between fluids with different concentrations

pain: An unpleasant sensory and emotional experience associated with actual or potential tissue damage or described in terms of such damage

paralysis: A state in which no active muscle contraction is possible; the loss of voluntary movement

paresis: Less severe reduction of active muscle contraction than paralysis; only weak muscular contraction can be elicited

passive motion: Movement produced entirely by an external force without voluntary muscle contraction by the subject

periosteum: Connective tissue covering all bones

peripheral vascular disease: General term for disease of the peripheral arteries or veins; usually used to describe narrowing of the arteries

phonophoresis: The application of ultrasound with a topical drug to facilitate transdermal drug delivery

physical agent: Various forms of energy and materials applied to patients and their means of application

physiological motion: The motion of one segment of the body relative to another

piezoelectric: The property of producing electricity in response to the application of mechanical pressure and of contracting and expanding in response to the application of an electrical current

plastic deformation: The elongation produced under loading that remains after the load is removed

power: The amount of energy per unit time; usually measured in Watts

precaution: Any condition for which special care should be taken prior to rendering a particular form of treatment

psoriasis: A common benign, acute, or chronic inflammatory skin disease characterized by bright red plaques with silvery scales, usually on the knees, elbows, and scalp, associated with mild itching

pulsed shortwave diathermy: The therapeutic use of pulsed shortwave radiation in which heat is not the mechanism of action

radiation: Exchange of energy directly without an intervening medium

range of motion: The amount of motion that occurs when one segment of the body moves in relation to an adjacent segment

referred pain: Pain that is felt at a location distant from its source

relative refractory period: Time after an action potential during which another action potential can occur only in response to a suprathreshold stimulus

resistance: Force opposing motion; may refer to the force of water against a patient or the force opposing the flow of electrical current

rheobase: The minimum current amplitude required to excite a particular type of nerve fiber when a pulse with an infinitely long duration is applied

shortwave diathermy: Electromagnetic radiation with a frequency of 10^7 to 10^8 cycles per second

spasm: An involuntary muscle contraction

spasticity: A type of muscle hypertonicity in which there is a velocity-dependent resistance to passive stretch of a muscle; the muscle resists quicker stretches more than slower stretches

specific heat: The amount of energy required to raise the temperature of a given weight of material by a given number of degrees

stratum corneum: The superficial cornified layer of the skin that acts as a protective barrier

strength-duration (S-D) curve: Illustration of the relationship between the current amplitude and pulse duration required to produce a threshold stimulus to create an action potential in different types of nerve fibers and directly in denervated skeletal muscle fibers

substance P: A peptide that is thought to be an important neurotransmitter for the transmission of painful stimuli

substantia gelatinosa: Lamina II of the gray matter of the spinal cord where afferent pain-transmitting fibers synapse with interneurons

tendinitis: Inflammation of tendons

tetany: Steady contraction of a muscle without twitching

thermal agent: A physical agent that can increase or decrease tissue temperature

thermal conductivity: Rate at which a material can conduct thermal energy

thermotherapy: The therapeutic use of heat

thrombophlebitis: A condition in which inflammation of the vein wall precedes the formation of a thrombus

thrombosis: The formation, development, or presence of a thrombus

thrombus: A clot in a vessel or in one of the cavities of the heart

traction: The application of a mechanical force to the body in a way that separates, or attempts to separate, the joint surfaces and elongate the surrounding soft tissues

transducer: A device that converts energy from one form to another

ultrasound: Sound with a frequency of greater than 20,000 cycles per second

ultraviolet radiation: Electromagnetic radiation with a frequency of 7.5×10^{14} to 10^{15} cycles per second

urticaria: Vascular skin reaction marked by the transient appearance of smooth, slightly elevated patches that are redder or paler than the surrounding skin and are often attended by severe itching

vasoconstriction: Diminution of the cross section of vessels, generally of the arterioles

vasodilation: Dilation of vessels, generally of the arterioles

venous stasis ulcer: An area of tissue breakdown and necrosis that occurs as the result of impaired venous circulation

viscoelastic: Having both viscous and elastic properties

viscosity: The physical property of resisting the force tending to cause a substance to flow, caused by friction between the molecules of a substance

waveform: The shape or visual representation of the change in energy intensity over time

wavelength: The distance between two successive points in a wave that are in the same phase of oscillation

Appendix B

Commonly Used Abbreviations and Acronyms

AC: Alternating current
AOTA: American Occupational Therapy Association
APTA: American Physical Therapy Association
ATP: Adenosine triphosphate
BNR: Beam nonuniformity ratio
CHF: Congestive heart failure
CNS: Central nervous system
CSF: Cerebrospinal fluid
CT: Computed tomography
CVA: Cardiovascular accident (stroke)
DC: Direct current
DOMS: Delayed onset muscle soreness
DVT: Deep venous thrombosis
EMG: Electromyography
ERA: Effective radiating area
ES: Electrical stimulation
FCC: Federal Communications Commission
FDA: Food and Drug Administration
FES: Functional electrical stimulation
HP: Hot pack
HVPC: High-volt pulsed current
ICIDH: International Classification of Impairments, Disabilities, and Handicaps
IP: Ice pack
IR: Infrared

L: Left
MED: Minimal erythemal dose (for UV treatment)
MRI: Magnetic resonance imaging
MVIC: Maximum voluntary isometric contraction
MWD: Microwave diathermy
NDT: Neurodevelopmental training
NMES: Neuromuscular electrical stimulation
PC: Pulsatile current
PEMF: Pulsed electromagnetic field
PNF: Proprioceptive neuromuscular facilitation
PSWD: Pulsed shortwave diathermy
PUVA: Psoralens with ultraviolet A
R: Right
RICE: Rest, ice, compression, elevation
ROM: Range of motion
SNS: Sympathetic nervous system
SWD: Shortwave diathermy
TENS: Transcutaneous electrical nerve stimulation
US: Ultrasound
UV: Ultraviolet
WHO: World Health Organization
′: Minutes
″: Seconds
#: pounds

Appendix C

Units

Unit (abbreviation): Measure of

Ampere (A): Electrical current. 1 Ampere = 1 Coulomb per second

Calorie (C): Energy. 1 calorie = energy required to increase the temperature of 1 g of water by 1°C

Coulomb (C): Electrical charge

Farad (F): Electrical capacitance

Gauss (G): Magnetic field strength

gram (g): Weight

Hertz (Hz): Frequency. 1 Hertz = 1 cycle per second

Joule (J): Energy. 1 J = 1 Wsecond

meter (m): Length, distance

Ohm (Ω): Electrical resistance. $1 \, \Omega = \frac{1 \, volt}{1 \, amp}$

Pounds per square inch (psi): Pressure

Pulses per second (pps): Frequency when the events are not cycles

Siemen (σ): Electrical conductance

Volt (V): Electrical potential difference

Watt (W): Power. 1 W = 1 J/sec

Watt per centimeter squared (W/cm^2): Intensity

Prefixes for Units

pico (p): 10^{-12}

nano (n): 10^{-9}

micro (μ): 10^{-6}

milli (m): 10^{-3}

Kilo (K): 10^3

Mega (M): 10^6

Giga (G): 10^9

Index